AF358720

Structural and Computational-Driven Molecule Design in Drug Discovery

Structural and Computational-Driven Molecule Design in Drug Discovery

Editors

Halil İbrahim Ciftci
Belgin Sever
Hasan Demirci

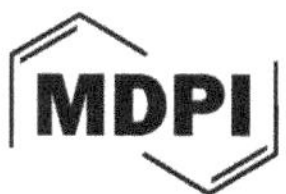

Basel • Beijing • Wuhan • Barcelona • Belgrade • Novi Sad • Cluj • Manchester

Editors

Halil İbrahim Ciftci
Department of
Bioengineering Sciences
Izmir Katip Celebi University
Izmir
Turkey

Belgin Sever
Department of
Pharmaceutical Chemistry
Anadolu University
Eskisehir
Turkey

Hasan Demirci
Department of Molecular
Biology and Genetics
Koc University
Istanbul
Turkey

Editorial Office
MDPI
St. Alban-Anlage 66
4052 Basel, Switzerland

This is a reprint of articles from the Special Issue published online in the open access journal *Pharmaceuticals* (ISSN 1424-8247) (available at: www.mdpi.com/journal/pharmaceuticals/special_issues/6GZO5SB951).

For citation purposes, cite each article independently as indicated on the article page online and as indicated below:

Lastname, A.A.; Lastname, B.B. Article Title. *Journal Name* **Year**, *Volume Number*, Page Range.

ISBN 978-3-7258-1014-7 (Hbk)
ISBN 978-3-7258-1013-0 (PDF)
doi.org/10.3390/books978-3-7258-1013-0

Contents

About the Editors ix

Preface xi

**Omur Guven, Belgin Sever, Faika Başoğlu-Ünal, Abdulilah Ece, Hiroshi Tateishi,
Ryoko Koga, et al.**
Structural Characterization of TRAF6 N-Terminal for Therapeutic Uses and Computational
Studies on New Derivatives
Reprinted from: *Pharmaceuticals* **2023**, *16*, 1608, doi:10.3390/ph16111608 1

Dony Ang, Cyril Rakovski and Hagop S. Atamian
De Novo Drug Design Using Transformer-Based Machine Translation and Reinforcement
Learning of an Adaptive Monte Carlo Tree Search
Reprinted from: *Pharmaceuticals* **2024**, *17*, 161, doi:10.3390/ph17020161 21

**Megha Krishnappa, Sindhu Abraham, Sharon Caroline Furtado, Shwetha Krishnamurthy,
Aynul Rifaya, Yahya I. Asiri, et al.**
An Integrated Computational and Experimental Approach to Formulate Tamanu Oil Bigels as
Anti-Scarring Agent
Reprinted from: *Pharmaceuticals* **2024**, *17*, 102, doi:10.3390/ph17010102 36

**Géssica Oliveira Mendes, Moysés Fagundes de Araújo Neto, Deyse Brito Barbosa,
Mayra Ramos do Bomfim, Lorena Silva Matos Andrade, Paulo Batista de Carvalho, et al.**
Identification of Potential Multitarget Compounds against Alzheimer's Disease through
Pharmacophore-Based Virtual Screening
Reprinted from: *Pharmaceuticals* **2023**, *16*, 1645, doi:10.3390/ph16121645 51

**Diana López-López, Rodrigo Said Razo-Hernández, César Millán-Pacheco,
Mario Alberto Leyva-Peralta, Omar Aristeo Peña-Morán, Jessica Nayelli Sánchez-Carranza
and Verónica Rodríguez-López**
Ligand-Based Drug Design of Genipin Derivatives with Cytotoxic Activity against HeLa
Cell Line: A Structural and Theoretical Study
Reprinted from: *Pharmaceuticals* **2023**, *16*, 1647, doi:10.3390/ph16121647 69

**Cleydson B. R. Santos, Cleison C. Lobato, Sirlene S. B. Ota, Rai C. Silva,
Renata C. V. S. Bittencourt, Jofre J. S. Freitas, et al.**
Analgesic Activity of 5-Acetamido-2-Hydroxy Benzoic Acid Derivatives and an In-Vivo
and In-Silico Analysis of Their Target Interactions
Reprinted from: *Pharmaceuticals* **2023**, *16*, 1584, doi:10.3390/ph16111584 96

**Juan Carlos Gomez-Verjan, Emmanuel Alejandro Zepeda-Arzate,
José Alberto Santiago-de-la-Cruz, Edgar Antonio Estrella-Parra
and Nadia Alejandra Rivero-Segura**
Unraveling the Neuroprotective Effect of Natural Bioactive Compounds Involved in the
Modulation of Ischemic Stroke by Network Pharmacology
Reprinted from: *Pharmaceuticals* **2023**, *16*, 1376, doi:10.3390/ph16101376 119

**Maximiliano Martínez-Cifuentes, Emmanuel Soto-Tapia, Camila Linares-Pipón,
Ben Bradshaw, Paulina Valenzuela-Hormazabal, David Ramírez, et al.**
Design of β-Keto Esters with Antibacterial Activity: Synthesis, In Vitro Evaluation, and
Theoretical Assessment of Their Reactivity and Quorum-Sensing Inhibition Capacity
Reprinted from: *Pharmaceuticals* **2023**, *16*, 1339, doi:10.3390/ph16101339 132

Swapnil P. Bhujbal and Jung-Mi Hah
An Innovative Approach to Address Neurodegenerative Diseases through Kinase-Targeted
Therapies: Potential for Designing Covalent Inhibitors
Reprinted from: *Pharmaceuticals* **2023**, *16*, 1295, doi:10.3390/ph16091295 . . . . **148**

Márton Ivánczi, Balázs Balogh, Loretta Kis and István Mándity
Molecular Dynamics Simulations of Drug-Conjugated Cell-Penetrating Peptides
Reprinted from: *Pharmaceuticals* **2023**, *16*, 1251, doi:10.3390/ph16091251 . . . . **162**

Shoukat Hussain, Ghulam Mustafa, Sibtain Ahmed and Mohammed Fahad Albeshr
Underlying Mechanisms of *Bergenia* spp. to Treat Hepatocellular Carcinoma Using an Integrated
Network Pharmacology and Molecular Docking Approach
Reprinted from: *Pharmaceuticals* **2023**, *16*, 1239, doi:10.3390/ph16091239 . . . . **184**

Katarzyna Stępnik, Wirginia Kukula-Koch, Wojciech Plazinski, Magda Rybicka
and Kinga Gawel
Neuroprotective Properties of Oleanolic Acid—Computational- Driven Molecular Research
Combined with In Vitro and In Vivo Experiments
Reprinted from: *Pharmaceuticals* **2023**, *16*, 1234, doi:10.3390/ph16091234 . . . . **204**

Violina T. Angelova, Borislav Georgiev, Tania Pencheva, Ilza Pajeva, Miroslav Rangelov,
Nadezhda Todorova, et al.
Design, Synthesis, In Silico Studies and In Vitro Evaluation of New Indole- and/or Donepezil-like
Hybrids as Multitarget-Directed Agents for Alzheimer's Disease
Reprinted from: *Pharmaceuticals* **2023**, *16*, 1194, doi:10.3390/ph16091194 . . . . **224**

César Millán-Pacheco, Lluvia Rios-Soto, Noé Corral-Rodríguez, Erick Sierra-Campos,
Mónica Valdez-Solana, Alfredo Téllez-Valencia and Claudia Avitia-Domínguez
Discovery of Potential Noncovalent Inhibitors of Dehydroquinate Dehydratase from
Methicillin-Resistant *Staphylococcus aureus* through Computational-Driven Drug Design
Reprinted from: *Pharmaceuticals* **2023**, *16*, 1148, doi:10.3390/ph16081148 . . . . **265**

José Antonio Mora-Melgem, Jesús Gilberto Arámburo-Gálvez,
Feliznando Isidro Cárdenas-Torres, Jhonatan Gonzalez-Santamaria,
Giovanni Isaí Ramírez-Torres, Aldo Alejandro Arvizu-Flores, et al.
Dipeptidyl Peptidase IV Inhibitory Peptides from Chickpea Proteins (*Cicer arietinum* L.):
Pharmacokinetics, Molecular Interactions, and Multi-Bioactivities
Reprinted from: *Pharmaceuticals* **2023**, *16*, 1109, doi:10.3390/ph16081109 . . . . **281**

Faez Ahmmed, Samiah Hamad Al-Mijalli, Emad M. Abdallah, Ibrahim H. Eissa, Ferdausi Ali,
Ajmal R. Bhat, et al.
Galactoside-Based Molecule Enhanced Antimicrobial Activity through Acyl Moiety Incorporation:
Synthesis and In Silico Exploration for Therapeutic Target
Reprinted from: *Pharmaceuticals* **2023**, *16*, 998, doi:10.3390/ph16070998 . . . . **296**

Alexandre Blanco-González, Alfonso Cabezón, Alejandro Seco-González, Daniel Conde-Torres,
Paula Antelo-Riveiro, Ángel Piñeiro and Rebeca Garcia-Fandino
The Role of AI in Drug Discovery: Challenges, Opportunities, and Strategies
Reprinted from: *Pharmaceuticals* **2023**, *16*, 891, doi:10.3390/ph16060891 . . . . **325**

Ali Irfan, Shah Faisal, Ameer Fawad Zahoor, Razia Noreen, Sami A. Al-Hussain, Burak Tuzun, et al.
In Silico Development of Novel Benzofuran-1,3,4-Oxadiazoles as Lead Inhibitors of *M. tuberculosis*
Polyketide Synthase 13
Reprinted from: *Pharmaceuticals* **2023**, *16*, 829, doi:10.3390/ph16060829 . . . . **336**

**Hizbullah Khan, Muhammad Sirajuddin, Amin Badshah, Sajjad Ahmad,
Muhammad Bilal, Syed Muhammad Salman, et al.**
Synthesis, Physicochemical Characterization, Biological Evaluation, In Silico and
Molecular Docking Studies of Pd(II) Complexes with P, S-Donor Ligands
Reprinted from: *Pharmaceuticals* **2023**, *16*, 806, doi:10.3390/ph16060806 . . . . **355**

**Mohammed Helmy Faris Shalayel, Ghassab M. Al-Mazaideh, Abdulkareem A. Alanezi,
Afaf F. Almuqati and Meshal Alotaibi**
Diosgenin and Monohydroxy Spirostanol from *Prunus amygdalus var amara* Seeds as
Potential Suppressors of EGFR and HER2 Tyrosine Kinases: A Computational Approach
Reprinted from: *Pharmaceuticals* **2023**, *16*, 704, doi:10.3390/ph16050704 . . . . **374**

**Shaker Ullah, Muhammad Sirajuddin, Zafran Ullah, Afifa Mushtaq, Saba Naz,
Muhammad Zubair, et al.**
Synthesis, Structural Elucidation and Pharmacological Applications of Cu(II)
Heteroleptic Carboxylates
Reprinted from: *Pharmaceuticals* **2023**, *16*, 693, doi:10.3390/ph16050693 . . . . **397**

**Ali Irfan, Shah Faisal, Sajjad Ahmad, Sami A. Al-Hussain, Sadia Javed,
Ameer Fawad Zahoor, et al.**
Structure-Based Virtual Screening of Furan-1,3,4-Oxadiazole Tethered *N*-phenylacetamide
Derivatives as Novel Class of hTYR and hTYRP1 Inhibitors
Reprinted from: *Pharmaceuticals* **2023**, *16*, 344, doi:10.3390/ph16030344 . . . . **417**

**Gema Lizbeth Ramírez Salinas, Alejandro López Rincón, Jazmín García Machorro,
José Correa Basurto and Marlet Martínez Archundia**
In Silico Screening of Drugs That Target Different Forms of E Protein for Potential
Treatment of COVID-19
Reprinted from: *Pharmaceuticals* **2023**, *16*, 296, doi:10.3390/ph16020296 . . . . **435**

About the Editors

Halil İbrahim Ciftci

Dr. Halilibrahim Ciftci received a BSc in Chemistry from Ege University, Turkey, in 2006, and an M.Sc. in Cancer Pharmacology from the Institute of Cancer Therapeutics, University of Bradford, UK, in 2008. He worked at major Turkish pharmaceutical companies (i.e., Neutec, Bilim, and Deva) as an R&D senior scientist to manage all technical aspects of the product development processes. After working for four years at major pharmaceutical companies, he returned to his academic career at the School of Pharmacy at Kumamoto University, Japan, in 2012, as a Japanese Government (MEXT) PhD scholar to develop anti-cancer and anti-HIV drug candidates. He received his PhD in Pharmaceutical Sciences in 2016; immediately after, he began working as a JSPS (Japanese Society for the Promotion of Science) postdoctoral fellowship at the same school. During his postdoctorate studies, he closely collaborated with the Stanford PULSE Institute for SFX-based drug development. His primary areas of research include chemical biology, drug design, and nanoparticles.

Belgin Sever

Dr. Belgin Sever is currently an Associate Professor at the Department of Pharmaceutical Chemistry, Faculty of Pharmacy, Anadolu University. Her research mainly focuses on the development of anticancer, antimicrobial, antidiabetic, anti-HIV, and anti-ALS drug candidates particularly based on medicinal chemistry and computational chemistry disciplines. She was awarded the first rank upon her graduation from Anadolu University, Faculty of Pharmacy, in 2013. She received her MSc and PhD in Pharmaceutical Chemistry from Anadolu University, Faculty of Pharmacy, in 2015 and 2019, respectively. During her PhD, she was a scholarship holder of The Scientific and Technological Research Council of Turkey (TUBITAK) 2211-A National Scholarship Programme. After her PhD, she was accepted as a fellow of the Takeda Science Foundation International Fellowship Program. As a post-doc fellow, she worked at Kumamoto University, Faculty of Life Sciences, Medicinal and Biological Chemistry Science Farm Joint Research Laboratory, Kumamoto, Japan, from November 2020 to May 2021. She has been also accepted for the TUBITAK 2219-International Postdoctoral Research Fellowship Program to work at the same research laboratory, Faculty of Life Sciences, Kumamoto University, from June 2022 to June 2023. She was selected as a "Young Woman Researcher" in the 7th Women Awards - Venus International Women Awards (VIWA) 2022" based on the VIWA 2022 Expert Committee Report and Apex Committee Recommendations. She was also awarded by the Turkish Pharmacists' Association- Academy of Pharmacy in 2022 for her contributions to pharmaceutical science. She has been an Editorial Board member of Open Chemistry, Plos One, Heliyon-Pharmaceutical Science, Current Topics in Medicinal Chemistry, Frontiers in Chemistry, Frontiers in Chemical Biology, and Oncology Research.

Hasan Demirci

Dr. Hasan DeMirci is a member of the Biosciences Division at SLAC National Accelerator Laboratory and is affiliated with the Non-Periodic Imaging group at the Stanford PULSE Institute. He completed his B.S. at Bosphorus University in 2002 and later obtained a Ph.D., in Molecular Biology, Cell Biology, and Biochemistry at Brown University in 2007. His research focuses on i) structural studies of bacterial ammonia monooxogenase (AMO) and ii) structural biology of mutant prokaryotic ribosomes, of which he is interested in characterizing the function and dynamics of these mutants, answering questions in the structure and dynamics of ribosomes that are resistant to some of today's most commonly used antibiotics. His current research efforts also include methodological developments for time-resolved ambient-temperature X-ray crystallography of large and challenging biomacromolecules of 4th-generation light sources, such as the Linac Coherent Light Source at SLAC.

Preface

Drug development is a complicated, high-risk, expensive, and lengthy process along with several stages, including target identification, lead discovery, and lead optimization. In this process, the congruence between the computational and experimental outcomes is a mainstay for the exploration of novel compounds. In silico studies, which were performed to define promising ligands in a target structure provide insights for further synthesis and evaluation of biological activities and, consequently, the identification of a three-dimensional (3D) structure of the ligand–receptor complex. The elucidation of key macromolecular drug targets using the cutting-edge technology of X-ray crystallography and spectroscopic methods in molecular and structural biology also results in a rise in diverse computational methods. Structure-based and ligand-based drug design strategies, including molecular docking, molecular dynamics, quantitative structure–activity relationship (QSAR) modeling, and pharmacophore generation, have been followed in computer-aided drug designs. Virtual screening is a versatile platform that enables the screening of a large number of compounds in a short period of time. Molecular docking is one of the virtual screening methods, which can anticipate the binding affinity of ligands and receptors. Thereafter, molecular dynamic simulations could be used to predict the stability of a ligand–receptor complex obtained from molecular docking assessment. Moreover, in the drug development process, many drug candidates could not pass the trials successfully due to inadequate ADMET (absorption, distribution, metabolism, excretion, and toxicity) properties. Therefore, in silico ADMET analysis is an attractive and cost-saving strategy for a large number of compounds before applying expensive and time-consuming in vitro and in vivo ADMET estimations.

This Special Issue aimed to provide deep mechanistic insights into strategies in structural dynamics studies and computational methods. The areas of research included but were not limited to the following: structural dynamics studies, computer-aided drug designs, molecular dynamic simulations, molecular docking, virtual screening, QSAR, and in silico ADMET analyses.

Halil İbrahim Ciftci, Belgin Sever, and Hasan Demirci
Editors

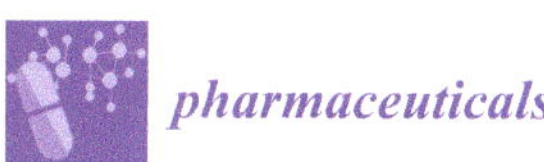

pharmaceuticals

Article

Structural Characterization of TRAF6 N-Terminal for Therapeutic Uses and Computational Studies on New Derivatives

Omur Guven [1], Belgin Sever [2,3], Faika Başoğlu-Ünal [4], Abdulilah Ece [5], Hiroshi Tateishi [2], Ryoko Koga [2], Mohamed O. Radwan [2], Nefise Demir [6], Mustafa Can [7], Mutlu Dilsiz Aytemir [8,9], Jun-ichiro Inoue [10], Masami Otsuka [2,11], Mikako Fujita [2], Halilibrahim Ciftci [1,2,11,*] and Hasan DeMirci [1,12,13,*]

[1] Department of Molecular Biology and Genetics, Koç University, Istanbul 34450, Turkey; oguven@ku.edu.tr
[2] Medicinal and Biological Chemistry Science Farm Joint Research Laboratory, Faculty of Life Sciences, Kumamoto University, Kumamoto 862-0973, Japan; belginsever@anadolu.edu.tr (B.S.); htateishi@kumamoto-u.ac.jp (H.T.); cherry9pichan@gmail.com (R.K.); motsuka@gpo.kumamoto-u.ac.jp (M.O.); mfujita@kumamoto-u.ac.jp (M.F.)
[3] Department of Pharmaceutical Chemistry, Faculty of Pharmacy, Anadolu University, Eskisehir 26470, Turkey
[4] Department of Pharmaceutical Chemistry, Faculty of Pharmacy, European University of Lefke, Northern Cyprus, TR-10, Mersin 99770, Turkey; fabasoglu@eul.edu.tr
[5] Department of Pharmaceutical Chemistry, Faculty of Pharmacy, Biruni University, Istanbul 34015, Turkey; aece@biruni.edu.tr
[6] Department of Nanoscience and Nanotechnology, Izmir Katip Celebi University, Izmir 35620, Turkey; demir.nefise53@gmail.com
[7] Faculty of Engineering and Architecture, Department of Engineering Sciences, Izmir Katip Celebi University, Izmir 35620, Turkey; mustafa.can@ikc.edu.tr
[8] Department of Pharmaceutical Chemistry, Faculty of Pharmacy, İzmir Katip Çelebi University, Izmir 35620, Turkey; mutlud@hacettepe.edu.tr
[9] Department of Pharmaceutical Chemistry, Faculty of Pharmacy, Hacettepe University, Ankara 6100, Turkey
[10] Research Platform Office, The Institute of Medical Science, The University of Tokyo, Tokyo 108-8639, Japan; jun-i@g.ecc.u-tokyo.ac.jp
[11] Department of Drug Discovery, Science Farm Ltd., Kumamoto 862-0976, Japan
[12] Koc University Isbank Center for Infectious Diseases (KUISCID), Koc University, Istanbul 34010, Turkey
[13] Stanford PULSE Institute, SLAC National Laboratory, Menlo Park, CA 94025, USA
* Correspondence: hiciftci@kumamoto-u.ac.jp (H.C.); hdemirci@ku.edu.tr (H.D.)

Citation: Guven, O.; Sever, B.; Başoğlu-Ünal, F.; Ece, A.; Tateishi, H.; Koga, R.; Radwan, M.O.; Demir, N.; Can, M.; Dilsiz Aytemir, M.; et al. Structural Characterization of TRAF6 N-Terminal for Therapeutic Uses and Computational Studies on New Derivatives. *Pharmaceuticals* **2023**, *16*, 1608. https://doi.org/10.3390/ph16111608

Academic Editor: Antonello Merlino

Received: 31 August 2023
Revised: 9 November 2023
Accepted: 9 November 2023
Published: 14 November 2023

Abstract: Tumor necrosis factor receptor-associated factors (TRAFs) are a protein family with a wide variety of roles and binding partners. Among them, TRAF6, a ubiquitin ligase, possesses unique receptor binding specificity and shows diverse functions in immune system regulation, cellular signaling, central nervous system, and tumor formation. TRAF6 consists of an N-terminal Really Interesting New Gene (RING) domain, multiple zinc fingers, and a C-terminal TRAF domain. TRAF6 is an important therapeutic target for various disorders and structural studies of this protein are crucial for the development of next-generation therapeutics. Here, we presented a TRAF6 N-terminal structure determined at the Turkish light source *"Turkish DeLight"* to be 3.2 Å resolution at cryogenic temperature (PDB ID: 8HZ2). This structure offers insight into the domain organization and zinc-binding, which are critical for protein function. Since the RING domain and the zinc fingers are key targets for TRAF6 therapeutics, structural insights are crucial for future research. Separately, we rationally designed numerous new compounds and performed molecular docking studies using this template (PDB ID:8HZ2). According to the results, 10 new compounds formed key interactions with essential residues and zinc ion in the N-terminal region of TRAF6. Molecular dynamic (MD) simulations were performed for 300 ns to evaluate the stability of three docked complexes (compounds 256, 322, and 489). Compounds 256 and 489 was found to possess favorable bindings with TRAF6. These new compounds also showed moderate to good pharmacokinetic profiles, making them potential future drug candidates as TRAF6 inhibitors.

Keywords: TRAF6; zinc finger; RING domain; cancer; X-ray crystallography; structural biology; Turkish light source *"Turkish DeLight"*; molecular modelling; pharmacokinetic determinants

1. Introduction

Zinc finger proteins are widely distributed transcription factors in the human genome with an array of biological functions. These functions include those associated with ubiquitin-mediated protein degradation, signal transduction, differentiation, metabolism, apoptosis, autophagy, migration, invasion, and a plethora of other processes. These functions arise from the capability of zinc finger proteins to interact with their particular DNA and RNA targets. Zinc finger proteins are dependent on Zn^{2+} cations, which can bind to cysteine and histidine residues. These proteins can be separated into distinct members of classical and non-classical types, referring to proteins whose zinc fingers contain the signature cys-cys-his-his (C_2H_2) motif and those that do not. Despite the great endeavors for the identification of the majority of zinc finger motifs, the structures of most of them have remained poorly characterized [1–4].

Tumor necrosis factor (TNF) receptor-associated factor (TRAF) family proteins are key regulatory molecules in the immune and inflammatory systems. They are the main signal transducers for the TNF receptor, the Interleukin-1 receptor/Toll-like receptor (IL-1/TLR), and NOD-like receptor (NLR) superfamilies. Until recently, TRAFs were classified as classical members (TRAF1-6) and a single nonclassical member (TRAF7) [5–7]. In general, TRAFs (TRAF1-7) adopt a common structure including the Really Interesting New Gene (RING) domain (except for TRAF1), zinc finger motifs, a coiled-coil domain, and a highly conserved C-terminal β-sandwich domain (TRAF-C or MATH domain). Apart from TRAF7, other TRAF proteins share a common structure at the TRAF-C domain. The RING domain is responsible for E3 ubiquitin ligase activity structurally supported by the zinc fingers. TRAF6 is a well-characterized E3 ubiquitin ligase, whereas the E3 activity of other TRAFs (TRAF2, TRAF3, and TRAF5) is not fully identified [8–10].

TRAF6, a non-conventional E3 ubiquitin ligase, attracts significant attention as the most studied TRAF member, differing from other TRAFs participating in the signal transduction of both the TNF receptor and the IL-1/TLR family proteins. TRAF6 is capable of activating a cascade of signaling events and upstream kinases, including kappa-B kinase (IKK), c-Jun NH_2-terminal kinase (JNK), and p38 mitogen-activated protein kinase, (MAPK) resulting in the stimulation of transcription factors including interferon-regulatory factor (IRF), the nuclear factor kappa B (NF-κB), and activator protein-1 (AP1) families [11–15]. In particular, NF-κB regulates the expression of a variety of genes involved in inflammatory responses, proliferation, differentiation, migration, cell adhesion, and apoptosis. Thus, NF-κB dysfunction can increase cancer cell proliferation and hamper apoptosis [16–18]. Moreover, TRAF6 has been reported to enhance the ubiquitination and activation of protein kinase B (AKT) and transforming growth factor activated kinase 1 (TAK1), leading to cell cycle progression, proliferation, and migration of cancer cells along with impairment of apoptosis in cancer cells. Therefore, the overexpression of TRAF6 is linked with inflammatory disorders and various types of cancers including pancreatic, liver, lung, head and neck, breast, colorectal, prostate, melanoma, and osteosarcoma [19–24]. On the other hand, it has also been reported that TRAF6 serves important roles in osteoclastogenesis, defective lymph node organogenesis, and hypohidrotic ectodermal dysplasia [15,25]. Recent studies also documented that high levels of TRAF6 were observed in serum patients with autoimmune diseases including systemic lupus erythematosus, rheumatoid arthritis, and myasthenia gravis [26]. Separately, the connection between upregulation and/or accumulation of TRAF6 and neurodegenerative disorders such as Alzheimer's disease, Parkinson's disease, and amyotrophic lateral sclerosis (ALS) has been reported since TRAF6 triggers neuronal apoptosis and central nervous system (CNS) disruption. In CNS, TRAF6 also contributes to inflammatory responses in stroke and neuropathic pain [27–30].

In this study, we investigated the N-terminal region of TRAF6 at atomic resolution to examine the structure. We designed 503 new compounds on the basis of SN-1, which was previously synthesized by our group and was determined to bind to TRAF6 decreasing long-chain poly-ubiquitination [31,32]. After we determined the structure (PDB ID: 8HZ2), we conducted molecular docking studies for our 503 new SN-1 derivatives using this template (PDB ID: 8HZ2) [33] compared to SN-1 and molecular dynamic (MD) simulations for three favorable docked complexes. We also conducted absorption, distribution, metabolism, and excretion (ADME) analysis to detect the most promising candidates with optimum pharmacokinetic profiles. Our findings have important implications for further pharmaceutical studies, particularly for the development of next-generation TRAF6 inhibitors to be effective as anti-inflammatory, anticancer, anti-osteoporosis, immunosuppressant or anti-neurodegenerative agents.

2. Results

2.1. TRAF6 N-Terminal Structure at 3.2 Å Resolution

TRAF6 is a 59.4 kDa protein consisting of 522 amino acids. Here, we structurally calculated the 18.14 kDa N-terminal region consisting of 157 amino acids. The crystal belongs to the P1 triclinic space group with a = 45.893, b = 51.6293, c = 54.3003, α = 91.064, β = 112.16, γ = 108.43. The dimerized structure of TRAF6 N-terminal region was determined to be 3.2 Å resolution at cryogenic temperature at the Turkish light source "*Turkish DeLight*" [34] (Figure 1). The determined structure was deposited to the PDB database with the ID: 8HZ2 [33].

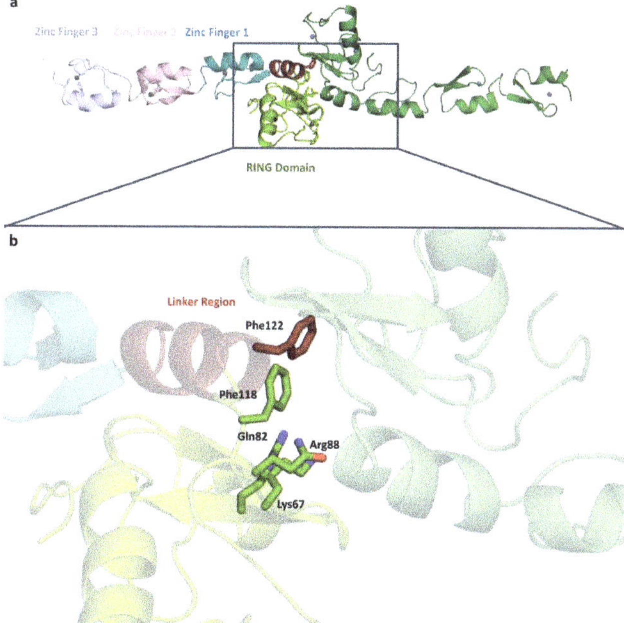

Figure 1. (**a**) Dimeric structure of TRAF6 N-terminal region at 3.2 Å (Chain A RING Domain: Splitpea, ZF1: Deepteal, ZF2: Lightpink, ZF3: Lightblue, Zn: Gray; Chain B: Forest, Zinc atoms: Gray) and domain organization of TRAF6 N-terminal region. (**b**) A close-up of the dimerization residues is shown at the dimerization surface.

Our study reveals the structure of TRAF6, which has dimerized at the N-terminal RING domain and linker region. Residues known to mediate the dimerization are shown in Figure 1. There are four residues in the RING domain (Lys67, Gln82, Arg88, and Phe118) and one residue in the linker region (Phe122) shown to be participating in dimerization.

TRAF6 N-terminal region consists of five domains, a RING domain, a linker helix, and three zinc fingers. Figure 1a shows the domain organization in detail, where the zinc atoms can be clearly seen at the center of the domains.

2.2. Detailed Analysis of RING Domain and Zinc Fingers

A closer look at the RING domain (Figure 2) and zinc fingers (Figure 3) was also taken. Every zinc atom and their interacting residues are visible within the refined *2Fo-Fc* density map. A clear repeating pattern among the zinc fingers can be observed in secondary structures. Each finger is made of a Sheet-Loop-Sheet-Helix-Loop pattern. Separately, there are always three Cys residues and one His residues forming the finger. While the two cysteine residues are located on the first loop, the third cysteine is located on the second loop and the histidine is located on the helix region. The distances between zinc and interacting residues are also conserved, ranging from 2.0 to 2.3 Å. We have generated the *2Fo-Fc* electron density maps of the zinc and the interacting residues, which show a continuation throughout and enclose the zinc atom and the residues.

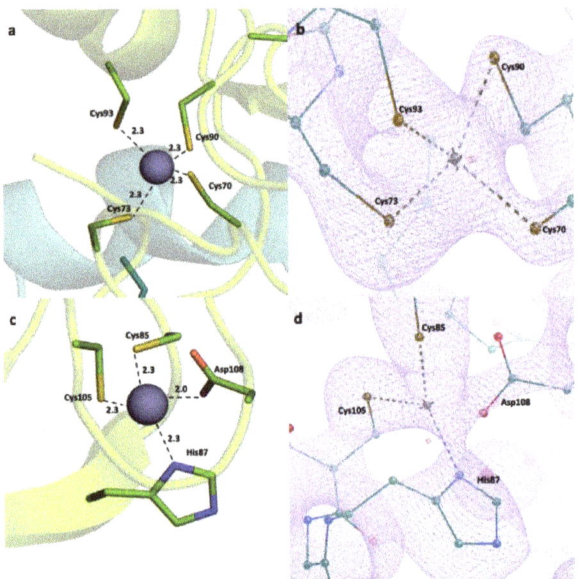

Figure 2. RING domain zinc-interacting residues. (**a,c**) Distances between residues and the bivalent zinc ions. (**b,d**) The *2Fo-Fc* electron density maps shown at sigma level of 1, with the root mean square deviation (RMSD) showing the interaction.

2.3. Structural Alignment with the Reference Protein

Our structure (PDB ID:8HZ2) and the reference structure (PDB ID:3HCS) [35] are aligned with the RMSD value of 1.09 and show minor differences within the loops (Figure 4). Also, we have looked at the zinc-interacting residues in both structures (Supplementary Figure S1). Although the residues have similar conformations, there are slight differences based on the loop movements. We have also checked the distances between the zinc binding residues and zinc ions. Here, we observe that these distances are similar in reference structure and our structure, although the former have a slightly larger range between 2.1 and 2.8 Å.

Our structure and the reported structure are almost identical sequence-wise, except for the Histidine tags. The reported structure has a Histidine tag at the C-terminal, while the Histidine tag is cleaved in our structure. Although we did not see a significant difference in the structures, it is an important note for future research.

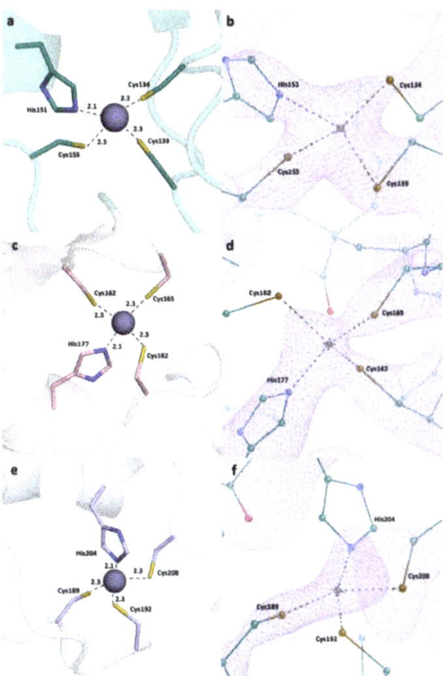

Figure 3. Zinc fingers and zinc-interacting residues. (**a**) Zinc finger 1 distances. (**b**) Zinc finger 1 electron density map at sigma level of 1 RMSD. (**c**) Zinc finger 2 distances. (**d**) Zinc finger 2 *2Fo-Fc* electron density map at sigma level of 1 RMSD. (**e**) Zinc finger 3 distances. (**f**) Zinc finger 3 *2Fo-Fc* electron density map at sigma level of 1 RMSD.

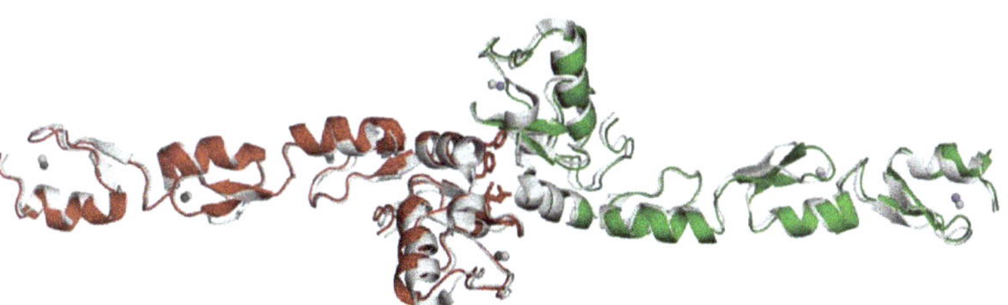

Figure 4. Structure alignment between the obtained data (PDB ID: 8HZ2) and the used model (PDB ID: 3HCS). Model structure is shown in gray.

2.4. Design of New Compounds

Over the years, our research group has pursued the discovery of small molecules with efficacy on zinc finger proteins. With great efforts in this area, we have discovered compounds with pyridine and histidine nuclei and proved their remarkable efficacy against zinc finger proteins such as human immunodeficiency virus type I enhancer binding protein 1 (HIV-EP1) [36,37]. Following these efforts, SN-1 (Figure 5), developed by our research group as an inhibitor of zinc finger transcription factor [38], was found to enhance steady-state expression level of antiviral apolipoprotein B mRNA-editing enzyme-catalytic polypeptide-like (APOBEC) 3G (A3G) bearing two zinc-binding domains in the presence of viral infectivity factor (Vif) protein [39]. In our other study, we reported that SN-1 bound to TRAF6, suppressing its auto-ubiquitination and downstream NF-κB signaling. Previous molecular docking study also pointed out that the pyridine ring and NH of the side chain of SN-1 interacted with His151, whereas the dithiol groups interacted with zinc ion and His141 separately in the N-terminal region of TRAF6 (Figure 5) [31]. We further demonstrated that SN-1 derivatives hold promise for developing new drug candidates targeting zinc proteins [32,40,41].

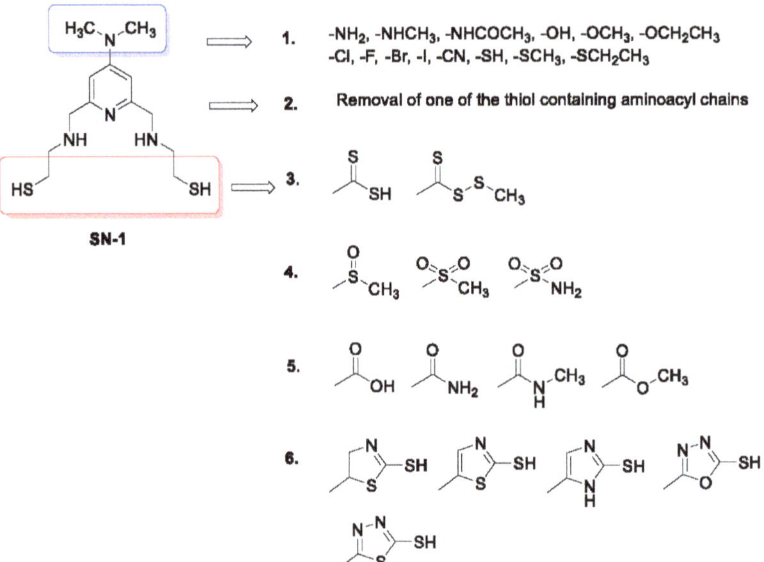

Figure 5. The chemical structure of SN-1 and its favorable interactions with key residues in the N-terminal region of TRAF6.

The potential binding mode of SN-1 to the N-terminal region of TRAF6 encouraged us to design 503 new SN-1 derivatives based on six design strategies (Figure 6) on the structural modification of dimethylamino groups on pyridine ring and thiol containing aminoacyl chains.

Figure 6. Design strategies for new SN-1 derivatives.

These strategies are as follows:

- Replacement of dimethylamino groups with amine, methylamine, acetamido, hydroxyl, methoxy, ethoxy, fluoro, chloro, bromo, iodo, cyano, thiol, thiomethyl, thioethyl groups;
- Removal of one of the thiols containing aminoacyl chains;
- Replacement of thiol group to methyl/ethyl (dithioperoxo)thioate, dithiocarbamates in aminoacyl chains;
- Replacement of thiol group to methylsulfinyl, methylsulfonyl, and sulfonamide groups in aminoacyl chains;
- Replacement of thiol group to amide, carboxylic acid, and ester groups in aminoacyl chains;
- Replacement of thiol group to thiol-substituted thiazoline, thiazole, imidazole, oxadiazole, thiadiazole, and pyridine rings in aminoacyl chains.

2.5. Molecular Docking Studies for New Compounds

The crystal structure of the TRAF6 elucidated in the current study was used (PDB IDs: 8HZ2) [33] for 503 new SN-1 derivatives to discover their binding affinities to TRAF6 by molecular docking studies. Results indicated that compounds 111, 115, 119, 129, 142, 168, 210, 256, 322, and 489 (Figure 7) exhibited the highest affinity to the N-terminal region of TRAF6 (Figure 8A,B). These compounds formed key π-π stacking, hydrogen bonding, and ionic bonds with important residues and zinc ion. Although all these compounds revealed a similar binding profile with SN-1 (Figure 8A,B), they showed less affinity compared to SN-1 associated with docking scores (Table 1). Among these derivatives, compounds 256, 322, and 489 were found to bind to TRAF6 more effectively through hydrogen bonding with His141, both π-π stacking, and hydrogen bonding with His151 and salt-bridge formation with zinc ion (Figure 9). Compounds 256, 322, and 489 also presented the highest docking scores as depicted in Table 1. The other compounds were sorted in order of their TRAF6 binding potential as compound 168 > compound 129 > compound 115 > compound 210 > compound 119 > H compound 142 > compound 111.

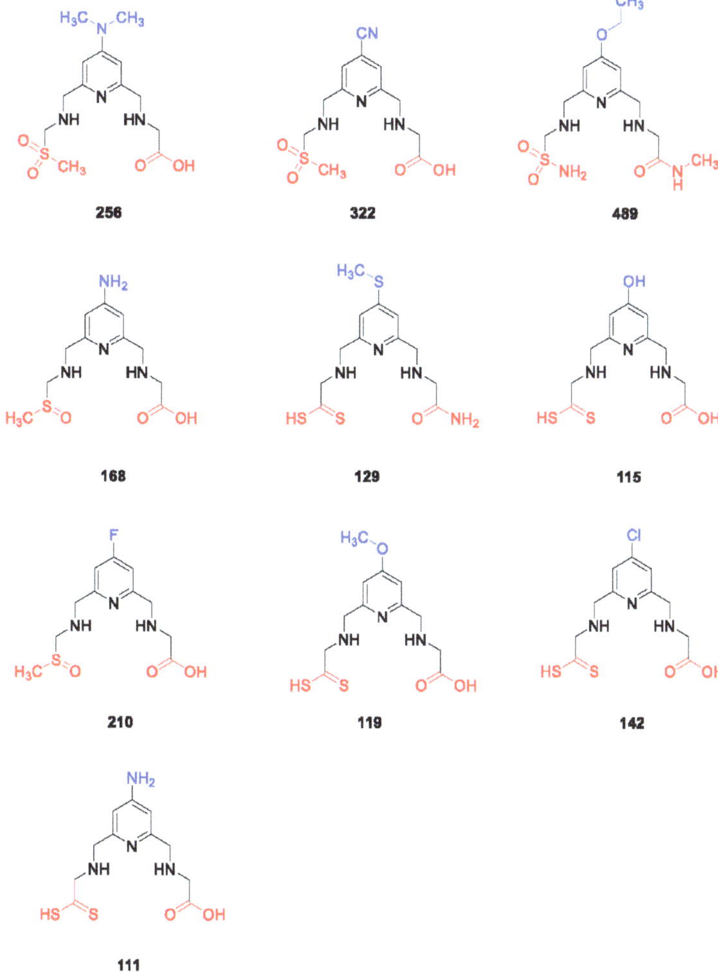

Figure 7. The chemical structures of the most effective new SN-1 derivatives.

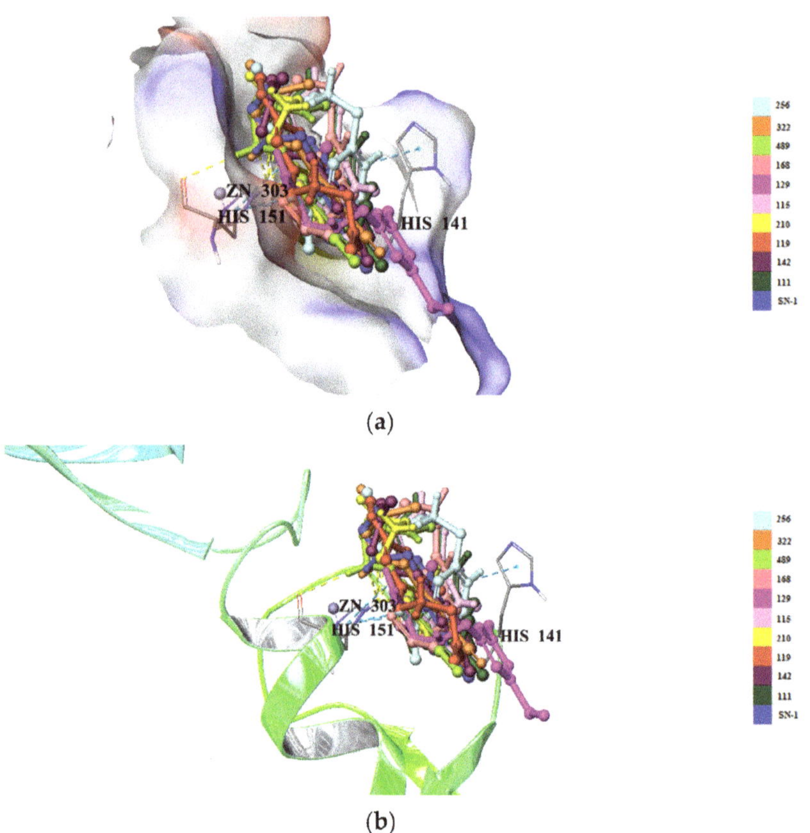

Figure 8. Docking poses of new SN-1 derivatives (yellow dashes: hydrogen bonding; blue dashes: π-π stacking) in the N-terminal region of TRAF6 (PDB ID: 8HZ2) (surface presentation) (**a**) (ribbon presentation) (**b**).

Table 1. Docking scores (kcal/mol) of the most effective new SN-1 derivatives and SN-1 in the N-terminal region of TRAF6.

Compound	8HZ2
	Docking Score
256	−6.889
322	−6.747
489	−6.259
168	−5.698
129	−5.647
115	−5.578
210	−5.570
119	−5.532
142	−5.526
111	−5.522
SN-1	−7.335

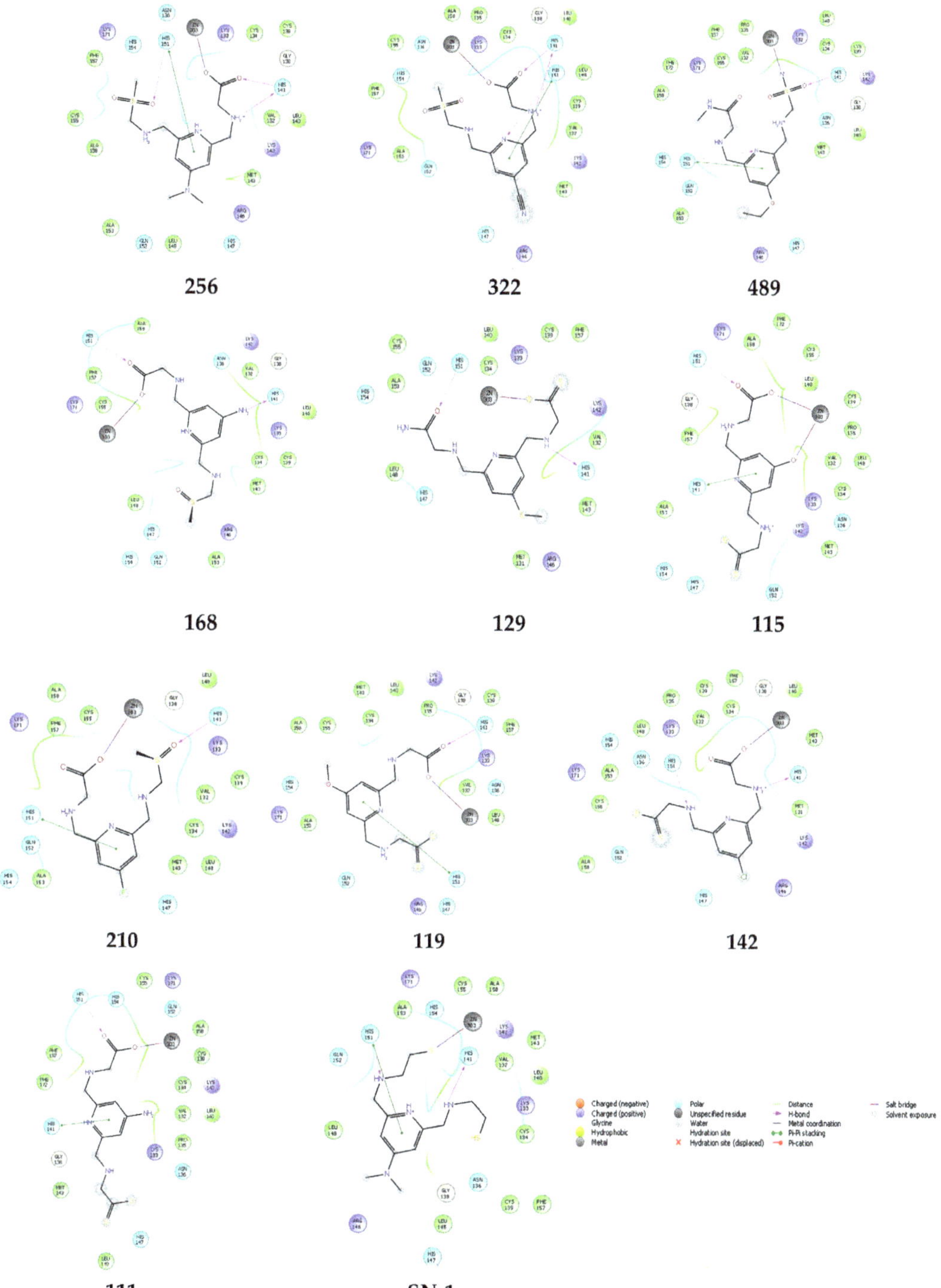

Figure 9. Docking interactions of compounds 256, 322, 489, 168, 129, 115, 210, 119, 142, 111, and SN-1 in the N-terminal region of TRAF6 (PDB ID: 8HZ2).

2.6. MD Simulations

MD simulations help us to study dynamics of ligand–protein complexes to elucidate binding interactions and the conformational changes of both protein and the ligands in a biologically simulated environment [42–44]. Three complexes (compounds 256, 322, and 489 docked complexes) were subjected to MD simulations to evaluate the stability of macromolecules and also to reveal critical binding interactions throughout the simulations.

Figure 10 right panels show ligand–protein contacts for both systems. Only amino acid residues that the ligands interact with for at least 30% of the simulation time are shown. Notably, compound 256 interacts with Zn metal during the whole course of the simulation. A hydrogen bond with His141 is preserved for 59% of the time while another hydrogen bond remains for 45% of all time. Compound 489 acts as a hydrogen bond acceptor and shows favorable interactions with the negatively charged Glu144 and polar His147.

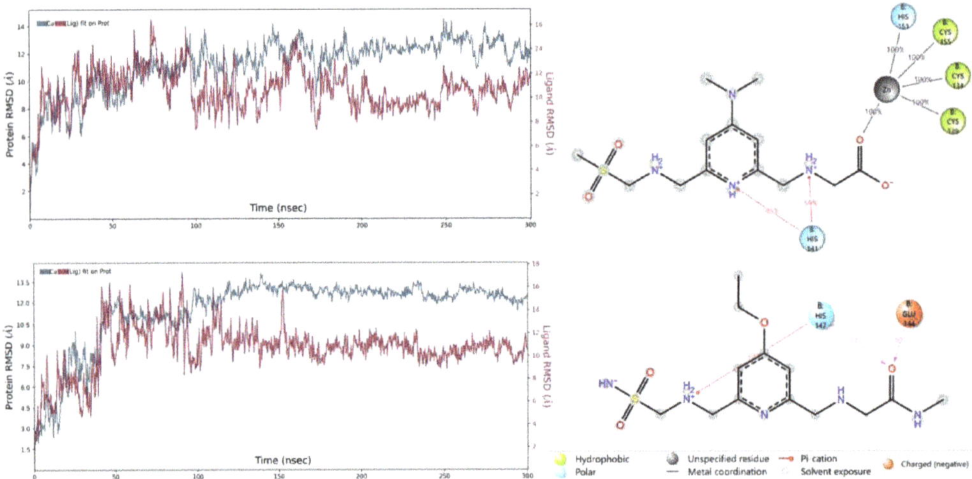

Figure 10. Protein and ligand RMSD (**left** panels) plots and ligand contacts of the compounds 256 (**top**) and 489 (**bottom**) with TRAF6 obtained for a 300 ns simulation.

2.7. ADME Prediction of New Compounds

Some pharmacokinetic descriptors and properties of these 10 new SN-1 derivatives were predicted using the QikProp algorithm [45] and SwissADME web service [46,47]. These properties involve aqueous solubility (QPlogS), octanol/water partition coefficient (QPlogPo/w), brain/blood partition coefficient (QPlogBB), human serum albumin binding (QPlogKhsa), and compliance to Lipinski's rule of five in the QikProp algorithm, whereas they involve the potential of several cytochrome P450 (CYP) enzyme inhibitors, P-glycoprotein (P-gp) substrate, BBB permeability, and druglikeness in SwissADME web service. Among all compounds, compound 256 was found to present the most acceptable pharmacokinetic profile. All compounds except for compound 168 exhibited acceptable aqueous solubility with QPlogS values of -1.822 to 0.258 (the limits are -6.5 to 0.5) and human serum albumin binding with QPlogKhsa of -1.194 to -0.244 (the limits are -1.5 to 1.5). The QPlogPo/w values of these derivatives were detected in the specified limits (-2 to 6.5) except for compounds 168, 210, and 322. The QPlogBB values of compounds were found as -2.084 to -0.211 (the limits are -3 to 1.2). However, these negative values and the BOILED-Egg model of SwissADME indicated that these compounds were not capable of crossing the blood brain barrier (BBB). Compounds showed no violation of Lipinski's rule of five (Table 2).

Table 2. Predicted ADME properties of new SN-1 derivatives.

Compound	QPlogS	QPlogPo/w	QPlogBB	QPlogKhsa	Rule of Five
111	−1.331	−1.943	−1.128	−0.978	0
115	−1.187	−1.972	−0.805	−0.965	0
119	−1.822	−0.885	−0.427	−0.798	0
129	−0.174	−0.024	−0.462	−0.942	0
142	−2.235	−0.552	−0.211	−0.730	0
168	0.638	−3.322	−1.680	−1.184	0
210	0.258	−2.265	−0.872	−1.059	0
256	−1.368	−2.015	−1.648	−0.957	0
322	−1.024	−3.418	−1.717	−1.194	0
489	0.345	−1.981	−2.084	−1.254	0
SN-1	−2.049	2.396	0.624	−0.244	0

According to SwissADME, the pink region of bioavailability radar (Figure 11) refers to the values of saturation (INSATU), size (SIZE), polarity (POLAR), solubility (INSOLU), lipophilicity (LIPO), and flexibility (FLEX) for oral bioavailability. The red lines for compounds 168, 210, and 256 and SN-1 were detected in the pink area. These compounds also demonstrated good gastrointestinal (GI) absorption. No compounds matched with CYP1A2, CYP2C19, CYP2C9, CYP2D6, and CYP3A4 inhibition. However, compounds 119, 129, 142, and 489 and SN-1 were identified as P-gp substrates.

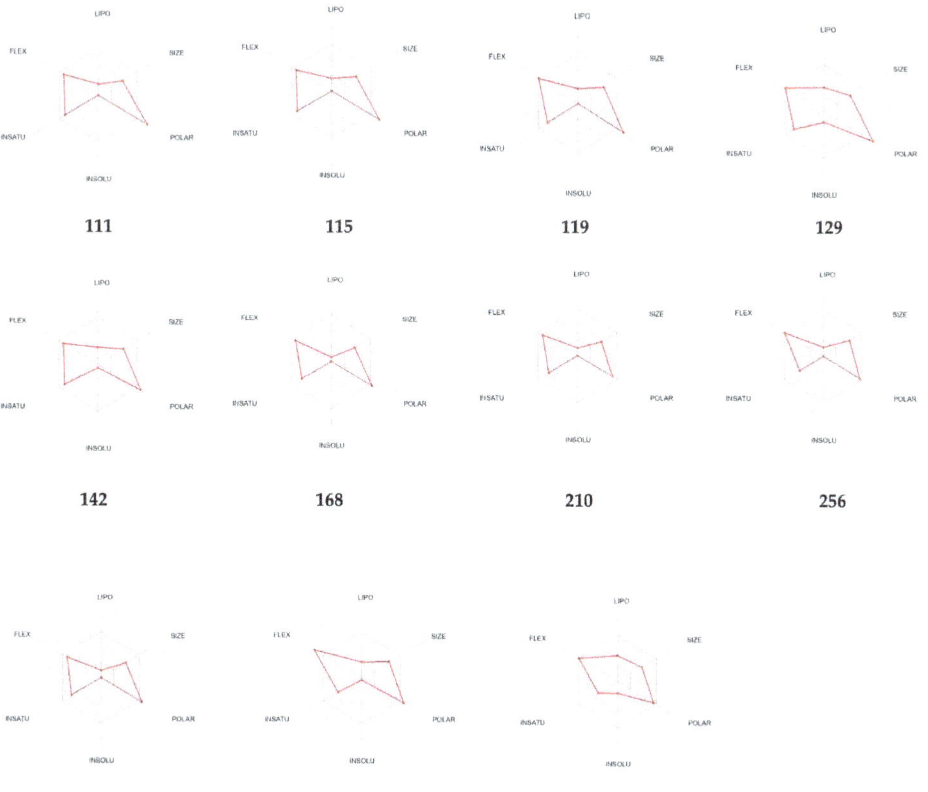

Figure 11. Bioavailability radars for compounds 111, 115, 119, 129, 142, 168, 210, 256, 322, 489, and SN-1 from the SwissADME web tool.

3. Discussion

TRAF6 is widely distributed in the brain, lung, liver, skeletal muscle, and kidney and is involved in a great number of immune and inflammatory reactions as a characteristic E3 ubiquitin ligase. TRAF6 plays a pivotal role in NF-κB stimulation, which triggers a vast array of cellular and organismal processes such as development, immunity, tissue homeostasis and inflammation regulating gene expression, apoptosis, and proliferation at molecular and cellular levels. Therefore, TRAF6 is associated with diverse abnormalities including different cancer types, autoimmune diseases, neurodegenerative disorders, and inflammatory diseases [48–50].

Having access to the structural details of TRAF6 provides insights that can support the development of new-generation anticancer therapeutics. Furthermore, the previously deposited structure used as a model (PDB ID: 3HCS) serves as a reference point from which we can observe that our structure is highly similar. The most significant characteristic of TRAF6 is the zinc interaction. Bivalent ions provide a structural scaffold around where the zinc fingers and the RING domain folds. Therefore, zinc has an important role in TRAF6 function, and altering the zinc interaction is a good starting point for inhibition The overall structure of the TRAF6 N-terminal region shows the dimerized structure with zinc atoms at the center of each domain. The domain organization shows, in addition to RING domain and zinc fingers, a linker region, consisting of a single helix (Figure 3). This region has a role in N-terminal dimerization, as a phenylalanine residue here is part of the dimerization surface.

RING domain and zinc fingers were analyzed in detail. Zinc fingers are one of the most abundant structural motifs observed in proteins [51]. As their name suggests, they are characterized around a bivalent zinc ion and they can interact with a wide range of molecules, such as nucleic acids and other proteins. Therefore, zinc finger proteins have a wide variety of functions, from transcriptional regulation to actin targeting. Zinc fingers have common patterns: for example, they consist mainly of cysteine and histidine residues, in different ratios [52]. Classical zinc fingers have two of each (Cys_2His_2); however, some cases show differences. Zinc finger domains have two β-sheets and one α-helix, although the number of loops change depending on the protein.

RING domain is a common domain in ubiquitin-ligase proteins (E3), with over 340 such proteins possessing this domain. It interacts with two bivalent zinc ions, forming RING fingers [53]. RING domains interact with DNA; therefore, the proteins including RING domain could mediate DNA transcription. The presented structure has a RING domain and three zinc fingers. Each zinc finger follows a conserved pattern: Sheet-Loop-Sheet-Helix-Loop. Moreover, each zinc finger has the same residue pattern: two cysteine residues in the first loop, one histidine residue in the helix, and a third cysteine residue in the second loop. This is an expected result, as the zinc fingers fold around bivalent zinc ions and they possess similar patterns. This is a classical zinc finger pattern in a way that it has two sheets and a helix; however, it differs as classical zinc finger in its Cys_2His_2 structure.

We have also investigated the distances between the zinc-interacting residues and the zinc ion. We observed that the distances are well within the range of strong bond formation at up to 2.4 Å. The cysteine residues interact with the zinc through the sulfur at the side chain while the histidines interact through their side chain nitrogens. We compared the distances in three zinc fingers, and we observed that they are similar as well, further showing that the zinc fingers have common characteristics. Moreover, it is confirmed that our structure has a RING finger, with its two bivalent zinc ions presenting thus, forming a RING domain. This domain mediates DNA interaction, and is crucial for the role of TRAF6 on NF-κB regulation. These four domains, all revolving around the central zinc atom, are great targets for TRAF6 therapeutics. The high number of cysteine residues results in disulfide bond formation, in addition to zinc interaction; therefore, altering these bonds with reducing agents (for example, dithiol compounds) will go a long way in modulating TRAF6 function.

Structural alignment with the model protein was performed. We used a deposited structure (PDB ID: 3HCS) as a model, and aligned it to the obtained structure (Figure 6). We observed that the structures aligned with high similarity (RMSD = 1.09), except for the loops. This is expected as loops are generally flexible, and the difference is based on the natural properties of the protein. We have also looked into the RING domain and zinc fingers in detail. We observed that the distances between zinc-interacting residues and zinc ions are very similar to that of obtained structure (PDB ID: 8HZ2), ranging between 2.1 and 2.8 Å. This is an expected result as the zinc fingers are conserved regions further confirmed by these distances.

We also applied molecular docking assessment for 503 new SN-1 derivatives. These new compounds were rationally designed for mimicking the binding effects of SN-1, which was previously synthesized and confirmed by our research group to bind to N-terminal region of TRAF6. We also observed that SN-1 and new derivatives presented the similar interactions with our previous study [31] such as hydrogen bonding with His141 and His151 residues and ionic bonding with zinc ion. This similarity confirmed the significance of certain residues in the binding site. Although new compounds revealed similar binding profile with SN-1 (Figure 8A,B), they showed less affinity compared to SN-1 associated with docking scores (Table 1). Among these derivatives, compounds 256, 322, and 489 were found to bind to TRAF6 more effectively through hydrogen bonding with His141, both π-π stacking and hydrogen bonding with His151 and salt-bridge formation with zinc ion These derivatives were designed following different strategies based on the fact that pyridine and amino groups in acyl chains were found critical for binding affinity. The docking assessment on these 503 new derivatives at the N-terminal region of TRAF6 (PDB ID: 8HZ2) supported our previous data. In general, the carboxylate, sulfonamide, and dithiocarbamate groups established salt-bridge formation with zinc ion as similar with the thiol group of SN-1. The replacement of dimethylaminogroup with the other groups did not make a huge impact in binding capacity of new derivatives. The π-π stacking interactions with His151 also played important roles in binding potential of compounds 256, 322 and 489.

The RMSD plot after MD simulations tells us the average changes in the positions of atoms with respect to a reference frame. At the end of 300 ns MD simulations, compound 322-TRAF6 complex did not stabilize and the ligand was observed to diffuse away from the binding site. The RMSD plots for the 256/TRAF6 and 489/TRAF6 complexes are shown in Figure 10. In both cases, relatively high RMSD values are observed. Compound 256-/TRAF6 complex stabilizes after 200 ns and fluctuations are mostly within 2 Å. Compound 489-/TRAF6 complex, on the other hand, reaches equilibrium after ~105 ns and remains relatively stable until the end of simulation. Visual inspection at the trajectories revealed that the relatively large RMSD values could be explained by fluctuations in the zinc finger regions of the protein that possessed a significant flexibility adopting different conformations. The ring domain and the binding site underwent much fewer fluctuations. We believe that such initial conformational changes were induced by the ligands upon binding. During reorganization and partial folding of the zinc finger regions, both ligands remained in the binding site.

The ADME calculation results signified that all compounds possessed moderate drug-likeness profiles with appropriate water solubility and lipophilicity values. As the human serum albumin binding is directly related to the volume of distribution and half-life of drugs, it can be concluded that all compounds showed adequate human serum albumin binding values. Although compounds revealed QPlogBB values in the limits, they failed to penetrate into the brain according to BOILED-Egg chart of Swiss ADME. Compounds exerted no inhibition against all tested CYP enzymes indicating a lower risk for drug–drug interactions. However, some compounds were found as P-gp substrates increasing the possibility of resistance by tumor cell lines through efflux. Compound 256 revealed the most prominent ADME values with optimum properties along with high GI absorption implying its drug-likeness potential.

4. Materials and Methods

4.1. Transformation and Expression

TRAF6 N-Terminal RING domain and 3 zinc fingers with the sequence "MAHHHHH-HHHHHVGTENLYFQSMEEIQGYDVEFDPPLESKYECPICLMALREAVQTPCGHRFCK-ACIIKSIRDAGHKCPVDNEILLENQLFPDNFAKREILSLMVKCPNEGCLHKMELRHL-E-DHQAHCEFALMDCPQCQRPFQKFHINIHILKDCPRRQVSCDNCAASMAFEDKEIHD-QNCPLA" was cloned into pRSF vector with an N-terminal decahistidine purification tag with a TEV cut site. As a cloning restriction enzyme cut sites, *Hind*III and *Kpn*I were chosen and the Kanamycin resistance gene was used as a selection marker. The constructed plasmid was transformed into competent *Escherichia coli (E. coli)* BL21 Rosetta-2 strain, with heat shock method. Transformed bacterial cells were grown in 18 L regular LB media containing 50 µg/mL kanamycin and 35 µL/mL chloramphenicol at 37 °C. At OD600 value of 0.8, the protein expression was induced by using β-D-1-thiogalactopyranoside (IPTG) at a final concentration of 0.4 mM for 18 h at 18 °C. Cell harvesting was done using Beckman Allegra 15 R desktop centrifuge at 4 °C at 3500 rpm for 45 min. Cell pellets were stored at −45 °C until protein purification.

4.2. Purification

The cells were dissolved in lysis buffer containing 500 mM NaCl, 50 mM Tris-HCl pH 8, 10% (*v*/*v*) Glycerol, 0.1% (*v*/*v*) Triton X-100, 2 mM BME, and 10 µM $ZnCl_2$. The homogenized cells were lysed using a Branson W250 sonifier (Brookfield, CT, USA). The cell lysate was centrifuged at 4 °C at 35000 rpm for 1 h with Beckman Optima™ L-80XP Ultracentrifuge equipped with Ti45 rotor (Beckman, Brea, CA, USA). The pellet containing membranes and cell debris was discarded. The supernatant containing the soluble protein was filtered through 0.2 micron hydrophilic membrane and loaded to a Ni-NTA column that was previously equilibrated with a wash buffer containing 150 mM NaCl, 20 mM Tris-HCl pH 8, 20 mM Imidazole, 10% (*v*/*v*) Glycerol, 2 mM BME, and 10 µM $ZnCl_2$. Unbound proteins were discarded by washing the column using a wash buffer. Then, the target protein (TRAF6 RING domain) was eluted using an elution buffer containing 250 mM NaCl, 20 mM Tris-HCl pH 8, 250 mM Imidazole, 10% (*v*/*v*) Glycerol, 2 mM BME and 10 µM $ZnCl_2$. Then, the eluted TRAF6 protein was dialyzed in a dialysis membrane (3 kDa MWCO) against a buffer with the same composition as the wash buffer for 3 h at 4 °C to remove excess imidazole. Dialyzed TRAF6 protein was cut using Tobacco Etch Virus nuclear inclusion-a endopeptidase (TEV) protease to remove the hexahistidine-tag overnight at 4 °C.

4.3. Crystallization

The crystallization screening of N-terminal decahistidine cleaved TRAF6 was performed using the sitting-drop microbatch under oil method against ~3000 commercially available sparse matrix crystallization screening conditions in a 1:1 volumetric ratio in 72-Terasaki plates (Greiner Bio-One, Kremsmünster, Austria) as described in Ertem 2021 et al. [54]. The mixtures were covered with 16.6 µL 100% paraffin oil (Tekkim Kimya, Istanbul, Türkiye). The crystallization plates were incubated at 4 °C and checked frequently under a stereo light microscope. The best TRAF6 crystals were grown within one month in Salt Rx-I condition #22 (Hampton Research, USA). This condition contains 1.2 M sodium citrate tribasic dihydrate and 0.1 M TRIS-HCl 8.5.

4.4. Crystal Harvesting and Delivery

The TRAF6 crystals were harvested using MiTeGen MicroLoops attached to a magnetic wand [55] while being monitored under microscope [56]. The obtained crystals were flash frozen by plunging in liquid nitrogen and placed in a cryo-cooled sample storage puck (Cat#M-CP-111-021, MiTeGen, USA). Then, the puck was placed into the *Turkish DeLight* liquid nitrogen-filled autosample dewar at 100 K.

4.5. Data Collection and Data Reduction

Collection of diffraction data from the TRAF6 crystal was performed by utilizing Rigaku's XtaLAB Synergy Flow XRD source *"Turkish DeLight"* at University of Health Sciences (Istanbul, Türkiye) with *CrysAlisPro* software 1.171.42.35a [57]. The crystals were kept cooled by the Cryostream 800 Plus system, which was set to 100 K. The PhotonJet-R X-ray generator operated at 30 mA, 1200.0 W, and 40 kV with 10% beam intensity. The data was collected at 1.54 Å wavelength and the detector distance was set to 47.00 mm. The crystal oscillation width was set to 0.25 degrees per image while exposure time was 20.0 min. CrysAlis Pro version 1.171.42.35a [57] was utilized to perform data reduction and an *.mtz file was obtained as the result.

4.6. Structure Determination and Refinement

The cryogenic TRAF6 structure was determined at 3.2 Å with the space group P1 utilizing *PHASER* 2.8.3 [58], an automated molecular replacement program within the *PHENIX* suite 1.20.1 [59]. The previously released TRAF6 structure with PDB ID: 3HCS was used as an initial search model for molecular replacement [35]. Simulated annealing and rigid-body refinements were performed during the first refinement cycle including individual coordinates and translation/liberates/screw (TLS) parameters were refined. The structure was checked by *COOT* [60] after each set of refinement and the solvent molecules were added into unfilled, appropriate electron density maps. The obtained final structure was examined by using *PyMOL* [61] 2.5.4 and *COOT* 0.9.8, and the figures were created. Data collection and refinement statistics were given in Table 3.

Table 3. Data collection and refinement statistics.

Dataset	TRAF6
Wavelength (Å)	1.54
Resolution range	20.58–3.231 (3.346–3.231)
Space group	P 1
Unit cell	a = 45.893 Å b = 51.693 Å c = 54.302 Å α = 91.064° β = 112.116° γ = 108.43°
Total reflections	6725 (639)
Unique reflections	4506 (545)
Multiplicity	1.5.(1.5)
Completeness (%)	88.28 (79.80)
Mean I/sigma (I)	7.48 (7.05)
Wilson B-factor	31.96
R-merge	0.6108 (0.6305)
R-meas	0.8208 (0.8537)
R-pim	0.5435 (0.5705)
CC1/2	0.0159 (−0.0765)
CC *	0.177 (−0.407)
Reflections used in refinement	6129 (545)
Reflections used for R-free	606 (56)
R-work	0.2708 (0.3092)
R free	0.3750 (0.3958)
CC (work)	−0.007 (−0.107)
CC (free)	0.066 (0.380)

Table 3. *Cont.*

Dataset	TRAF6
Number of non-hydrogen atoms	2537
proteins	2518
ligands	10
solvent	9
Protein residues	314
RMS(bonds)	0.008
RMS(angles)	1.07
Ramachandran favored (%)	90.00
Ramachandran allowed (%)	9.68
Ramachandran outliers (%)	0.32
Rotamer outliers (%)	12.24
Clashscore	19.22
Average B-factor	41.64
macromolecules	41.69
ligands	44.54
solvent	25.02
Number of TLS groups	13

* Statistics for the highest-resolution shell are shown in parentheses.

4.7. Molecular Docking Studies

The crystal structure of the TRAF6 was obtained from the RSCB database (PDB ID 8HZ2) [33]. The PrepWizard module of Maestro was used for preparing the raw file for the docking analysis. The missing chains were added automatically by Prime and the protonation state was calculated by PropKa at physiological pH. The receptor–ligand complex was minimized by Optimized Potential Liquid Simulations (OPLS_2005) force field. Grid generation of Maestro was used to determine the docking grid. The enclosing box and ligand diameter midpoint box were defined to involve the specified residues (His141, His147, His151 Zn303, Cys134, Cys139, Cys155, Glu156). The generated grid was used for the further docking experiments. Compounds were drawn and cleaned in Maestro workspace and were prepared with energy minimization using OPLS_2005 force field at physiological pH using the LigPrep module. Metal binding states were generated using EpiK. Then, the best minimized structures were submitted to the docking experiments without further modifications. Self-docking experiment was performed to validate the docking protocol. SN-1 was prepared and minimized by the LigPrep module of Maestro using EpiK at physiological pH. The optimum structure (lowest energy) was used for the self-docking procedure. After the obtained ligand was submitted to Glide/SP docking protocols, the same docking procedures were carried out for all designed compounds [62,63].

4.8. MD Simulations

The docked complexes of the compounds 256, 322, and 489 were simulated by subjecting to MD simulations using Desmond Software implemented in Schrödinger small molecule drug discovery program [64]. Each complex was put in an orthorhombic box and solvated with the reparameterized transferable intermolecular potential with 4 points model (TIP4P/2005 [65] water model. After neutralizing systems with sodium ions, 0.15 M NaCl was added to meet physiological condition. Those ion and salt additions were excluded within 20 Å of the ligand. Default relaxation protocol and NPT ensemble was selected and finally, 300 ns MD simulation was conducted with the recording interval of 200 ps yielding approximately 1000.

4.9. In Silico ADME Studies

Some crucial pharmacokinetic properties of new SN-1 derivatives were estimated by QikProp module of Maestro [45] and the SwissADME web tool [46,47].

5. Conclusions

RING domain and zinc fingers of TRAF6 mediate the activation of nuclear factor kappa B (NF-κB), which has essential roles in the regulation of inflammatory responses, proliferation, differentiation, migration, cell adhesion, and apoptosis. Therefore, it has been found that TRAF6 is overexpressed in various types of cancer including pancreatic, liver, lung, head and neck, breast, colorectal cancers, and melanoma along with inflammatory, autoimmune and neurodegenerative disorders. Therefore, examining and knowing the accurate protein structure can guide us in understanding the exact mechanism of action. The current research manifested the characteristics of the RING domain organization and zinc-binding of TRAF6, shedding light on the crucial functions of the protein. This study encouraged us to carry out further molecular docking studies with TRAF6 and new SN-1 derivatives based on the fact that SN-1 is a potential TRAF6 inhibitor developed by our research group. Results showed that in particular methylsulfonyl and carboxylate carrying compound 256 showed remarkable binding efficacy to the N-terminal region of TRAF6. MD simulations revealed that compound 322 did not form a stable complex while compounds 256 and 489 had favorable bindings with TRAF6. Compound 256 also exhibited appropriate pharmakinetic profile making it as a potential drug-like TRAF6 inhibitor. Overall, the results of this study will lead us for further structural studies including SN-1 and most effective SN-1 derivatives. Based on our continuous endeavors, we aim to develop TRAF6-specific drug candidates to be effective against various disorders.

Supplementary Materials: The following supporting information can be downloaded at: https://www.mdpi.com/article/10.3390/ph16111608/s1, Figure S1: A close up of zinc-binding pockets in aligned structure.

Author Contributions: Conceptualization, O.G., R.K., H.C. and H.D.; methodology, O.G., H.C., B.S., F.B.-Ü., A.E. and H.D.; software, O.G, B.S., F.B.-Ü., A.E., H.C. and H.D.; validation, O.G., H.C., B.S., F.B.-Ü., A.E. and H.D.; formal analysis, O.G., H.C. and H.D.; investigation, O.G., B.S., F.B.-Ü., A.E., J.-i.I., H.C. and H.D.; resources, O.G., H.C. and H.D.; data curation, O.G., B.S., F.B.-Ü., A.E., H.C. and H.D; writing—original draft preparation, O.G, B.S., F.B.-Ü., A.E., H.C. and H.D; writing—review and editing, O.G., B.S., F.B.-Ü., A.E., H.T., R.K., M.O.R., N.D., M.C., M.D.A., J.-i.I., M.O., M.F., H.C. and H.D.; visualization, O.G., B.S., F.B.-Ü., A.E., H.C. and H.D.; supervision, H.C. and H.D.; project administration, H.C. and H.D.; funding acquisition, H.C. and H.D. All authors have read and agreed to the published version of the manuscript.

Funding: This project and the experiments are funded by TÜBİTAK 1001 program with a project number 120Z520. This publication has been produced benefiting from the 2232 International Fellowship for Outstanding Researchers and 2236 CoCirculation2 Programs of the TÜBİTAK (Project No. 118C270 and 121C063). However, the entire responsibility of the publication belongs to the authors of the publication. The financial support received from TÜBİTAK does not mean that the content of the publication is approved in a scientific sense by TÜBİTAK.

Institutional Review Board Statement: Not applicable.

Informed Consent Statement: Not applicable.

Data Availability Statement: The Traf6 N-terminal presented in this manuscript has been deposited to the Protein Data Bank under the accession number 8HZ2 Any remaining information can be obtained from the corresponding author upon request.

Acknowledgments: Authors would like to dedicate this manuscript to the memory of Albert E. Dahlberg and Nizar Turker. The authors gratefully acknowledge the use of the services and Turkish Light Source (Turkish DeLight) X-ray facility at the University of Health Sciences, Experimental Medicine Application & Research Center, Validebag Research Park. Coordinates of the TRAF6 N-terminal structure have been deposited in the Protein Data Bank under accession codes 8HZ2.

Conflicts of Interest: The authors declare no conflict of interest with Science Farm Ltd.

References

1. Laity, J.H.; Lee, B.M.; Wright, P.E. Zinc finger proteins: New insights into structural and functional diversity. *Curr. Opin. Struct. Biol.* **2001**, *11*, 39–46. [CrossRef] [PubMed]
2. Jen, J.; Wang, Y.C. Zinc finger proteins in cancer progression. *J. Biomed. Sci.* **2016**, *23*, 53. [CrossRef]
3. Gibson, T.J.; Postma, J.P.; Brown, R.S.; Argos, P. A model for the tertiary structure of the 28 residue DNA-binding motif ('zinc finger') common to many eukaryotic transcriptional regulatory proteins. *Protein Eng.* **1988**, *2*, 209–218. [CrossRef] [PubMed]
4. Bu, S.; Lv, Y.; Liu, Y.; Qiao, S.; Wang, H. Zinc Finger Proteins in Neuro-Related Diseases Progression. *Front. Neurosci.* **2021**, *15*, 760567. [CrossRef] [PubMed]
5. Zhao, L.; Hao, Y.; Song, Z.; Fan, Y.; Li, S. TRIM37 negatively regulates inflammatory responses induced by virus infection via controlling TRAF6 ubiquitination. *Biochem. Biophys. Res. Commun.* **2021**, *556*, 87–92. [CrossRef]
6. Li, J.; Liu, N.; Tang, L.; Yan, B.; Chen, X.; Zhang, J.; Peng, C. The relationship between TRAF6 and tumors. *Cancer Cell Int.* **2020**, *20*, 429. [CrossRef]
7. Chen, Y.; Li, Y.; Li, P.T.; Luo, Z.H.; Zhang, Z.P.; Wang, Y.L.; Zou, P.F. Novel Findings in Teleost TRAF4, a Protein Acts as an Enhancer in TRIF and TRAF6 Mediated Antiviral and Inflammatory Signaling. *Front. Immunol.* **2022**, *13*, 944528. [CrossRef]
8. Lamothe, B.; Campos, A.D.; Webster, W.K.; Gopinathan, A.; Hur, L.; Darnay, B.G. The RING domain and first zinc finger of TRAF6 coordinate signaling by interleukin-1, lipopolysaccharide, and RANKL. *J. Biol. Chem.* **2008**, *283*, 24871–24880. [CrossRef]
9. He, X.; Li, Y.; Li, C.; Liu, L.J.; Zhang, X.D.; Liu, Y.; Shu, H.B. USP2a negatively regulates IL-1β- and virus-induced NF-κB activation by deubiquitinating TRAF6. *J. Mol. Cell Biol.* **2013**, *5*, 39–47. [CrossRef]
10. Lalani, A.I.; Zhu, S.; Gokhale, S.; Jin, J.; Xie, P. TRAF molecules in inflammation and inflammatory diseases. *Curr. Pharmacol. Rep.* **2018**, *4*, 64–90. [CrossRef]
11. Bradley, J.R.; Pober, J.S. Tumor necrosis factor receptor-associated factors (TRAFs). *Oncogene* **2001**, *20*, 6482–6491. [CrossRef] [PubMed]
12. Wang, P.H.; Wan, D.H.; Gu, Z.H.; Deng, X.X.; Weng, S.P.; Yu, X.Q.; He, J.G. Litopenaeus vannamei tumor necrosis factor receptor-associated factor 6 (TRAF6) responds to Vibrio alginolyticus and white spot syndrome virus (WSSV) infection and activates antimicrobial peptide genes. *Dev. Comp. Immunol.* **2011**, *35*, 105–114. [CrossRef] [PubMed]
13. Walsh, M.C.; Lee, J.; Choi, Y. Tumor necrosis factor receptor- associated factor 6 (TRAF6) regulation of development, function, and homeostasis of the immune system. *Immunol. Rev.* **2015**, *266*, 72–92. [CrossRef]
14. Inoue, J.I.; Ishida, T.; Tsukamoto, N.; Kobayashi, N.; Naito, A.; Azuma, S.; Yamamoto, T. Tumor necrosis factor receptor-associated factor (TRAF) family: Adapter proteins that mediate cytokine signaling. *Exp. Cell Res.* **2000**, *254*, 14–24. [CrossRef]
15. Yamamoto, M.; Gohda, J.; Akiyama, T.; Inoue, J.I. TNF receptor-associated factor 6 (TRAF6) plays crucial roles in multiple biological systems through polyubiquitination-mediated NF-κB activation. *Proc. Jpn. Acad. Ser. B Phys. Biol. Sci.* **2021**, *97*, 145–160. [CrossRef]
16. Hayden, M.S.; Ghosh, S. Signaling to NF-kappaB. *Genes Dev.* **2004**, *18*, 2195–2224. [CrossRef]
17. Park, M.H.; Hong, J.T. Roles of NF-κB in Cancer and Inflammatory Diseases and Their Therapeutic Approaches. *Cells* **2016**, *5*, 15. [CrossRef] [PubMed]
18. Soleimani, A.; Rahmani, F.; Ferns, G.A.; Ryzhikov, M.; Avan, A.; Hassanian, S.M. Role of the NF-κB signaling pathway in the pathogenesis of colorectal cancer. *Gene* **2020**, *726*, 144132. [CrossRef]
19. Middleton, A.J.; Budhidarmo, R.; Das, A.; Zhu, J.; Foglizzo, M.; Mace, P.D.; Day, C.L. The activity of TRAF RING homo- and heterodimers is regulated by zinc finger 1. *Nat. Commun.* **2017**, *8*, 1788. [CrossRef]
20. Qi, Y.; Pradipta, A.R.; Li, M.; Zhao, X.; Lu, L.; Fu, X.; Wei, J.; Hsung, R.P.; Tanaka, K.; Zhou, L. Cinchonine induces apoptosis of HeLa and A549 cells through targeting TRAF6. *J. Exp. Clin. Cancer Res.* **2017**, *36*, 35. [CrossRef]
21. Khusbu, F.Y.; Zhou, X.; Roy, M.; Chen, F.Z.; Cao, Q.; Chen, H.C. Resveratrol induces depletion of TRAF6 and suppresses prostate cancer cell proliferation and migration. *Int. J. Biochem. Cell Biol.* **2020**, *118*, 105644. [CrossRef] [PubMed]
22. Li, N.; Luo, L.; Wei, J.; Liu, Y.; Haque, N.; Huang, H.; Qi, Y.; Huang, Z. Identification of a new TRAF6 inhibitor for the treatment of hepatocellular carcinoma. *Int. J. Biol. Macromol.* **2021**, *182*, 910–920. [CrossRef] [PubMed]
23. Guangwei, Z.; Zhibin, C.; Qin, W.; Chunlin, L.; Penghang, L.; Ruofan, H.; Hui, C.; Hoffman, R.M.; Jianxin, Y. TRAF6 regulates the signaling pathway influencing colorectal cancer function through ubiquitination mechanisms. *Cancer Sci.* **2022**, *113*, 1393–1405. [CrossRef]
24. Zhao, X.; Ren, L.; Wang, X.; Han, G.; Wang, S.; Yao, Q.; Qi, Y. Benzoyl-xanthone derivative induces apoptosis in MCF-7 cells by binding TRAF6. *Exp. Ther. Med.* **2022**, *23*, 181. [CrossRef]

25. Bai, S.; Zha, J.; Zhao, H.; Ross, F.P.; Teitelbaum, S.L. Tumor necrosis factor receptor-associated factor 6 is an intranuclear transcriptional coactivator in osteoclasts. *J. Biol. Chem.* **2008**, *283*, 30861–30867. [CrossRef]

26. Li, T.; Li, Y.; Li, J.W.; Qin, Y.H.; Zhai, H.; Feng, B.; Li, H.; Zhang, N.N.; Yang, C.S. Expression of TRAF6 in peripheral blood B cells of patients with myasthenia gravis. *BMC Neurol.* **2022**, *22*, 302. [CrossRef]

27. Semmler, S.; Gagné, M.; Garg, P.; Pickles, S.R.; Baudouin, C.; Hamon-Keromen, E.; Destroismaisons, L.; Khalfallah, Y.; Chaineau, M.; Caron, E.; et al. TNF receptor-associated factor 6 interacts with ALS-linked misfolded superoxide dismutase 1 and promotes aggregation. *J. Biol. Chem.* **2020**, *295*, 3808–3825. [CrossRef]

28. Huang, H.; Xia, A.; Sun, L.; Lu, C.; Liu, Y.; Zhu, Z.; Wang, S.; Cai, J.; Zhou, X.; Liu, S. Pathogenic Functions of Tumor Necrosis Factor Receptor-Associated Factor 6 Signaling Following Traumatic Brain Injury. *Front. Mol. Neurosci.* **2021**, *14*, 629910. [CrossRef] [PubMed]

29. Lu, Y.; Cao, D.L.; Ma, L.J.; Gao, Y.J. TRAF6 Contributes to CFA-Induced Spinal Microglial Activation and Chronic Inflammatory Pain in Mice. *Cell Mol. Neurobiol.* **2022**, *42*, 1543–1555. [CrossRef]

30. Masperone, L.; Codrich, M.; Persichetti, F.; Gustincich, S.; Zucchelli, S.; Legname, G. The E3 Ubiquitin Ligase TRAF6 Interacts with the Cellular Prion Protein and Modulates Its Solubility and Recruitment to Cytoplasmic p62/SQSTM1-Positive Aggresome-Like Structures. *Mol. Neurobiol.* **2022**, *59*, 1577–1588. [CrossRef]

31. Koga, R.; Radwan, M.O.; Ejima, T.; Kanemaru, Y.; Tateishi, H.; Ali, T.F.S.; Ciftci, H.I.; Shibata, Y.; Taguchi, Y.; Inoue, J.I.; et al. A Dithiol Compound Binds to the Zinc Finger Protein TRAF6 and Suppresses Its Ubiquitination. *ChemMedChem* **2017**, *12*, 1935–1941. [CrossRef]

32. Radwan, M.O.; Koga, R.; Hida, T.; Ejima, T.; Kanemaru, Y.; Tateishi, H.; Okamoto, Y.; Inoue, J.I.; Fujita, M.; Otsuka, M. Minimum structural requirements for inhibitors of the zinc finger protein TRAF6. *Bioorg. Med. Chem. Lett.* **2019**, *29*, 2162–2167. [CrossRef]

33. Guven, O.; Ciftci, H.; DeMirci, H. Tumor Necrosis Factor Receptor Associated Factor 6 (TRAF6) N-terminal Domain. PDB Entry—8HZ2. 2023. Available online: https://doi.org/10.2210/pdb8HZ2/pdb (accessed on 8 November 2023).

34. Gul, M.; Ayan, E.; Destan, E.; Johnson, J.A.; Shafiei, A.; Kepceoglu, A.; Yilmaz, M.; Ertem, F.B.; Yapici, I.; Tosun, B.; et al. Rapid and efficient ambient temperature X-ray crystal structure determination at Turkish Light Source. *Sci. Rep.* **2023**, *13*, 8123. [CrossRef]

35. Yin, Q.; Lin, S.C.; Lamothe, B.; Lu, M.; Lo, Y.C.; Hura, G.; Zheng, L.; Rich, R.L.; Campos, A.D.; Myszka, D.G.; et al. E2 interaction and dimerization in the crystal structure of TRAF6. *Nat. Struct. Mol. Biol.* **2009**, *16*, 658–666. [CrossRef]

36. Otsuka, M.; Fujita, M.; Aoki, T.; Ishii, S.; Sugiura, Y.; Yamamoto, T.; Inoue, J. Novel zinc chelators with dual activity in the inhibition of the kappa B site-binding proteins HIV-EP1 and NF-kappa. *Br. J. Med. Chem.* **1995**, *38*, 3264–3270. [CrossRef]

37. Otsuka, M.; Fujita, M.; Sugiura, Y.; Yamamoto, T.; Inoue, J.; Maekawa, T.; Ishii, S. Synthetic inhibitors of regulatory proteins involved in the signaling pathway of the replication of human immunodeficiency virus 1. *Bioorg. Med. Chem.* **1997**, *5*, 205–215. [CrossRef] [PubMed]

38. Fujita, M.; Otsuka, M.; Sugiura, Y. Metal-chelating inhibitors of a zinc finger protein HIV-EP1. Remarkable potentiation of inhibitory activity by introduction of SH groups. *J. Med. Chem.* **1996**, *39*, 503–507. [CrossRef] [PubMed]

39. Ejima, T.; Hirota, M.; Mizukami, T.; Otsuka, M.; Fujita, M. An anti-HIV-1 compound that increases steady-state expression of apoplipoprotein B mRNA-editing enzyme-catalytic polypeptide-like 3G. *Int. J. Mol. Med.* **2011**, *28*, 613–616. [CrossRef] [PubMed]

40. Tanaka, A.; Radwan, M.O.; Hamasaki, A.; Ejima, A.; Obata, E.; Koga, R.; Tateishi, H.; Okamoto, Y.; Fujita, M.; Nakao, M.; et al. A novel inhibitor of farnesyltransferase with a zinc site recognition moiety and a farnesyl group. *Bioorg. Med. Chem. Lett.* **2017**, *27*, 3862–3866. [CrossRef] [PubMed]

41. Tateishi, H.; Tateishi, M.; Radwan, M.O.; Masunaga, T.; Kawatashiro, K.; Oba, Y.; Oyama, M.; Inoue-Kitahashi, N.; Fujita, M.; Okamoto, Y.; et al. A new inhibitor of ADAM17 composed of a zinc-binding dithiol moiety and a specificity pocket-binding appendage. *Chem. Pharm. Bull.* **2021**, *69*, 1123–1130. [CrossRef] [PubMed]

42. Ece, A. Computer-aided drug design. *BMC Chem.* **2023**, *17*, 26. [CrossRef]

43. Güleç, Ö.; Türkeş, C.; Arslan, M.; Demir, Y.; Dincer, B.; Ece, A.; Beydemir, Ş. Novel beta-lactam substituted benzenesulfonamides: In vitro enzyme inhibition, cytotoxic activity and in silico interactions. *J. Biomol. Struct. Dyn.* **2023**, 1–19. [CrossRef]

44. Çelik Onar, H.; Özden, E.M.; Taslak, H.D.; Gülçin, İ.; Ece, A.; Erçağ, E. Novel coumarin-chalcone derivatives: Synthesis, characterization, antioxidant, cyclic voltammetry, molecular modelling and biological evaluation studies as acetylcholinesterase, α-glycosidase, and carbonic anhydrase inhibitors. *Chem. Biol. Interact.* **2023**, *383*, 110655. [CrossRef]

45. *Schrödinger Release 2016-2: QikProp*, Schrödinger, LLC.: New York, NY, USA, 2016.

46. SwissADME. Available online: http://www.swissadme.ch (accessed on 30 August 2023).

47. Daina, A.; Michielin, O.; Zoete, V. SwissADME: A free web tool to evaluate pharmacokinetics, drug-likeness and medicinal chemistry friendliness of small molecules. *Sci. Rep.* **2017**, *7*, 42717. [CrossRef]

48. Dou, Y.; Tian, X.; Zhang, J.; Wang, Z.; Chen, G. Roles of TRAF6 in Central Nervous System. *Curr. Neuropharmacol.* **2018**, *16*, 1306–1313. [CrossRef]

49. Min, Y.; Kim, M.J.; Lee, S.; Chun, E.; Lee, K.Y. Inhibition of TRAF6 ubiquitin-ligase activity by PRDX1 leads to inhibition of NFKB activation and autophagy activation. *Autophagy* **2018**, *14*, 1347–1358. [CrossRef] [PubMed]

50. Lin, Y.; Bai, L.; Chen, W.; Xu, S. The NF-kappaB activation pathways, emerging molecular targets for cancer prevention and therapy. *Expert Opin. Ther. Targets* **2010**, *14*, 45–55. [CrossRef] [PubMed]

51. Cassandri, M.; Smirnov, A.; Novelli, F.; Pitolli, C.; Agostini, M.; Malewicz, M.; Melino, G.; Raschella, G. Zinc-finger proteins in health and disease. *Cell Death Discov.* **2017**, *3*, 17071. [CrossRef] [PubMed]

52. Krishna, S.S.; Majumdar, I.; Grishin, N.V. Structural classification of zinc fingers: Survey and summary. *Nucleic Acids Res.* **2003**, *31*, 532–550. [CrossRef] [PubMed]
53. Cai, C.; Tang, Y.-D.; Zhai, J.; Zheng, C. The RING finger protein family in health and disease. *Signal Transduct. Target. Ther.* **2022**, *7*, 300. [CrossRef]
54. Ertem, F.B.; Guven, O.; Buyukdag, C.; Gocenler, O.; Ayan, E.; Yuksel, B.; Gul, M.; Usta, G.; Cakılkaya, B.; Johnson, J.A.; et al. Protocol for structure determination of SARS-CoV-2 main protease at near-physiological-temperature by serial femtosecond crystallography. *STAR Protoc.* **2022**, *3*, 101158. [CrossRef]
55. Garman, E.F.; Owen, R.L. Cryocooling and radiation damage in macromolecular crystallography. *Acta Crystallogr. Sect. D Biol. Crystallogr.* **2006**, *62*, 32–47. [CrossRef]
56. Atalay, N.; Akcan, E.K.; Gul, M.; Ayan, E.; Destan, E.; Ertem, F.B.; Tokay, N.; Çakilkaya, B.; Nergiz, Z.; Karakadioğlu, G.; et al. Cryogenic X-ray crystallographic studies of biomacromolecules at Turkish Light Source "Turkish DeLight". *Turk. J. Biol.* **2022**, *47*, 1–13. [CrossRef]
57. Rigaku. CrysAlisPro Software System, Version 1.171.42.35a. 2021. Rigaku Oxford Diffraction. Available online: https://www.rigaku.com (accessed on 8 November 2023).
58. McCoy, A.J.; Grosse-Kunstleve, R.W.; Adams, P.D.; Winn, M.D.; Storoni, L.C.; Read, R.J. Phaser crystallographic software. *J. Appl. Crystallogr.* **2007**, *40*, 658–674. [CrossRef] [PubMed]
59. Adams, P.D.; Afonine, P.V.; Bunkoczi, G.; Chen, V.B.; Davis, I.W.; Echols, N.; Headd, J.J.; Hung, L.W.; Kapral, G.J.; Grosse-Kunstleve, R.W.; et al. PHENIX: A comprehensive Python-based system for macromolecular structure solution. *Acta Crystallogr. D Biol. Crystallogr.* **2010**, *66*, 213–221. [CrossRef]
60. Emsley, P.; Cowtan, K. Coot: Model-building tools for molecular graphics. *Acta Crystallogr. D Biol. Crystallogr.* **2004**, *60*, 2126–2132. [CrossRef] [PubMed]
61. *The PyMOL Molecular Graphics System, Version 2.5.2*, Schrödinger, LLC.: New York, NY, USA, 2023.
62. *Schrödinger Release 2016-2*, Schrödinger, LLC.: New York, NY, USA, 2016.
63. Ciftci, H.; Sever, B.; Ayan, E.; Can, M.; DeMirci, H.; Otsuka, M.; TuYuN, A.F.; Tateishi, H.; Fujita, M. Identification of New L-Heptanoylphosphatidyl Inositol Pentakisphosphate Derivatives Targeting the Interaction with HIV-1 Gag by Molecular Modelling Studies. *Pharmaceuticals* **2022**, *15*, 1255. [CrossRef] [PubMed]
64. *Schrödinger Release 2023-3*, Schrödinger, LLC.: New York, NY, USA, 2023.
65. Abascal, J.L.; Vega, C. A general purpose model for the condensed phases of water: TIP4P/2005. *J. Chem. Phys.* **2005**, *123*, 234505. [CrossRef]

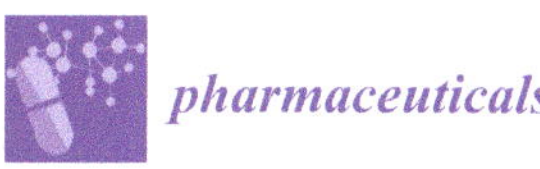 *pharmaceuticals*

Article

De Novo Drug Design Using Transformer-Based Machine Translation and Reinforcement Learning of an Adaptive Monte Carlo Tree Search

Dony Ang [1,2], Cyril Rakovski [1,2] and Hagop S. Atamian [2,3,*]

[1] Computational and Data Sciences Program, Chapman University, Orange, CA 92866, USA; doang@chapman.edu (D.A.); rakovski@chapman.edu (C.R.)
[2] Schmid College of Science and Technology, Chapman University, Orange, CA 92866, USA
[3] Biological Sciences Program, Chapman University, Orange, CA 92866, USA
* Correspondence: atamian@chapman.edu

Citation: Ang, D.; Rakovski, C.; Atamian, H.S. De Novo Drug Design Using Transformer-Based Machine Translation and Reinforcement Learning of an Adaptive Monte Carlo Tree Search. *Pharmaceuticals* 2024, 17, 161. https://doi.org/10.3390/ph17020161

Academic Editors: Halil İbrahim Ciftci, Belgin Sever and Hasan Demirci

Received: 30 October 2023
Revised: 24 January 2024
Accepted: 25 January 2024
Published: 27 January 2024

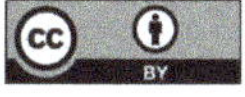

Abstract: The discovery of novel therapeutic compounds through de novo drug design represents a critical challenge in the field of pharmaceutical research. Traditional drug discovery approaches are often resource intensive and time consuming, leading researchers to explore innovative methods that harness the power of deep learning and reinforcement learning techniques. Here, we introduce a novel drug design approach called drugAI that leverages the Encoder–Decoder Transformer architecture in tandem with Reinforcement Learning via a Monte Carlo Tree Search (RL-MCTS) to expedite the process of drug discovery while ensuring the production of valid small molecules with drug-like characteristics and strong binding affinities towards their targets. We successfully integrated the Encoder–Decoder Transformer architecture, which generates molecular structures (drugs) from scratch with the RL-MCTS, serving as a reinforcement learning framework. The RL-MCTS combines the exploitation and exploration capabilities of a Monte Carlo Tree Search with the machine translation of a transformer-based Encoder–Decoder model. This dynamic approach allows the model to iteratively refine its drug candidate generation process, ensuring that the generated molecules adhere to essential physicochemical and biological constraints and effectively bind to their targets. The results from drugAI showcase the effectiveness of the proposed approach across various benchmark datasets, demonstrating a significant improvement in both the validity and drug-likeness of the generated compounds, compared to two existing benchmark methods. Moreover, drugAI ensures that the generated molecules exhibit strong binding affinities to their respective targets. In summary, this research highlights the real-world applications of drugAI in drug discovery pipelines, potentially accelerating the identification of promising drug candidates for a wide range of diseases.

Keywords: artificial intelligence; drug design; novel molecules; encoder–decoder; transformer; quantitative estimate of drug-likeness (QED); virtual screening; validity; reinforcement learning; molecular docking

1. Introduction

The task of finding molecules that bind to specific biological targets is challenging due to the vast molecular space [1]. Despite recent advancements in high-throughput screening methods, screening millions of molecules for their binding to proteins of interest remains a costly and time-consuming process [2]. The possible promiscuity of the identified molecules poses yet another challenge that is receiving increasing attention in drug discovery [3]. Molecules can bind to multiple off targets, leading to undesirable and sometimes even life-threatening side effects [4]. Yet, molecules that target multiple biological targets simultaneously, could be needed for treating complex illnesses such as cancer and cardiovascular disease. Such promiscuous drugs, such as aspirin, are very rare but very effective [5]. This biological complexity could be addressed by the integration of cutting-edge data science that incorporates AI-driven approaches and by encouraging collaboration between academia, pharmaceutical companies, and the biotechnology industry.

Computational methods have played a pivotal role in accelerating drug discovery and reducing associated costs [6]. By combining ligand- and structure-based virtual screening methods, researchers can efficiently screen large chemical databases to identify potential drug candidates in a short time [7]. Furthermore, scientists can employ molecular dynamics simulations to predict how molecules will interact with specific biological targets [8]. These methods, although effective, have limitations as they rely on existing molecules, whether synthetic or natural. As part of the recent wave of advancements in artificial intelligence, generative AI models have emerged as a powerful tool in the field of drug discovery, particularly for de novo drug design, which involves creating novel molecular structures [9].

Generative AI models used in drug discovery can be broadly categorized into two main groups based on their use of target information. The models in the first category are trained on a large dataset of known molecules, allowing them to efficiently explore the chemical space and generate molecules with properties similar to known compounds. However, this focus on similarity to known molecules may limit their ability to produce entirely novel chemical structures and optimize interactions with specific targets. In the second category, models rely on the 3D structure or binding site characteristics of the target, enabling the generation of molecules tailored for interaction with specific targets. Nevertheless, a major drawback of such models is the limited availability of high-quality structural data for many drug targets [10]. To leverage the advantages of both categories, a combination of these models is often used.

Self-supervised pretraining, which involves training models on large amounts of unlabeled data, has become a dominant paradigm in Natural Language Processing (NLP) and has been successfully used in the two influential NLP technologies GPT and BERT [11,12]. Researchers have adapted the principles of NLP pretraining to develop "chemical language models" given the analogies between human language and the "language" of chemical structures represented by SMILES (Simplified Molecular Input Line Entry System) strings. In natural languages, grammatical rules and syntax govern the arrangement of words in sentences, which affects the meaning and interpretation of text [13]. The chemical language follows similar specific rules and syntax to those in natural language for representing chemical structures, where the order and arrangement of symbols in SMILES strings convey information about the chemical structure and properties of a molecule. By treating chemical structures like sentences, where each symbol or combination of symbols represents a chemical entity (atom, bond, or group), chemical language models can be pre-trained on large datasets of SMILES strings. These models learn to generate SMILES strings by predicting each symbol or subsequent symbols [14]. Such chemical language models have been shown to obtain promising results on downstream tasks.

This research drew inspiration from Machine Translation (MT) using the sequence-to-sequence model [15] and from the rapid success of applying transformation architecture [16] in various NLP use cases. Greedy and beam search methods have traditionally been common approaches for decoding auto-regressive machine translation models in NLP [17,18]. Recently, the Monte Carlo Tree Search (MCTS)-based method has been demonstrated to outperform the greedy and beam search methods in generic language applications [19]. The MCTS is a probabilistic and heuristic-driven search algorithm that enables multiple constraint optimization steps. Moreover, this MCTS-based method has been successfully applied in Large Language Models (LLM) [20].

In this work, we introduce an innovative de novo drug design engine named drugAI, which marks the first integration of a decoder transformer model with the MCTS in the fields of bioinformatics and cheminformatics. At the core of drugAI, we employ an encoder–decoder transformer model coupled with a MCTS algorithm. This novel approach enabled us to implement multiple constraint optimization steps during the protein sequence to small molecule (SMILES string) generation. The drugAI engine, which was extensively trained on protein–ligand pairs, filtered from the comprehensive BindingDB [21], takes target protein sequences as input and generates small molecules (SMILES strings) as candidate inhibitors for these protein targets. Notably, drugAI surpasses traditional greedy and beam search methods by enabling multi-constrained optimization of the generated molecules. It evaluates their (1) validity; (2) pharmacological or biological properties for orally active drugs in humans [22]; (3) quantitative estimate of drug-likeness (QED) to gouge the compounds' potential as drug candidates [23], and binding affinity to their targets. The molecules generated by drugAI were consistently valid with a validity rate of 100%. They showed 42% and 75% higher QED scores compared to those obtained through greedy and beam search methods, respectively. Furthermore, by integrating the binding affinity between the ligand and the target into the reinforcement learning process, the molecules generated by drugAI demonstrated strong binding affinities towards their respective targets. These affinities were comparable to those identified by traditional virtual screening approaches.

2. Results

2.1. Effectiveness of DrugAI

To assess the effectiveness of our proposed approach (drugAI) in generating small molecules with desired qualities for potential future drug candidates, we employed drugAI, alongside two other commonly used methods, greedy and beam, to train on the same dataset. We then conducted a comparative analysis of the results produced by these three methods by calculating various benchmarks within the GuacaMol codebase [24] using the Distributed-learning GuacaMol function. It is worth noting that the quantitative estimate of drug-likeness (QED) was not included in the standard GuacaMol benchmarks and was calculated separately using the RDKit package. DrugAI outperformed the greedy and beam methods by generating a significantly higher proportion of valid molecules (Table 1). In fact, all the molecules generated by drugAI were valid, whereas the greedy and beam methods produced 0.83 and 0.62 proportions of valid molecules, respectively. The uniqueness and novelty parameters of the generated molecules by drugAI were comparable to the greedy method but significantly higher than the beam method (Table 1). DrugAI demonstrated outstanding performance in terms of generating molecules with a high measure of drug-likeness, as assessed by the quantitative estimate of drug-likeness (QED). The molecules generated by drugAI achieved a significantly higher QED score (0.73) compared to greedy (0.41) and beam (0.18) (Table 1). The distribution of the QED scores also exhibited substantial differences. DrugAI did not produce QED scores below 0.3, while greedy search displayed scores spanning the entire spectrum. In contrast, the beam search predominantly lacked scores above 0.5 (Figure 1).

Table 1. Summary of the GuacaMol evaluations of the SMILES strings generated by three different decoding algorithms. The reported values represent the averages of ten independent runs. Significant differences are denoted by different letters, as determined by the Kruskal–Wallis test ($p < 0.05$). The values based on a 95% confidence interval are presented in parentheses.

Benchmark	DrugAI	Greedy	Beam (K = 2)
Validity	1.00 [a] (1)	0.83 [b] (0.82–0.84)	0.62 [c] (0.61–0.63)
Uniqueness	0.84 [a] (0.83–0.85)	0.87 [a] (0.86–0.88)	0.37 [b] (0.36–0.38)
Novelty	1.00 [a] (1)	1.00 [a] (1)	0.47 [b] (0.46–0.48)
Mean QED	0.73 [a] (72.95–73.05)	0.41 [b] (0.41)	0.18 [c] (0.18)

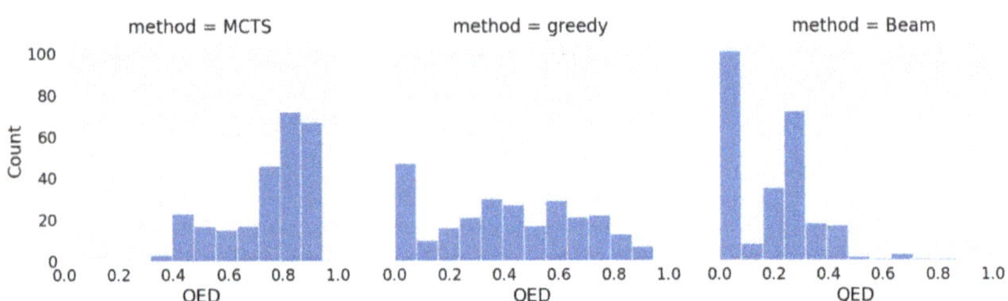

Figure 1. Distribution of QED drug-likeness of the generated molecules across the different decoding algorithms.

2.2. Physicochemical Properties of the Generated Molecules

One of the available methods for assessing the drug-likeness of a compound is Lipinski's Rule of Five (also known as RO5). In addition to its effectiveness against a target protein, newly designed drugs should be suitable for oral administration. Therefore, RO5 predicts whether a chemical compound has favorable pharmacokinetic properties based on criteria such as Molecular Weight (MW < 500), Lipophilicity (LogP < 5), Hydrogen Bond Donors (HBD < 5), and Hydrogen Bond Acceptors (HBA < 10). Compounds meeting these criteria have a high likelihood of being orally bioavailable. However, it is worth mentioning that in drug discovery, no rule is absolute, as up to 10% of approved oral drugs violate RO5 [25]. Another key feature of drugAI, in addition to its ability to generate 100% valid molecules with high QED values, is its adherence to the RO5 criteria while generating molecules. This adherence serves as a valuable initial filter for identifying compounds with the potential for oral drug development. To evaluate the performance in terms of generating molecules that conform to the RO5 criteria, we calculated these metrics and assessed the physicochemical properties of the molecules generated by the three methods. Figure 2 presents the data regarding the compliance of the generated molecules from all three methods with the aforementioned rules. All the molecules generated by drugAI had logP values less than or equal to 5, whereas nearly one third of the molecules generated by greedy and beam searches exceeded this threshold, reaching as high as 15. Similarly, the molecular weight of the compounds generated by drugAI did not exceed the 500 threshold while greedy and beam searches generated molecules with molecular weights of up to 800. Interestingly, unlike drugAI, both the greedy and beam methods produced a large number of very small molecules. Regarding HBD and HBA, drugAI strictly adhered to the RO5 criteria, producing molecules with values no higher than 5 for HBD and 10 for HBA, respectively. While HBA values rarely exceeded 10 in the greedy and beam methods, HBD values were more varied and often went beyond 5. The number of rotatable bonds was significantly smaller in the molecules generated by drugAI compared to the other two methods. There were no significant differences in terms of the number of rings among the three methods. In summary, these findings illustrate how drugAI can significantly enhance future de novo drug design efforts by generating drug-like molecules.

2.3. Demonstrating the Flexibility of DrugAI and Comparing It to Traditional Virtual Screening Approaches

Our findings conclusively demonstrated that drugAI outperforms two benchmark methods in terms of generating 100% valid molecules with high QED scores that are suitable for oral application. To further improve the model and showcase its adaptability and flexibility, we incorporated binding affinity (measured in kcal/mol) as an additional reward function in drugAI's reinforcement learning. The binding affinity, which describes the binding strength between a drug molecule and its target, plays a significant role in early drug development. Thus, adding this fourth reward function would further enhance the quality of the molecules produced as potential drugs by ensuring that the generated molecules strongly bind to the target protein.

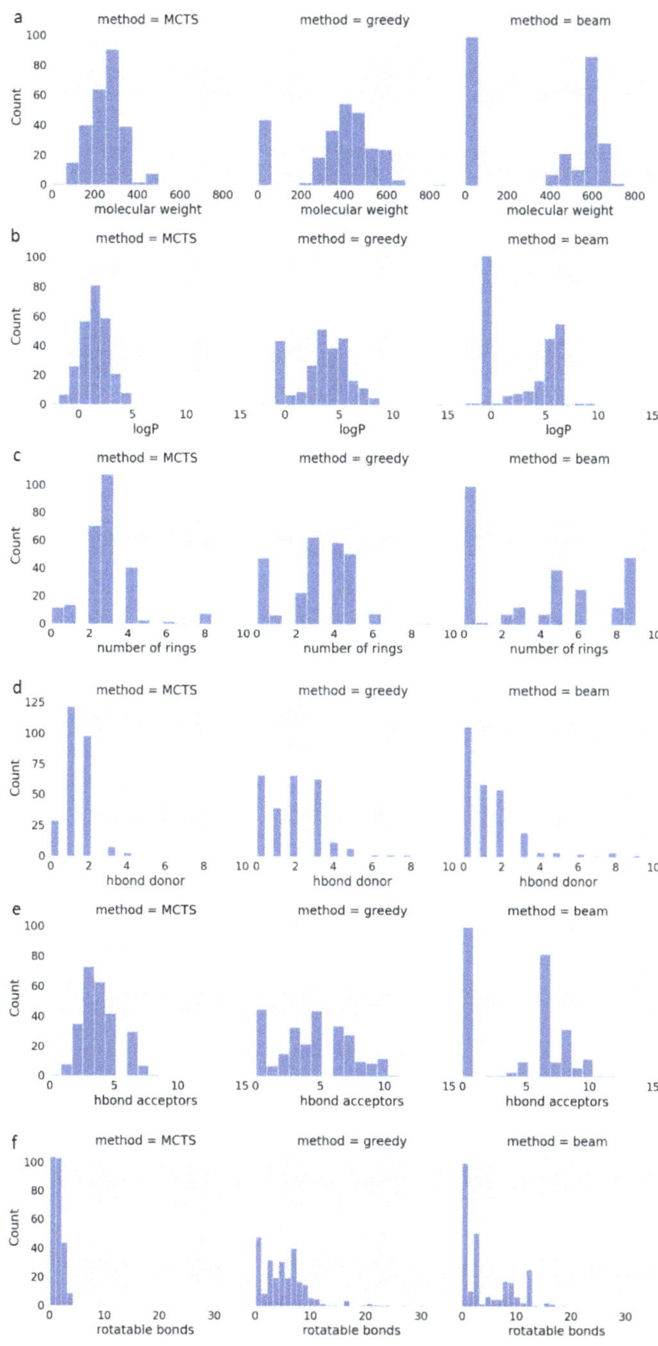

Figure 2. Distribution of properties for the generated molecules across the different decoding algorithms. (**a**) Molecular weight; (**b**) water–octanol partition coefficient (logP); (**c**) the number of rings; (**d**) the number of H donors; (**e**) the number of H acceptors; (**f**) the number of rotatable bonds.

We previously discovered natural products that bind to the SARS-CoV-2 Main Protease (M^{pro}) and inhibit its protease activity using a combined Ligand-based and Structure-based Virtual Screening (LBVS + SBVS) approach [26]. As a proof of concept, we used drugAI to generate small molecules targeting the same SARS-CoV-2 M^{pro} target protein. For consistency, both LBVS + SBVS and drugAI were configured to scan and utilize the same cavity coordinates and the same docking search area sizes [26]. As shown in Table 2, the average binding affinity for the top 10 generated molecules by drugAI is −9.4 (kcal/mol), which is comparable to the −9.37 (kcal/mol) obtained in [26]. The molecules generated by drugAI belonged to different chemical classes such as Benzenes, Isoindoles, Flavonoids, and Quinoles (Table S1). In conclusion, drugAI generated valid molecules with drug-like characteristics that are optimized to bind efficiently to their target in just two hours, with results comparable to widely used virtual screening methods, which take weeks to perform molecular docking on a large number of ligands.

Table 2. Molecules generated by drugAI against SARS-CoV-2 M^{pro} target protein.

Generated Molecule (SMILES)	Validity	Adherence to RO5	Binding Affinity (kcal/mol)	QED Score
O=C1c2cc(N3CCNCC3)ccc2C(OC2CCc3ccccc32)c2ccccc21	1	1	−9.87	0.69
O=C1c2cc(N3CCN(c4cnc5ncccc5c4)CC3)ccc2CCCc2ccccc21	1	1	−9.59	0.46
O=C1c2cc(N3CCNCC3)cc(-c3cccc(/C=C/C(=O)Nc4ccccc4)c3)c2C(=O)N1	1	1	−9.56	0.41
O=C1c2cc(N3CCNC(c4ncc(C(F)(F)F)cc4Cl)CC3)ccc2COC1O	1	1	−9.45	0.74
O=C1c2cc(N3CCNCC3)ccc2OC(COc2cccc([N+](=O)[O-])c2)Cc2ccccc21	1	1	−9.39	0.46
O=C1c2cc(N3CCNCC3)nc-c3ccc(C(=O)c4cc(F)cc(F)c4)cc3c2CCC1=O	1	1	−9.39	0.56
O=C1c2cc(N3CCNC4C3CC5CC(C4)OC5)ccc2C(=O)c2ccc(Cl)cc2N1	1	1	−9.30	0.61
O=C1c2cc(N3CCNCC3)nc(-c3cccc(C(F)(F)F)c3)c2CCc2ccccc21	1	1	−9.24	0.64
O=C1c2cc(N3CCNCC3)ccc2C(OC2Cc3ccccc3C2)=C2C(=O)CCC(O)C(F)(F)C21	1	1	−9.22	0.68
O=C1c2cc(N3CCNCC3)ccc2OC/C1=C(\O)c1cccc(-c2ccncc2)c1	1	1	−9.21	0.50
Average	1	1	−9.42	0.58

3. Discussion

Generative machine learning models are designed to learn patterns and structures within existing data and create new, previously unseen data [27]. These models have gained popularity in drug discovery in recent years and are expected to revolutionize the future of pharmaceutical engineering [28]. The Encoder–Decoder Transformer architecture, which takes an input sequence and generates an output sequence, has been widely used in natural language processing (NLP) [16]. Recently, this Encoder–Decoder Transformer architecture has been adapted in the field of drug discovery, where it takes molecular structures or protein sequences as input and generates novel molecules or sequences. At the decoding step, which involves the process of generating new sequences or molecules by adding amino acids or atoms one at a time, a decision-making strategy is needed to make the best choice at each step based on selecting the token with the highest probability as the next token in the output sequence [29]. The two most popular decoding algorithms in sequence-to-sequence models are the greedy search and the beam search. Both are heuristic search algorithms that seek to find the most likely output sequence. While greedy search simply selects the token with the highest probability as the next token in the output sequence, beam search considers multiple candidates at each time step and retains a diverse set of candidates throughout the decoding process [17,18].

However, the challenge with these types of decoding algorithms in drug design is to ensure that the newly generated molecules adhere to certain constraints or properties that could make them successful drugs. Reinforcement learning (RL) has been successfully applied in fields such as speech recognition and formal languages to address this challenge by introducing value functions into the decoding mechanisms [30]. These value functions reward desired behaviors and penalize undesired ones [31]. In our approach, we employed the Monte Carlo Tree Search (MCTS) method to overcome some of the limitations of deep generative models that use greedy and beam searches. By utilizing value functions to assess validity, binding to target, and adherence to Lipinski's Rule of Five (RO5), our generative model produced molecules that were both 100% valid and had significantly higher quantitative estimates of drug-likeness (QED) scores. Ensuring the generation of SMILES strings that are 100% chemically valid is crucial because it guarantees that all molecules to be investigated in the future can be chemically synthesized.

The QED, introduced almost a decade ago [23], is one of the most commonly used quantitative assessments of drug efficacy. Studies have shown that the average QED within the top cluster of human drug targets is 0.693. When focusing exclusively on the highest-ranked cluster of oral drug targets, the average QED increases to 0.766 [23]. This demonstrates that drugAI, with a mean QED of 0.73, is capable of generating molecules with properties suitable for potential oral drug candidates. In line with these findings, the analysis of the individual criteria within the RO5 showed that drugAI was able to accurately adhere to those criteria, which was not the case with other search methods. This, in itself, explains the superior QED scores of drugAI. In the future, additional benchmarks could be employed to further evaluate the molecules generated by drugAI.

Yet, another crucial advantage of drugAI is its ability to generate 100% novel molecules with very high QED scores. When computational programs aim to generate molecules with high drug-likeness, they tend to avoid exploring unconventional or entirely new chemical structures and often prioritize well-known molecular structures and properties that are associated with existing drugs. This often leads to difficulties in generating truly novel molecules because the algorithms tend to have a biased output toward known chemical patterns in the training set. The results from drugAI were remarkable in terms of balancing the generation of molecules with known drug-likeness properties (high QED value) and the exploration of novel chemical space as it generated 100% novel molecules, which shows that the model did not generate any molecules present in the training set. Thus, drugAI efficiently addressed the common challenge of "overfitting" in de novo drug design as it generated 100% novel SMILES strings, a result comparable to the greedy search. Deep learning models can sometimes memorize existing chemical structures rather than generate new ones, which often results in overfitting. In our case, drugAI was able to learn and generalize the chemical space to generate novel molecules.

Moreover, the model avoided generating the same molecule multiple times, as shown by the 84% uniqueness.

Many molecular docking techniques are available that can predict how molecules will bind to biomolecular targets and the affinity of this binding [32]. These virtual screening techniques have proven effective in finding new hits from extensive collections of chemical compounds, and in predicting their modes and affinities of binding [33]. Presently, molecular docking is a leading approach in the discovery of new compounds that act against target proteins. The flexibility of the MCTS-based reinforcement learning enabled us to incorporate this important matrix in the model. Accordingly, drugAI was able to generate molecules that showed strong binding affinity against the target comparable to those identified through virtual screening of large chemical databases. This showcases the capability of drugAI in the proficient and successful creation of potential drugs for various diseases in the future.

4. Materials and Methods

4.1. Data

The model was trained using experimentally determined protein–ligand binding affinities obtained from the BindingDB database. The complete database comprises over 2.4 million data records, offering a valuable source of information. To curate a focused dataset for training, we implemented selection criteria to extract the most relevant records. The following criteria were applied to filter the raw dataset:

1. The field "Target Source Organism According to Curator or DataSource" equals "Homo sapiens";
2. The record has an IC50 value less than 100 nm; if the IC50 is missing, then Kd is less than 100 nm; if both are missing, then EC50 is less than 100 nm;
3. The record has SMILES representation.

This resulted in a dataset comprising 319,030 entries, consisting of 1298 unique amino acid sequences and 198,490 distinct ligand SMILES strings. To ensure uniformity and consistency, all SMILES strings used in this study were canonicalized using RDKit. The dataset was then randomly divided into two subsets: a training set, which comprised 70% of the data, and a test set, which made up the remaining 30%. The training subset consisted of 223,321 pairs of protein sequences and ligands, representing 1038 unique proteins. The test subset, on the other hand, contained 95,709 pairs of protein sequences and ligands, representing 260 unique proteins.

4.2. High-Level Architecture of DrugAI

The high-level architecture of the Encoder–Decoder Transformer, coupled with a Monte Carlo Tree Search (MCTS) for molecule generation, represents a state-of-the-art framework specifically designed for the discovery of highly effective lead molecule candidates targeted at specific receptor proteins in drug discovery, as illustrated in Figure 3.

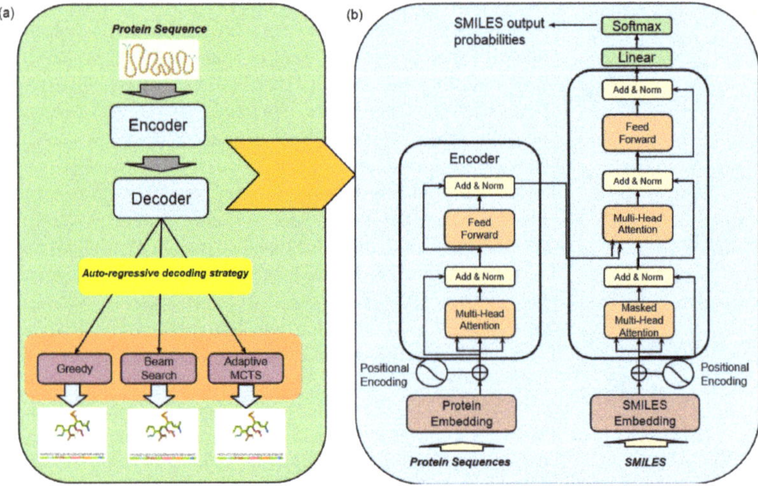

Figure 3. Machine translation—drugAI overview: (**a**) the workflow of the translation task of drugAI; (**b**) the encoder–decoder transformer architecture (modified from [16]).

This architecture combines two fundamental components to accelerate the process of identifying promising drug candidates:

- *Encoder–Decoder Transformer*
  At its core, this architecture employs a transformer model, which comprises an encoder and a decoder. The encoder takes input data in the form of protein sequences and transforms them into latent representations. Subsequently, the decoder utilizes these representations to systematically generate molecular sequences. The transformer model used in this study was trained with six layers of transformer blocks, each having a size of 512, a learning rate of 0.0001, and eight attention heads. The training process employed the Adam Optimizer with a batch size of five and a total of 25 epochs.
- *Monte Carlo Tree Search (MCTS)*
  The MCTS is a heuristic search algorithm used in conjunction with the transformer model. It facilitates the exploration of the vast and complex chemical space by consid-

ering different molecular modifications iteratively. The MCTS simulates the potential outcomes of these modifications, allowing for efficient decision making.

Altogether, this architecture integrates the transformer's generative capabilities with the MCTS's exploitation and exploration techniques in order to optimize the discovery of promising drug candidates that can meet multiple optimization goals. This architecture is designed to make sure the generated molecules are valid, show high bioactivity against target receptors, and can be administered orally.

4.3. Encoder–Decoder Transformer

At the core of our drugAI engine is the transformer model, as shown in Figure 3. We selected this deep-learning model for the following reasons:

a. Transformers excel at modeling sequential data. We see molecule generation as a machine translation task that needs to follow a sequence-to-sequence model (seq-to-seq).
b. Transformers are parallelizable, and this makes it efficient to parallelize the training and inference steps against Graphics Processing Units (GPUs) and Tensor Processing Units (TPUs).
c. Transformers can capture distant or long-range contexts and dependencies in the data between distant positions in the input or output sequences. Thus, longer connections can be learned, which makes it ideal for learning and capturing amino acid sequences whose residues can be hundreds or even thousands in length.
d. Transformers make no assumptions about the temporal/spatial relationships across the data.

For machine translation tasks that need to be modeled as seq-to-seq, the suitable transformer architecture is the encoder–decoder model. The encoder consists of encoding layers that process the amino acids iteratively one layer after another, while the decoder consists of decoding layers that iteratively process the encoder's output as well as the decoder output's SMILES strings in an auto-regressive manner.

The purpose of having an encoder layer is to generate a context representation of the protein (protein context), where each amino acid residue is represented by a "protein vector". It combines information from other amino acid residues via the self-attention mechanism. On the other hand, the decoder is responsible for generating the corresponding atoms that make up the small molecule in the SMILES notation. Each of the decoder layers consists of two sub-layers: (1) cross attention to incorporate the outputs of the encoder (also known as protein context); and (2) self-attention, which implements a teacher-forcing mechanism, feeding the decoder model with the previously predicted atoms to predict the probability distributions of the next atom from the vocabulary of SMILES notations. Both the cross-attention and self-attention layers also include an additional feed-forward layer and layer normalization for further processing of the outputs.

The building blocks of the transformer are self-attention, where each attention unit learns three weight matrices: the query weights W_Q, the key weights W_K, and the value weights W_V.

For each residue i, the input protein representation x_i is multiplied with each of the three weight matrices to produce a query vector $q_i = x_i W_Q$, a key vector $k_i = x_i W_K$, and a value vector $v_i = x_i W_V$.

Attention weights are calculated using the query and key vectors: the attention weight a_{ij} from amino acid i to amino acid j is the dot product between q_i and k_j. The attention weights are divided by $\sqrt{d_k}$ to stabilize gradients during training, and pass through a softmax layer, which normalizes the weights.

In summary, self-attention can be represented by the formula

$$Attention\,(Q, K, V) = softmax\frac{QK^T}{\sqrt{d_k}}$$

A set of (W_Q, W_K, W_V) matrices is called an attention head and each layer in a transformer model can have multiple attention heads. While each attention head attends to the amino acids that are relevant to each residue, multiple attention heads allow the model to do this for different definitions of relevance.

4.4. SMILES Decoding Strategies

4.4.1. Greedy Search

The greedy algorithm is one of the most common decoding algorithms, especially in Natural Language Processing. For drug design purposes, it simply generates one SMILE token at a time, iteratively. At each step, the model predicts the next token in the sequence based on the context of previously generated tokens. Note that in greedy decoding, the model selects the token with the highest probability as the next token to generate. This means that at each step, the model does not consider the global context or explore alternative token choices but simply chooses the most likely token according to its learned probabilities. This process continues until a predefined end-of-sequence token (e.g., <eos> for "end of SMILES") is generated or a maximum sequence length is reached. While greedy decoding is straightforward and computationally efficient, it may not always produce the best possible sequence, as it tends to favor local optimal choices at each step.

4.4.2. Beam Search

Beam search is another commonly used decoding algorithm. This decoder generates a set of candidate SMILES tokens for the next step in the sequence based on the current state (also known as teacher forcing). Each candidate is assigned a score based on its likelihood that is typically calculated using a combination of the model's output probabilities and a length normalization factor. The candidates with the highest scores are retained, while the rest are discarded. The retained candidates become the new set of states for the next step. These states are expanded further by generating new candidates for the subsequent step until a predefined end-of-sequence token is generated or a maximum sequence length is reached.

4.4.3. Monte Carlo Tree Search

The Monte Carlo Tree Search (MCTS) is a heuristic search algorithm that is often used in decision-making processes, particularly in the domain of artificial intelligence and game-playing software. It is commonly employed in software designed to play board games and other strategy games that require complex and branching decision trees to explore all possible moves and outcomes exhaustively. As the name suggests, it uses random sampling for deterministic problems that are difficult to solve using other traditional approaches due to the vast search space. The popularity of the algorithm increased after Google's DeepMind adopted it to build a program called AlphaGo [34] that became the first computer Go program to beat a professional human Go player.

The MCTS offers a promising solution for navigating the expansive and intricate landscape of chemical space in the context of molecule generation, as shown in Figure 4. This algorithmic framework, originally developed for game-playing AI, has found a novel application in the field of Natural Language Processing [19]. The MCTS leverages the principles of exploration and exploitation to efficiently sample and evaluate molecular candidates. By iteratively building a tree of possible chemical sequences and selecting the most promising branches evaluated via a reward function, the MCTS enables the exploration of diverse regions within the vast chemical space while maintaining a focus on regions likely to yield valuable molecules. This innovative approach holds the potential to revolutionize drug discovery, materials science, and other domains by aiding researchers in the rapid and intelligent exploration of uncharted territories within the complex realm of molecular design.

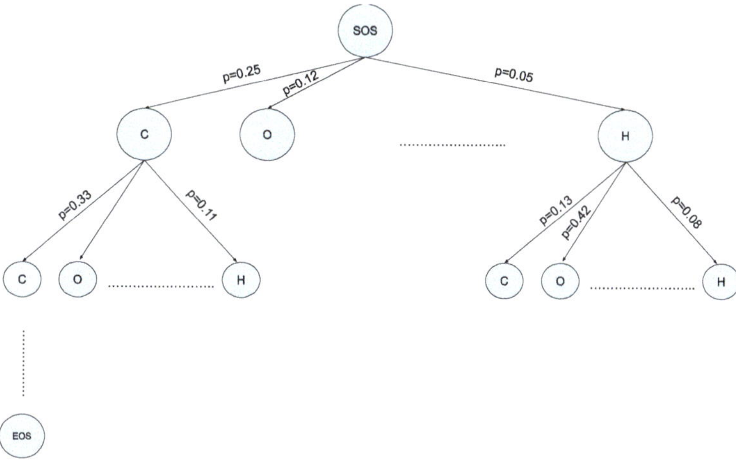

Figure 4. Vast chemical space in the tree structure format—V^d where V is the size of the SMILES vocabulary and d is the max depth of small molecules in SMILES notation.

To apply this powerful approach in drug design, we modified the original MCTS algorithm as described below and provide a summary in Figure 5:

1. Selection

   The MCTS traverses the SMILES tree structure from the root node using a strategy called the Upper Confidence Bound (UCB) to optimally select the subsequent nodes with the highest estimated value of UCB. Values derived by UCB balance the exploration-exploitation trade-off, and during the tree traversal, a node is selected based on some parameters that return the maximum value. The formula of UCB is described as follows:

$$UCB = \frac{r_i}{n_i} + c\sqrt{\frac{lnN_i}{n_i}}$$

   r_i is total cumulative rewards.
   n_i is the number of simulations for the node considered after i-th move.
   N_i is the total number of simulations after i-th move.
   c is the exploration parameter (default value set to 2).
   In summary, the first term of the equation will help determine when the MCTS should prioritize making the most of what it knows (exploitation) and the second term of the equation will determine when it should focus on trying out new options (exploration). This ensures that the algorithm is balanced between ensuring that it explores new possibilities and also exploiting known good choices.

2. Expansion

   During the traversal of a SMILES tree as part of the selection process in the Monte Carlo Tree Search (MCTS), the child node that yields the highest value from the equation will be chosen for further exploration. If this selected node is also a leaf node and not a terminal node, the MCTS will proceed with the expansion process. This involves creating all possible children of this leaf node based on the SMILES vocabulary.

3. Simulation

   The posterior distribution is derived by using the distribution supplied by the decoder as an informative prior (in contrast to using uniform distribution as a prior where a large proportion of the posterior samples are in the invalid form).

4. Back propagation

   When the terminal node is reached, the complete SMILES string can be finalized by concatenating all the traversed and simulated nodes from the root until the terminal and the reward is calculated by running the reward function based on the newly constructed SMILES string. Thus, the MCTS needs to update the traversed nodes with this new reward by performing a back-propagation process where it back-propagates from the selected leaf node as a result of step 2 all the way back up to the root node. During this process, the number of simulations stored in each node is also incremented.

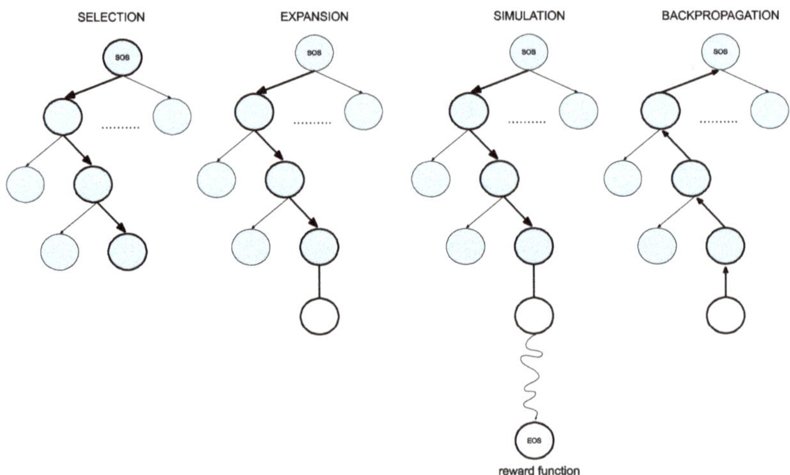

Figure 5. Four steps of Monte Carlo Tree Search (adapted from [20]).

In our emphasis on developing an effective reward function tailored for the drug design use case, we considered various options that could be employed as the reward function. Below, we describe the choices we used for the reward function.

1. Valid SMILES
   This binary variable is a straightforward check that assesses the validity of the newly generated SMILES string resulting from the simulation. The check is carried out by executing a basic function provided by RDKit, a toolkit commonly used in cheminformatics and drug discovery [35].
2. Lipinski's Rule of Five (Ro5)
   Another binary variable that checks to see if the newly constructed SMILES string passes all the 5 conditions set forth in the Ro5 [22].
3. Quantitive Estimation of Drug-likeness (QED)
   A floating-point variable that reflects the underlying distribution of molecular properties. This metric is intuitive, transparent, and straightforward to implement in many practical settings and allows compounds to be ranked by their relative merit. Medicinal chemists often consider a compound to exhibit characteristics and properties typically desired in drug candidates if the correlation coefficient of the QED value falls within the range of 0.5 to 0.6 [23].
4. Binding Affinity (kcal/mol)
   A floating-point variable that refers to the strength by which two molecules interact or bind. The smaller its value, the greater the affinity between two molecules. This binding affinity score is generated by AutoDock Vina [36], a commonly used open source program for doing molecular docking.

5. Conclusions and Future Perspectives

In conclusion, drugAI outperformed models using greedy and beam searches regarding the validity, QED, and adherence of the generated molecules to RO5. We further improved the drug design capabilities by adding a binding affinity reward function in drugAI's reinforcement learning. This proof of concept, combining the Encoder–Decoder Transformer architecture with the flexibility of the MCTS-based reinforcement learning, has the potential to significantly improve the quality of generated drugs by incorporating even more reward functions.

Future research could enhance the reinforcement learning of drugAI by supplementing the model with additional functions, such as the following:

1. pChEMBL values, including pKi, pKd, pIC50, or pEC50 [37];
2. ADMET-related properties, such as acute oral toxicity, Ames mutagenicity, and Caco-2 permeability;
3. Adherence to Oprea's rules of drug-likeness [38];
4. Avoidance of functional groups with toxic, reactive, or otherwise undesirable moieties defined by the REOS (Rapid Elimination of Swill) rules [39].

Such a multi-objective optimization reinforcement learning approach could potentially yield valuable molecules. This approach would enable the model to simultaneously optimize multiple properties or functions rather than focusing on a single objective. By optimizing across multiple criteria, it may be possible to create molecules that are not only effective as potential drugs but also meet various safety and efficacy requirements. However, the success of this approach will depend on the specific objectives and constraints defined, as well as the quality of data used to train the model.

Supplementary Materials: The following supporting information can be downloaded at: https://www.mdpi.com/article/10.3390/ph17020161/s1, Table S1: Annotation of the molecules generated by drugAI.

Author Contributions: Conceptualization, D.A.; methodology, D.A.; formal analysis, D.A.; investigation, D.A., C.R., and H.S.A.; writing—original draft preparation, H.S.A.; writing—review and editing, H.S.A. and D.A.; visualization, D.A. and H.S.A.; supervision, H.S.A. and C.R.; project administration, H.S.A.; funding acquisition, H.S.A. All authors have read and agreed to the published version of the manuscript.

Funding: D.A. was supported by a scholarship from the Computational and Data Sciences Program at Chapman University.

Institutional Review Board Statement: Not applicable.

Informed Consent Statement: Not applicable.

Data Availability Statement: The complete code used in this research is publicly available at https://github.com/dangjaya/drugAI. A standalone more user-friendly executable version of drugAI is available for download at https://atamianlab.com/software/.

Acknowledgments: We thank the research systems administrator, James Kelly, and Brett Fisher in Research Computing at Chapman University for their help with computing resources.

Conflicts of Interest: The authors declare no conflicts of interest.

References

1. Walters, W.P. Virtual chemical libraries: Miniperspective. *J. Med. Chem.* **2018**, *62*, 1116–1124. [CrossRef] [PubMed]
2. Dreiman, G.H.; Bictash, M.; Fish, P.V.; Griffin, L.; Svensson, F. Changing the HTS paradigm: AI-driven iterative screening for hit finding. *SLAS Discov.* **2021**, *26*, 257–262. [CrossRef] [PubMed]
3. Senger, M.R.; Fraga, C.A.; Dantas, R.F.; Silva, F.P., Jr. Filtering promiscuous compounds in early drug discovery: Is it a good idea? *Drug Discov. Today* **2016**, *21*, 868–872. [CrossRef] [PubMed]
4. Gupta, M.N.; Alam, A.; Hasnain, S.E. Protein promiscuity in drug discovery, drug-repurposing and antibiotic resistance. *Biochimie* **2020**, *175*, 50–57. [CrossRef] [PubMed]
5. Frantz, S. Drug discovery: Playing dirty. *Nature* **2005**, *437*, 942. [CrossRef]
6. Lin, X.; Li, X.; Lin, X. A review on applications of computational methods in drug screening and design. *Molecules* **2020**, *25*, 1375. [CrossRef]
7. Sharma, V.; Wakode, S.; Kumar, H. Structure- and ligand-based drug design: Concepts, approaches, and challenges. In *Chemoinformatics and Bioinformatics in the Pharmaceutical Sciences*; Sharma, N., Ojha, H., Raghav, P.K., Goyal, R.K., Eds.; Academic Press: Cambridge, MA, USA, 2021; pp. 27–53.

8. Salo-Ahen, O.M.; Alanko, I.; Bhadane, R.; Bonvin, A.M.; Honorato, R.V.; Hossain, S.; Juffer, A.H.; Vanmeert, M. Molecular dynamics simulations in drug discovery and pharmaceutical development. *Processes* **2020**, *9*, 71. [CrossRef]
9. Cheng, Y.; Gong, Y.; Liu, Y.; Song, B.; Zou, Q. Molecular design in drug discovery: A comprehensive review of deep generative models. *Brief. Bioinform.* **2021**, *22*, bbab344. [CrossRef]
10. Xie, W.; Wang, F.; Li, Y.; Lai, L.; Pei, J. Advances and challenges in de novo drug design using three-dimensional deep generative models. *J. Chem. Inf. Model.* **2022**, *62*, 2269–2279. [CrossRef]
11. Brown, T.; Mann, B.; Ryder, N.; Subbiah, M.; Kaplan, J.D.; Dhariwal, P.; Neelakantan, A.; Amodei, D. Language models are few-shot learners. In Proceedings of the Advances in Neural Information Processing Systems 33 (NeurIPS 2020), Virtual, 6–12 December 2020; pp. 1877–1901.
12. Devlin, J.; Chang, M.W.; Lee, K.; Toutanova, K. Bert: Pre-training of deep bidirectional transformers for language understanding. *arXiv* **2018**, arXiv:1810.04805.
13. Chowdhary, K.R. Natural language processing. In *Fundamentals of Artificial Intelligence*; Springer: New Delhi, India, 2020; pp. 603–649.
14. Kell, D.B.; Samanta, S.; Swainston, N. Deep learning and generative methods in cheminformatics and chemical biology: Navigating small molecule space intelligently. *Biochem. J.* **2020**, *477*, 4559–4580. [CrossRef] [PubMed]
15. Sutskever, I.; Vinyals, O.; Le, Q.V. Sequence to sequence learning with neural networks. In Proceedings of the Advances in Neural Information Processing Systems 27 (NIPS 2014), Montreal, QC, Canada, 8–13 December 2014.
16. Vaswani, A.; Shazeer, N.; Parmar, N.; Uszkoreit, J.; Jones, L.; Gomez, A.N.; Kaiser, L.; Polosukhin, I. Attention is all you need. In Proceedings of the Neural Information Processing Systems 30 (NIPS 2017), Long Beach, CA, USA, 4–9 December 2017.
17. Chickering, D.M. Optimal structure identification with greedy search. *J. Mach. Learn. Res.* **2002**, *3*, 507–554.
18. Wiseman, S.; Rush, A.M. Sequence-to-sequence learning as beam-search optimization. *arXiv* **2016**, arXiv:1606.02960.
19. Leblond, R.; Alayrac, J.B.; Sifre, L.; Pislar, M.; Lespiau, J.B.; Antonoglou, I.; Simonyan, K.; Vinyals, O. Machine translation decoding beyond beam search. *arXiv* **2021**, arXiv:2104.05336.
20. Chaffin, A.; Claveau, V.; Kijak, E. PPL-MCTS: Constrained textual generation through discriminator-guided MCTS decoding. *arXiv* **2021**, arXiv:2109.13582.
21. Gilson, M.K.; Liu, T.; Baitaluk, M.; Nicola, G.; Hwang, L.; Chong, J. BindingDB in 2015: A public database for medicinal chemistry, computational chemistry and systems pharmacology. *Nucleic Acids Res.* **2016**, *44*, D1045–D1053. [CrossRef]
22. Lipinski, C.A. Lead-and drug-like compounds: The rule-of-five revolution. *Drug Discov. Today Technol.* **2004**, *1*, 337–341. [CrossRef] [PubMed]
23. Bickerton, G.R.; Paolini, G.V.; Besnard, J.; Muresan, S.; Hopkins, A.L. Quantifying the chemical beauty of drugs. *Nat. Chem.* **2012**, *4*, 90–98. [CrossRef]
24. Brown, N.; Fiscato, M.; Segler, M.H.; Vaucher, A.C. GuacaMol: Benchmarking models for de novo molecular design. *J. Chem. Inf. Model.* **2019**, *59*, 1096–1108. [CrossRef]
25. Benet, L.Z.; Hosey, C.M.; Ursu, O.; Oprea, T.I. BDDCS, the Rule of 5 and drugability. *Adv. Drug Deliv. Rev.* **2016**, *101*, 89–98. [CrossRef]
26. Ang, D.; Kendall, R.; Atamian, H.S. Virtual and In Vitro Screening of Natural Products Identifies Indole and Benzene Derivatives as Inhibitors of SARS-CoV-2 Main Protease (Mpro). *Biology* **2023**, *12*, 519. [CrossRef] [PubMed]
27. Harshvardhan, G.M.; Gourisaria, M.K.; Pandey, M.; Rautaray, S.S. A comprehensive survey and analysis of generative models in machine learning. *Comput. Sci. Rev.* **2020**, *38*, 100285.
28. Martinelli, D.D. Generative machine learning for de novo drug discovery: A systematic review. *Comput. Biol. Med.* **2022**, *145*, 105403. [CrossRef] [PubMed]
29. Grechishnikova, D. Transformer neural network for protein-specific de novo drug generation as a machine translation problem. *Sci. Rep.* **2021**, *11*, 321. [CrossRef] [PubMed]
30. Latif, S.; Cuayáhuitl, H.; Pervez, F.; Shamshad, F.; Ali, H.S.; Cambria, E. A survey on deep reinforcement learning for audio-based applications. *Artif. Intell. Rev.* **2023**, *56*, 2193–2240. [CrossRef]
31. Mouchlis, V.D.; Afantitis, A.; Serra, A.; Fratello, M.; Papadiamantis, A.G.; Aidinis, V.; Lynch, I.; Greco, D.; Melagraki, G. Advances in de novo drug design: From conventional to machine learning methods. *Int. J. Mol. Sci.* **2021**, *22*, 1676. [CrossRef] [PubMed]
32. Fan, J.; Fu, A.; Zhang, L. Progress in molecular docking. *Quant. Biol.* **2019**, *7*, 83–89. [CrossRef]
33. Parenti, M.D.; Rastelli, G. Advances and applications of binding affinity prediction methods in drug discovery. *Biotechnol. Adv.* **2012**, *30*, 244–250. [CrossRef]
34. Silver, D.; Huang, A.; Maddison, C.J.; Guez, A.; Sifre, L.; van den Driessche, G.; Schrittwieser, J.; Antonoglou, I.; Panneershelvam, V.; Lanctot, M.; et al. Mastering the game of Go with deep neural networks and tree search. *Nature* **2016**, *529*, 484–489. [CrossRef]
35. RDKit: Open-Source Cheminformatics. Available online: https://www.rdkit.org (accessed on 20 September 2023).
36. Trott, O.; Olson, A.J. AutoDock Vina: Improving the speed and accuracy of docking with a new scoring function, efficient optimization, and multithreading. *J. Comput. Chem.* **2010**, *31*, 455–461. [CrossRef]
37. Bento, A.P.; Gaulton, A.; Hersey, A.; Bellis, L.J.; Chambers, J.; Davies, M.; Kruger, F.A.; Overington, J.P. The ChEMBL bioactivity database: An update. *Nucleic Acids Res.* **2014**, *42*, D1083–D1090. [CrossRef] [PubMed]

38. Oprea, T.I. Property distribution of drug-related chemical databases. *J. Comput. Aided Mol. Des.* **2020**, *14*, 251–264. [CrossRef] [PubMed]
39. Walters, W.P.; Namchuk, M. Designing screens: How to make your hits a hit. *Nat. Rev. Drug Discov.* **2003**, *2*, 259–266. [CrossRef] [PubMed]

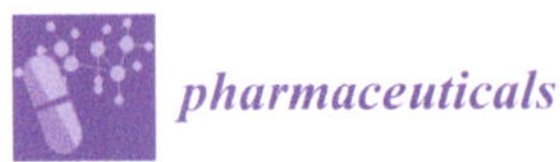

pharmaceuticals

Article

An Integrated Computational and Experimental Approach to Formulate Tamanu Oil Bigels as Anti-Scarring Agent

Megha Krishnappa [1], Sindhu Abraham [1,*], Sharon Caroline Furtado [1], Shwetha Krishnamurthy [1], Aynul Rifaya [2], Yahya I. Asiri [3], Kumarappan Chidambaram [3,*] and Parasuraman Pavadai [4,*]

[1] Department of Pharmaceutics, Faculty of Pharmacy, M.S. Ramaiah University of Applied Sciences, Gnanagangothri Campus, Bengaluru 56054, Karnataka, India; meghakrishnappa23@gmail.com (M.K.); sharongonsalves2006@gmail.com (S.C.F.); shwek2014@gmail.com (S.K.)

[2] Department of Chemical Engineering, Erode Sengunther Engineering College, Erode 638057, Tamil Nadu, India; aynulbioinfo@gmail.com

[3] Department of Pharmacology, College of Pharmacy, King Khalid University, Abha 61421, Asir Province, Saudi Arabia; yialmuawad@kku.edu.sa

[4] Department of Pharmaceutical Chemistry, Faculty of Pharmacy, M.S. Ramaiah University of Applied Sciences, Gnanagangothri Campus, Bengaluru 560054, Karnataka, India

* Correspondence: sindhusa@gmail.com (S.A.); ctkumarrx@gmail.com (K.C.); pvpram@gmail.com (P.P.)

Abstract: Tamanu oil has traditionally been used to treat various skin problems. The oil has wound-healing and skin-regenerating capabilities and encourages the growth of new skin cells, all of which are helpful for fading scars and hyperpigmentation, as well as promoting an all-around glow. The strong nutty odor and high viscosity are the major disadvantages associated with its application. The aim of this study was to create bigels using tamanu oil for its anti-scarring properties and predict the possible mechanism of action through the help of molecular docking studies. In silico studies were performed to analyze the binding affinity of the protein with the drug, and the anti-scarring activity was established using a full-thickness excision wound model. In silico studies revealed that the components inophyllum C, 4-norlanosta-17(20),24-diene-11,16-diol-21-oic acid, 3-oxo-16,21-lactone, calanolide A, and calophyllolide had docking scores of -11.3 kcal/mol, -11.1 kcal/mol, -9.8 kcal/mol, and -8.6 kcal/mol, respectively, with the cytokine TGF-β1 receptor. Bigels were prepared with tamanu oil ranging from 5 to 20% along with micronized xanthan gum and evaluated for their pH, viscosity, and spreadability. An acute dermal irritation study in rabbits showed no irritation, erythema, eschar, or edema. In vivo excisional wound-healing studies performed on Wistar rats and subsequent histopathological studies showed that bigels had better healing properties when compared to the commercial formulation (Murivenna™ oil). This study substantiates the wound-healing and scar reduction potential of tamanu oil bigels.

Keywords: bigel; *Calophyllum inophyllum*; calanolide A; piscean collagen; tamanu oil; molecular docking; ADMET

Citation: Krishnappa, M.; Abraham, S.; Furtado, S.C.; Krishnamurthy, S.; Rifaya, A.; Asiri, Y.I.; Chidambaram, K.; Pavadai, P. An Integrated Computational and Experimental Approach to Formulate Tamanu Oil Bigels as Anti-Scarring Agent. *Pharmaceuticals* **2024**, *17*, 102. https://doi.org/10.3390/ph17010102

Academic Editor: Roberta Rocca

Received: 17 November 2023
Revised: 25 December 2023
Accepted: 9 January 2024
Published: 11 January 2024

1. Introduction

Damaged skin is repaired through wound healing, a complex biological process that includes hemostasis, inflammation, proliferation, and remodeling. The final three steps are essential in determining if healing is taking place naturally or if it is causing excessive extracellular matrix (ECM) protein production and fibrosis, which would indicate an aberrant healing [1]. The restoration of skin barrier function after wounding or damage plays a major role in preventing further damage to the skin. Extended wound healing may even hinder normal wound healing, resulting in scarring [1]. Scars are the normal and inevitable outcome of mammalian tissue repair. Tissue regeneration, as well as the formation of new tissue similar to the original undamaged skin, is the ideal endpoint [2]. Scar formation may be due to the overproduction of connective tissue (collagen) and differences during the wound-healing process. Millions of people experience scarring annually as a result of burns, trauma, or skin injury following surgery, which has an impact on mental health [3]. Keloid and hypertrophic scars are a prevalent issue as wound healing progresses. Clinically, they are distinguished by an excessive buildup of collagen due to damage to the dermis and subcutaneous regions. Growth factors and cytokines include transforming growth factor β (TGF-β), epidermal growth factor (EGF), fibroblast growth factor (FGF), and platelet-derived growth factor (PDGF) that control this process [4].

The cytokine transforming growth factor β (TGF-β), which is released by many cell types involved in wound healing, is essential for the healing process. TGF-β comprises three isomers, TGF-β1, TGF-β2, and TGF-β3, which together influence fibroblast proliferation, angiogenesis, and ECM synthesis by promoting the infiltration of inflammatory cells. In addition, TGF-β prevents re-epithelialization [5,6]. The effects of various TGF-β isoforms on wound healing may vary depending on the environment. TGF-β3 has also been reported to facilitate reduced scarring, but TGF-β1 may also mediate fibrosis in adult wounds. In order to treat both acute and chronic wounds as well as fibrosing illnesses, TGF-β3 may provide a scar-reducing therapy [7].

Since ancient times, tamanu oil, which is extracted from the nuts of the tamanu tree (*Calophyllum inophyllum* Linn.), has been used for a variety of skin-care purposes. The plant is found primarily in Australia, East Africa, India, Malaysia, and the Pacific Ocean. The oil is dark green in color, with a nutty odor and disagreeable taste. Owing to the non-fatty constituents present in the oil, it is not edible. Tamanu oil has limited scientific evidence, although it is widely used to treat scars, burns, diabetic wounds, and abrasions [8]. The oil is reported to contain constituents such as calophyllolide, inophyllum C, inophyllum D, inophyllum E, inophyllum P, tamanolide D, tamanolide P, calanolide A, calanolide B, and calanolide D. Calophyllolide, the major constituent, is responsible for anti-coagulant, anti-inflammatory, anti-aging, wound-healing, and antioxidant and anti-microbial properties [9–13]. Tamanu oil is also effective in scar removal, reduction of stretch marks, and treatment of psoriasis, eczema, skin allergies, sunburn, and acne. Extracts of the stem bark and seeds of *Calophyllum inophyllum* have also shown promising anti-arthritic activity in a Freund's-complete-adjuvant-induced arthritis model in rats [14]. Calophyllolide, calophyllic acid, and inophyllum, as well as polyphenols with antioxidant properties, are components of *Calophyllum inophyllum* that are responsible for the ability of the plant to promote wound healing. However, the medicinal benefits of tamanu oil have only been reported and quantified in a small number of scientific investigations [15–19]. The oil has wound-healing and skin-regenerating capabilities and encourages the growth of new skin cells, all of which are helpful for fading scars and hyperpigmentation, as well as promoting an all-around glow [20].

Oleogels and hydrogels, two distinctive solid-like formulations with useful qualities for cosmetic and medicinal applications, are combined to create a bigel. Bigel exhibits superior qualities to individual gels and is capable of delivering both hydrophilic and lipophilic active substances [2,21]. They are different when compared to creams and ointments as they are devoid of surfactants, enhance hydration of the stratum corneum, resulting in cooling and moisturizing effects, enhance permeability of drugs, can be prepared easily, and are water-washable [22,23].

The purpose of this study was to investigate the potential of tamanu oil as an active ingredient for the development of bigels with significant scar-reducing properties. An in silico study elucidating its interaction with 5E8W (TGF-β receptor type-1), a membrane-bound TGF beta receptor protein, was performed to demonstrate its clinical potential. The scar-free wound-healing potential of tamanu oil was compared with that of Ayurvedic murivenna oil, which is recommended by Ayurvedic physicians for its wound-healing and anti-inflammatory properties [24–26].

2. Results and Discussion

2.1. GC-MS Characterization of Tamanu Oil

The chemical composition of tamanu oil was determined by GC-MS and compared with previously reported data. The analysis revealed the presence of the main components calanolide A, calophyllolide (inophyllum derivative), inophyllum C, 4-norlanosta-17(20),24-diene-11,16-diol-21-oic acid, 3-oxo-16,21-lactone (steroid lactone), along with fatty acids palmitic acid, oleic acid, linoleic acid, stearic acid, and hyenic acid (Table 1 and Figure S1). The retention times of the components were identified by comparison with reported literature [18]. The gas chromatogram and corresponding mass spectra are shown in Figure S1. These constituents have been reported to possess anti-microbial, anti-inflammatory, antioxidant, wound-healing, anti-HIV, and anti-tumor activities [27–30]. Calophyllolide exhibits wound-healing activity by reducing myeloperoxidase (MPO) activity and regulating inflammatory cytokines (IL-1β, IL-6, and TNF-α). The pro-inflammatory cytokines IL-1β, IL-6, and TNF-α are downregulated, whereas the anti-inflammatory cytokine IL-10 is upregulated by calophyllolide [18].

Table 1. Components identified in GC-MS analysis of tamanu oil.

Sl.No.	Compounds	Component RT (Min)	SMILES	Percentage
1	Calanolide A	31.03	CCCC1=CC(=O)OC2=C1C3=C(C=CC(O3)(C)C)C4=C2[C@H]([C@@H]([C@H](O4)C)C)O	2.02
2	Calophyllolide	33.52	CC=C(C)C(=O)C1=C(C2=C(C3=C1OC(=O)C=C3 C4=CC=CC=C4)OC(C=C2)(C)C)OC	1.92
3	Inophyllum C	24.91	C[C@@H]1[C@H](OC2=C(C1=O)C3=C(C(=CC(=O)O3)C4=CC=CC=C4)C5=C2C=CC(O5)(C)C)C	3.65
4	Oleic acid	26.16	CCCCCCCC/C=C\CCCCCCCC(=O)O	0.85
5	Linoleic acid	26.16	CCCCC/C=C\C/C=C\CCCCCCCC(=O)O	0.64
6	Palmitic acid	23.27	CCCCCCCCCCCCCCCC(=O)O	0.23
7	Stearic acid	26.38	CCCCCCCCCCCCCCCCCC(=O)O	0.98
8	4-Norlanosta-17(20),24-diene-11,16-diol-21-oic acid, 3-oxo-16,21-lactone	29.66	CC1C2CCC3(C(C2(CCC1=O)C)C(CC4C3(CC5C4=C(C(=O)O5)CCC=C(C)C)C)O)C	2.3
9	Pentacosanoic acid	25.28	CCCCCCCCCCCCCCCCCCCCCCCCC(=O)O	0.66

2.2. In Silico Studies—Molecular Modeling

The extracellular matrix (ECM) is modulated by transforming growth factor beta (TGF-β), which increases collagen synthesis and controls the expression of numerous genes encoding the extracellular-matrix-degrading matrix metalloproteinases (MMPs) [31]. Transforming growth factor beta 1 (TGF-β1) is a polypeptide member of the TGF-β superfamily of cytokines that contributes to the progress of scar formation through its stimulatory effects on the manifestation of key ECM components and its inhibitory effects on the expression of MMPs in fibroblasts. Additionally, it stimulates collagen production in fibroblasts [32].

Initially, molecular docking studies were carried out to explore the possible synergetic mechanism of tamanu oil ingredients with the various protein targets that play a major role in scar formation. Binding energy for the selected targets is shown in Table S1. A comprehensive investigation of binding energy and binding interactions drove the eventual choice of the target molecule. The goal of this critical evaluation was to determine the strength and specificity of molecular interactions between the target molecule and its anticipated binding partners. Binding energy was the most important factor in determining the stability of these interactions, ensuring that the selected target (TGF protein) had strong and favorable binding features. Furthermore, a careful investigation of binding interactions revealed information about the kind of bonds produced between the target molecule and its binding partners. This thorough review sought to discover a target molecule with appropriate binding characteristics, focusing on both the affinity and specificity of molecular interactions with TGF protein. Hence, TGF protein was selected for further analysis. To analyze the binding and molecular interactions of the active constituents of tamanu oil with the potential therapeutic target TGF-β type 1 kinase domain (T204D) in complex with staurosporine (PDB ID:5E8W) [33], molecular docking studies were performed using PyRx 0.8 [34–37]. The predicted binding affinities of all identified constituents, as well as the staurosporine standard, was found to be −5.0 kcal/mol to −11.3 kcal/mol for test compounds and -8.6 kcal/mol for standard, as presented in Table 2.

Table 2. Binding affinities of constituents of tamanu oil with TGF-β type 1 kinase (5E8W).

Compounds	Docking Score kcal/mol	H-Bond Interactions Residue	H-Bond Interactions Distance (Å)	Hydrophobic Interactions	External Bond Interactions
Calophyllolide	−8.6	Ser287	2.3	Val219, Lys337	-
Inophyllum C	−11.3	His283	2.47	Val219, Ala230, Lys232, Leu260, Leu340, Ala350, Asp351	-
Calanolide A	−9.8	Ser280, His283	2.88 2.31	Ile211, Val219, Lys232, Leu260, Leu340	-
Oleic acid	−5.3	Ser280	2.56	Ile211, Val219, Leu260, Leu340, Ala350, Asp351	-
Linoleic acid	−6.4	Ser280, His283	3.25 1.87	Ile211, Val219, Lys232, Tyr249, Leu260, Phe262, Asp351	-
Palmitic acid	−5.9	His283	2.9	Lys232, Tyr249, Phe262, Leu278, Leu340, Lys232	-
4-Norlanosta-17(20),24-diene-11,16-diol-21-oic acid, 3-oxo-16,21-lactone	−11.1	Ser287	3.08	Ile211, Val219, Ala230, Leu260, Tyr282, Lys337, Leu340, Ala350, Asp351	Lys232 (salt bridge)
Hyenic acid	−5	Val231	3.29	Ile211, Val219, Lys232, Leu260, Lys337, Leu340, Ala350, Asp351	
Staurosporine	−8.6	Ser280, Asp281, His 283	2.57 2.76 1.94	Ile 211, Gly212, Lys337	Val219, Ala230, Lys232, Leu340, Ala350 π stacking

In accordance with the findings of the molecular docking experiments, the chosen standard staurosporine and the bioactive compounds inophyllum C, 4-norlanosta-17(20),24-diene-11,16-diol-21-oic acid, 3-oxo-16,21-lactone, calanolide A, and calophyllolide exhibited distinct patterns of interaction with the target protein. Staurosporine, with a binding score of −8.6 kcal/mol, exhibited many interactions. These included hydrophobic contacts with amino acids Ile 211, Gly212, and Lys337; hydrogen bond interactions with Ser280, Asp281, and His 283; and π-stacking interactions with Val219, Ala230, Lys232, Leu340, and Ala350. Inophyllum C demonstrated improved binding, including H-bond interactions with His283 and hydrophobic interactions with Val219, Ala230, Lys232, Leu260, Leu340, Ala350, and Asp351. Furthermore, 4-norlanosta-17(20), 24-diene-11,16-diol-21-oic acid, 3-oxo-16,21-lactone had a significant binding score of −11.0 kcal/mol. Salt bridges, hydrophobic contacts, and hydrogen bond interactions were all generated as a result of these interactions. Both calanolide A and calophyllolide exhibited distinct interactions, such as hydrophobic and H-bond interactions, with binding scores of −9.8 kcal/mol and −8.6 kcal/mol when compared to one another. In addition to providing substantial insights into the binding processes and probable pharmacological importance of these chemicals, these findings also pave the way for further study and the possibility of therapeutic uses. Figure 1a–j illustrates the visualization of the interactions that occurred between the chosen bioactive chemicals and the standard with the protein. This visualization was carried out with the help of Discovery Studio Visualizer.

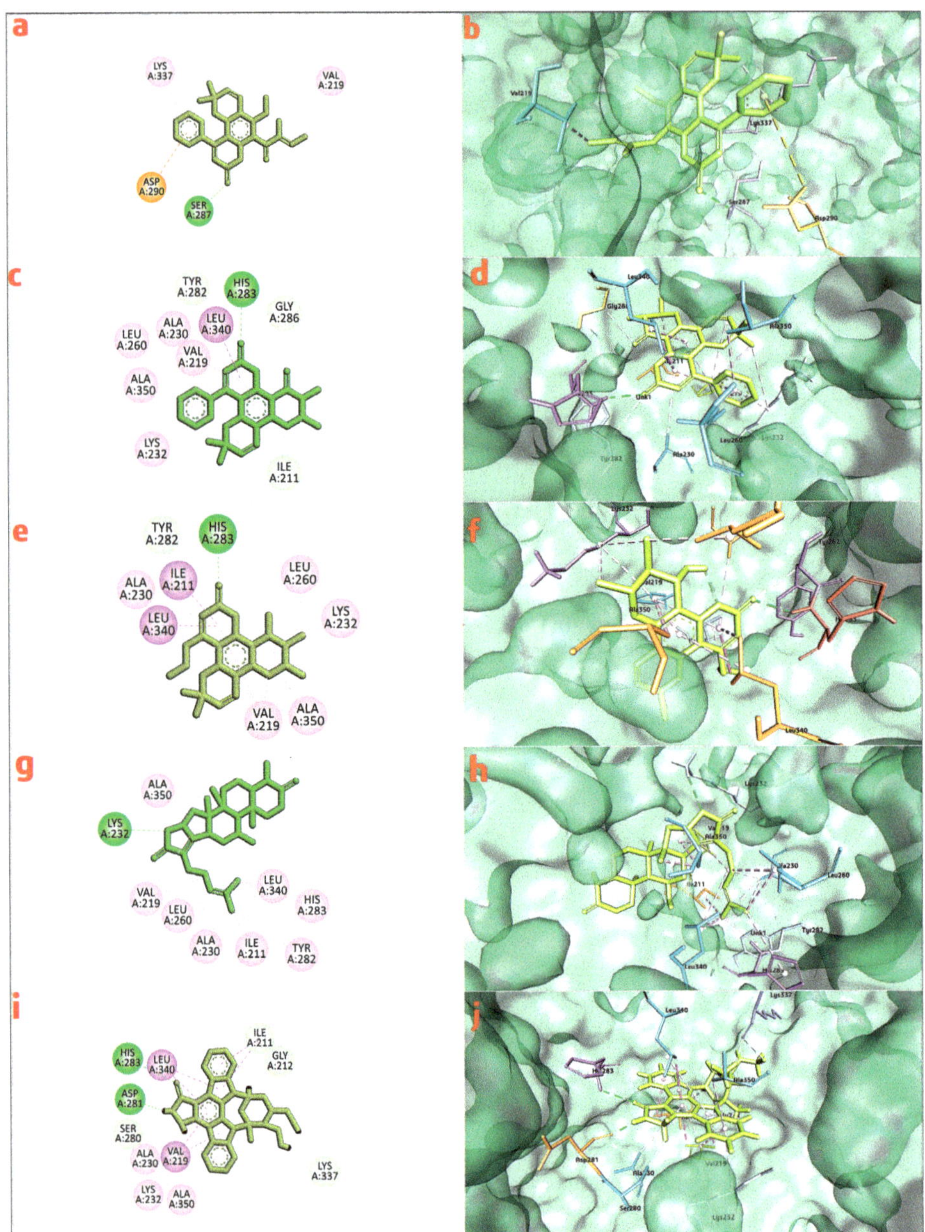

Figure 1. Binding interaction of calophyllolide with 5E8W, (**a**) 2D and (**b**) 3D interaction; binding interaction of inophyllum C, (**c**) 2D and (**d**) 3D interaction; binding interaction of calanolide A with 5E8W, (**e**) 2D and (**f**) 3D interaction; binding interaction of norlanosta-17(20),24-diene-11,16-diol-21-oic acid, 3-oxo-16,21-lactone ring with 5E8W, (**g**) 2D and (**h**) 3D interaction; binding interaction of staurosporine with 5E8W, (**i**) 2D and (**j**) 3D interaction.

According to Lipinski's rule of five, molecules with poor permeation will have molecular weight > 500, $\log p$ > 5, hydrogen bond donors > 5, and hydrogen bond acceptors > 10. Among all the ligands investigated, calanolide A showed a molecular weight of 370.445, $\log p$ of 4.3801, one hydrogen bond donor, and five hydrogen bond acceptors, suggesting good permeation characteristics (Table S2).

The absorption, distribution, metabolism, excretion, and toxicity (ADMET) of the constituents of tamanu oil were predicted using in silico methods (Table S3) [38].

2.3. Formulation of Bigels

Eight formulations containing 5–20% tamanu oil were prepared. Formulations BG1–BG4 contained 1% micronized xanthan gum in the hydrogel phase, whereas BG5–BG8 contained 2% micronized xanthan gum in the hydrogel phase. The concentrations of Tween 20 and Geogard® ECT were maintained at 3% and 1%, respectively, for all the formulations. The nutty odor of tamanu oil was masked with vanilla fragrance oil.

2.4. Evaluation of Bigel

All formulations were pastel green with a mild nutty odor, non-greasy, shiny texture, and easy washability and were homogenous with good consistency. The fragrances of topical products can significantly affect customer acceptance and satisfaction. As a result, smell is an essential characteristic of cosmetics that consumers consider and appreciate during their selection [39]. The strong odor of the oil was masked by vanilla fragrance.

2.4.1. pH

The regular use of cosmetics can help maintain skin health by controlling the pH of skin. In some skin disorders, topical products that correct skin pH should be part of the treatment plan. Therefore, it is crucial to carefully consider the pH and buffering capacity of topically applied products [40]. The pH of all formulations was found to be in the range of 5.58–6.04 (Table 3). All reported values are close to the pH of the skin and can be safely used topically without causing irritation or any other skin reactions [41].

Table 3. Evaluation of bigels.

Parameters	BG1	BG2	BG3	BG4	BG5	BG6	BG7	BG8
pH	5.82 ± 0.05	5.96 ± 0.06	5.92 ± 0.12	6.04 ± 0.07	5.96 ± 0.17	5.58 ± 0.03	5.62 ± 0.13	5.76 ± 0.10
Spreadability (cm)	6.50 ± 0.36	6.10 ± 0.26	5.93 ± 0.25	5.63 ± 0.30	5.46 ± 0.40	5.36 ± 0.05	5.30 ± 0.10	5.26 ± 0.15
Viscosity (cps)	220.4 ± 0.96	238.9 ± 0.85	252.9 ± 0.65	273.8 ± 0.05	313.0 ± 0.15	337.4 ± 0.25	378.4 ± 0.05	391.5 ± 0.28

2.4.2. Viscosity

The viscosities of all bigel formulations were in the range 220.4 to 391.5 cps. An increase in viscosity was observed with an increase in oil concentration, as reported in Table 3.

2.4.3. Spreadability

The spreadability of all bigel formulations was 5.30–6.50 cm (Table 3). Spreadability is a function of the structural viscosity, with lower viscosity meaning better spreadability. The results confirmed a strong correlation between spreadability and viscosity values, signifying good application characteristics [42].

2.4.4. SEM Analysis

Scanning electron microscopic examination was performed to analyze the surface characteristics of the bigel. The micrographs of formulations BG4 and BG8 at 270× and 50× magnification, as shown in Figure 2, revealed the presence of fibrous structures, which could be attributed to the entrapment of the oleogel within the hydrogel phase [43].

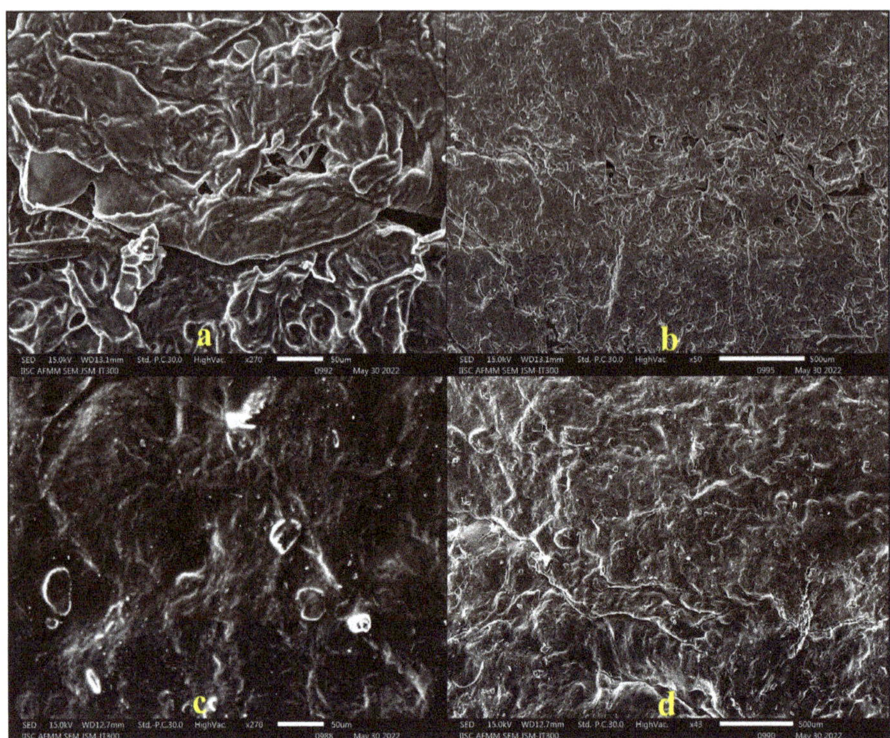

Figure 2. SEM micrographs of (**a**) BG4 at 270×, (**b**) BG4 at 50×, (**c**) BG8 at 270×, (**d**) BG8 at 50×.

2.5. In Vivo Studies

2.5.1. Acute Dermal Irritation Studies

Formulations BG4 and BG8 containing the highest concentration of tamanu oil (20%) were selected for the test. The results of dermal irritation studies are shown in Figure 3. No responses, such as erythema, eschar, or edema, were visible on the rabbits after exposure to the bigels for 4 h. Thus, these formulations can be considered non-irritant and safe for topical application [44].

2.5.2. In Vivo Wound-Healing Studies

Based on the results obtained from the evaluation studies, formulations BG1, BG4, and BG8 were selected for the in vivo studies. An excision wound with a diameter of 6 mm was created in all the rats and they were further segregated for treatment. Five groups were treated with pure tamanu oil, commercial formulation (Murivenna™), and test formulations separately, while the control group did not receive any treatment. Treatment was started 24 h post-wound induction and continued daily until complete healing was observed. The wound area was measured on days 3, 6, 9, 12, and 15 of the treatment. The excised wound treated with bigels showed significant wound contraction over a period of 12 days, indicating an accelerated re-epithelialization process compared to the untreated wound (control). The animals did not show any signs of necrosis, inflammation, or hemorrhage and survived throughout the study period. Although the BG4 and BG8 formulations significantly increased wound healing, the best results were observed with BG8 (100% wound contraction on day 12). Overall, the wounds healed and were completely sealed within 15 days post-wound induction, with no evidence of scars [45]. Representative images of wound healing and contraction data are presented in Figure 4, Figure S2 and Table 4, respectively.

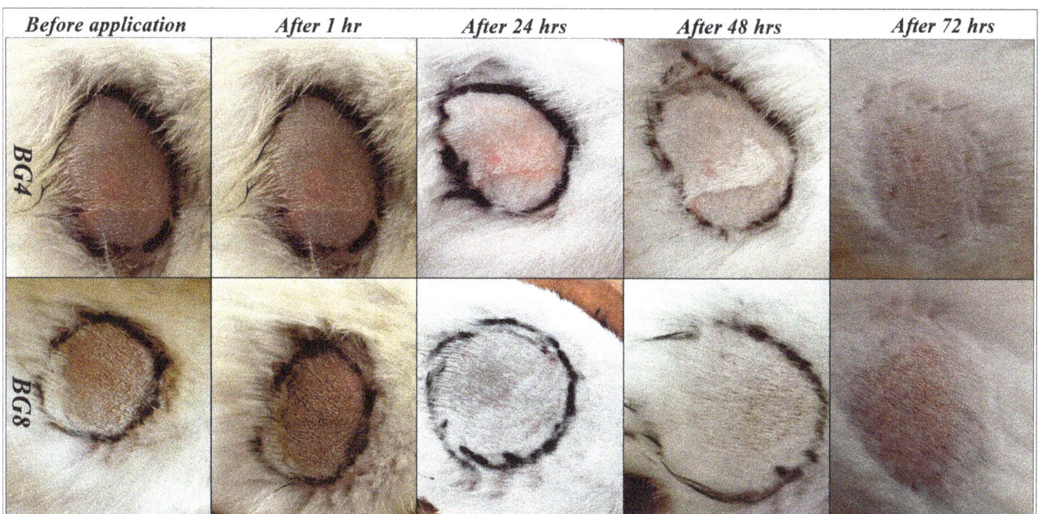

Figure 3. Photographs of dermal irritation studies carried out on rabbits.

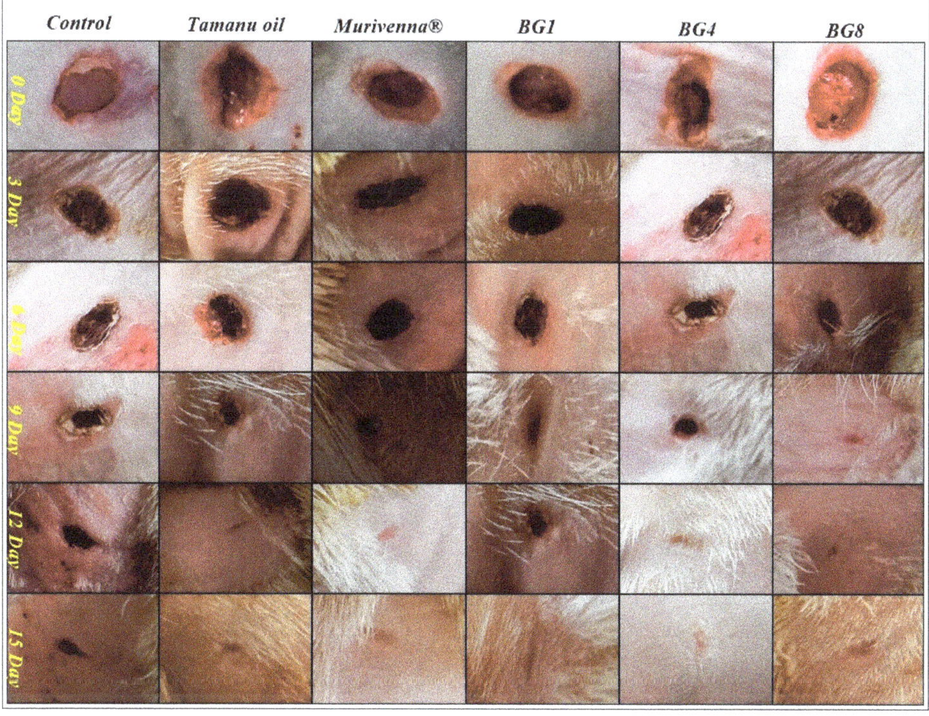

Figure 4. Representative images of wound control and wounds treated with standard and bigels for 15 days in rats.

Table 4. Statistical analysis of wound contraction.

Group	Control	Tamanu Oil	Murivenna	BG1	BG4	BG8
Day 3	0.573 ± 0.0049	0.538 ± 0.0047 **	0.555 ± 0.0042 [ns]	0.561 ± 0.0094 [ns]	0.511 ± 0.0060 **	0.505 ± 0.0042 **
Day 6	0.470 ± 0.0057	0.460 ± 0.0051 [ns]	0.451 ± 0.0047 *	0.463 ± 0.0042 [ns]	0.415 ± 0.00428 **	0.405 ± 0.0042 **
Day 9	0.418 ± 0.0094	0.350 ± 0.0036 **	0.358 ± 0.0095 **	0.380 ± 0.0057 **	0.273 ± 0.0066 **	0.248 ± 0.0095 **
Day 12	0.251 ± 0.0104	0.112 ± 0.0107 **	0.098 ± 0.0047 **	0.1283 ± 0.0060 **	0.0833 ± 0.0066 **	0.00 ± 0.00 **
Day 15	0.083 ± 0.0025	0.00 ± 0.00 **	0.00 ± 0.00 **	0.00 ± 0.00 **	0.00 ± 0.00 **	0.00 ± 0.00 **

All values represent the diameter of the wound (in cm) on different days of measurement and are expressed as mean $\pm$ SEM ($n = 6$); one-way ANOVA followed by Dunnett's test where ns $p > 0.05$, * $p < 0.05$, ** $p < 0.01$, in comparison to control. (ns = non-significant, * moderately significant, ** highly significant).

Epithelialization was observed on the wound area until the eschar had fallen off, without leaving any traces of a raw wound. The period of epithelialization was faster in the BG8 group as the eschar had fallen off on after an average of 6.66 days (Table S4).

2.6. Histopathological Studies

Re-epithelialization and collagen production in full-thickness wounds was assessed by H&E and Masson's trichome staining. The microscopic examination of all skin specimens revealed successful wound healing in all commercial- and bigel-treated animals (Figures 5 and S3). The control group showed the presence of inflammatory cells, irregular connective tissues, poor collagen deposition, and incomplete epithelial layer formation, in comparison to the treated groups. Tamanu-oil- and murivenna-treated groups showed more collagen fiber deposition, reduced inflammatory cells, and partially developed connective tissues. Bigel-treated groups exhibited normal architecture with a well-developed epidermal layer and an abundance of collagen fibers [46].

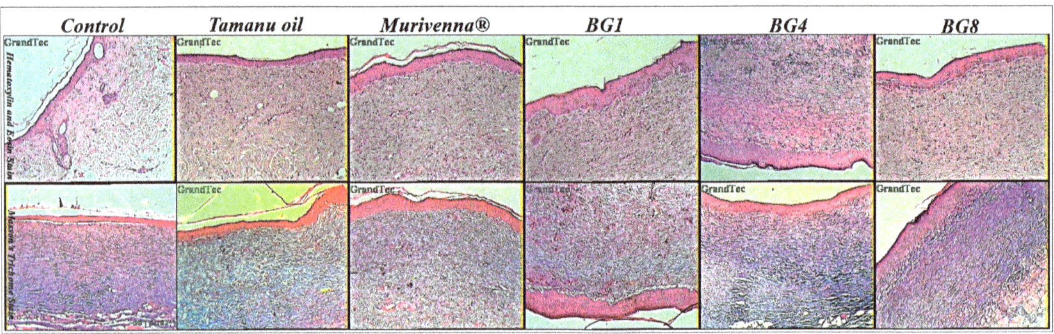

Figure 5. Photomicrographs (100×) showing H&E stain and MT stain section of skin tissues at day 15 for control, standard-, and formulation-treated groups of rats.

3. Materials and Methods

3.1. Materials

Tamanu oil and Geogard® ECT were purchased from Moksha Lifestyle Products (Delhi, India). Piscean collagen was procured from Himrishi Herbals (Delhi, India) and xanthan gum from Shakthi enterprises (Mumbai, India).

3.2. GC-MS Characterization of Tamanu Oil

The chemical composition of tamanu oil was determined using an Agilent 7890B Series gas chromatograph linked with a 5977A Series mass selective detector (Agilent Technologies, Santa Clara, CA, USA). The chromatographic column was HP-5 ms (5% phenyl-methylpolysiloxane; Agilent Technologies, USA) of 30 m length; 0.25 mm internal diameter; and 0.25 μm film thickness. The flow rate of the carrier gas (99.99% pure helium) was maintained at 2.0 mL/min. A 1.0 μL sample (oil diluted with hexane) was injected in split mode (split ratio of 50:1; injector temperature, 290 °C). The oven was programmed at 60 °C as the initial temperature for 2 min, increased to 270 °C at a rate of 4 °C/min and then to 290 °C at a rate of 10 °C/min for a total duration of 65 min. The mass selective detector was operated at an ion source temperature of 270 °C, with electron ionization at 70 eV. The peak areas are represented by the percentage of each compound and their retention times were compared to the calibration curves of the internal standards for compound identification.

3.3. In Silico Studies

3.3.1. Preparation of Ligand and Selection of Protein

Ligands selected from the GC-MS report were downloaded in sdf format (3D structures) from PubChem (https://pubchem.ncbi.nlm.nih.gov/, accessed on 16 November 2023) and they were also optimized using the Avogadro tool (https://avogadro.cc/, accessed on 16 November 2023). The structure of the protein target was selected and extracted from Research Collaboratory for Structural Bioinformatics Protein Data Bank (https://www.rcsb.org/, accessed on 16 November 2023). The protein fibronectin (PDB: 5KF4), transforming growth factor beta (TGF-β) (PDB: 5E8W), matrix metalloproteinases (MMPs) (PDB: 3UTZ), tissue inhibitors of metalloproteinases (TIMPs) (PDB: 3V96), platelet-derived growth factor (PDGF) (PDB: 5K5X), vascular endothelial growth factor (VEGF) (PDB: 6T9D), insulin-like growth factor (IGF) (PDB: 4D2R), and various cytokines, such as interleukin-1 (IL-1) (PDB: 7SZL) and IL-6 (PDB: 2L3Y), were selected and downloaded in the pdb format.

3.3.2. Preparation of Protein

Hetero atoms and ligands in the downloaded protein were removed using BIOVIA Discovery Studio (v4.5). The protein target was prepared by the addition of hydrogen atoms and saved in pdb format using Swiss-Pdb Viewer (v4.1).

3.3.3. Molecular Modeling Studies

In order to analyze the binding and molecular interactions of identified active constituents of tamanu oil with therapeutic targets, molecular docking studies were carried out using PyRx with default settings and parameters. The X-ray-resolved crystal structures of the potential were retrieved from the PDB with good resolution and R-free factor. The ligand was uploaded, minimized, and converted to pdbqt format. The molecular docking was performed using PyRX 0.8 software which runs on the Autodock Vina algorithm, the grid box was calculated from the co-crystal ligands, and for pure protein the grid box was generated using the PRANK webserver (https://prankweb.cz/, accessed on 16 November 2023) for carrying out active pocket docking (Figure S4). All complex binding affinity energies were calculated on the basis of ligand conformation at the active binding site, with the root mean square deviation (RMSD) between the original and then the structures taken into account. The number of hydrogen bonds and non-covalent interactions for each complex was calculated using Discovery Studio Visualizer (http://accelrys.com/products/collaborative-science/biovia-discovery-studio/, accessed on 16 November 2023), which produced details, compound images, and interaction images (2D and 3D). We used web-based pkCSM-pharmacokinetic tools to determine the pharmacokinetics (absorption, distribution, metabolism, and excretion); safety; and physicochemical properties of the selected bioactive molecules [43,47].

ADMET profile was analyzed using the pkCSM ADMET descriptors algorithm.

3.4. Formulation of Bigels

Micronized xanthan gum was dispersed in 10 mL water for 1h to obtain a gel-like consistency. Geogard® ECT was added along with vanilla fragrance to the above gel to form hydrogel phase. Tamanu oil and Tween 20 were mixed together and heated to 75 °C to obtain an oleogel phase. The oleogel phase was slowly blended with the hydrogel phase to form a bigel.

Eight formulations were prepared containing 5–20% tamanu oil (Table S5). Formulations BG1–BG4 were prepared with 1% micronized xanthan gum as the hydrogel and formulations BG5–BG8 contained 2% micronized xanthan gum in the hydrogel phase. The concentration of Tween 20 and Geogard® ECT (preservative) was maintained constant at 3% and 1%, respectively, for all formulations. Geogard ECT is a water-soluble, low-odor and low-color, broad spectrum preservative that offers broad spectrum protection in a variety of personal care products. It is a combination of benzyl alcohol, salicylic acid, and sorbic acid. Vanilla fragrance was used to mask the nutty odor of tamanu oil.

3.5. Evaluation of Bigels

3.5.1. Organoleptic Evaluation

The bigels were evaluated for their organoleptic properties like color, odor, homogeneity, consistency, phase separation, and texture.

3.5.2. pH

The pH of all formulations was tested using a digital pH meter (MK VI, Systronics, Ahmedabad, India). First, 1g of the bigel was dissolved in 100 mL of water and tested. The measurements were taken in triplicate, and the standard deviation was determined.

3.5.3. Spreadability

A good topical formulation should spread evenly during application. This was evaluated by preparing a thin smear of the bigel on a glass slide with the aid of another glass slide. A weight of 100 g was placed over the glass plate for 5 min to obtain an even smear. The time taken to separate the slides was considered and the spreadability was calculated using the following formula [48].

$$S = M \times L/T$$

where S is the spreadability, M is the weight applied, L is the length moved by the glass slide during separation and T is the time taken to separate the slides from each other.

3.5.4. Viscosity

The viscosity of all formulations was determined using a Brookfield viscometer (Model DV-II+, Middleboro, MA, USA) with a spindle number of 4 at 10 rpm.

3.5.5. Scanning Electron Microscopic Analysis

The surface characteristics of bigels were observed using scanning electron microscopy (JSM-IT300, Peabody, MA, USA). Dried bigel specimens were coated with a thin layer of gold in an argon atmosphere, glued to aluminum stubs, and observed at $50\times$ and $270\times$ magnification [41].

3.6. In Vivo Studies

3.6.1. Acute Dermal Irritation Studies

The likelihood of bigels to cause dermal irritation was investigated on healthy female New Zealand white rabbits in accordance with OECD 404 [40] test guidelines. The experimental protocol was executed after obtaining prior approval from the Institutional Animal Ethical Committee (IAEC Ref No.: XXV/MSRFPH/CEU/M-017/21.10.2021). All the rabbits were acclimatized to the facilities for 2 weeks and individually housed under controlled environmental conditions (20 ± 3 °C/50–60% RH) with a 12 h light and 12 h dark cycle and maintained on a pellet diet and unrestricted supply of drinking water. The fur on the dorsal area of rabbits was carefully shaved 24 h before the test. The animals were distributed into groups of six randomly with one group for control and the others for the formulations. The formulations were applied on the shaved area and secured with gauze and non-irritating tapes. After the exposure period of 4 h, the formulation was removed by rinsing the area with water and the exposed area was closely monitored for any visible change (erythema, redness, and edema). Observations were scored on a scale of 0–4, with 0 indicating the absence of erythema/edema and 4 indicating severe erythema/edema. Scoring was carried out 60 min after removal of formulation, as well as 24, 48, and 72 h later.

3.6.2. In Vivo Wound-Healing Studies

The scar-free wound-healing potential of bigels was determined by an excisional wound model on male albino Wistar rats (weight range of 200–350 g). The fasted rats were weighed and anaesthetized with a mixture of ketamine (80 mg/kg) and xylazine (20 mg/kg) prior to wounding. The dorsal area was depilated and disinfected with 70% ethanol. A full-thickness wound of 6 mm diameter was made using a sterile biopsy punch. The wounded rats were segregated into six groups ($n = 6$) and treatment was carried out with tamanu oil, commercial formulation (Murivenna™), and test formulations BG1, BG4, and BG8 while the control group did not receive any treatment. On the 3rd, 6th, 9th, 12th, and 15th day, the wound area was measured using a scale and the % closure calculated [45].

$$\% \text{ Wound closure} = \frac{\text{Initial wound area} - \text{Specific day wound area}}{\text{Initial wound area}} \times 100$$

The number of days from the day of wound induction till the falling off of eschar without leaving any raw wound behind was considered to be the period of epithelialization.

3.7. Histopathological Studies

At the end of the 15-day treatment period, one animal from each group was anaesthetized with a mixture of ketamine and xylazine (80 mg/kg and 20 mg/kg, i.p., respectively) and sacrificed. Restored skin samples from each group were carefully isolated and stored in 10% v/v formalin solution. The specimens were embedded in paraffin, divided into sections of 4 μm thickness, and stained with hematoxylin and eosin (H&E) and Masson's trichrome for microscopic evaluation of epithelization, fibroblast proliferation, keratinization, and collagen formation [49].

3.8. Statistical Analysis

The wound contraction data were statistically analyzed by one-way ANOVA followed by comparisons with the control group using Dunnett's test. GraphPad Instat 3.1 software was employed for statistical interpretations. Values with $p > 0.05$ were considered not significant (ns), $p < 0.05$ moderately significant (*), and $p < 0.01$ as highly significant (**).

4. Conclusions

The main objective of the present study was to develop bigels of tamanu oil and assess its anti-scarring activity. Bigels were prepared with 5 to 20% tamanu oil and 1–2% micronized xanthan gum. In silico studies were performed and it was found that the components calanolide A, inophyllum C, and 4-norlanosta-17(20),24-diene-11,16-diol-21-oic acid, 3-oxo-16,21-lactone had a docking score of −9.8 kcal/mol, −11.3 kcal/mol, and −11.1 kcal/mol, respectively, with 5E8W, a cytokine TGF-β1 receptor. The standard staurosporine reported a docking score of −8.3 kcal/mol. Acute dermal irritation performed on rabbits showed no irritation, erythema, eschar, or edema. In vivo wound-healing studies were performed to compare the effectiveness of bigel formulations and standard (Murivenna oil) in healing and scar reduction. Based on the results obtained, formulation BG8 was found to be better compared to all other formulations and the standard as it was able to heal the wound within 12 days without leaving behind a scar. Thus, the present study concludes that bigels of tamanu oil are a promising topical product with good scar-healing activity.

Supplementary Materials: The following supporting information can be downloaded at: https://www.mdpi.com/article/10.3390/ph17010102/s1, Figure S1: Representative GC chromatogram of tamanu oil components; Figure S2: Graphical representation of % Wound Contraction; Figure S3: Photomicrographs (100×) showing H&E stain and MT stain section of skin tissues at day 15 for control, standard-, and formulation-treated groups; Figure S4: TGF-β type 1 kinase (5E8W) with binding site; Table S1: Molecular docking results (kcal/mol); Table S2: Molecular properties of selected Ligands; Table S3: Predicted ADMET properties of compounds; Table S4: Period of epithelialization in all groups; Table S5: Formulation of Bigels.

Author Contributions: Conceptualization and initiation—S.A.; Methodology, data collection, and analysis—M.K., P.P., S.C.F., S.K., A.R., Y.I.A. and K.C.; Original draft preparation—S.A. Review and editing—P.P. All authors have read and agreed to the published version of the manuscript.

Funding: This research received no external funding.

Institutional Review Board Statement: All procedures involving experimental animals were performed after obtaining prior approval from the Institutional Animal Ethical Committee (IAEC Ref No.: XXV/MSRFPH/CEU/M-017/21.10.2021).

Data Availability Statement: Data are available in the article and the Supplementary Materials.

Acknowledgments: The authors would like to thank M.S. Ramaiah University of Applied Sciences for supporting this project by providing necessary facilities. The authors thank IISc, Bangalore and IIT Bombay for extending instrumentation facilities to conduct SEM and GCMS studies. The authors extend their appreciation to the Deanship of Scientific Research at King Khalid University for funding this work through Large Group Research Project under grant number RGP2/131/44.

Conflicts of Interest: The authors declare no conflicts of interest.

References

1. Guo, S.; DiPietro, L.A. Factors Affecting Wound Healing. *J. Dent. Res.* **2010**, *89*, 219–229. [CrossRef] [PubMed]
2. Andonova, V.; Peneva, P.; Georgiev, G.V.; Toncheva, V.T.; Apostolova, E.; Peychev, Z.; Dimitrova, S.; Katsarova, M.; Petrova, N.; Kassarova, M. Ketoprofen-Loaded Polymer Carriers in Bigel Formulation: An Approach to Enhancing Drug Photostability in Topical Application Forms. *Int. J. Nanomed.* **2017**, *12*, 6221–6238. [CrossRef]
3. Kamolz, L.-P.; Griffith, M.; Finnerty, C.C.; Kasper, C. Skin Regeneration, Repair, and Reconstruction. *BioMed Res. Int.* **2015**, *2015*, 892031. [CrossRef] [PubMed]
4. Shi, H.; Lin, C.; Lin, B.; Wang, Z.; Zhang, H.; Wu, F.; Cheng, Y.; Xiang, L.; Guo, D.-J.; Luo, X.; et al. The Anti-Scar Effects of Basic Fibroblast Growth Factor on the Wound Repair In Vitro and In Vivo. *PLoS ONE* **2013**, *8*, e59966. [CrossRef] [PubMed]
5. Ramirez, H.; Patel, S.; Pastar, I. The Role of TGFB Signaling in Wound Epithelialization. *Adv. Wound Care* **2014**, *3*, 482–491 [CrossRef] [PubMed]
6. Stoica, A.-I.; Grumezescu, A.M.; Hermenean, A.; Andronescu, E.; Vasile, B.S. Scar-Free Healing: Current Concepts and Future Perspectives. *Nanomaterials* **2020**, *10*, 2179. [CrossRef] [PubMed]
7. Lichtman, M.K.; Otero-Viñas, M.; Falanga, V. Transforming Growth Factor Beta (TGF-β) Isoforms in Wound Healing and Fibrosis *Wound Repair Regen.* **2016**, *24*, 215–222. [CrossRef]
8. Dweck, A.C.; Meadows, T.T. Tamanu (*Calophyllum inophyllum*)—The African, Asian, Polynesian and Pacific Panacea. *Int. J. Cosmet. Sci.* **2002**, *24*, 341–348. [CrossRef]
9. Cassien, M.; Mercier, A.; Thétiot-Laurent, S.; Culcasi, M.; Ricquebourg, E.; Asteian, A.; Herbette, G.; Bianchini, J.-P.; Raharivelomanana, P.; Pietri, S. Improving the Antioxidant Properties of *Calophyllum inophyllum* Seed Oil from French Polynesia Development and Biological Applications of Resinous Ethanol-Soluble Extracts. *Antioxidants* **2021**, *10*, 199. [CrossRef]
10. Ginigini, J.; Lecellier, G.; Nicolas, M.; Nour, M.; Hnawia, E.; Lebouvier, N.; Herbette, G.; Lockhart, P.J.; Raharivelomanana, P. Chemodiversity of *Calophyllum inophyllum* L. Oil Bioactive Components Related to Their Specific Geographical Distribution in the South Pacific Region. *PeerJ* **2019**, *7*, e6896. [CrossRef]
11. Prasad, J.S.; Shrivastava, A.; Khanna, A.; Bhatia, G.; Awasthi, S.K.; Narender, T. Antidyslipidemic and Antioxidant Activity of the Constituents Isolated from the Leaves of *Calophyllum inophyllum*. *Phytomedicine* **2012**, *19*, 1245–1249. [CrossRef] [PubMed]
12. Pribowo, A.; Girish, J.; Gustiananda, M.; Nandhira, R.G.; Hartrianti, P. Potential of Tamanu (*Calophyllum inophyllum*) Oil for Atopic Dermatitis Treatment. *Evid. Based Complement. Altern. Med* **2021**, *2021*, 6332867. [CrossRef]
13. Saki, E.; Murthy, V.; Khandanlou, R.; Wang, H.; Wapling, J.; Weir, R. Optimisation of *Calophyllum inophyllum* Seed Oil Nanoemulsion as a Potential Wound Healing Agent. *BMC Complement. Med. Ther.* **2022**, *22*, 285. [CrossRef]
14. Perumal, S.; Ekambaram, S.; Dhanam, T. In Vivo Antiarthritic Activity of the Ethanol Extracts of Stem Bark and Seeds of *Calophyllum inophyllum* in Freund's Complete Adjuvant Induced Arthritis. *Pharm. Biol.* **2017**, *55*, 1330–1336. [CrossRef] [PubMed]

15. Erdogan, S.S.; Gur, T.; Terzi, N.K.; Dogan, B. Evaluation of the Cutaneous Wound Healing Potential of Tamanu Oil in Wounds Induced in Rats. *J. Wound Care* **2021**, *30* (Suppl. S9a), Vi–Vx. [CrossRef] [PubMed]
16. Léguillier, T.; Lecsö-Bornet, M.; Lemus, C.; Rousseau-Ralliard, D.; Lebouvier, N.; Hnawia, E.; Nour, M.; Aalbersberg, W.G.L.; Ghazi, K.; Raharivelomanana, P.; et al. The Wound Healing and Antibacterial Activity of Five Ethnomedical *Calophyllum inophyllum* Oils: An Alternative Therapeutic Strategy to Treat Infected Wounds. *PLoS ONE* **2015**, *10*, e0138602. [CrossRef] [PubMed]
17. Liu, W.-H.; Liu, Y.-W.; Chen, Z.-F.; Chiou, W.-F.; Tsai, Y.-C.; Chen, C.-C. Calophyllolide Content in *Calophyllum inophyllum* at Different Stages of Maturity and Its Osteogenic Activity. *Molecules* **2015**, *20*, 12314–12327. [CrossRef] [PubMed]
18. Nguyen, V.-L.; Truong, C.-T.; Nguyen, B.C.Q.; Van Vo, T.-N.; Dao, T.-T.; Nguyen, V.-D.; Trinh, D.-T.T.; Huynh, H.K.; Bui, C.-B. Anti-Inflammatory and Wound Healing Activities of Calophyllolide Isolated from *Calophyllum inophyllum* Linn. *PLoS ONE* **2017**, *12*, e0185674. [CrossRef]
19. Tsai, S.C.; Yu, L.; Chiang, J.-H.; Liu, F.C.; Lin, W.-H.; Chang, S.-Y.; Lin, W.; Wu, C.H.; Weng, J.R. Anti-Inflammatory Effects of *Calophyllum inophyllum* L. in RAW264.7 Cells. *Oncol. Rep.* **2012**, *28*, 1096–1102. [CrossRef]
20. Ansel, J.-L.; Lupo, E.; Mijouin, L.; Guillot, S.; Butaud, J.-F.; Ho, R.; Lecellier, G.; Raharivelomanana, P.; Pichon, C. Biological Activity of Polynesian *Calophyllum inophyllum* Oil Extract on Human Skin Cells. *Planta Medica* **2016**, *82*, 961–966. [CrossRef]
21. Shakeel, A.; Farooq, U.; Gabriele, D.; Marangoni, A.G.; Lupi, F.R. Bigels and Multi-Component Organogels: An Overview from Rheological Perspective. *Food Hydrocoll.* **2021**, *111*, 106190. [CrossRef]
22. Baltuonytė, G.; Eisinaitė, V.; Kazernavičiūtė, R.; Vinauskienė, R.; Jasutienė, I.; Leskauskaitė, D. Novel Formulation of Bigel-Based Vegetable Oil Spreads Enriched with Lingonberry Pomace. *Foods* **2022**, *11*, 2213. [CrossRef] [PubMed]
23. Martín-Illana, A.; Notario-Pérez, F.; Cazorla-Luna, R.; Ruiz-Caro, R.; Bonferoni, M.C.; Tamayo, A.; Veiga, M.D. Bigels as Drug Delivery Systems: From Their Components to Their Applications. *Drug Discov. Today* **2022**, *27*, 1008–1026. [CrossRef]
24. Keerthy, P.; Patil, S.B. A Clinical Study to Evaluate the Efficacy of Murivenna Application on Episiotomy Wound. *J. Ayurveda Integr. Med. Sci.* **2020**, *5*, 65–71. [CrossRef]
25. Hepsibah, P.T.; Rosamma, M.P.; Prasad, N.B.; Kumar, P.S. Standardisation of murivenna and hemajeevanti taila. *Anc. Sci. Life* **1993**, *12*, 428–434. [PubMed]
26. Manikandan, A.; Mani, M.P.; Jaganathan, S.K.; Rajasekar, R.; Mani, M.P. Formation of Functional Nanofibrous Electrospun Polyurethane and Murivenna Oil with Improved Haemocompatibility for Wound Healing. *Polym. Test.* **2017**, *61*, 106–113. [CrossRef]
27. Itoigawa, M.; Ito, C.; Tan, H.T.W.; Kuchide, M.; Tokuda, H.; Nishino, H.; Furukawa, H. Cancer Chemopreventive Agents, 4-Phenylcoumarins from *Calophyllum inophyllum*. *Cancer Lett.* **2001**, *169*, 15–19. [CrossRef]
28. Saravanan, R.; Dhachinamoorthi, D.; Senthilkumar, K.; Thamizhvanan, K. Antimicrobial activity of various extracts from various parts of *Calophyllum inophyllum* L. *J. Appl. Pharm. Sci.* **2011**, *1*, 12.
29. Creagh, T.; Ruckle, J.; Tolbert, D.T.; Giltner, J.; Eiznhamer, D.A.; Dutta, B.; Flavin, M.T.; Xu, Z. Safety and Pharmacokinetics of Single Doses of (+)-Calanolide A, a Novel, Naturally Occurring Nonnucleoside Reverse Transcriptase Inhibitor, in Healthy, Human Immunodeficiency Virus-Negative Human Subjects. *Antimicrob. Agents Chemother.* **2001**, *45*, 1379–1386. [CrossRef]
30. Saechan, C.; Kaewsrichan, J.; Leelakanok, N.; Petchsomrit, A. Antioxidant in Cosmeceutical Products Containing *Calophyllum inophyllum* Oil. *OCL* **2021**, *28*, 28. [CrossRef]
31. White, L.A.; Mitchell, T.; Brinckerhoff, C.E. Transforming Growth Factor β Inhibitory Element in the Rabbit Matrix Metalloproteinase-1 (Collagenase-1) Gene Functions as a Repressor of Constitutive Transcription. *Biochim. Et Biophys. Acta* **2000**, *1490*, 259–268. [CrossRef] [PubMed]
32. Pakyari, M.; Farrokhi, A.; Maharlooei, M.K.; Ghahary, A. Critical Role of Transforming Growth Factor Beta in Different Phases of Wound Healing. *Adv. Wound Care* **2013**, *2*, 215–224. [CrossRef] [PubMed]
33. Tebben, A.J.; Ruzanov, M.; Gao, M.; Xie, D.; Kiefer, S.E.; Yan, C.; Newitt, J.A.; Zhang, L.; Kim, K.; Lu, H.; et al. Crystal structures of apo and inhibitor-bound TGFβR2 kinase domain: Insights into TGFβR isoform selectivity. *Acta Cryst.* **2016**, *D72*, 658–674. [CrossRef]
34. Kalimuthu, A.K.; Pavadai, P.; Panneerselvam, T.; Babkiewicz, E.; Pijanowska, J.; Mrówka, P.; Rajagopal, G.; Deepak, V.; Sundar, K.; Maszczyk, P.; et al. Cytotoxic Potential of Bioactive Compounds from Aspergillus flavus, an Endophytic Fungus Isolated from Cynodon dactylon, against Breast Cancer: Experimental and Computational Approach. *Molecules* **2022**, *27*, 8814. [CrossRef] [PubMed]
35. Kalimuthu, A.K.; Panneerselvam, T.; Pavadai, P.; Pandian SR, K.; Sundar, K.; Murugesan, S.; Ammunje, D.N.; Kumar, S.; Arunachalam, S.; Kunjiappan, S. Pharmacoinformatics-based investigation of bioactive compounds of Rasam (South Indian recipe) against human cancer. *Sci. Rep.* **2021**, *11*, 21488. [CrossRef] [PubMed]
36. Gade, A.C.; Murahari, M.; Pavadai, P.; Kumar, M.S. Virtual Screening of a Marine Natural Product Database for In Silico Identification of a Potential Acetylcholinesterase Inhibitor. *Life* **2023**, *13*, 1298. [CrossRef]
37. Hua, I.; Anjum, F.; Shafie, A.; Ashour, A.A.; Almalki, A.A.; Alqarni, A.A.; Banjer, H.J.; Almaghrabi, S.A.; He, S.; Xu, N. Identifying Promising GSK3β Inhibitors for Cancer Management: A Computational Pipeline Combining Virtual Screening and Molecular Dynamics Simulations. *Front. Chem.* **2023**, *11*, 1200490. [CrossRef] [PubMed]
38. Han, Y.; Zhang, J.; Hu, C.Q.; Zhang, X.; Ma, B.; Zhang, P. In Silico ADME and Toxicity Prediction of Ceftazidime and Its Impurities. *Front. Pharmacol.* **2019**, *10*, 434. [CrossRef]

39. Sharmeen, J.B.; Mahomoodally, F.; Zengin, G.; Maggi, F. Essential Oils as Natural Sources of Fragrance Compounds for Cosmetics and Cosmeceuticals. *Molecules* **2021**, *26*, 666. [CrossRef]
40. Lukić, M.; Pantelić, I.; Savić, S. Towards Optimal PH of the Skin and Topical Formulations: From the Current State of the Art to Tailored Products. *Cosmetics* **2021**, *8*, 69. [CrossRef]
41. Sandeep, D.S. Development, Characterization, and In vitro Evaluation of Aceclofenac Emulgel. *Asian J. Pharm.* **2020**, *14*, 1–7.
42. Szulc-Musioł, B.; Dolińska, B.; Kołodziejska, J.; Ryszka, F. Influence of Plasma on the Physical Properties of Ointments with Quercetin. *Acta Pharm.* **2017**, *67*, 569–578. [CrossRef] [PubMed]
43. Ilomuanya, M.O.; Hameedat, A.T.; Akang, E.E.U.; Ekama, S.O.; Silva, B.O.; Akanmu, A.S. Development and Evaluation of Mucoadhesive Bigel Containing Tenofovir and Maraviroc for HIV Prophylaxis. *Future J. Pharm. Sci.* **2020**, *6*, 81. [CrossRef] [PubMed]
44. OECD. *Test No. 404: Acute Dermal Irritation/Corrosion*; OECD: Paris, France, 2015.
45. Nagar, H.; Srivastava, A.; Srivastava, R.; Kurmi, M.L.; Chandel, H.S.; Ranawat, M.S. Pharmacological Investigation of the Wound Healing Activity of *Cestrum nocturnum* (L.) Ointment in Wistar Albino Rats. *J. Pharm.* **2016**, *2016*, 9249040. [CrossRef] [PubMed]
46. Balakrishnan, B.; Mohanty, M.; Fernandez, A.C.; Mohanan, P.V.; Jayakrishnan, A. Evaluation of the Effect of Incorporation of Dibutyryl Cyclic Adenosine Monophosphate in an in Situ-Forming Hydrogel Wound Dressing Based on Oxidized Alginate and Gelatin. *Biomaterials* **2006**, *27*, 1355–1361. [CrossRef]
47. Artanti, N.; Dewijanti, I.D.; Muzdalifah, D.; Windarsih, A.; Suratno, S.; Handayani, S. Alpha glucosidase inhibitory activity of combination of *Caesalpinia sappan* L. and *Garcinia mangostana* extract. *J. Appl. Pharm. Sci.* **2023**, *13*, 189–198. [CrossRef]
48. Vellur, S.; Pavadai, P.; Babkiewicz, E.; Ram Kumar Pandian, S.; Maszczyk, P.; Kunjiappan, S. An In Silico Molecular Modelling-Based Prediction of Potential Keap1 Inhibitors from *Hemidesmus indicus* (L.) R.Br. against Oxidative-Stress-Induced Diseases. *Molecules* **2023**, *28*, 4541. [CrossRef]
49. Sabale, V.; Kunjwani, H.K.; Sabale, P.M. Formulation and in Vitro Evaluation of the Topical Antiageing Preparation of the Fruit of Benincasa Hispida. *J. Ayurveda Integr. Med.* **2011**, *2*, 124–128. [CrossRef]

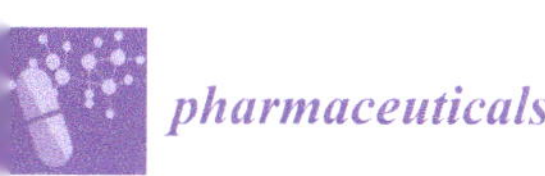

pharmaceuticals

Article

Identification of Potential Multitarget Compounds against Alzheimer's Disease through Pharmacophore-Based Virtual Screening

Géssica Oliveira Mendes [1], Moysés Fagundes de Araújo Neto [1], Deyse Brito Barbosa [1], Mayra Ramos do Bomfim [1], Lorena Silva Matos Andrade [2], Paulo Batista de Carvalho [3], Tiago Alves de Oliveira [4,5], Daniel Luciano Falkoski [4], Eduardo Habib Bechelane Maia [5], Marcelo Siqueira Valle [6], Laila Cristina Moreira Damázio [7], Alisson Marques da Silva [5], Alex Gutterres Taranto [4] and Franco Henrique Andrade Leite [1,*]

[1] Laboratory of Molecular Modeling, Department of Health, State University of Feira de Santana, Feira de Santana 44036-900, BA, Brazil; gomendes05@gmail.com (G.O.M.); moysesfagundes@gmail.com (M.F.d.A.N.); deyse.brito@hotmail.com (D.B.B.); mayramosbonfim@hotmail.com (M.R.d.B.)

[2] Laboratory of Chemoinformatics and Biological Assessment, Department of Health, State University of Feira de Santana, Feira de Santana 44036-900, BA, Brazil; lorena.pharm@gmail.com

[3] Feik School of Pharmacy, University of the Incarnate Word, San Antonio, TX 78212, USA; pcarvalh@uiwtx.edu

[4] Department of Bioengineering, Federal University of São João del-Rei, São João del-Rei 36301-160, MG, Brazil; tiago@cefetmg.br (T.A.d.O.); dlfalkoski@yahoo.com.br (D.L.F.); proftaranto@hotmail.com (A.G.T.)

[5] Department of Informatics, Management and Design, Federal Center for Technological Education of Minas Gerais (CEFET-MG), Divinópolis 35503-822, MG, Brazil; habib@cefetmg.br (E.H.B.M.); alisson@cefetmg.br (A.M.d.S.)

[6] Department of Natural Sciences, Federal University of São João del-Rei, São João del-Rei 36301-160, MG, Brazil; marcelovalle@gmail.com

[7] Department of Medicine, Federal University of São João del-Rei, São João del-Rei 36301-160, MG, Brazil; lailacmdamazio@gmail.com

* Correspondence: fhenrique@uefs.br

Citation: Mendes, G.O.; Araújo Neto, M.F.d.; Barbosa, D.B.; Bomfim, M.R.d.; Andrade, L.S.M.; Carvalho, P.B.d.; Oliveira, T.A.d.; Falkoski, D.L.; Maia, E.H.B.; Valle, M.S.; et al. Identification of Potential Multitarget Compounds against Alzheimer's Disease through Pharmacophore-Based Virtual Screening. *Pharmaceuticals* 2023, 16, 1645. https://doi.org/10.3390/ph16121645

Academic Editors: Halil İbrahim Ciftci, Belgin Sever and Hasan Demirci

Received: 11 August 2023
Revised: 11 October 2023
Accepted: 17 October 2023
Published: 23 November 2023

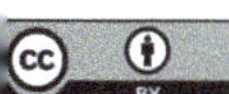

Abstract: Alzheimer's disease (AD) is a neurodegenerative disease characterized by progressive loss of cognitive functions, and it is the most prevalent type of dementia worldwide, accounting for 60 to 70% of cases. The pathogenesis of AD seems to involve three main factors: deficiency in cholinergic transmission, formation of extracellular deposits of β-amyloid peptide, and accumulation of deposits of a phosphorylated form of the TAU protein. The currently available drugs are prescribed for symptomatic treatment and present adverse effects such as hepatotoxicity, hypertension, and weight loss. There is urgency in finding new drugs capable of preventing the progress of the disease, controlling the symptoms, and increasing the survival of patients with AD. This study aims to present new multipurpose compounds capable of simultaneously inhibiting acetylcholinesterase (AChE), butyrylcholinesterase (BChE)—responsible for recycling acetylcholine in the synaptic cleft—and beta-secretase 1 (BACE-1)—responsible for the generation of amyloid-β plaques. AChE, BChE, and BACE-1 are currently considered the best targets for the treatment of patients with AD. Virtual hierarchical screening based on a pharmacophoric model for BACE-1 inhibitors and a dual pharmacophoric model for AChE and BChE inhibitors were used to filter 214,446 molecules by $QFIT_{BACE} > 0$ and $QFIT_{DUAL} > 56.34$. The molecules selected in this first round were subjected to molecular docking studies with the three targets and further evaluated for their physicochemical and toxicological properties. Three structures: ZINC45068352, ZINC03873986, and ZINC71787288 were selected as good fits for the pharmacophore models, with ZINC03873986 being ultimately prioritized for validation through activity testing and synthesis of derivatives for SAR studies.

Keywords: Alzheimer's disease; human acetylcholinesterase; human butyrylcholinesterase; human beta-secretase 1

1. Introduction

Alzheimer's disease (AD) is a progressive and irreversible neurodegenerative disease that causes memory loss and several cognitive disorders [1]. AD is responsible for 70% of all cases of dementia and affects approximately 50 million people worldwide [2]. Those numbers are expected to double by 2050 [2].

1.1. Pathogenesis of Alzheimer's Disease

Alzheimer's pathogenesis involves three main factors: the first is characterized by a deficiency in cholinergic transmission due to the selective loss of cholinergic neurons, the second is related to extracellular deposits of β-amyloid protein due to the catalytic action of beta-secretase 1 (BACE-1; EC 3. 4. 23. 46), and the third occurs through the formation of neurofibrillary clumps of a phosphorylated form of the TAU protein [1,3].

The cholinergic hypothesis is described as one of the main causes of AD [1]. Since the decline of cholinergic neurons induces a lack of acetylcholine (ACh), one way to compensate for this is to reduce the postsynaptic destruction of ACh by cholinesterases. Cholinesterases are a family of enzymes responsible for catalyzing the hydrolysis of ACh into choline and acetic acid to be reused into neuronal processes and are divided into two types: acetylcholinesterase (AChE; EC 3.1.1.7), and butyrylcholinesterase (BChE; EC 3.1.1.8). These enzymes are found mainly in the central nervous system, and their inhibition would lead to an increase in the available ACh at the synaptic cleft, promoting cognitive improvement [3].

The hypothesis of extracellular deposits of β-amyloid protein is noteworthy as it can explain the neurodegeneration process. This hypothesis states that the catalytic action of beta-secretase 1 generates, through the amyloidogenic pathway, the accumulation of insoluble β-amyloid peptide plaques in neurons. This pathophysiological process begins with the enzyme β-secretase (BACE1), which initiates the cleavage of the transmembrane protein called APP (Amyloid Precursor Protein). This cleavage is completed by another enzyme, γ secretase, generating the β-amyloid peptide (Aβ), which aggregates into oligomers, forming plaques that are deposited in different parts of the brain, mainly in the hippocampal neurons, basal nucleus, cortex entorhinal, and associative cortex [4].

1.2. Current Pharmacotherapy for Alzheimer's Disease

The therapeutic resources currently available for AD include cholinesterase inhibitors (donepezil, rivastigmine, and galantamine), N-methyl-D-aspartate (NMDA) receptor antagonists (memantine), chelating agents (deferiprone), and metal–protein attenuating compounds (MPACs) (clioquinol) [1]. These drugs are essentially prescribed for symptomatic treatment and cannot prevent neurodegeneration. They also present serious adverse effects (e.g., hepatotoxicity, hypertension, and weight loss) and low therapeutic efficacy [4], giving urgency to the search for new drugs capable of preventing the disease's progression and controlling its symptoms.

1.3. Multitarget Inhibitors

An approach that has been attracting interest for the treatment of multifactorial diseases such as AD is the identification and/or design of multitarget inhibitors, compounds capable of simultaneously acting on two or more biological targets, enhancing the therapeutic efficiency with lower doses. Previous studies show that treatment with multi-active drugs or molecular hybrids has greater efficacy and fewer adverse events [5] when compared with drug combination therapy in patients with complex diseases. This approach of using molecular hybrids has good potential to achieve the goal of slowing down the progression of AD [6].

One way to identify lead compounds with multitarget inhibition properties involves the use of computational strategies capable of prioritizing promising molecules for biological assays and accelerating the discovery of new, safe, and effective drugs. The ligand-based approach of computer-aided drug design can help to identify promising inhibitors with triple activity by defining the main stereo-electronic requirements of pharmacophore models for compounds with activity against each of the three molecular targets [7]. Ligand-based approaches have shown high efficiency in screening large datasets with low computational costs [8]. The selected compounds can be further subjected to structure-based approaches (e.g., molecular docking), and those showing complementarity with the target site are refined, helping to hypothesize the binding modes responsible for biological activity [9].

This study aimed to build and validate pharmacophore models of BACE-1, AChE, and BChE inhibitors and use them for a joint hierarchical virtual screening, followed by molecular docking virtual screening. Those models were used to identify promising multitarget inhibitors of beta-secretase 1, acetylcholinesterase, and butyrylcholinesterase in a Sigma-Aldrich® (St. Louis, MO, USA) dataset.

2. Results and Discussion

Computational methods used to mine for potentially active compounds have presented a quicker enrichment rate of potential candidate molecules for biological testing than random methods. Their capacity for building pharmacophore models can quickly identify essential stereo-electronic requirements for inhibition of specific targets and help to prioritize potentially active compounds.

2.1. Pharmacophore Model Generation and Evaluation

The search parameters for potential BACE-1 inhibitors were based on the main pharmacophore features of known active inhibitors and were used to identify molecules sharing the same stereo-electronic features. In total, 56 inhibitors were chosen with an IC_{50} equal or lower than 1000 nM, with 14 of them being used to generate the model and the remaining 42 for the validation stage.

The heuristic of the Genetic Algorithm (GA) generated ten pharmacophore models, and their parameters are presented in Table 1. Those internal statistical parameters are expected to fit a strain energy criterion lower than 100.0 kcal/mol [10], as high energy values (>100.00 Kcal/mol) reflect a high conformational tension, building energetically unfavorable conformers [11]. Therefore, models 05, 06, 07, and 10 were discarded.

Table 1. Internal statistical parameters of each pharmacophore model for the BACE-1 inhibitors provided by GALAHAD.

Model	Energy (Kcal/mol)	Sterics	H_Bond	Mol_qry	Pareto
01	21.74	756.00	155.60	9.09	00
02	42.36	746.60	151.50	15.59	00
03	20.65	687.30	157.00	14.42	00
04	50.89	713.40	161.20	8.47	00
05	1043.58	746.90	153.00	14.40	00
06	783.55	738.00	161.30	6.34	00
07	151,768.74	779.70	152.30	15.64	00
08	64.82	750.30	161.20	2.92	00
09	25.54	693.90	155.80	9.04	00
10	254.77	723.20	153.60	10.54	00

All models were evaluated for the PARETO value, which considers the listed parameters Mol_qry, H_bond, Sterics, and Energy. The conformers are overlapped and the pharmacophore agreement for the generation of the models is directly linked to the quality of pharmacophoric models [12]. All models, even the rejected ones, had PARETO = 0, meaning all the models were statistically similar. The parameters provided by GALAHAD were not sufficient to define the best model, and another metric, the Receiver Operation Characteristic (ROC) curves, was calculated to assess the ability of the models to differentiate between real and false positives.

A dataset with 42 BACE-1 inhibitors (IC$_{50} \leq$ 1000 nM) and 2100 decoys was aligned to each pharmacophore model. Their superposition value (QFIT value; 0–100) was employed to calculate the ROC curves, and their respective areas (area under the curve—AUC-ROC) were calculated [13]. The results are presented in Figure 1.

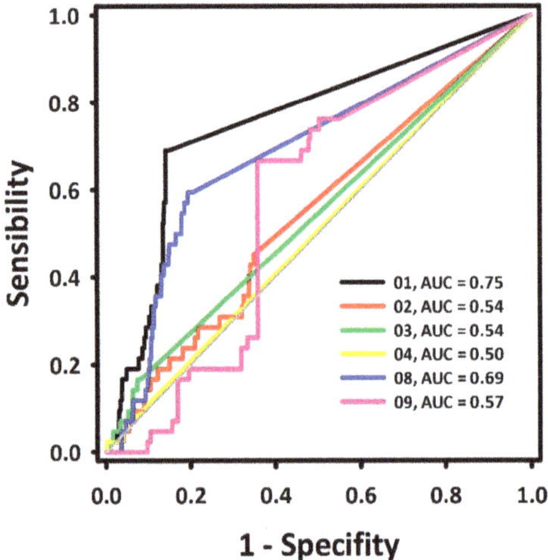

Figure 1. ROC curves for the BACE-1 inhibitor pharmacophore models.

The ROC curve displays the recognition of assets (represented by the Y coordinate) and false positives (represented by the X coordinate). An ideal curve first runs vertically along the Y axis, recognizing all assets, and then horizontally along the X axis continuously, which represents the recognition of all assets from the aligned molecule bank without any false positive recognition with its area under the curve (AUC) equal to 1.0 [13]. The diagonal line represents the ROC curve of a randomized trial, where pharmacophoric models with AUC < 0.50 are associated with models that perform worse than a random selection. In contrast, models with AUC > 0.70 are moderately predictive [14]. Previous research [15] describes hydrogen donor centers as essential requirements for the inhibition of BACE-1, while hydrogen acceptor centers define the potency of those inhibitors.

Based on the AUC values, pharmacophore model 1 (Figure 2) was chosen for further pharmacophore-based virtual screening. Its AUC-ROC was higher than 0.7, which characterized it to be the model with the highest potential capacity to correctly recognize active compounds.

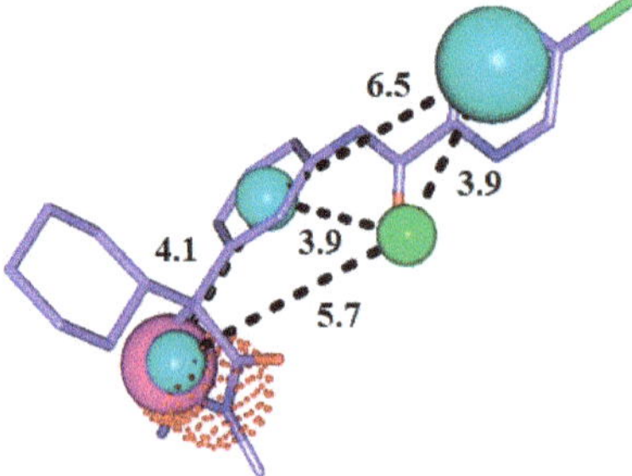

Figure 2. Representation of the pharmacophore model for BACE-1 inhibitors superimposed with a potent inhibitor. Cyan = hydrophobic centers (HY), red = positive centers, green = hydrogen acceptors (HBA), and magenta = hydrogen donors (HBD). The size of the spheres varies according to the tolerance radii calculated by GALAHAD™ (Seattle, WA, USA).

2.2. Pharmacophore-Based Virtual Screening

After identifying a useful pharmacophore model, successive filtering of 214,446 molecules from a Sigma Aldrich® dataset was performed. In total, 14,273 molecules showed QFIT > 0 when aligned to the BACE-1 inhibitor pharmacophore model 1. Subsequently, those molecules were filtered through the dual pharmacophore model previously built [7], with 119 molecules showing QFIT > 56.34 (Scheme 1), suggesting that they have stereo-electronic features important to biological activity. After virtual screening through pharmacophore models and based on alignment values, the selected structures were submitted to molecular docking studies with AChE, BChE, and BACE-1.

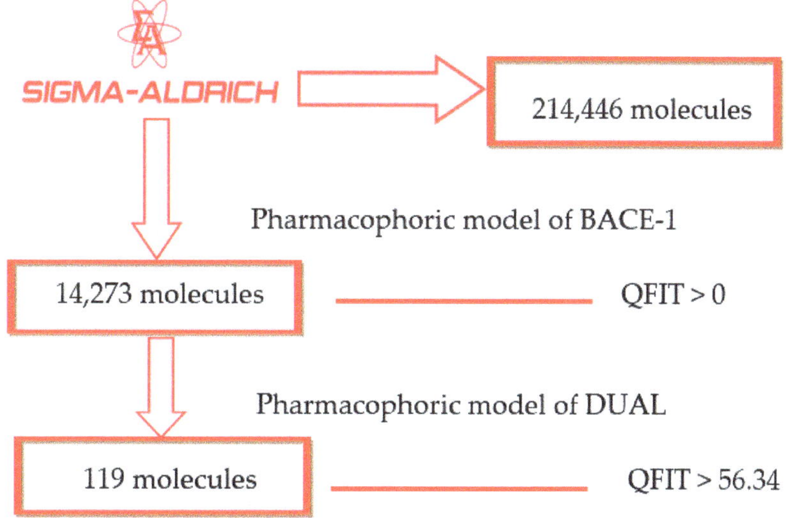

Scheme 1. Virtual screening by the pharmacophore model.

Although the pharmacophore model is helpful in searching for and selecting molecules that meet essential molecular requirements for biological activity [16], it has some limitations, such as the lack of information on how the molecules bind to the target site, as well as the limit imposed by the volume of the site. Those gaps in knowledge can be filled when the three-dimensional structure of the macromolecular target is available. The optimized application of molecular docking can also be used to assist in prioritizing bioactive molecules [17].

2.3. Molecular-Docking-Based Virtual Screening

Structures selected through pharmacophore model virtual screening (n = 119) were subjected to molecular docking against AChE, BChE, and BACE-1 using two different systems. AutoDock Vina, selected for molecular docking to AChE and BChE [7], scores structures by mapping intermolecular forces in kcal/mol, with lower energy indicating better docking. GOLD (ASP score function) was selected for molecular docking to BACE-1 [18]. It assigns a dimensionless number to each pose generated, and unlike AutoDock Vina, higher numbers indicate better docking.

The docking of the cholinesterases presented an average of the AChE energy values of −9.1, with 55 molecules showing lower affinity energy values. The BChE showed mean values of −10.02, with 67 molecules showing lower affinity energy values. The docking of BACE-1 showed mean energy values of 36.06, with 66 molecules presenting higher affinity energy values.

Then, the 22 molecules presenting the best values overall were selected and analyzed in order to exclude enantiomers. They were further evaluated based on their molecular coupling (or bonding) and on the presence of chiral centers. Three compounds, presenting the best values overall, were selected for further evaluation (Table 2).

Table 2. Scores of the three best compounds selected through molecular docking.

Molecule	AChE *	BChE *	BACE-1 **
ZINC45068352	−9.6	−10.4	43.32
ZINC03873986	−10.6	−11.2	41.54
ZINC71787288	−9.6	−10.6	41.91

* AutoDock Vina 1.1.2—kcal/mol—lower energy indicates better docking. ** GOLD—dimensionless—Higher numbers indicate better docking.

In order to confirm our results, we re-ran the molecular docking of those three compounds against the three targets using the same programs. In other words, we ran ZINC45068352, ZINC03873986, and ZINC71787288 against AChE, BChE, and BACE-1 using AutoDock Vina 1.1.2 (despite it not being validated for BACE-1) and again, using GOLD 5.8.1, despite it not being validated for cholinesterases. The results, presented in the Supplementary Materials (Tables S1 and S2) confirm all three compounds present good scores in both programs, justifying their prioritization.

2.4. Application of Physicochemical Filters

Good scores in molecular docking do not guarantee the selected molecules will have the physicochemical requirements to reach the target site. Therefore, the best candidates were further screened for their physicochemical properties according to Lipinski's Rules and Veber's parameters [19,20], which are capable of virtually predicting oral bioavailability quickly and at a low computational cost. The results are presented in Table 3.

Table 3. Physicochemical analysis of the best candidates for triple inhibition according to Lipinski's Rule and Veber's parameters.

Molecule	MW (g/mol)	HBD	HBA	cLogP	PSA ($\mathring{A}^2$)	RB	HBD + HBA
ZINC45068352	486.58	0	7	4.77	89.45	5	7
ZINC03873986	442.43	2	6	4.15	100.27	0	8
ZINC71787288	444.44	0	7	5.38	61.53	3	7

MW = molecular weight; HBD = hydrogen bond donor; HBA = hydrogen bond acceptor; cLogP = calculated octanol–water partition coefficient; PSA = Polar surface area; RB = Rotatable bonds.

Table 3 shows that the selected structures (ZINC45068352, ZINC03873986, ZINC71787288) satisfy all parameters for oral bioavailability according to Lipinski's and Veber's criteria, with only one suffering a penalty (ZINC71787288, with a cLogp value > 5). This penalty, however, does not justify eliminating the structure from consideration, as about 6% of the drugs orally bioavailable, currently in use, do not fully obey the accepted parameters for bioavailability [21].

2.5. Analysis of Intermolecular Interactions

Despite the importance of a selected structure overlapping the pharmacophore model, obtaining a good score in molecular docking, and having the physicochemical requisites for oral bioavailability, these metrics do not identify the bonds between potential inhibitors and their targets. Three-dimensional complexes were generated based on the known crystallographic structures of AChE, BChE, and BACE-1 to study the molecular bonds and mode of interaction of the three best-ranked compounds with the enzymatic active sites.

2.5.1. AChE Complexes

The analysis of the interactions performed by the AChE crystallographic inhibitor (Figure 3) can be useful in understanding the interactions important for biological activity and mapping those interactions for the subsequent analysis of the drug candidates screened by previous computational methods.

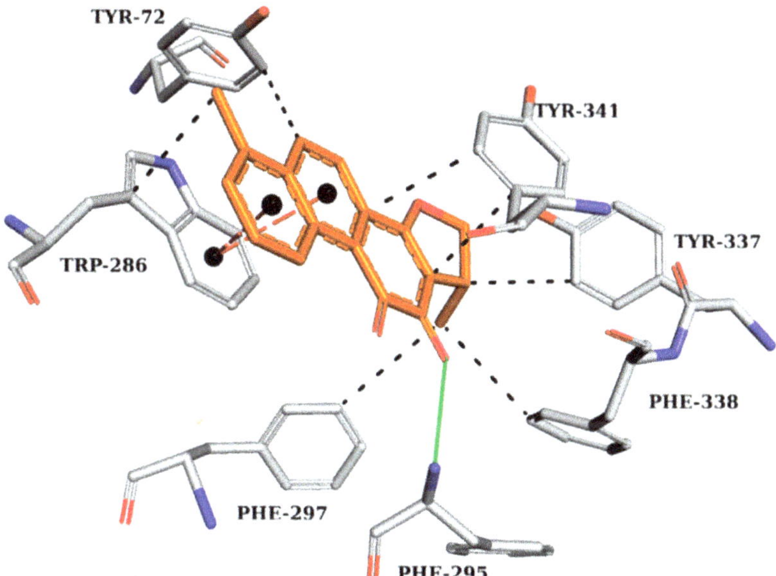

Figure 3. Interaction map of AChE crystallographic ligand (1YL—Dihydrotanshinone I) in the active site from PDB (4M0E), generated by the Protein–Ligand Interaction Profiler online server. Hydrogen bond as donor in solid green line, π stacking interactions in dashed red lines, and hydrophobic interactions in dashed black lines. (Orange: carbon of the ligand; blue: nitrogen; red: oxygen; gray: carbon of the amino acids; red: oxygen).

The AChE crystallographic ligand forms a hydrogen bond with PHE295, a π-stacking interaction with TRP286, and hydrophobic interactions with TYR72, TRP286, PHE297, TYR337, PHE338, and TYR341 (Figure 3).

Based on this figure, interaction maps were generated for ZINC45068352 (Figure 4A), ZINC03873986 (Figure 4B), and ZINC71787288 (Figure 4C) in the AChE active site to observe whether the prioritized molecules maintained the same intermolecular interaction profile as the crystallographic ligand.

ZINC45068352 (Figure 4A) showed hydrophobic interactions at the AChE active site with TRP286 and TYR341, similar to the crystallographic ligand and additionally with the residue GLU292. ZINC03873986 (Figure 4B) repeated important interactions established by the crystallographic ligand, such as the hydrogen donor to PHE295, π-stacking interaction with TRP286, and hydrophobic interactions with TRP286, TYR337, PHE338, and TYR341. Furthermore, this molecule established π-stacking interactions with TYR341 and hydrophobic interactions with LEU76. ZINC71787288 (Figure 4C) made hydrophobic interactions with residues TYR72, TRP286, and TYR341, hydrogen bonding with TYR72, and π-stacking interactions with TRP286. Notably, the binding with TRP286 is related to potent compounds at the nanomolar scale, which also interact with the PHE 338 residue and participate in the binding of the substrate to the enzyme, ensuring catalytic efficiency [22–24].

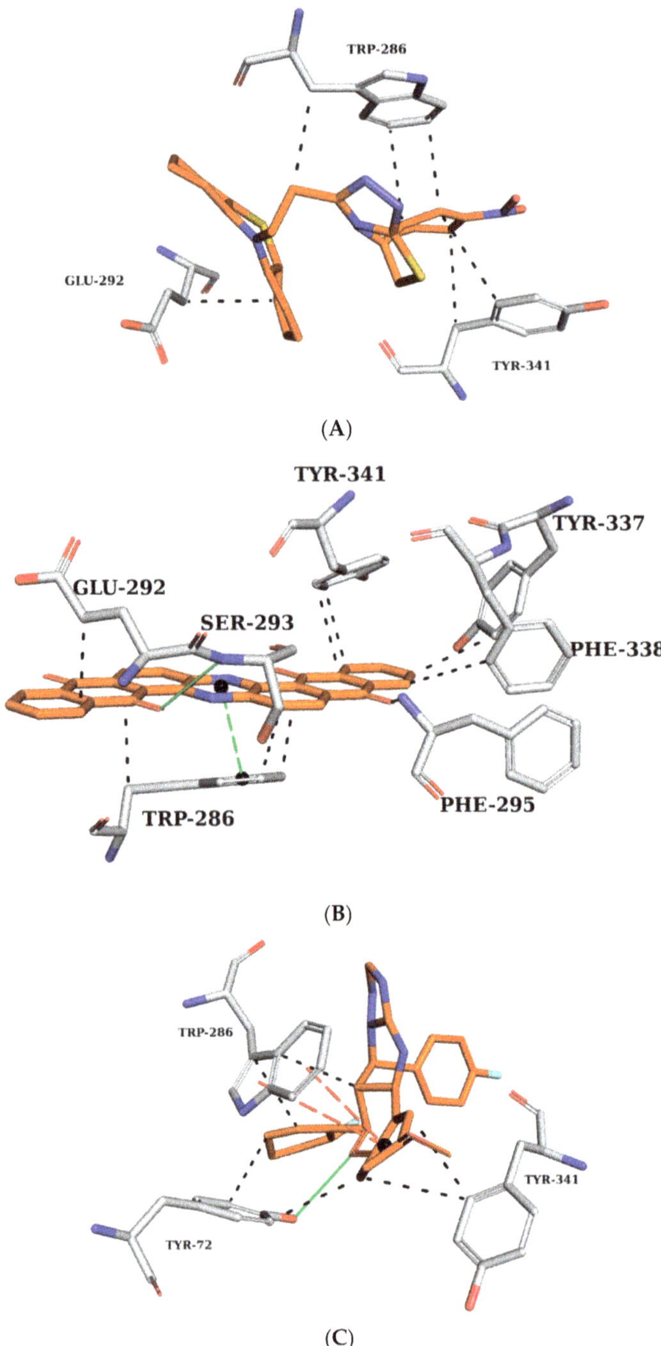

Figure 4. Interaction map of ZINC45068352 (**A**), ZINC03873986 (**B**), and ZINC71787288 (**C**) in the AChE active site generated by the Protein–Ligand Interaction Profiler online server. (The information is contained in Figure 3).

2.5.2. BChE Complexes

The crystallographic structure of BChE with its inhibitor was analyzed to highlight the requirements for the proper interactions of the three best-ranked compounds. The interaction map of the BChE crystallographic ligand shows π-stacking interactions with TRP82 and hydrophobic interactions with TRP82, ALA328, and TRP430 (Figure 5).

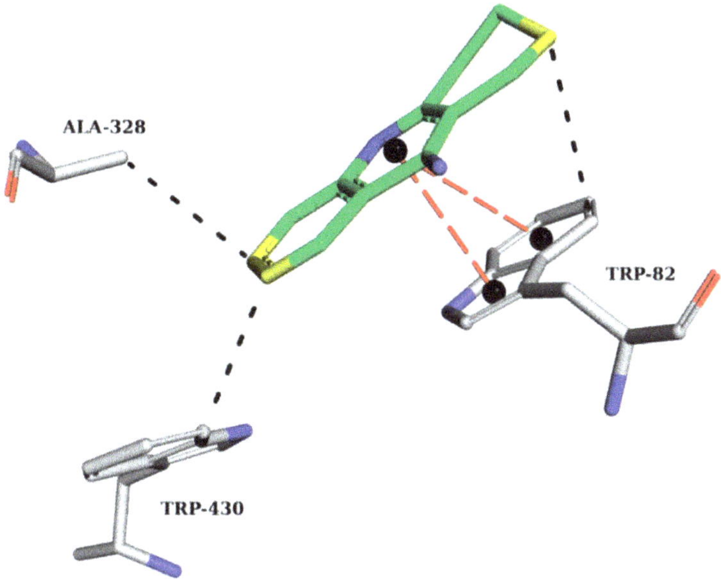

Figure 5. Interaction map of the BChE crystallographic ligand (THA) in the active site from PDB (4BDS). (The information is contained in Figure 3). (Green: carbon of the ligand; blue: nitrogen; red: oxygen; gray: carbon of the amino acids; red: oxygen).

Interaction maps were subsequently generated for ZINC45068352 (Figure 6A), ZINC03873986 (Figure 6B), and ZINC71787288 (Figure 6C) to compare the interactions observed with the crystallographic ligand with the expected interactions with the selected molecules.

ZINC45068352 forms hydrogen bonds with GLY116, GLY117, HIS438, π-stacking interaction with HIS438, and hydrophobic interactions with residues ASP70, TRP82, THR120, TRP430, and TYR440 (Figure 6A). ZINC03873986 forms hydrophobic interactions with residues ASN68, ASP70, TRP82, and THR120 (Figure 6B). ZINC71787288 forms hydrogen bonds with HIS438 and hydrophobic interactions with ASP70, TRP82, THR120, ALA328, TYR332, and TRP430 (Figure 6C). The interactions observed with the TRP82 residues in the anionic site prevent the substrate from reaching the catalytic site. In the interaction maps, it is also possible to observe binding with residue ASP70, which is part of the peripheral site. This interaction is also important for inhibitory activity against BChE since it also prevents the entry of the substrate [25]. Interactions with residues THR120, GLY116, and GLY117 were observed in potent BChE inhibitors [26,27].

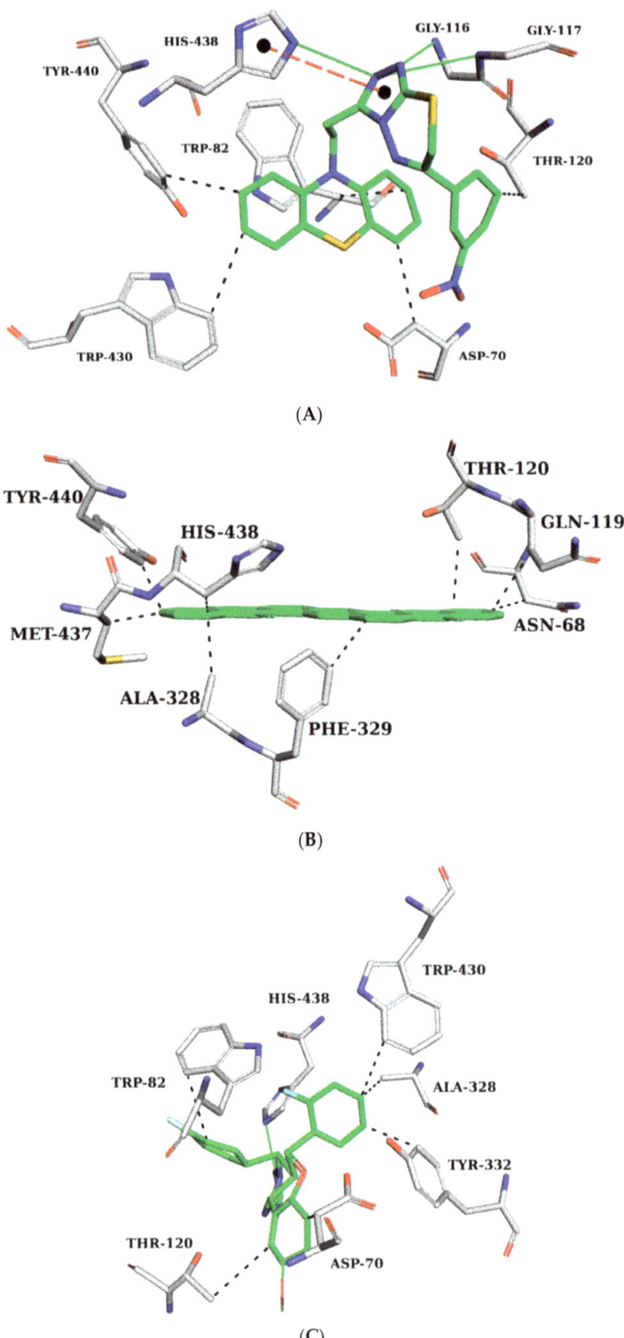

Figure 6. Interaction map of ZINC45068352 (**A**), ZINC03873986 (**B**), and ZINC71787288 (**C**) with the BChE active site generated by the Protein–Ligand Interaction Profiler online server. (The information is contained in Figure 5).

2.5.3. BACE-1 Complexes

The BACE-1 crystallographic ligand (Figure 7) forms hydrogen bonds with TRP76, ASP32, ASP228, and GLY230 and hydrophobic interactions with LEU30, VAL69, TYR71, ILE118, and ARG128 [18]. Figure 8 shows the analysis of the complexes generated between BACE-1 and ZINC45068352, ZINC03873986, and ZINC71787288.

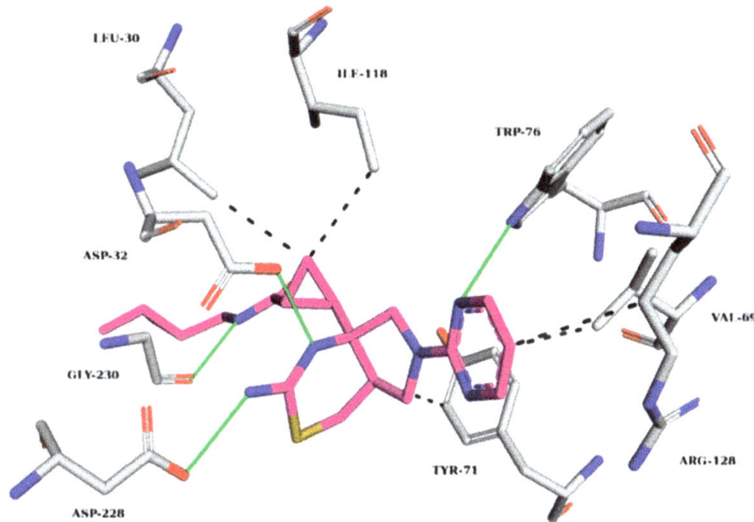

Figure 7. Interaction map of the BACE-1 crystallographic ligand (QKA) in the active site from PDB (6UWP). (The information is contained in Figure 3). (Margin: carbon of the ligand; blue: nitrogen; red: oxygen; gray: carbon of the amino acids; red: oxygen).

At the BACE-1 active site, ZINC45068352 held π-stacking interactions with TYR71, hydrophobic interactions with residues TYR71, PHE108, TRP115, ILE118, and ILE226, and π-cation interactions with ARG35 (Figure 8A). As for ZINC03873986, it formed a hydrogen bond with TRP76, π-stacking interactions with TYR71, hydrophobic interactions with residues VAL69, TYR71, TRP76, PHE108, ILE118, and ARG128, and π-cation interactions with ARG35 (Figure 8B). ZINC71787288, displayed π-stacking interactions with TYR71, hydrogen bonding with TYR71, and hydrophobic interactions with residues LEU30, VAL69, TYR71, PHE108, ILE110, and TRP115 (Figure 8C). The published data showed that the observed interactions with the amino acid residue TYR71 are essential for inhibiting activity, as they promote conformational changes and prevent the substrate from reaching the catalytic site [28,29]. Interactions with amino acid residues VAL69, ILE118, and TRP115 are cited as important for BACE-1 inhibition, which has been observed in the molecular dynamics simulations already described [30].

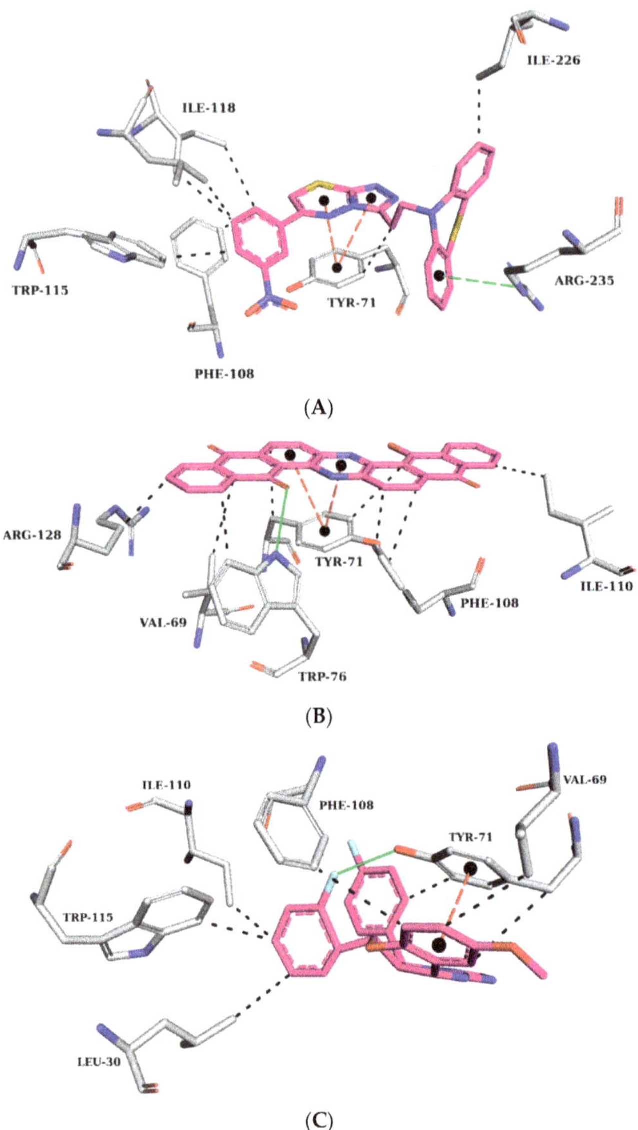

Figure 8. Interaction map of ZINC45068352 (**A**), ZINC03873986 (**B**), and ZINC71787288 (**C**) in the BACE-1 active site generated by the Protein–Ligand Interaction Profiler online server. (The information is contained in Figure 7).

2.6. Analysis of AMES Test (Cytotoxicity) and Other Parameters of Toxicity

After the molecular docking stage and the evaluation of their interactions with the three target enzymatic sites, the three compounds ZINC45068352, ZINC03873986, and ZINC71787288 were subjected to an in silico AMES test, using the online server pkCSM [29]. The AMES test is an essay originally performed on *Salmonella typhimurium* and *Escherichia coli*. It is based on the knowledge that if a substance is mutagenic for these bacteria, it also presents a risk of developing cancer in humans [31]. In silico mutagenicity screening tools were later developed and optimized to screen drug candidates, yielding comparable results to the original AMES test [32–34].

ZINC03873986 and ZINC71787288 were negative for the AMES test, but ZINC45068352 was positive and discarded from future steps. Additional simulations were performed for the structures ZINC03873986 and ZINC71787288 to characterize other aspects of their toxicity profile. According to our analysis, presented in the Supplementary Materials (Table S3), ZINC71787288 is hepatotoxic, which leaves ZINC0387398 as our lead compound.

3. Materials and Methods

3.1. Dataset

A dataset of 56 compounds (Supplementary Materials Tables S4 and S5) with $IC_{50} \leq 1000$ nM for human BACE-1 was obtained from the literature [35]. The 2D structures and most reliable tautomers (pH = 4.5) were drawn using Marvin® Sketch 15.4.20 [36]. Subsequently, the structures were converted to 3D format using the CONCORD module, implemented in the SYBYL®-X 2.0 package [37]. Partial atomic charges were calculated using the Gasteiger–Hückel method, as available on the SYBYL platform. Energy minimization was performed through Conjugate Gradient (CG) with a convergence criterion of 0.001 kcal/mol and Tripos force field (dielectric constant $\varepsilon = 80.0$ and a maximum number of iterations = 50.000) [12]. Four compounds with the best IC_{50} values were selected, two for the construction and two for the validation stage of the pharmacophore model (Figure 9).

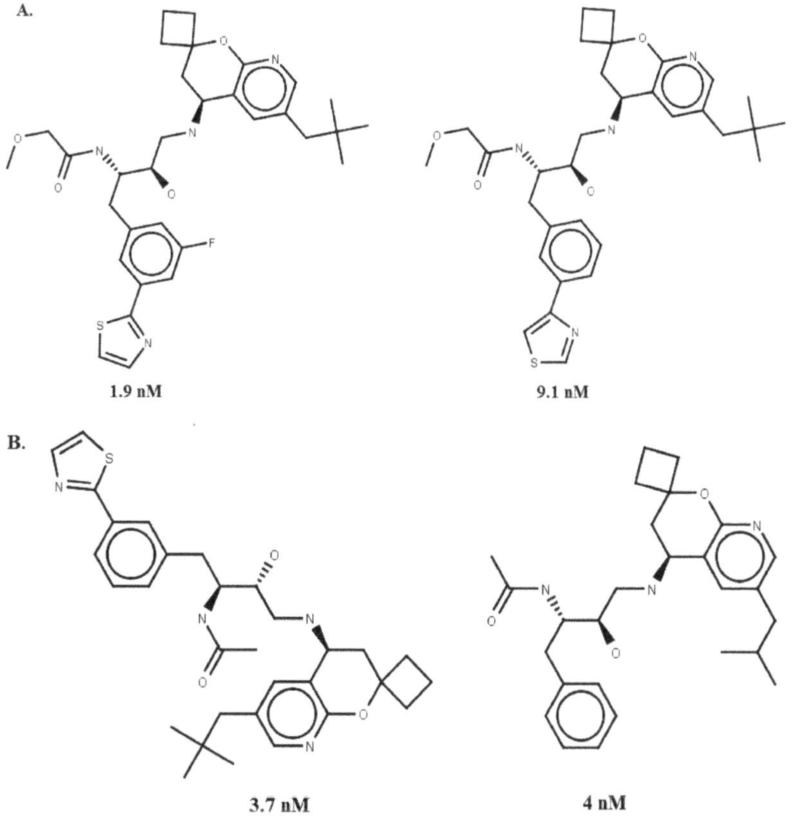

Figure 9. The four chemical structures and biological activities of inhibitors against BACE-1 that were used in generating (**A**) and evaluating (**B**) the pharmacophore models.

3.2. Pharmacophore Model Generation

The GALAHAD (Genetic Algorithm Linear Algorithm for Hyper molecular Alignment of Data sets) implemented on the SYBYL platform was used to obtain the conformers. The flexibly superimposed training set compounds generated the pharmacophore features to create hyper molecular alignments. The Genetic Algorithm (GA) employed in this step starts with 80 conformations (population size) of each compound that evolves through a maximum of 830 generations. The other parameters (CROSSING = 1.0 and MUTATION = 1.0) were maintained at their default values, as implemented in the GALAHAD module from SYBYL-X$^{®}$ 2.0 [37].

3.3. Pharmacophore Model Evaluation

The statistical parameters of GALAHAD (ENERGY < 100 Kcal/mol and PARETO $\neq$ 00) were used to select the pharmacophore models. The discriminatory power to recognize active compounds and decoys evaluated the remaining models. Thus, the DUD-E server [38] was used to build decoys, and the SigmaPlot$^{®}$ program v. 12.0 [39] was used to calculate the area under the curve of each receiver operating characteristic (AUC-ROC curve). The model that attained an AUC-ROC > 0.7 was chosen as the best BACE-1 inhibitor pharmacophore model.

3.4. Pharmacophore-Based Virtual Screening

The best BACE-1 pharmacophore model was used to filter the database Sigma-Aldrich$^{®}$ (n = 214,446) (http://zinc15.docking.org/catalogs/sialbb accessed on 5 September 2020) available on the ZINC15 platform [40] by using the UNITY module of SYBYL-X 2.0. This step was implemented through the option "3D flexible alignment", available in the UNITY 3D module. The quality of the alignment of the molecules was expressed by the value of QFIT, which can vary from 0 to 100.

The superimposed compounds in the BACE-1 model (QFIT > 0) were then flexibly aligned with a dual AChE and BChE inhibitors pharmacophore model [7], available in the GALAHAD™ module. To prioritize the best-superimposed compounds in this model, the mathematical equation of average plus the standard deviation of QFIT values (Equation (1)) was employed as a cutoff. Compounds showing QFIT > $\underline{x}$ + σ were then selected for molecular docking with AChE, BChE, and BACE-1. Equation (1) was used to select the compounds best fitting the dual pharmacophore model:

$$X \geq \underline{x} + \sigma, \tag{1}$$

where X = QFIT value, $\underline{x}$ = average, and σ = standard deviation.

3.5. Molecular Docking

The crystallographic structures of AChE (PDB ID: 4M0E) [22], BChE (PDB ID: 4BDS) [41], and BACE-1 (PDB ID: 6UWP) [42] were prepared with Biopolymer implemented on SYBYL-X 2.0 [37], where ions and water molecules were removed. Hydrogen atoms were inserted to optimize the hydrogen bonds. For the AChE and BChE target structures, the protonation state of the receptors was adjusted to pH 7.4 through the PropKa [43] server, and the conformational search and scoring were performed by AutoDock Vina 1.1.2 [44], according to previously validated parameters [7]. As for the BACE-1 structure, the receptor had its protonation state evaluated by the H++ 1.0 server [http://newbiophysics.cs.vt.edu/H++/ accessed on 24 September 2020] program, and pKa was corrected at pH 4.5 [45]. Validation methods were used, and the program selected for molecular docking with BACE-1 was GOLD 5.8.1 [46]; the score was provided by the Astex Scoring Potential (ASP, knowledge-based function derived from a database of protein–ligand complexes) function with the parameters previously validated [18].

3.6. Physicochemical Filters

The designed molecules were characterized using the pkCSM server [34] for the physicochemical descriptors for Lipinski's [19] and Veber's [20] descriptors. For reference:

- Lipinski's: Molecular Weight (MW) $\leq$ 500 Da; Hydrogen Bond Donors (HBD) $\leq$ 5; Hydrogen Bond Acceptors (HBA) $\leq$ 10; and cLog$p$ $\leq$ 5.
- Veber's: Polar Surface Area (PSA) $\leq$ 140 $\mathring{A}^2$; Rotatable Bonds (RB) $\leq$ 10; Sum of HBD and HBA $\leq$ 12.

3.7. Evaluation of Intermolecular Interactions

Molecules having one or fewer penalties were selected for evaluation of the intermolecular interaction through the Protein–Ligand Interaction Profiler (PLIP) server and PyMOL v. 2.4.0 [47,48].

3.8. AMES Test (Cytotoxicity) and Other Parameters of Toxicity

After the molecular docking stage and evaluation of active-site interactions, the three higher-scoring compounds were subjected to the AMES test [31] to predict their potential cytotoxicity using the pkCSM server [34]. The results led to ZINC45068352 being discarded. The same pkCSM server was used to analyze other parameters of toxicity, such as oral rat acute toxicity (LD_{50}), hepatotoxicity, and skin sensitization, among others. The results, presented in Table S3 of the Supplementary Materials, indicated that ZINC71787288 was hepatotoxic, leading to it also being discarded.

4. Conclusions

The use of multitarget drugs is relatively recent in the history of therapy, with those few showing distinct advantages over a combination of separate drugs. We expect a multitarget treatment against AD would need lower doses, present fewer drug–drug interactions, and encourage higher patient compliance.

The virtual screening strategy associated with the individual pharmacophore models for AChE, BChE, and BACE1 allowed the generation and evaluation of models evaluated for recovery rate of true inhibitors versus false positives, resulting in the selection of a pharmacophore model with discriminatory power (AUC > 0.7). This approach, aligned with a dual pharmacophore model and docking, allowed the identification of possible hybrid triple-inhibitors against AChE, BChE, and BACE1. Computational techniques employed in a hierarchical process enabled the selection of molecules with proper stereo-electronic requirements for triple-target inhibition.

ZINC03873986 was selected as a good fit for the pharmacophore models with low cytotoxic potential, which makes it a potential multitarget hybrid compound for the treatment of Alzheimer's disease. Our next steps aim to validate these computational results through enzymatic testing on the targets and synthesis of derivatives of those lead compounds for SAR studies.

Supplementary Materials: The following supporting information can be downloaded at: https://www.mdpi.com/article/10.3390/ph16121645/s1, Table S1. Scores of the three best compounds selected through molecular docking by AutoDock Vina 1.1.2. Table S2. Scores of the three best compounds selected through molecular docking by GOLD. Table S3. Toxicological analysis of the remaining molecules. Table S4. Chemical structure and biological activity of inhibitors against BACE-1 used in generating pharmacophore models. Table S5. Chemical structure and biological activity of inhibitors against BACE-1 that were used in evaluating pharmacophore models.

Author Contributions: All authors contributed to the conception and design of the study. Material preparation and data analysis were performed by G.O.M., M.F.d.A.N. and F.II.A.L. D.B.B. and M.R.d.B. performed the molecular docking step. A.G.T. and P.B.d.C. contributed to the review of the manuscript. All authors commented on previous versions of the manuscript. All authors have read and agreed to the published version of the manuscript.

Pharmaceuticals **2023**, 16, 1645

Funding: This work was supported by the FAPESB under grant 4902; Fundação de Amparo à Pesquisa do Estado de Minas Gerais—FAPEMIG, grants APQ-02741-17, APQ-00855-19, APQ-01733-21, and APQ-04559-22; Conselho Nacional de Desenvolvimento Científico e Tecnológico—CNPq-Brazil, grants 305117/2017-3, 426261/2018-6; and grant 310108/2020-9.

Institutional Review Board Statement: Not applicable.

Informed Consent Statement: Not applicable.

Data Availability Statement: Data is contained within the article and supplementary material.

Acknowledgments: We thank the State University of Feira de Santana (UEFS), Federal University of São João del-Rei (UFSJ), Programa de Pós-graduação em Bioengenharia (PPBE/UFSJ), and the Federal Center for Technological Education of Minas Gerais (CEFET-MG) for providing the physical infrastructure and human resources.

Conflicts of Interest: The authors declare no conflict of interest.

References

1. de Falco, A.; Cukierman, D.S.; Hauser-Davis, R.A.; Rey, N.A. Doença de Alzheimer: Hipóteses etiológicas e perspectivas de tratamento. *Química Nova* **2016**, *39*, 63–80. [CrossRef]
2. World Health Organization. *Dementia. [S. L.]*; WHO: Geneva, Switzerland, 2019. Available online: https://www.who.int/es/news-room/fact-sheets/detail/dementia (accessed on 5 January 2020).
3. Johnson, K.A.; Schultz, A.; Betensky, R.A.; Becker, J.A.; Sepulcre, J.; Rentz, D.; Mormino, E.; Chhatwal, J.; Amariglio, R.; Papp, K.; et al. Tau positron emission tomographic imaging in aging and early Alzheimer disease. *Ann. Neurol.* **2016**, *79*, 110–119. [CrossRef] [PubMed]
4. Najafi, Z.; Mahdavi, M.; Saledi, M.; Karimpour-Razkenari, E.; Asatouri, R.; Vafadarnejad, F.; Moghadam, F.H.; Khanavi, M.; Shariffadeh, M.; Akbarzadeh, T. Novel tacrine-1,2,3-triazole hybrids: In vitro, in vivo biological evaluation and docking study of cholinesterase inhibitors. *Eur. J. Med. Chem.* **2017**, *125*, 1200–1212. [CrossRef] [PubMed]
5. Zhou, J.; Jiang, X.; He, S.; Jiang, H.; Feng, F.; Liu, W.; Qu, W.; Sun, H. Rational design of multitarget-directed ligands: Strategies and emerging paradigms. *J. Med. Chem.* **2019**, *62*, 8881–8914. [CrossRef]
6. Dias, K.S.T.; de Paula, C.T.; Riquiel, M.M.; Lago, S.T.; Costa, K.C.M.; Vaz, S.M.; Machado, R.P.; Lima, L.M.S.; Viegas Junior, C. Aplicações recentes da abordagem de fármacos multialvo para o tratamento da Doença de Alzheimer. *Virtual Química* **2015**, *7*, 609–648. [CrossRef]
7. Mascarenhas, A.M.S.; de Almeida, R.B.M.; Araujo, M.F.N.; Mendes, G.O.; da Cruz, J.N.; dos Santos, C.B.R.; Botura, M.B.; Leite, F.H.A. Pharmacophore-based virtual screening and molecular docking to identify promising dual inhibitors of human acetylcholinesterase and butyrylcholinesterase. *J. Biomol. Struct. Dyn.* **2020**, *39*, 6021–6030. [CrossRef]
8. Rodrigues, R.P.; Mantoani, S.P.; de Almeida, J.R.; Pinseta, F.R.; Semighini, E.P.; da Silva, V.B.; da Silva, C.H.P. Estratégias de Triagem Virtual no Planejamento de Fármacos. *Rev. Virtual Química* **2012**, *4*, 739–776. [CrossRef]
9. Ballester, P.J.; Mangold, M.; Howard, N.I.; Robinson, R.L.M.; Abell, C.; Blumberger, J.; Mitchell, J.B. Hierarchical virtual screening for the discovery of new molecular scaffolds in antibacterial hit identification. *J. R. Soc.* **2012**, *9*, 3196–3207.
10. Liu, K.P.Y.; Chan, C.C.H.; Chu, M.M.L.; Ng, T.Y.L.; Chu, L.W.; Hui, F.S.L.; Yuen, H.K.; Fisher, A.G. Activities of daily living performance in dementia. *Acta Neurol. Scand.* **2007**, *116*, 91–95. [CrossRef]
11. Sterling, T.; Irwin, J. Zinc 15—Ligand Discovery for Everyone. *J. Chem. Inf. Model.* **2015**, *55*, 2324–2337.
12. Clark, R.D.; Abrahamian, E. Using a staged multi-objective optimization approach to find selective pharmacophore models. *J. Comput. -Aided Mol. Des.* **2009**, *23*, 765–771. [CrossRef] [PubMed]
13. Shepphird, J.K.; Clark, R.D. A marriage made in torsional space using GALAHAD models to drive pharmacophore multiplet searches. *J. Comput. -Aided Mol. Des.* **2006**, *20*, 763–771. [CrossRef]
14. Metz, C.E. Basic principles of ROC analysis. *Semin. Nucl. Med.* **1978**, *8*, 283–298.
15. Prati, F.; Bottegoni, G.; Bolognesi, M.L.; Cavalli, A. BACE-1 Inhibitors: From Recent Single-Target Molecules to Multitarget Compounds for Alzheimer's Disease. *J. Med. Chem.* **2017**, *61*, 619–637. [CrossRef] [PubMed]
16. Kothandan, G.; Madhavan, T.; Gadhe, C.G.; Cho, S.J. A combined 3D QSAR and pharmacophore-based virtual screening for the identification of potent p38 MAP kinase inhibitors: An in silico approach. *Med. Chem. Res.* **2013**, *22*, 1773–1787. [CrossRef]
17. Leite, F.H.A. Planejamento e Avaliação de Novos Inibidores de Pteridina Redutase 1 (Ptr1) de Leishmania Major. Ph.D. Thesis, Universidade Estadual de Feira de Santana, Feira de Santana, Brazil, 2015.
18. Bomfim, M.R.; Barbosa, D.B.; Carvalho, P.B.; Silva, A.M.; Oliveira, T.A.; Taranto, A.G.; Leite, F.H.A. Identification of potential human beta-secretase 1 inhibitors by hierarchical virtual screening and molecular dynamics. *J. Biomol. Struct. Dyn.* **2022**, *41*, 4560–4574. [CrossRef] [PubMed]

19. Lipinski, C.A.; Lombardo, F.; Dominy, B.W.; Feeney, P.J. Experimental and computational approaches to estimate solubility and permeability in drug discovery and development settings. *Adv. Drug Deliv. Rev.* **1997**, *23*, 3–26. [CrossRef]

20. Veber, D.F.; Johnson, S.R.; Cheng, H.Y.; Smith, B.R.; Ward, K.W.; Kopple, K.D. Molecular Properties That Influence the oral bioavailability of Drug Candidates. *J. Med. Chem.* **2002**, *45*, 2615–2623. [CrossRef]

21. Degoey, D.A.; Chen, H.-J.; Cox, P.B.; Wendt, M.D. Beyond the Rule of 5: Lessons Learned from AbbVie's Drugs and Compound Collection. *J. Med. Chem.* **2018**, *61*, 2636–2651. [CrossRef]

22. Cheung, J.; Gary, E.N.; Shiomi, K.; Rosenberry, T.L. Structures of human acetylcholinesterase bound to dihydrotanshinone I and territrem B show peripheral site flexibility. *ACS Med. Chem. Lett.* **2013**, *4*, 1091–1096.

23. Munoz-Torrero, D.; Camps, P. Dimeric and hybrid anti-Alzheimer drug candidates. *Curr. Med. Chem.* **2006**, *13*, 399–422. [CrossRef] [PubMed]

24. Türkeş, C.; Arslan, M.; Demir, Y.; Çoçaj, L.; Nixha, A.R.; Beydemir, Ş. Synthesis, biological evaluation and in silico studies of novel N-substituted phthalazine 103 sulfonamide compounds as potent carbonic anhydrase and acetylcholinesterase inhibitors. *Bioorg. Chem.* **2019**, *89*, 103004. [CrossRef]

25. Senol, F.S.; Ślusarczyk, S.; Matkowski, A.; Pérez-Garrido, A.; Girón-Rodríguez, F.; Cerón-Carrasca, J.P.; Den-Haan, H.; Pena-García, J.; Pérez-Sánchez, H.; Domaradzki, K. Selective in vitro and in silico butyrylcholinesterase inhibitory activity of diterpenes and rosmarinic acid isolated from *Perovskia atriplicifolia* Benth. and *Salvia glutinosa* L. *Phytochemistry* **2016**, *133*, 33–44. [CrossRef]

26. Wajid, S.; Khatoon, A.; Khan, M.A.; Zafar, H.; Kanwal, S.; Atta-Ur-Rahman; Choudhary, M.I.; Basha, F.Z. Microwave-assisted organic synthesis, structure-activity relationship, kinetics and molecular docking studies of non-cytotoxic benzamide derivatives as selective butyrylcholinesterase inhibitors. *Bioorg. Med. Chem.* **2019**, *27*, 4030–4040. [CrossRef] [PubMed]

27. Kumar, V.; Saha, A.; Roy, K. In silico modeling for dual inhibition of acetylcholinesterase (AChE) and butyrylcholinesterase (BuChE) enzymes in Alzheimer's disease. *Comput. Biol. Chem.* **2020**, *88*, 4030–4040. [CrossRef]

28. Dhanjal, J.K.; Goyal, S.; Sharma, S.; Hamid, R.; Grover, A. Mechanist insights into mode of action of potent natural antagonists of BACE-1 for checking Alzheimer's plaque pathology. *Biochem. Biophys. Res. Commun.* **2014**, *443*, 1054–1059. [CrossRef] [PubMed]

29. Semighini, E.P. In silico design of beta-secretase inhibitors in Alzheimer's disease. *Chem. Biol. Drug Des.* **2014**, *86*, 284–290. [CrossRef]

30. Dhanabalan, A.K.; Kesherwani, M.; Velmurugan, D.; Gunasekaran, K. Identification of new BACE1 inhibitors using pharmacophore and molecular dynamics simulations approach. *J. Mol. Graph. Model.* **2017**, *76*, 56–69. [CrossRef]

31. Barbezan, A.B.; Martins, R.; Bueno, J.B.; Villavicencio, A.L.C.H. Ames test to detect mutagenicity of 2-alkylcyclobutanones: A review. *J. Food Sci.* **2017**, *82*, 1518–1522. [CrossRef]

32. Modi, S.; Li, J.; Malcomber, S.; Moore, C.; Scott, A.; White, A.; Carmichael, P. Integrated in silico approaches for the prediction of Ames test mutagenicity. *J. Comput. -Aided Mol. Des.* **2012**, *26*, 1017–1033. [CrossRef]

33. Vian, M.; Raitano, G.; Roncaglioni, A.; Benfenati, E. In silico model for mutagenicity (Ames test), taking into account metabolism. *Mutagenesis* **2019**, *34*, 41–48. [CrossRef] [PubMed]

34. Pires, D.E.; Blundell, T.L.; Ascher, D.B. pkCSM: Predicting small-molecule pharmacokinetic and toxicity properties using graph-based signatures. *J. Med. Chem.* **2015**, *58*, 4066–4072. [CrossRef] [PubMed]

35. Palakurti, R.; Vadrevu, R. Pharmacophore based 3D-QSAR modeling, virtual screening and docking for identification of potential inhibitors of B-secretase. *Comput. Biol. Chem.* **2017**, *68*, 107–117. [CrossRef] [PubMed]

36. Chemaxon. *Marvin Sketch*, Version 15.4.20; Chemaxon: Budapest, Hungary, 2015.

37. Tripos. *SYBYL-X 2.0*.; Tripos: St Louis, MO, USA, 2010; Volume 190.

38. Mysinger, M.M.; Carchia, M.; Irwin, J.J.; Shoichet, B.K. DUD Enhanced: Better ligands and decoys for better benchmarking. *J. Med. Chem.* **2012**, *55*, 6582–6594. [CrossRef]

39. Systat. *SigmaPlot™*, versão 12.0; A Scientific Data Management Company: Palo Alto, CA, USA, 2014.

40. Manoharan, P.; Ghoshal, N. Fragment-based virtual screening approach and molecular dynamics simulation studies for identification of BACE1 inhibitor leads. *J. Biomol. Struct. Dyn.* **2017**, *36*, 1878–1892. [CrossRef] [PubMed]

41. Nachon, F.; Carletti, E.; Ronco, C.; Trovaslet, M.; Nicolet, Y.; Jean, L.; Renard, P. Crystal structures of human cholinesterases in complex with Huprine W and Tacrine: Elements of specificity for anti-Alzheimer's drugs targeting acetyl- and butyrylcholinesterase. *Biochem. J.* **2013**, *453*, 3393–3399. [CrossRef]

42. Winneroski, L.L.; Erickson, J.A.; Green, S.J.; Lopez, J.E.; Stout, S.L.; Porter, W.J.; Timm, D.E.; Audia, J.E.; Barberis, M.; Beck, J.P.; et al. Preparation and Biological Evaluation of BACE1 Inhibitors: Leveraging trans-Cyclopropyl Moieties as Ligand Efficient Conformational Constraints. *Bioorg. Med. Chem.* **2019**, *28*, 115–119. [CrossRef]

43. Sondergaard, C.R.; Olsson, M.H.; Rostkowski, M.; Jensen, J.H. Improved Treatment of Ligands and Coupling Effects in Empirical Calculation and Rationalization of pKa Values. *J. Chem. Theory Comput.* **2011**, *7*, 2284–2295. [CrossRef]

44. Trott, O.; Olson, A.J.; Vina, A. Improving the speed and accuracy of docking with a new scoring function, efficient optimization, and multithreading. *J. Comput. Chem.* **2009**, *31*, 455–461. [CrossRef]

45. Yang, S.Y. Pharmacophore modeling and applications in drug discovery: Challenges and recent advances. *Drug Discov. Today* **2010**, *15*, 444–450. [CrossRef]

46. Cole, J.C.; Nissink, J.W.M.; Taylor, R. Protein-ligand docking and virtual screening with GOLD. In *Virtual Screening in Drug Discovery*; Shoichet, B., Alvarez, J., Eds.; Taylor & Francis CRC Press: Boca Raton, FL, USA, 2005.

47. Salentin, S.; Schreiber, S.; Haupt, V.J.; Adasme, M.F.; Schroeder, M. PLIP: Fully automated protein–ligand interaction profiler. *Nucleic Acids Res.* **2015**, *43*, W443–W447. [CrossRef] [PubMed]
48. Schrödinger, LLC. *The PyMOL Molecular Graphics System*; Schrödinger, LLC: New York, NY, USA, 2015.

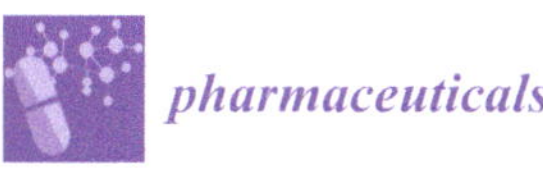

pharmaceuticals

Article

Ligand-Based Drug Design of Genipin Derivatives with Cytotoxic Activity against HeLa Cell Line: A Structural and Theoretical Study

Diana López-López [1,†], Rodrigo Said Razo-Hernández [2,*], César Millán-Pacheco [1], Mario Alberto Leyva-Peralta [3], Omar Aristeo Peña-Morán [4], Jessica Nayelli Sánchez-Carranza [1] and Verónica Rodríguez-López [1,*]

[1] Facultad de Farmacia, Universidad Autónoma del Estado de Morelos, Cuernavaca 62209, Mexico; diana.lopezl@uaem.edu.mx (D.L.-L.); cmp@uaem.mx (C.M.-P.); jessica.sanchez@uaem.mx (J.N.S.-C.)
[2] Laboratorio de Quimioinformática y Diseño de Fármacos, Centro de Investigación en Dinámica Celular, Instituto de investigación en Ciencias Básicas y Aplicadas, Universidad Autónoma del Estado de Morelos, Cuernavaca 62209, Mexico
[3] Departamento de Ciencias Químico Biológicas y Agropecuarias, Universidad de Sonora, H. Caborca, Sonora 83621, Mexico; mario.leyva@unison.mx
[4] Departamento de Ciencias Farmacéuticas, División de Ciencias de la Salud, Universidad Autónoma del Estado de Quintana Roo, Chetumal 77019, Mexico; omar.moran@uqroo.edu.mx
* Correspondence: rodrigo.razo@uaem.mx (R.S.R.-H.); veronica_rodriguez@uaem.mx (V.R.-L.)
† Taken in part from the Ph.D. thesis of Diana López-López.

Citation: López-López, D.; Razo-Hernández, R.S.; Millán-Pacheco, C.; Leyva-Peralta, M.A.; Peña-Morán, O.A.; Sánchez-Carranza, J.N.; Rodríguez-López, V. Ligand-Based Drug Design of Genipin Derivatives with Cytotoxic Activity against HeLa Cell Line: A Structural and Theoretical Study. *Pharmaceuticals* **2023**, *16*, 1647. https://doi.org/10.3390/ph16121647

Academic Editors: Halil İbrahim Ciftci, Belgin Sever and Hasan Demirci

Received: 9 October 2023
Revised: 20 November 2023
Accepted: 21 November 2023
Published: 23 November 2023

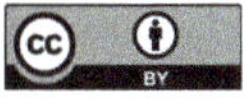

Abstract: Cervical cancer is a malignant neoplastic disease, mainly associated to HPV infection, with high mortality rates. Among natural products, iridoids have shown different biological activities, including cytotoxic and antitumor effects, in different cancer cell types. Geniposide and its aglycone Genipin have been assessed against different types of cancer. In this work, both iridoids were evaluated against HeLa and three different cervical cancer cell lines. Furthermore, we performed a SAR analysis incorporating 13 iridoids with a high structural similarity to Geniposide and Genipin, also tested in the HeLa cell line and at the same treatment time. Derived from this analysis, we found that the dipole moment (magnitude and direction) is key for their cytotoxic activity in the HeLa cell line. Then, we proceeded to the ligand-based design of new Genipin derivatives through a QSAR model (R^2 = 87.95 and Q^2 = 62.33) that incorporates different quantum mechanic molecular descriptor types (ρ, ΔPSA, ΔPolarizability^2, and logS). Derived from the ligand-based design, we observed that the presence of an aldehyde or a hydroxymethyl in C4, hydroxyls in C1, C6, and C8, and the lack of the double bond in C7–C8 increased the predicted biological activity of the iridoids. Finally, ten simple iridoids (D9, D107, D35, D36, D55, D56, D58, D60, D61, and D62) are proposed as potential cytotoxic agents against the HeLa cell line based on their predicted IC$_{50}$ value and electrostatic features.

Keywords: cytotoxic iridoids; SAR; DFT; dipole moment; QSAR; ligand-based design

1. Introduction

Cancer is a group of diseases characterized by abnormal cells that grow uncontrollably, and do not recognize cell death signaling [1]. Then, these abnormal cells can invade adjoining tissues and spread to other body organs in a process named metastasis. In 2020, 19 million new cases were diagnosed and 9.9 million deaths by cancer worldwide were reported for men and women, being the second cause of death [2].

Cervical cancer is a malignant neoplastic disease, originating in women's cervixes. It is the fourth cause of incidence and death in women between 0 and 85 years globally, with 604 127 new cases and 341 831 deaths reported in 2020 [2]. Human papillomavirus (HPV) infection is the principal cause of cervical cancer. HPV16 and HPV18 are the two main high-risk HPVs related to cervical cancer development, and they are present in 70–75% of cervical cancer patient biopsies, with HPV16 the most carcinogenic subtype [3].

Since the actual chemotherapeutic treatments are not selective and, in many cases, cancer cells have developed resistance to them, finding new anti-cancer compounds with desirable selectivity toward cancer cells is crucial nowadays [4].

Vincristine, irinotecan, etoposide, and paclitaxel are plant-derived drugs used to treat cervical cancer clinically, alone, and as neoadjuvant chemotherapy with other chemotherapeutics such as cisplatin [5–9]; natural products are essential molecules since they comprise 50% of anti-tumor drugs [10,11]. Iridoids, a diverse class of secondary metabolites, are present in numerous plant families, with a prevalent occurrence in Apocynaceae, Loganiaceae, Scrophulariaceae, and others [12,13]. Across cultures and civilizations, iridoid-rich plants have been employed for their medicinal properties [12,13].

Structurally, iridoids are atypical monoterpenoids and are generally described as cyclopentane [C]-pyran. The cyclopentane is fused to a six-member oxygenated ring, forming the iridoid skeleton as a bicycle system [14,15]. The cyclopentane is fused to a six-member oxygenated ring, forming the iridoid skeleton as a bicycle system [14]. Over 2500 known iridoids are derived from nature, distinguished by the iridoid skeleton's type and number of substituents [15]. The present work is related to two principal groups: simple iridoids and iridoid glycosides. Simple iridoids are iridoids that have a simple modification of the cyclopentane ring, and such modifications could be hydroxyl, acyloxy, keto, epoxy, chlorine, and olefins. Iridoid glycosides comprise a cyclopentane ring linked to a dihydropyran ring, with a sugar moiety commonly in R1; mainly, they are β-D-glucosides, and could have many different substituents in the sugar moiety such as coumaroyl, feruloyl, caffeoyl, and cinnamoyl groups [13] (Figure S1). Iridoid glycosides are sources of lead molecules as they share high modifiability and rapid absorption [12].

Iridoids have demonstrated significant bioactivity, with a growing body of research suggesting their potential in the prevention and treatment of cancer [12,16,17]. These compounds exhibit a range of pharmacological effects, including anti-inflammatory, antioxidant, and anti-proliferative activities, making them intriguing candidates for anticancer interventions. Studies have delved into the specific mechanisms through which iridoids exert their anticancer effects. In vitro studies about Geniposide and Genipin as potential compounds against different types of cancer cells have been reported [18–25]. Iridoids appear to target various hallmarks of cancer; these include inhibiting uncontrolled cell growth, promoting apoptosis, and impeding angiogenesis. The ability of iridoids to modulate multiple pathways involved in cancer development and progression makes them attractive candidates for further investigation [17]. The exploration of iridoids as anticancer agents represents a dynamic and evolving field within cancer research. While challenges exist, the multifaceted pharmacological activities of iridoids make them promising candidates for further investigation and potential development into novel cancer therapeutics.

Molecular similarity analysis is important in drug discovery because it helps to identify new drug candidates based on the structural and/or functional similarity of other drugs [26]. Moreover, ligand-based drug design is a method that combines mathematical modeling, and the physicochemical and structural properties, of a variety of biologically active chemical structures, to find the key elements that trigger their biological activity. This information is employed for the discovery of new structurally different drug candidates or for the optimization of lead compounds. Quantitative structure activity relationships (QSAR) in cancer are a powerful tool that considers strict statistical parameters to generate an equation or an algorithm that describes the relationship between the biological activity and one or more properties of the compounds [27].

The aim of the present work was to evaluate Geniposide and Genipin against different cervical cancer cells. From the obtained results, a molecular similarity analysis was undertaken using several active iridoids to explain the biological activity of Geniposide and Genipin. This molecular similarity analysis was undertaken by comparing the electronic properties (molecular potential maps and dipole moment) of all the iridoids. We found that the dipole moment is crucial for the biological activity of simple iridoids. Finally, after generating a QSAR model, we carried out a ligand-based drug design of new simple iridoids with potential cytotoxic activity.

2. Results and Discussion

2.1. In Vitro Cytotoxic Activity of Geniposide and Genipin

Table 1 shows the IC_{50} values of Geniposide and Genipin in three cervical cancer cell lines. Geniposide exhibited no activity in these cell lines. Genipin exerted a similar effect in the CaSki and CaLo cell lines and exhibited less potency in the INBL cell line. Although these cancer cell lines are from the cervix, they exhibit different molecular characteristics. CaSki is associated with HPV16 and derived from metastasis, while both CaLo and INBL are associated with HPV18. However, CaLo represents an early stage (stage IIB), while INBL represents a metastatic stage (stage IVB) according to the FIGO classification [28]. This suggests that Genipin could potentially affect cervical cancer cells from both high-risk HPV types (16 and 18) and from different stages of the disease.

Table 1. Cytotoxic activity of Geniposide and Genipin in cervical cancer cell lines (IC_{50}: μM).

Cell Lines	Geniposide	Genipin	Cisplatin	Podophyllotoxin
CaSki	>1000	65.930 ± 4.420	0.640 ± 0.080	0.025 ± 0.001
CaLo	>1000	58.970 ± 9.040	0.240 ± 0.020	0.014 ± 0.002
INBL	>1000	178.800 ± 12.990	1.340 ± 0.160	0.011 ± 0.001
HaCaT [1]	>1000	106.250 ± 9.290	1.150 ± 0.140	0.050 ± 0.006

[1] HaCaT is a non-tumorigenic cell line of immortalized keratinocytes and was used as control.

In the literature, there is a vast number of glycosylated iridoids against various types of cancer in vitro. However, in this study, Geniposide did not exert any cytotoxic effects in any of the cell lines tested. On the contrary, Genipin emerged as an active compound against all the tested cell lines. Similar findings regarding the effects of Geniposide and its aglycone, Genipin, have been reported in relation to other types of cancer cell lines: *MCF-7 breast, HT-29 colon, K562 leukemia, U251 glioma, 786-0 renal,* and *PC-3 prostate* [29]. Some iridoid glycosides do not inherently possess antiproliferative activity; instead, they exhibit effects on human cancer cells once they undergo hydrolysis [30]. Our objective was to investigate the relationship between the chemical structure, molecular features, and the cytotoxic activity of both iridoids.

2.2. Cytotoxic Iridoids Assessed against the HeLa Cell Line

To understand the lack of activity of Geniposide and the low activity of Genipin, both of which were tested against cervical cancer cells, we conducted a search for reported iridoids with cytotoxic effects against cervical cancer in vitro. We identified forty-four iridoids (Figure S2), primarily evaluated in cervical cancer cell lines, including HeLa, KB-3-1, and HeLa-S3, with exposure times of 24, 48, and 72 h [31–43]. Table 2 lists the 13 iridoids that were selected because they were assessed in the same cell line (HeLa) and for the same treatment duration (48 h). Additionally, these iridoids exhibited structural similarities to Geniposide and Genipin, with minor variations in their substituents over the core of the iridoid skeleton; iridoids with greater modification on the sugar core were not considered.

Table 2. Cytotoxic iridoids against cervical cancer HeLa cells.

Compound	Cell Line	Exposure Time (h)	IC_{50} (μM)
Euphrasin [1]	HeLa	48	0.20
Campsinol [1]	HeLa	48	1.90
Artselaenin B [1]	HeLa	48	12.30
Artselaenin A [1]	HeLa	48	13.80

Table 2. *Cont.*

Compound	Cell Line	Exposure Time (h)	IC$_{50}$ (μM)
Pulchelloside I [2]	HeLa	48	25.22
Catalpol [3]	HeLa	48	28.20
Lamiide [2]	HeLa	48	31.96
Spinomannoside [2]	HeLa	48	38.89
5-deoxypulchelloside I [2]	HeLa	48	42.47
Geniposidic acid [4]	HeLa	48	43.60
10-O-(E)-*p*-coumaroylgeniposidic acid [3]	HeLa	48	48.10
Genipin	HeLa	48	419.00 [5]
Geniposide	HeLa	48	NA [5]

[1] Compounds from [31]; [2] compounds from [39]; [3] compounds from [32]; [4] compounds from [33]; [5] experimental data. NA: not active.

As there was no reported cytotoxic activity of Geniposide and Genipin against the HeLa cell line in the literature, as indicated by its IC$_{50}$ at 48 h [34], we conducted our own test using the MTS method. The IC$_{50}$ for Genipin at this time of treatment was found to be 419 $\pm$ 27.25 μM, with paclitaxel used as the positive control (IC$_{50}$: 15.8 $\pm$ 0.67 nM).

The structures of the 13 iridoids listed in Table 2 are depicted in Figure 1. Among these, five iridoids are simple (non-glycosylated, including Genipin), and eight iridoids are glycosylated (including Geniposide). All these iridoids were tested against the HeLa cell line under the same treatment condition of 48 h. The chemical structures of these iridoids typically featured substituents such as: methyl, hydroxyl, hydroxymethyl, ester, acid, aldehyde, and glucose. In some specific cases, mannose, epoxy, and *p*-coumaroyl substituents were also present. The iridoid skeleton (as shown in Figure S1) in certain instances exhibited a double bond between C7 and C8, like Genipin and geniposide.

Subsequently, to obtain more precise geometry and energy values of the molecules, a reoptimization process was undertaken using the density functional theory (DFT) approach. The objective was to analyze the structure–activity relationship of the iridoids (Figure 1) based on their electronic distribution and derived properties (polarizability, hardness, molecular electrostatic potential, and dipole moment).

2.3. Structural and Molecular Analysis of Genipin and Other Simple Iridoids

As an initial step, Euphrasin, Campsinol, Artselaenin A, and Artselaenin B [31] were compared in terms of their structure, activity, and molecular descriptors against Genipin. Table 3 presents the IC$_{50}$ experimental values, and molecular descriptors calculated with Spartan'20, for the lowest-energy conformer of each simple iridoid, such as dipole moment, area, volume, polar surface area (PSA), ovality, LogP, polarizability, and the number of hydrogen bond donors (HBD) and acceptors (HBA). The first four simple iridoids demonstrated the highest potency, with their IC$_{50}$ values being less than 14 μM, compared to Genipin. Genipin, in contrast, was 30- to 2000-fold less active. Artselaenin A had a GAP$_{\text{HOMO-LUMO}}$ value more like that of Genipin. However, they differ in terms of polarity, as evidenced by the polar surface area values. Genipin had a higher value for this descriptor (64.589 Å^2) compared to the others (ranging from 26.808 to 46.922 Å^2).

Table 3. Molecular descriptors of simple iridoids with reported cytotoxic activity (IC$_{50}$) against the HeLa cell line.

Ligand	IC$_{50}$ (μM)	GAP$_{\text{HOMO-LUMO}}$ (kcal)	Dipole moment (debye)	Area (Å^2)	Volume (Å^3)	PSA (Å^2)	Ovality	LogP	Polarizability	HBD Count	HBA Count
Euphrasin	0.20	−123.01	4.81	234.27	216.65	44.645	1.34	−0.10	57.69	1	4
Campsinol	1.90	−122.30	5.78	236.86	216.59	46.922	1.36	−0.10	57.69	1	4
Artselaenin B	12.3	−125.40	4.67	227.13	208.64	26.808	1.34	1.11	57.01	0	3
Artselaenin A	13.8	−121.90	4.20	228.14	209.46	27.236	1.34	1.11	57.11	0	3
Genipin	419.00	−126.18	1.26	239.61	219.74	64.589	1.36	−0.26	57.91	2	5

The dipole moment of the remaining simple iridoids was higher, ranging from 4.2 to 5.78 debye, compared to Genipin, which exhibited a lower dipole moment of 1.26 debye

The dipole moment is a measure of the polarity of a molecule, established when there is an unequal distribution of electrons due to differences in electronegativity within the molecule. Consequently, the degree of electron distribution inequality is greater in simple iridoids than in Genipin, which appears to favor their biological activity. Additionally, Euphrasin and Campsinol exhibited hydrophilic properties like those of Genipin, while Artselaenin A and B displayed greater hydrophobicity than the others. Genipin also featured more HBD and HBA. The first iridoids closely resembled Genipin in terms of size (area and volume) and shape, as evidenced by their ovality values (ranging from 1.34 to 1.36). Furthermore, they shared similar polarizability values (ranging from 57.01 to 57.91).

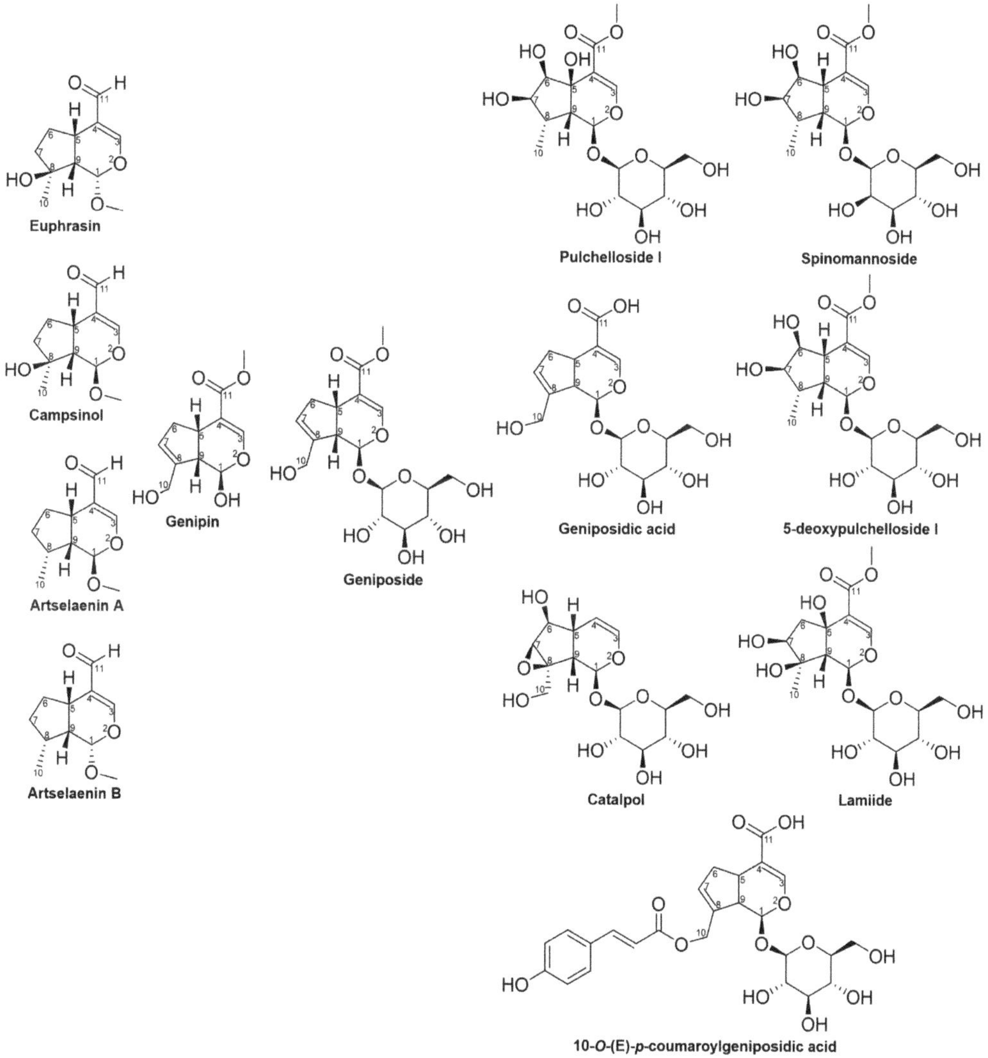

Figure 1. Chemical structures of iridoids tested against the HeLa cell line; Genipin and Geniposide are the central iridoids in this study marked in yellow color.

The 2D and 3D structures of simple iridoids are presented in Figure 2. Genipin has several structural differences compared to the other simple iridoids: it has a carbomethoxy group at C11, while the others have an aldehyde group. It has a double bond between C7 and C8 and the others lack this structural feature. In addition, it has a hydroxyl group at C10 instead of a hydroxyl group at C8. Genipin presents a free hydroxyl at C1, while in the other iridoids there is a methoxy group. Furthermore, the dipole angle in Genipin differs from that of Euphrasin, Campsinol, Artselaenin A, and Artselaenin B (Figure 2).

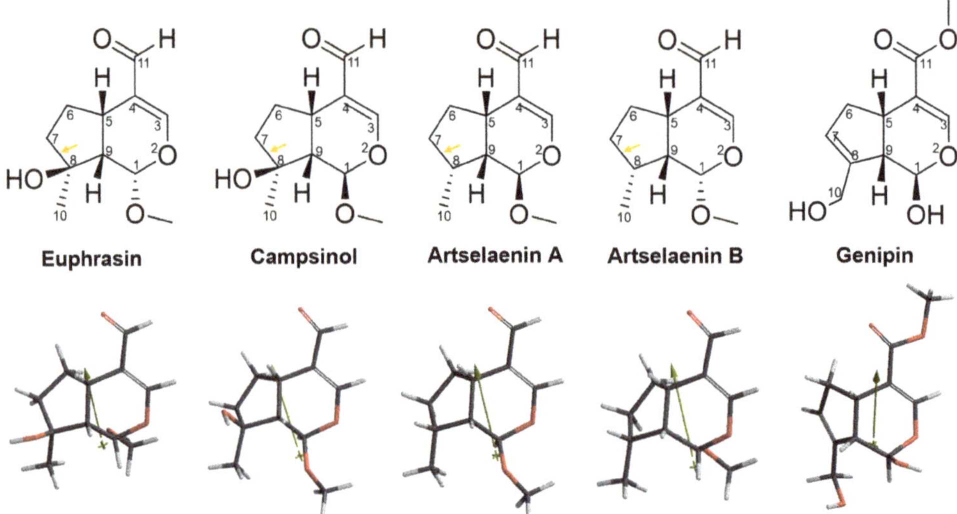

Figure 2. The 2D and 3D structures of simple iridoids including Genipin. The yellow rectangles indicate the change or addition of some substituents with respect to Genipin, the arrows indicate the lack of the double bond in cyclopentane respect to Genipin. The dipole vector is shown as a gold arrow over the 3D structures.

After analyzing the dipole orientation and magnitude, our interest turned to the electrostatic potential distribution of each iridoid. For that reason, an iso-surface of −10 kcal/mol value of MEP was obtained (see Figure 3). It is noteworthy that the most cytotoxic iridoids (Figure 3A,B) exhibit a higher electrostatic distribution in the aldehydic substituent at C4, which also features a hydroxyl at C8. Genipin, on the other hand, shows a divided electrostatic distribution on its substituent in C4 (partially over the sp2 and sp3 oxygens) and a greater electrostatic distribution in the pyran ring, along with the hydroxyl at C1 and C10. These observations revealed specific regions where the simple iridoids could interact with positively charged species at an energy level of −10 kcal/mol. The higher electron density over the aldehydic group and the hydroxyl group in C8 allows a better interaction with the possible target of these iridoids.

Then, the MEP map was obtained (Figure 4), indicating the regions more susceptible to an electrophilic attack (yellow to red color) and those more susceptible to a nucleophilic attack (blue color). The regions with more electronic density are located at the oxygen of the aldehydic group at C4, and the oxygen of the hydroxyl at C8. In the case of Genipin, these zones of higher electron density also correspond to the sp2 and sp3 oxygens, the oxygen of the hydroxyl at C1, and the oxygen of the hydroxyl at C10, correlating with our earlier observations regarding molecular electrostatic distributions.

These molecular descriptors and structural features affect the reactivity of the simple iridoids, particularly the substituent at C4 (aldehyde or ester), added to the forward hydroxyl at C8. Now, we are interested in studying the physicochemical differences between the conformer of lower energy of Geniposide and Genipin.

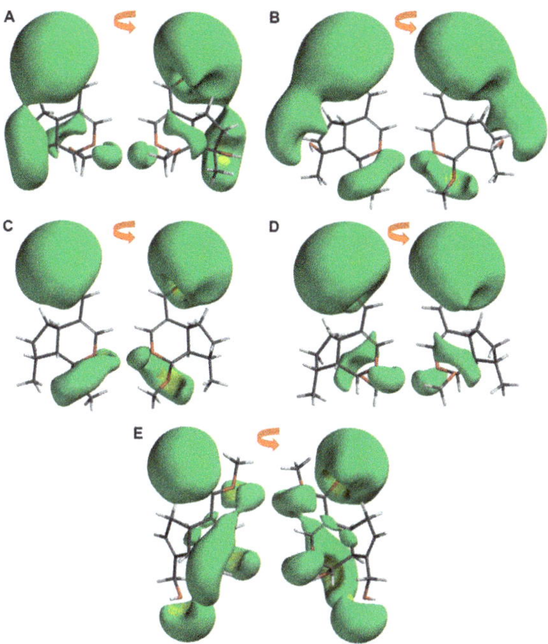

Figure 3. Molecular electrostatic potential iso-surface of −10 kcal/mol of simple iridoids. (**A**) Euphrasin, (**B**) Campsinol, (**C**) Artselaenin A, (**D**) Artselaenin B, (**E**) Genipin.

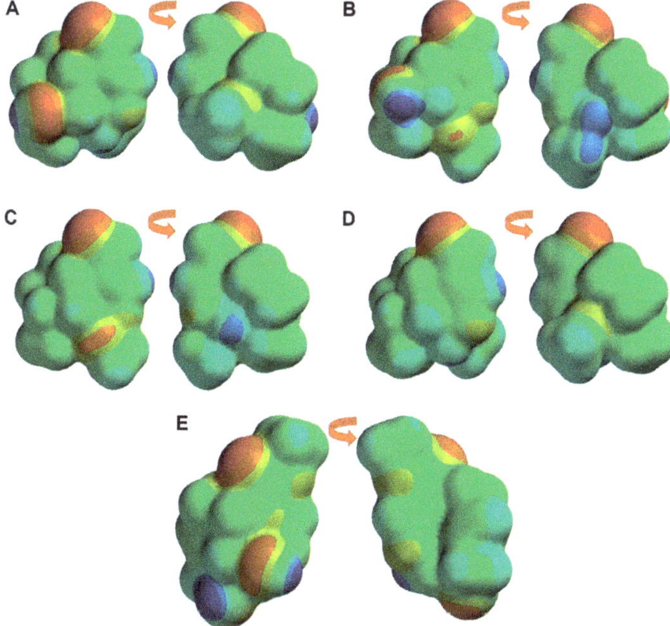

Figure 4. Molecular electrostatic potential map of simple iridoids: (**A**) Euphrasin, (**B**) Campsinol, (**C**) Artselaenin A, (**D**) Artselaenin B, (**E**) Genipin. Zero, negative, and positive values of MEP are depicted as green, red, and blue colored regions, respectively.

2.4. Structural and Molecular Analysis of Genipin and Geniposide

Genipin and Geniposide descriptors are presented in Table 4. Geniposide was inactive against cervical cancer cells, but Genipin was cytotoxic against the HeLa cell line. Both iridoids differ in the $GAP_{HOMO-LUMO}$, LogP, and dipole moment. Due to the presence of a glucose unit in Geniposide, the size and the volume increased considerably compared to the Genipin 132 and 136 units, respectively. Also, the molecular shape is different between them, as we can see from the ovality parameter (1.36 for Genipin and 1.53 for Geniposide). The polarity of Geniposide was 2.5-fold higher than Genipin, based on the molecular charge and the polar surface area.

Table 4. Molecular descriptors of simple iridoids with reported cytotoxic activity against the HeLa cell line.

Ligand	IC_{50} (μM)	$GAP_{HOMO-LUMO}$ (kcal)	Dipole Moment (debye)	Area (Å^2)	Volume (Å^3)	PSA (Å^2)	Ovality	LogP	Polarizability	HBD Count	HBA Count
Genipin	419.00	−126.18	1.26	239.61	219.74	64.589	1.36	−0.26	57.91	2	5
Geniposide	NA	−128.37	3.41	371.47	355.38	119.843	1.53	−2.00	68.89	5	9

Moreover, the Genipin and Geniposide 2D and 3D structures are displayed in Figure 5. The only structural difference between them is the glucose moiety at C1. We can observe the contrary direction of the vector dipole, that in Genipin is directed to the carbonyl at C11, and in Geniposide is directed to the glucose moiety, specifically to two hydroxyl groups in the sugar.

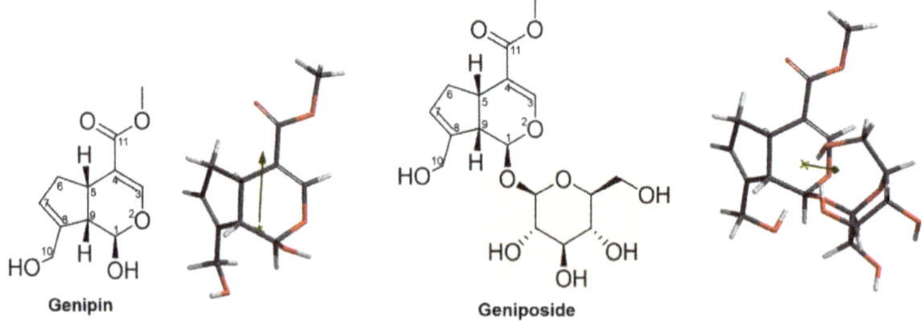

Figure 5. The 2D and 3D structures of Genipin and Geniposide. Yellow rectangle indicates the addition of the glucose with respect to Genipin. The dipole vector is shown as a gold arrow over the 3D structures.

After analyzing the dipole orientation and magnitude, we obtained the molecular electrostatic potential iso-surface of −10 kcal/mol showing the electrostatic profile of both iridoids (Figure 6). A higher electronic distribution in the carbonyl at C11 until the 3′ and 6′ hydroxyls of the sugar is observed in Geniposide, while in Genipin a different pattern is presented. In these green zones, intermolecular interactions could take place, such as hydrogen bonds or electrostatic interactions with a positively charged group.

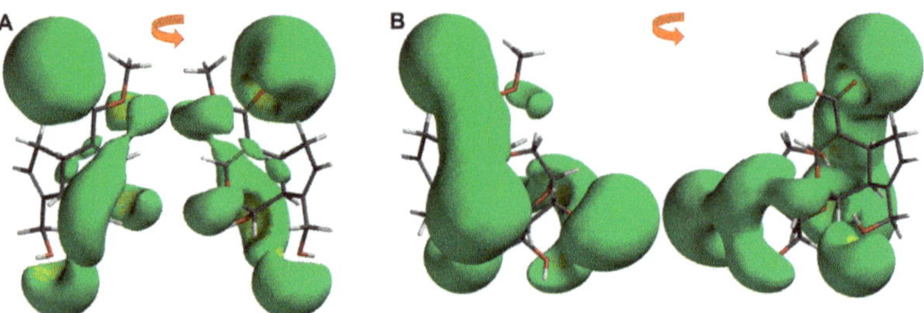

Figure 6. Molecular electrostatic potential iso-surface of −10 kcal/mol of (**A**) Genipin, (**B**) Geniposide.

The regions with more electron density of both iridoids are displayed in Figure 7. In Geniposide, these regions are located mainly at the oxygen of the carbonyl at C11, the oxygen of the hydroxyl at C10, and the 3′, 4′, and 6′ hydroxyls in the sugar. In Genipin these zones of more electron density also correspond to the carbonyl at C11, the sp3 oxygen of the ester at C11, the oxygen of the hydroxyl at C1, and the hydroxyl at C10.

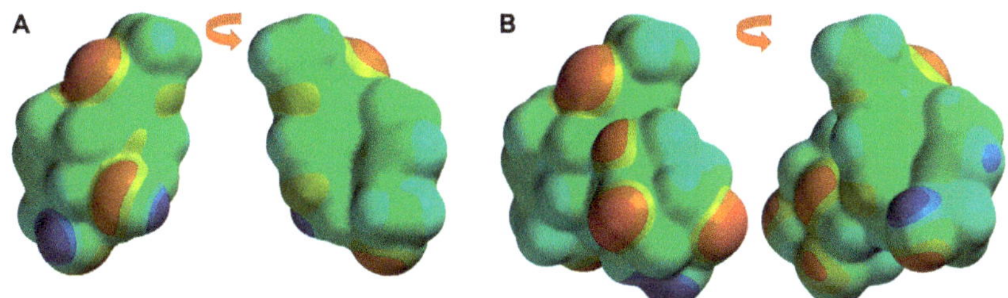

Figure 7. Molecular electrostatic potential map of (**A**) Genipin, (**B**) Geniposide. Zero, negative, and positive values of MEP are depicted as green, red, and blue colored regions, respectively.

Finally, intramolecular hydrogen bonds are observed in Figure 8. These intramolecular interactions were displayed and obtained with the Discovery Studio 2021 software [44]. In Genipin, two non-conventional hydrogen bonds are present, while in Geniposide there is one non-conventional and three conventional hydrogen bonds. Sugar conformation in Geniposide causes the formation of these types of strong interactions that confer stability to the iridoid.

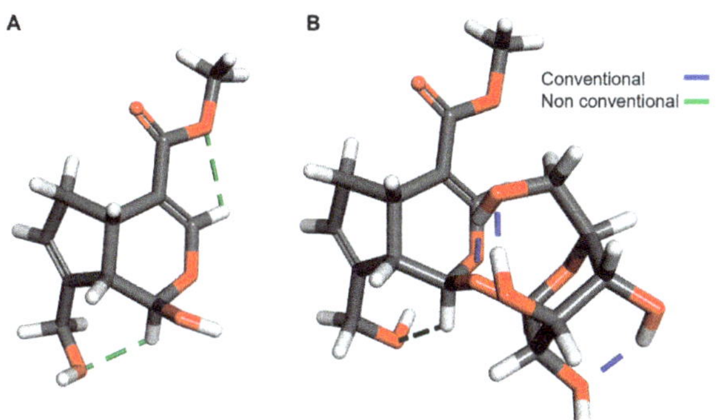

Figure 8. Intramolecular H bonds in (**A**) Genipin, (**B**) Geniposide.

The increased polarity of Geniposide due to the incorporation of the glucose in C1, and the distribution of this molecular charge, impact on the electronic distribution, and finally on the inactivity of the iridoid, unlike Genipin. Now, our interest is turned to comparing the physicochemical differences between Geniposide and active iridoid glycosides.

2.5. Structural and Molecular Analysis of Geniposide and Other Iridoid Glycosides

In Table 5 are listed some descriptors related to the reactivity, solubility, shape, and size of active iridoid glycosides and Geniposide. The iridoid glycosides Pulchelloside I, Catalpol, Lamiide, Spinomannoside, 5-deoxypulchelloside I, geniposidic acid, and 10-O-(E)-p-coumaroylgeniposidic acid have a similar cytotoxic activity against the HeLa cell line (25.22–48.10 μM). However, compared to the inactive Geniposide, all of them are different in size, and in HBD and HBA. Conversely, Geniposide was similar in form, as given by the ovality parameter, and in the polarizability, but it was quite different in the molecular charge distribution given by the dipole moment, and it was less polar compared to the rest of the iridoids (less hydrophilic). The anion forms of geniposidic acid and 10-O-(E)-p-coumaroylgeniposidic acid were considered since these charged forms exist predominantly at physiologic pH (7.4). The pKa value of the acids are shown in Table S2.

Table 5. Calculated molecular descriptor values and experimental biological activity (IC_{50}) of iridoid glycosides and Geniposide tested against the HeLa cell line.

Ligand	IC_{50} (μM)	$GAP_{HOMO\text{-}LUMO}$ (kcal)	Dipole Moment (debye)	Area (Å^2)	Volume (Å^3)	PSA (Å^2)	Ovality	LogP	Polarizability	HBD Count	HBA Count
Pulchelloside I	25.22	−121.84	5.95	383.69	372.30	148.544	1.53	−3.30	70.33	7	11
Catalpol	28.20	−144.80	2.50	324.51	320.55	126.832	1.43	−3.24	65.89	6	10
Laamide	31.96	−116.96	7.99	392.42	373.46	158.057	1.56	−3.48	70.47	7	11
Spinomannoside	38.89	−124.51	4.28	381.33	367.08	140.269	1.54	−2.51	69.87	5	10
5-deoxypulchelloside I	42.47	−125.49	3.32	374.98	365.07	134.805	1.52	−2.51	69.70	6	10
Geniposidic acid *	43.60	−85.84	12.02	353.50	335.17	139.852	1.51	--	67.68	5	10
10-O-(E)-p-coumaroylgeniposidic acid *	48.10	−61.97	16.64	481.01	476.36	147.201	1.63	--	79.38	5	11
Geniposide	NA	−128.37	3.41	371.47	355.38	119.843	1.53	−2.00	68.89	5	9

* These iridoids were analyzed in their anion form.

The 2D structures of iridoid glycosides are presented in Figure 9. These iridoids have a glucose moiety at C1, except Spinomannoside, which contains a mannosyl at C1 instead of the glucosyl. The 5-deoxypulchelloside has two extras' hydroxyls at C6 and C7, lacks the double bond in C7–C8, and has a methyl instead of the hydroxymethyl at C8. Pulchelloside I, in addition to these structural differences compared to Geniposide, also presents an extra hydroxyl at C5. Spinomannoside, which is structurally very similar to 5-deoxypulchelloside, contains a mannose at C1 instead of the glucose. Lamiide presents a hydroxyl at C5, C7, and C8, lacks the double bond in C7–C8, and has a methyl instead of the hydroxymethyl at C8. Catalpol presents an epoxy in C7–C8, lacks the double bond in C7–C8, contains a hydroxyl at C6, and lacks the ester at C4 compared to Geniposide. Geniposidic acid has an acid at C4, just like 10-O-(E)-p-coumaroylgeniposidic acid (this last one additionally presents a p-coumaroyl group at C10), contrary to Geniposide, which presents an ester at C4. These structural changes, compared to Geniposide, seem to confer cytotoxic activity against the HeLa cell line.

The 3D structures of the iridoid glycosides, showing the dipole vector, are displayed in Figure S3. The most similar to Geniposide is Catalpol, although the conformation of the sugar is very different compared to Geniposide. In Pulchelloside I and Spinomannoside, the conformation of the sugar was more like the one displayed in Geniposide. It is noteworthy how the conformation of the iridoids impacted on their size and shape, as is noted in the area, volume, and ovality values. For example, Pulchelloside I and Lamiide, although they have the same number and type of substituents, the conformation of the glucose increased the area in Lamiide (Figure S3).

Moreover, we were interested in visualizing the regions where the intermolecular interactions can occur. For this reason, an iso-surface of −10 kcal/mol value of MEP was obtained (Figure S4). It can be observed that the most cytotoxic glycosylated iridoid (Figure S4f) has a higher electrostatic distribution, principally on the region rich in hydroxyls on the cyclopentane, which are excellent acceptors of hydrogen bonds. This electrostatic distribution is also present on the oxygen of the carbonyl at C11 and is extended until the hydroxyl at C6. In the case of geniposidic acid (Figure S4a), a similar region and electrostatic distribution is present, principally due to the hydroxymethyl at C8. The rest of iridoid glycosides show several and similar electron density regions where the intermolecular interactions could occur.

In addition, we obtained the MEP map of the glycosylated iridoids (Figure S5). The regions with more electron density in Geniposide are located mainly at the oxygen of the carbonyl at C11, the oxygen of the hydroxyl at C10, and the 3', 4', and 6' hydroxyls of the sugar. A greater number of susceptible regions to electrophilic and nucleophilic attacks are observed in glycosylated iridoids. Additionally, we performed molecular similarity analysis of the most cytotoxic iridoids and the central iridoids of this study.

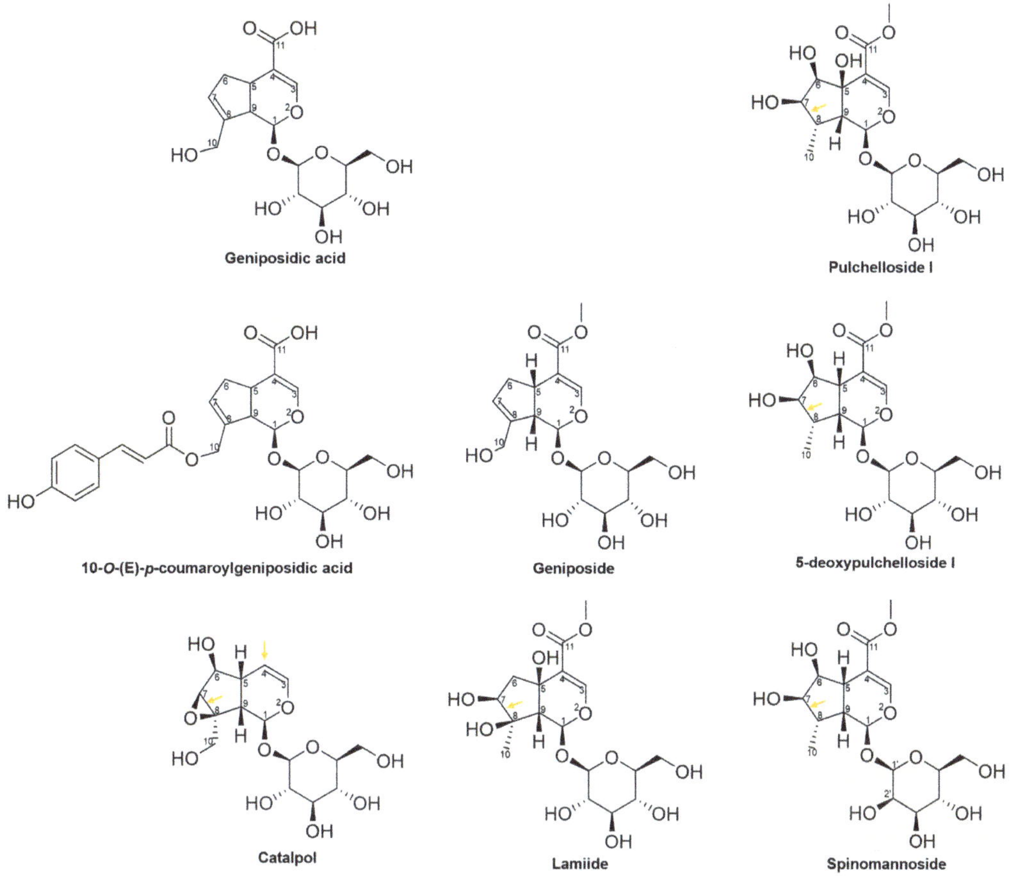

Figure 9. The 2D chemical structures of iridoid glycosides. The yellow rectangles indicate the change or addition of some substituents with respect to Geniposide, the arrows indicate the lack of the double bond in cyclopentane, and the lack of the substituent at C4 with respect to Geniposide.

2.6. Molecular Similarity Analysis of Iridoids

Molecular similarity analysis of the simple iridoids with Genipin was performed based on the chemical function descriptors (CFDs). The alignment and the dipole vector of the five iridoids are presented in Figure 10. Five CFDs were selected in Genipin as they were common with the other four simple iridoids (Euphrasin, Campsinol, Artselaenin A, and Artselaenin B). The most active iridoids, Euphrasin and Campsinol, did not align well with Genipin (Figure 10C,D); their alignment scores were 0.50 and 0.49, respectively. Otherwise, Artselaenin A and Artselaenin B, in which the only difference is the stereochemistry of the methoxy group at C1, had parallel dipole vectors that present a different orientation to the dipole vector of Genipin (Figure 10E); their alignment scores were 0.56 and 0.50, respectively.

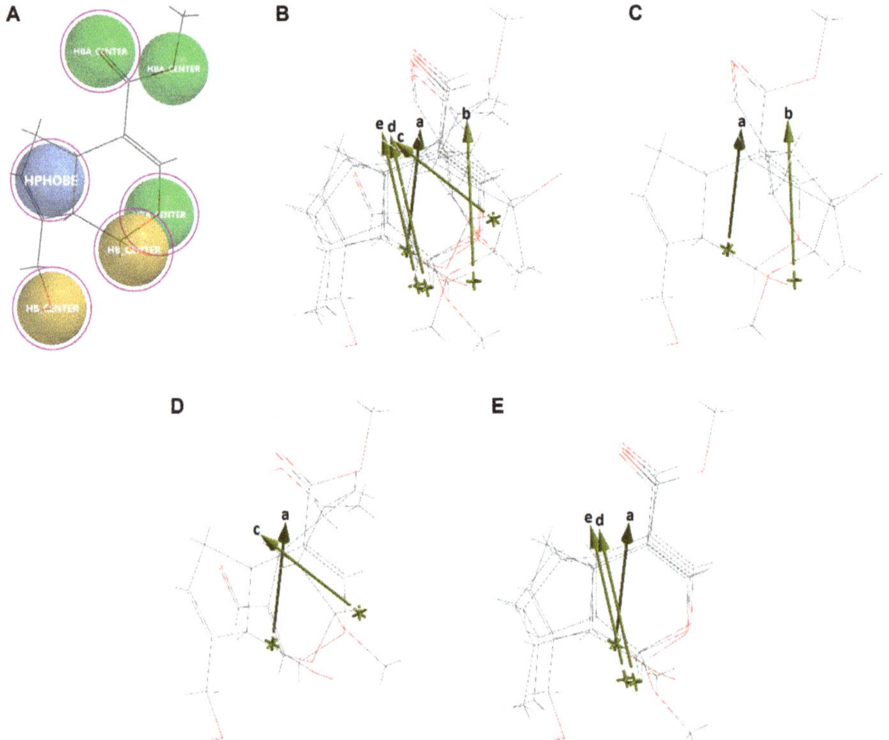

Figure 10. Alignment of Genipin with simple iridoids Euphrasin, Campsinol, Artselaenin A, and Artselaenin B. (**A**) Common similarity centers by CFDs of Genipin (purple circles represent the CFDs selected for the alignment). (**B**) Alignment of Genipin with simple iridoids. (**C**) Alignment of Artselaenin A with Euphrasin. (**D**) Alignment of Artselaenin A with Campsinol. (**E**) Alignment of Artselaenin A with Artselaenin A and Artselaenin B. Dipole vector represented by gold arrows of each iridoid aligned is shown (a: Genipin, b: Euphrasin, c: Campsinol, d: Artselaenin A, e: Artselaenin B).

Additionally, to verify the difference in the chemical natures between Geniposide and its aglycone Genipin, we performed a molecular similarity analysis by the CFD alignment that is shown in Figure S6. Six CFDs were selected in Genipin as they were also common to Geniposide; the alignment score was 0.65. Although Geniposide and Genipin share those selected CFDs, it is evident that there is a difference in their orientation and the direction of the dipole vector, which could explain the lack of biological activity of Geniposide (Figure S6).

2.7. Ligand-Based Drug Design of Genipin Derivatives

Afterward, we were interested in designing iridoids based on Genipin's structure. We noticed that the dipole vector correlated with the biological activity of the most cytotoxic iridoids (Table 3). Therefore, we obtained the dimensional components of the dipole vector of these simple iridoids. The Cartesian coordinates of the dipole vector were transformed to polar spherical coordinates and their values are presented in Table 6, where ρ corresponds to the dipole moment magnitude, θ is the angle in the polar coordinates, and φ is the azimuthal angle.

Table 6. Magnitude and polar spherical coordinates of the dipole vector of simple active iridoids and their experimental biological activity values (IC_{50}).

Ligand	ρ (debye)	θ	φ	IC_{50} (μM)
Euphrasin	4.81	0.8097	1.6749	0.20
Campsinol	5.78	-1.0080	1.3527	1.90
Artselaenin B	4.67	0.9716	1.3933	12.3
Artselaenin A	4.20	-1.3515	1.1341	13.8
Genipin	1.26	1.5078	2.2265	419.00

Derived from this set of data, a multilinear regression analysis considering the azimuthal angle (φ), the dipole moment magnitude (ρ), and the potency of the iridoids ($-logIC_{50}$), was performed and we obtained a mathematical model that describes the biological activity of simple iridoids:

$$-LogIC_{50} = 1.5425(\varphi) + 0.8941(\rho) - 6.9922 \tag{1}$$

$$R = 0.89; \ R^2 = 0.79; \ s = 0.79; \ F = 3.69; \ n = 5$$

According to this equation and its statistical parameters, the potency of simple iridoids will increase proportional to the magnitude of the dipole moment and the azimuthal angle φ. Then, we plotted the linear correlation between the calculated and the experimental activity, which is displayed in Figure 11. The squared correlation (R^2), which explain the variance of the description model, is shown in the plot. The plot of Figure 11 shows that the mathematical model has an acceptable descriptive ability, considering the limited number of compounds employed for the model.

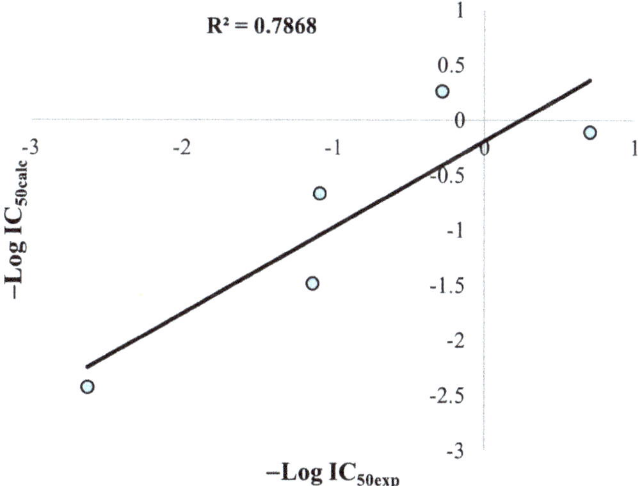

Figure 11. Linear correlation of the calculated activity (IC_{50calc}) versus experimental activity (IC_{50exp}).

Derived from this analysis we observed that the dipole moment was crucial for the activity of the iridoids, but the model considering the magnitude and the angle φ of the dipole vector was only descriptive, and not predictive for other iridoids. For this reason, we considered all 13 iridoids to perform a QSAR study using molecular descriptors related to the electronic nature of the compounds. QSAR models of a small set of molecules have been successfully employed to help explain their biological activity.

2.8. QSAR Analysis

The final QSAR model indicates once again the influence of the dipole moment on the activity of the iridoids, as shown in Equation (2). Moreover, the difference of the polar surface area of the iridoids with respect to Genipin (ΔPSA), the solubility of the iridoids in water (LogS), and the difference in the polarizability of the iridoids with respect to Genipin (ΔPolarizability) are relevant for the biological activity.

$$-LogIC_{50} = 0.1118(\rho) - 0.07433(\Delta PSA) + 2.56022(LogS) + 0.02923\left(\Delta Polarizability^2\right) + 1.26184 \qquad (2)$$

$$R = 93.781; \ R^2 = 87.95; \ R^2_{ADJ} = 81.07; \ s = 0.3563 \ F = 12.78; \ n = 13$$

$$R^P = 0.622; \ R^N = -0.208; \ Q^2_{LOO} = 62.33$$

The values of the molecular descriptors considered in the QSAR model are listed in Table 7. In addition, all the experimental values of the cytotoxic activity against the HeLa cell line (IC_{50}) are shown. From Table 7, it can be seen that the most potent iridoids (simple iridoids) have a lower PSA value than Genipin, since its difference (ΔPSA) is negative. This agrees with our QSAR equation since the negative coefficient indicates that increasing the PSA value of the iridoids compared to Genipin will negatively affect its cytotoxic activity against the HeLa cell line. On the contrary, an increase in the solubility or the polarizability of the iridoids will favor the cytotoxic activity of iridoids according to their coefficient positive sign. These descriptors can work as counterweights of each other, specially ΔPSA and LogS. It is worth mentioning that all the iridoids used for the construction of the QSAR model have a LogS negative value, that reflects their hydrophobic nature. This feature affects the positive contributions of the dipole moment and the ΔPolarizability, descriptors related to the electron density distribution over the iridoid framework. Iridoids glycoside have higher values for the dipole moment, ΔPSA, and ΔPolarizability. Nevertheless, some of them have a lower LogS value than Genipin, and this can be related to their sugar moiety and its ability to form intramolecular hydrogen bonds, making the iridoid glycosides more hydrophobic.

Table 7. Values of the molecular descriptors present in the QSAR model and the biological activity (IC_{50}) of simple and glycosylated iridoids.

Ligand	ρ (debye)	ΔPSA(Å^2)	LogS	ΔPolarizability^2	IC_{50}(µM)
Euphrasin	4.81	−19.944	−1.21	0.048	0.20
Campsinol	5.78	−17.667	−1.21	0.048	1.90
Artselaenin B	4.67	−37.781	−2.23	0.810	12.30
Artselaenin A	4.20	−37.353	−2.23	0.640	13.80
Pulchelloside I	5.95	83.955	−0.50	154.256	25.22
Catalpol	2.50	62.243	−0.19	63.680	28.20
Lamiide	7.99	93.468	−0.69	157.754	31.96
Spinomannoside	4.28	75.680	−0.73	143.042	38.89
5-deoxypulchelloside I	3.32	70.216	−0.73	139.004	42.47
Geniposidic acid [1]	12.02	75.260	−1.22	95.453	43.60
10-*O*-(E)-*p*-coumaroylgeniposidic acid [1]	16.64	82.610	−2.86	460.961	48.10
Genipin	1.26	0	−1.50	0	419.00

[1] These iridoids were analyzed in their anion form.

All the experimental biological activities ($-Log \ IC_{50exp}$ is represented as Y_{exp}), the calculated and predicted biological activities ($-Log \ IC_{50calc}$ is represented as Y_{calc} and $-Log \ IC_{50pred}$ is represented as Y_{pred}) by the QSAR model, and leverage values (Hat) of iridoids are presented in Table 8. Also, the calculation error and prediction error values that state the differences between Y_{exp} and both Y_{calc} and Y_{pred}, are presented by the residual$_{calc}$ and the residual$_{pred}$ terms, respectively.

Table 8. Values of the cytotoxic experimental Y_{exp}, calculated Y_{calc}, and predicted Y_{pred} activities, and residual$_{calc}$ and residual$_{pred}$ values are shown.

Ligand	Y_{exp}	Y_{calc}	Y_{pred}	Hat	residual$_{calc}$	residual$_{pred}$
Euphrasin	0.70	0.19	−0.24	0.451	−0.51	−0.93
Campsinol	−0.28	0.12	0.40	0.403	0.40	0.68
Artselaenin B	−1.09	−1.09	−1.10	0.389	0	−0.01
Artselaenin A	−1.14	−1.18	−1.21	0.377	−0.04	−0.07
Pulchelloside I	−1.40	−1.09	−0.95	0.305	0.32	0.46
Catalpol	−1.45	−1.71	−2.00	0.524	−0.26	−0.55
Lamiide	−1.50	−1.95	−2.25	0.407	−0.44	−0.75
Spinomannoside	−1.59	−1.57	−1.57	0.231	0.02	0.02
5-deoxypulchelloside I	−1.63	−1.39	−1.32	0.244	0.24	0.31
Geniposidic acid [1]	−1.64	−1.59	−1.56	0.387	0.05	0.08
10-*O*-(E)-*p*-coumaroylgeniposidic acid [1]	−1.68	−1.62	−1.51	0.656	0.06	0.17
Genipin	−2.62	−2.44	−2.13	0.627	0.18	0.49

[1] These iridoids were analyzed in their anion form.

Figure 12 displays the descriptive and predictive ability of the QSAR model, according to the squared regression coefficient (R^2)–that corresponds to the value of the explained variance in the description and the prediction (Q^2)–our model has an acceptable ability to predict biological activity. Campsinol and Lamiide were the outliers of the correlation prediction, since the polar surface area of Lamiide was higher than the PSA value for other similar iridoids, and consequently the difference with the PSA of Genipin did not permit a reasonable adjustment.

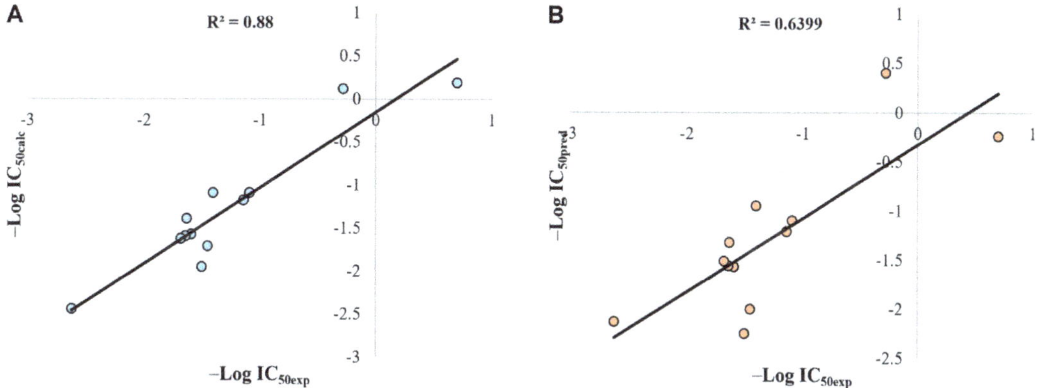

Figure 12. (**A**) Linear correlation of calculated activity (Y_{calc}) versus experimental activity (Y_{exp}). (**B**) Linear correlation of predicted activity (Y_{pred}) versus experimental activity (Y_{exp}).

William's plot, based on the prediction residuals and the leverage values, was used to define the applicability domain of the model (Figure 13). Structural (h > h*) and response outliers (residual$_{pred}$ > 3SDEP) can be observed outside the area limited by the three dashed black lines. These lines represent the warning leverage (h*, dashed horizontal line), and three times the standard deviation in the prediction error (3×SDEP, dashed vertical lines). All the iridoids fell within the applicability domain of the model, suggesting the application of the model for predicting the cytotoxic activity of new iridoids with remarkably high molecular and structural similarity.

Now, we proceed to design iridoids based on the principal structural characteristics of Genipin. As Genipin is an active molecule with low potency, it could be considered as the lead compound in anticancer drug development.

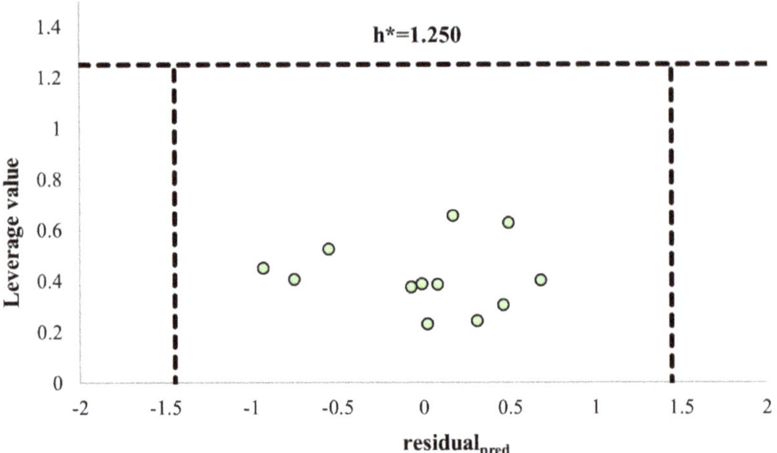

Figure 13. The William plot of prediction residuals versus leverage values of iridoids. The horizontal dashed line shows the warning leverage (h* = 3 p/n, n is the number of iridoids, and p is the number of descriptors in the model plus one), and the two vertical dashed lines indicate the limits within which all residuals should lie (3×SDEP = 1.444).

The 2D structures of a set of iridoids based on the structure of Genipin, including some derived from glycosylated iridoids, are shown in Figure 14. The hydroxyl at C1 of Genipin was conserved in these proposed iridoids, due to its crucial role for the cytotoxic activity of Genipin derivatives, as reported by Yang et al. [45] for a pancreatic cancer cell line (Panc-1). Some structural elements of simple active iridoids (Euphrasin, Campsinol, Artselaenin A, and Artselaenin B) were considered. First, we decided to change the functional group of C4, as we saw its effect on simple and glycosylated iridoids in an increased biological activity, following this order: ester (Genipin), carboxylic acid (D1), and aldehyde (D2). We also considered primary amide (D21-D23) and ketone (D24-D26) as substituents of C4. Then, we evaluated the effect of the lack of the double bond in C7–C8 in the biological activity, plus the effect of the functional group present in C4, with both stereoisomers of the hydroxymethyl at C8 (see Figure 14). We also evaluated the introduction of fluorine in position 3 of the iridoid skeleton in three cases. For those Genipin derivatives we also modified the substituent of C10, represented by R_1. These Genipin derivatives are comprised from D1-D8, and D12-D26. The rest of the iridoids were based on the simple iridoids reported in the literature, some present in iridoid biosynthetic pathways [46,47], such as 7-deoxyloganetic alcohol (D27, also named 7-deoxyloganetol), 7-deoxyloganetic aldehyde (D28, also named iridotrial), 7-deoxyloganetic acid (D29), and 7-deoxyloganetin (D30). These iridoids include D9-D11, D27-D59, D63-D90, with diverse structural modifications in C4, conserving the carbonyl and adding methyl groups over the cyclopentyl. Finally, we include a third set of three iridoids, which are derived from glycosylated iridoids (D60-D62), that have shown inhibitory activity against Taq DNA polymerase [48].

The molecular descriptors of all the 86 designed iridoids were calculated and are presented in Table S3. We applied the QSAR model for the designed iridoids with these values and predicted the biological activity (IC_{50pred}) for all the compounds. The results for the best candidates are presented in Table 9. Finally, the best results are: 0.053, 0.002, 0.006, 0.011, 0.146, 0.103, 0.011, 0.029, and 0.021 μM for D9, D10, D35, D36, D55, D56, D58, D60, D61, and D62, respectively.

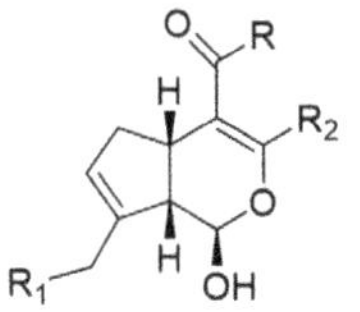

Figure 14. Chemical structures of designed simple iridoids based on Genipin.

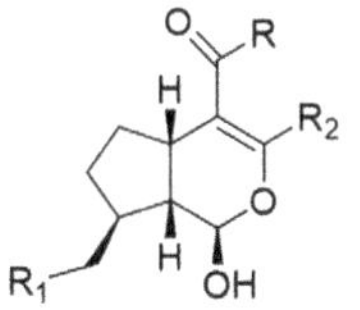

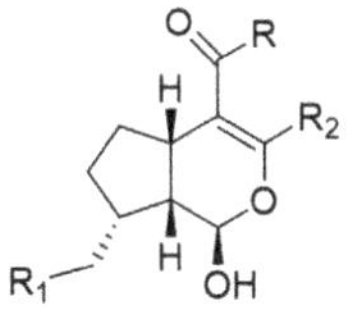

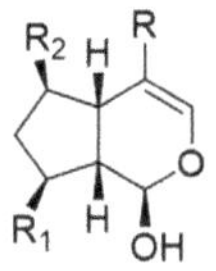

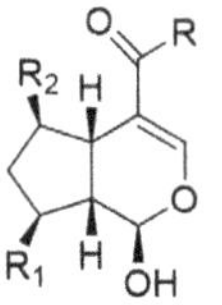

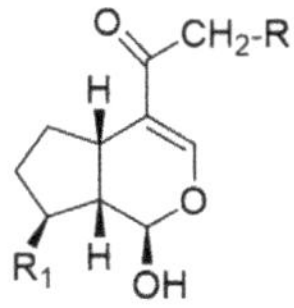

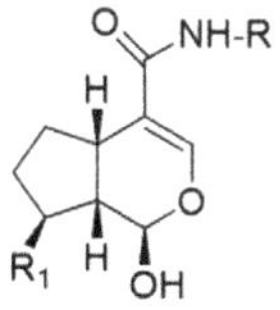

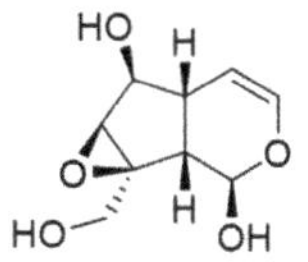

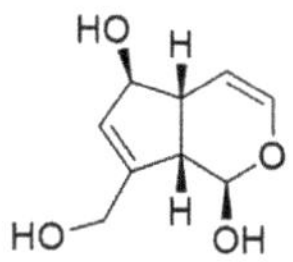

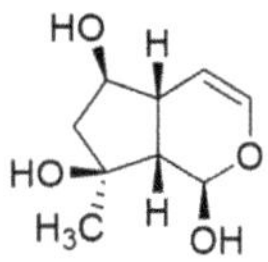

Table 9. Molecular descriptors of the best designed iridoids.

Ligand	GAP$_{HOMO\text{-}LUMO}$ (kcal)	Dipole Moment (debye)	Area (Å²)	Volume (Å³)	PSA (Å²)	Ovality	LogP	Polarizability	HBD Count	HBA Count
D9	−123.61	4.80	187.58	170.55	42.052	1.26	0.42	53.94	1	3
D10 [1]	−599.13	12.32	190.51	175.42	54.222	1.26	--	54.14	1	4
D35	−123.99	3.36	197.34	178.62	60.872	1.29	−0.67	54.59	2	4
D36	−138.78	0.69	196.25	176.32	47.478	1.29	0.55	54.25	2	3
D55	−139.52	1.70	196.35	176.4	47.351	1.29	0.61	54.25	2	3
D56	−118.90	4.81	213.74	196.37	57.202	1.31	−0.41	56.08	2	4
D58	−140.01	1.99	219.39	201.1	61.709	1.32	−0.28	56.25	3	4
D60	−144.58	2.30	201.54	184.95	73.770	1.28	−1.50	54.89	3	5
D61	−145.63	3.19	207.72	190.41	80.817	1.30	−1.25	55.33	4	5
D62	−135.25	0.86	196.11	178.97	61.665	1.28	−0.79	54.50	3	4

[1] These iridoids were analyzed in their anion form.

After applying the QSAR model of Equation (2), a set of ten iridoids had a higher predicted biological activity than the experimental activity of Euphrasin (Figure 15), IC$_{50pred}$ lower than 0.2 µM. Most of these designed iridoids had an aldehyde or an hydroxymethyl in C4, but four of them lacked a substituent in this position. Only one of them had an acid in this position D10. All of them conserved the hydroxyl in C1, and others featured a methyl or a hydroxyl in C8, or both, and a hydroxyl in C6. Only two iridoids, D60 and D62, presented an hydroxymethyl in C8, as with Genipin, but D60 had an epoxy group between C7 and C8. D62 was the only iridoid with a double bond in C7–C8, as with Genipin.

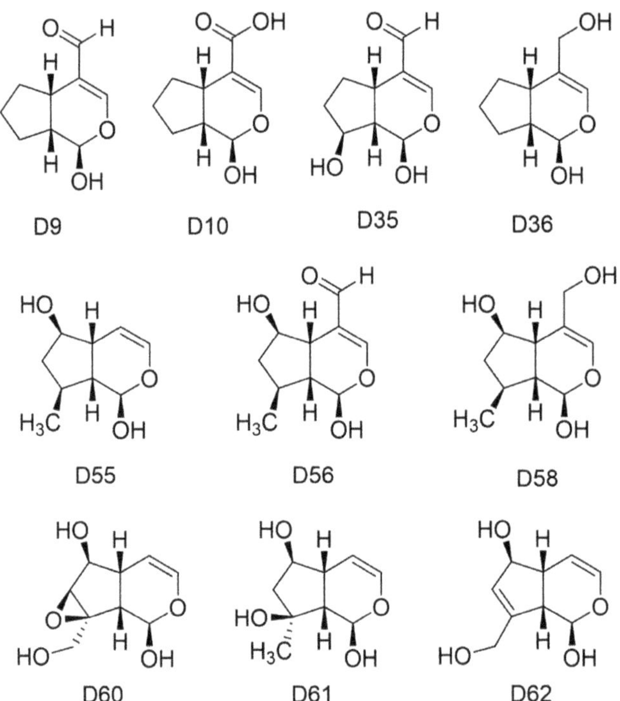

Figure 15. Chemical structures of the best designed iridoids based on Genipin.

In Table 9, the descriptors of these ten designed ligands are presented. The ligands with an aldehyde in C4 (D9, D35, and D56) had similar GAP$_{HOMO\text{-}LUMO}$ to Genipin; those having an acid or an hydroxymethyl, or no substituent in C4, had a less negative GAP$_{HOMO\text{-}LUMO}$. D9, D10, and D56 had the highest values of dipole moment, but D36 and D62 had lower values of the dipole moment than that of Genipin (see Table 3). D9 and D10 were smaller in area and volume than the most cytotoxic iridoids. D60, D61, and D62 were more polar than Genipin, and the rest of the iridoids were less polar compounds compared to Genipin, with PSA values in the range 42–61 Å^2. All the proposed iridoids had a higher affinity for water, except D36 and D55, which present a higher affinity for a lipidic phase, as with Artselaenin A and Artselaenin B. Almost all compounds were *less* polarizable molecules than Genipin and the other simple iridoids presented in Table 3. These iridoids had a variable number of hydrogen bond donors and acceptors, ranging from 1 to 4, and 3 to 5, respectively.

The 3D structures of the *best* designed iridoids based on the structure of Genipin, with their respective dipole vectors, are displayed in Figure S7. Curiously, only D9, D10, D36, and D56 present a dipole vector with a similar direction to the most active simple iridoids (Euphrasin, Campsinol, Artselaenin A, and Artselaenin B); this could be attributed to the aldehyde in C4, that was common to these four designed iridoids. The rest of the iridoids presented a dipole vector with a different orientation. This was influenced by the presence of other substituents in C4, or the lack of anyone.

It is noteworthy that the change of the ester for the carboxylic acid at C4 increased the potency of the iridoid compared to Genipin, but the change of the carboxylic acid by an aldehyde decreased the potency of the iridoid compared to the IC$_{50exp}$ of Genipin. The elimination of the double bond in C7–C8 also increased the potency of the iridoids. In addition to the lack of the double bond in C7–C8 of Genipin, the absence of any substituent in the cyclopentane ring increased the biological activity, and the incorporation of a hydroxyl in C8, or an extra hydroxyl in C6 (D60-D62) increased the potency of the compound. In some cases, the reactivity order of the compound related to the substitutions in C4 is as follows: any > hydroxymethyl > aldehyde (D55, D56, and D58).

Next, the alignment of the three best designed iridoids (D9, D10, D35, D36, D55, D56, D58, D60, D61, and D62) and the most structurally similar active iridoid (Artselaenin A) is shown in Figure 16. All four CFDs were selected since they are in common with the designed iridoids and Artselaenin A. The highest alignment scores were those between the designed iridoids D9, D10, and D36 with Artselaenin A, and their values were 0.78, 0.77, and 0.99, respectively. The best alignment score was obtained with D36, comparing the structure of the iridoid skeleton, but its dipole vector was not parallel to that of Artselaenin A (Figure 16F). The alignment with D9 had a lowest score of 0.78, but the orientation of the dipole vector was parallel to that of Artselaenin A (Figure 16D). These iridoids have not been evaluated against cervical cancer cells to our knowledge.

Finally, we analyzed the MEP graphics of the best candidates of the designed iridoids to evaluate the principal differences and similarities to explain their reactivity. The MEP isosurface of −10 kcal/mol shows the electrostatic profile of the designed iridoids (Figure S8). The increased calculated activity of the designed iridoids could be attributed to the higher electron density over the carboxylic acid or aldehyde at C4, the hydroxyl at C1, and the sp3 oxygen in the pyran. Also, this higher electron density is observed on the oxygen of the hydroxymethyl in C4, and on the hydroxyls in C6, and C8. This electron density pattern is observed in Artselaenin A, which was the most similar to D9, D35, and D56 (Figure S8A,C,F). D61 and D62 also present a higher electron density over the hydroxymethyl at C8 (Figure S8I,J).

In Figure S9, regions most susceptible to an electrophilic attack (yellow to red color) and those to a nucleophilic attack (blue color) are displayed. In all iridoids the regions with more electronic density are located at the oxygen of the carbonyl at C4, and the oxygen of the hydroxyl at C1, C6, C8, and C10, correlating with the previous MEP distributions. The regions with less electron density were located principally over the hydrogen of the aldehyde at C4, and the other hydrogens of the hydroxyls at C1 and C10, which correlated to the other surface graphics, and were like the regions of the MEP map of Artselaenin A, principally D9, D35, and D56 (this last with an extra electron distribution on the sp2 oxygen). Iridoids such as D60 and D61 presented a greater electron distribution due to the hydroxyls present on their structures, and in the case of D60, due to the presence of the epoxy group.

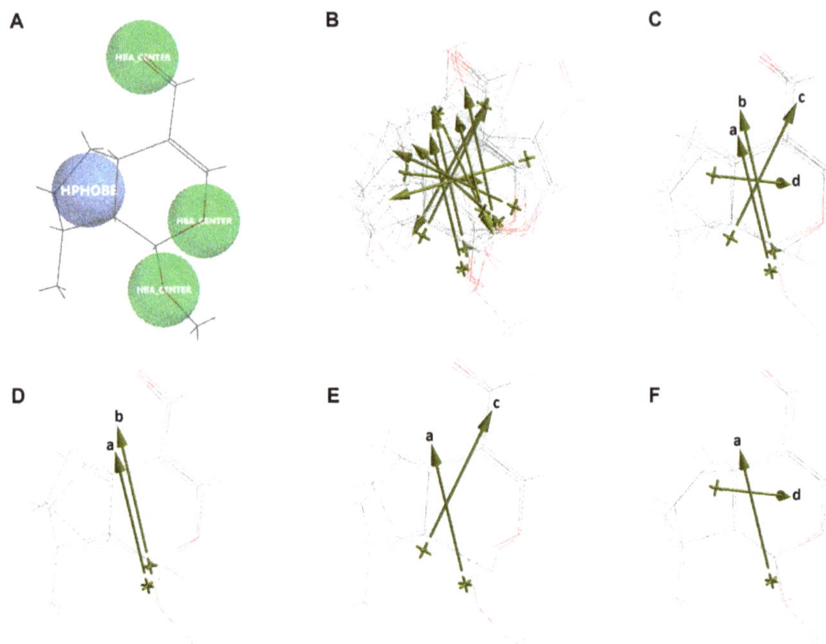

Figure 16. Alignment of Artselaenin A with the best designed iridoids. (**A**) Common similarity centers by CFDs of Artselaenin A (purple circles represent the CFDs selected for the alignment). (**B**) Alignment of Artselaenin A with D9, D10, D35, D36, D55, D56, D58, D60, D61, and D62. (**C**) Alignment of Artselaenin A with D9, D10, D36. (**D**) Alignment of Artselaenin A with D9. (**E**) Alignment of Artselaenin A with D10. (**F**) Alignment of Artselaenin A with D36. Dipole vector represented by gold arrows for each iridoid aligned is shown (a: Artselaenin A, b: D9, c: D10, d: D36).

3. Materials and Methods

3.1. In Vitro Cytotoxic Activity of Geniposide and Genipin

In vitro cytotoxicity activity of Geniposide and Genipin was measured using the sulforhodamine B (SRB) (MP Biomedicals, Irvine, CA, USA) protein staining assay [49–51], using three different cervical cancer cell lines CaSki, CaLo, and INBL; and the immortalized keratinocytes HaCaT, as a non-tumorigenic cell line. The CaLo and INBL cell lines [28] were donated by Profesor María de Lourdes Gutiérrez Xicoténcatl from Centro de Investigación sobre Enfermedades Infecciosas, Instituto Nacional de Salud Pública. Briefly, cells were cultured in RPMI-1640 medium supplemented with 10% fetal bovine serum, and seeded in a 96-well microtiter plate at a cellular density of 5000 cells/mL, and placed in an incubator (5% CO_2 and 37 °C) for 5 h. Afterward, different concentrations of pure iridoids (0.04128, 0.2064, 1.032, 5.16, 25.8, and 129 µM), of podophyllotoxin positive control (0.00303, 0.00606, 0.01213, 0.02425, 0.04850, and 0.09700 µM), and of cisplatin positive control (0.10400, 0.20781, 0.41563, 0.83125, 1.6625, and 3.325 µM) were added in triplicate and incubated for 72 h. The assays were conducted in three independent experiments.

Afterward, cells were fixed with cold trichloroacetic acid (30% in water) and stained with SRB (0.4% in a 1% of acetic acid solution). Cells were washed with a cold 1% acetic acid solution. Finally, the bound colorant was solubilized with Tris base to obtain the optical density (ODsample). The bound colorant was proportional to either total protein or cells amount. DMSO (final concentration of 0.5%) was used as vehicle and blank (ODblank) in Genipin experiments, and only deionized water was employed as vehicle and blank in Geniposide experiments. The total protein concentration in a single plate with cells at the assay's beginning was considered zero (ODzero). Microtiter plates were incubated for 72 h, after which the total protein concentration was determined with Equation (3). Using an ELISA-Reader spectrophotometer, this assay measures the respective absorbance at 490 nm (Molecular Devices, SPECTRA max plus 384). Results were expressed as the concentration that inhibits 50% of control growth after the treatment period (IC_{50}), using the statistical program GraphPad Prism, version 8.00 (GraphPad Software, Inc, La Jolla, CA, USA).

$$\%Survival = \frac{OD_{sample} - OD_{zero}}{OD_{blank} - OD_{zero}} \times 100 \qquad (3)$$

Cytotoxic activity assays with Geniposide and Genipin against the HeLa cell line were performed by the MTS method [52]. For this assay, 5000 cells were seeded in a 96-well cell culture plate and treated for 48 h using 882, 441, 220.50, 110.25, 55.125, 27.5625, and 13.78125 µM of Genipin or Geniposide, and 50, 25, 12.5, 6, and 3 nM of paclitaxel as positive control. DMSO (final concentration of 0.5%) was used as a vehicle and blank. We used CellTiter 96® Aqueous One Solution Cell Proliferation Assay kit (Promega, Madison, WI, USA) to determine the number of viable cells, following the manufacturer's instruction. Cell viability was estimated by measuring the absorbance at 450 nm using an automated ELISA reader (Promega, Madison, WI, USA). Data were analyzed in the Prism 5.0 statistical program (GraphPad Software, Inc, La Jolla, CA, USA), and the IC_{50} values were determined by regression analysis.

3.2. Searching of Cytotoxic Reports of Iridoids in Cervical Cancer

The information about the cytotoxicity of iridoids in cervical cancer cells in vitro was collected by searching on databases and websites such as PubMed, SciFinder, Google Scholar, Elsevier, ScienceDirect, and Web of Science. The following words or phrases were used in diverse combinations for searching: "cytotoxic iridoids in cervical cancer", "iridoids against cervical cancer", "antiproliferative iridoids in cervical cancer", "cervical cancer", "in vitro", "cytotoxic iridoids", "cell death". More than 30 scientific works of literature were consulted from 2004 to the date, gathering forty-four iridoids with reported cytotoxic activity in a cervical cancer cell line.

Eleven of the forty-four iridoids were selected to analyze their similarity on their structure, molecular descriptors, and the reported cytotoxic activities to understand the absence of Geniposide activity and the low Genipin activity. The iridoids were selected based on the two following criteria: (1) they were assessed in the same cell line, and (2) they were evaluated at the same time of treatment.

3.3. Conformation Analysis, Geometry Optimization, and Energy Calculation

A conformational analysis of all the simple and glycosides iridoids in their neutral and anionic form using the MMFF94 molecular mechanism model was performed [53]. The minimum energy conformer was submitted to a geometry optimization without symmetry constraints, employing the PM6 semiempirical method [54]. A harmonic frequency analysis was performed to ensure that the structure corresponds to a minimum on the potential energy surface. Furthermore, to acquire a more precise energy value and electronic density characteristics, a geometry reoptimization, at a density functional theory level, with the B3LYP hybrid functional [55] and the 6-31G* basis set [56], was performed. These systems were evaluated in water within the SM8 model [57].

Additionally, a single-point calculation using the B3LYP functional and 6-311 + G** basis set [58] in vacuum (in water for 10-*O*-(E)-*p*-coumaroylgeniposidic acid) was performed.

3.4. Molecular Descriptors

The following global chemical reactivity descriptors: Energy of the Highest Occupied Molecular Orbital (E_{HOMO}), Energy of the Lowest Unoccupied Molecular Orbital (E_{LUMO}), dipole moment (ρ), polarizability, polar surface area (PSA), Hydrogen Bond Donnor (HBD), and Hydrogen Bond Acceptor (HBA) counts, and some related to their size and form: area, volume, ovality, and their solubility: LogP (1-octanol/water calculation) were obtained from the quantum calculations performed with SPARTAN'20 program [59].

3.5. Molecular Representation of Electron Density Properties

The molecular electrostatic potential (MEP) mapped onto an iso-density surface $(0.002 \, e\text{-}/\text{Å}^3)$ for each compound was obtained. The MEP map provides a perception of the molecular size and the location of electron-rich and -deficient zones on a compound. In addition, to evaluate the electronic effect caused by the substituents in the iridoid skeleton, a molecular electrostatic potential surface with a value of -10 kcal/mol was obtained. All the molecular graphics were performed in the SPARTAN'20 program.

3.6. Molecular Similarity Analysis of Iridoids

Molecular similarity analysis was performed by comparing the skeleton base of the iridoids and detecting the substituents that are changed or added between them to the central iridoid of the comparison (Genipin or Geniposide). A molecular similarity analysis of three groups was performed: (1) Genipin with other simple iridoids, (2) Genipin with Geniposide, and (3) designed iridoids with one of the most cytotoxic iridoids.

3.7. QSAR Construction and Validation

Molecular Descriptors

The following global chemical reactivity descriptors were considered to construct the QSAR model: Energy of the Highest Occupied Molecular Orbital (E_{HOMO}), Energy of the Lowest Unoccupied Molecular Orbital (E_{LUMO}), chemical hardness (η) expressed by equation 4, electronegativity (χ) expressed by Equation (5), dipole moment (ρ), polarizability, Δpolarizability, polar surface area (PSA), ΔPSA, Hydrogen Bond Donnor (HBD), and Hydrogen Bond Acceptor (HBA) counts, and some related to their size and form: area, Δarea, volume, Δvolume, ovality, Δovality, and their solubility: LogP (1-octanol/water calculation), ΔLogP, and LogP^2. All the Δ are the differences in the values between the descriptor of the iridoid in case and the descriptor of Genipin. All the calculations were performed in the SPARTAN'20 program. LogS (aqueous solubility calculation) was an extra descriptor and was obtained from Virtual Computational Chemistry Laboratory [60]. The energy corresponding to E_{HOMO} represents the ionization potential of the molecule and E_{LUMO} the corresponding electron affinity value, according to the Koopmans approximation.

$$\eta = \frac{E_{HOMO} - E_{LUMO}}{2} \tag{4}$$

$$\chi = \frac{E_{HOMO} + E_{LUMO}}{2} \tag{5}$$

3.8. Mathematical Model Generation

To construct our mathematical model, the multilinear regression by minimum quadratic differences was employed, using Excel Microsoft Office 365. All the molecular descriptors and the biological activity (IC$_{50}$) of the iridoids were used as the independent variables (X) and the dependent variable (Y), respectively.

3.9. Statistical Validation

For the validation of our QSAR model, we employed the coefficient of determination (R^2) (Equation (6)), cross-validated R^2 (Q^2), standard deviation (s), and Fisher test (F) [61]. The last two parameters gave information about how the correlation between the experimental and calculated activities is affected by the number of compounds in the study (Equation (7)), and what the probability is for the mathematical model to casually occur (Equation (8)).

$$R^2 = \frac{\sum_{i=1}^{n}(\hat{y}_i - y_i)^2}{\sum_{i=1}^{n}\left(y_i - \bar{y}\right)^2} \tag{6}$$

$$s = \frac{\sum_{i=1}^{n}(\hat{y}_i - y_i)^2}{n - 2} \tag{7}$$

$$F = \frac{\sum_{i=1}^{n}\left(\hat{y}_i - \bar{y}\right)^2 / df_M}{\sum_{i=1}^{n}(\hat{y}_i - y_i)^2 / df_E} \tag{8}$$

where $\hat{y}_i$, $\bar{y}$, and y_i refer to the calculated, average, and experimental values of activities, respectively. Also, df_M and df_E (Equation (9)) refer to the degrees of freedom of the model and error, respectively.

$$df_E = n - p - 1 \tag{9}$$

In the mathematical model, R^2 must possess high values ($R^2 \geq 80$), while s and F should have the smallest and largest possible values, respectively, to ensure that the QSAR model is reliable.

Also, to undertake a more sophisticated validation, we used redundancy (R^P) and overfitting (R^N) rules [62]. From the Pearson correlation matrix, we corroborated that the molecular descriptors are not linearly correlated (Table S1).

The goal of the redundancy rule is to detect models with an excess of good molecular descriptors (R^P) and establish that, if $R^P < t^P$, the model is rejected. Depending on the data, t^P values range from 0.01 to 0.1. R^P is defined by Equation (10).

$$R^P = \prod_{j=1}^{P^+}\left(1 - M_j\left(\frac{p}{p-1}\right)\right); \; M_j > 0 \;\; and \;\; 0 \leq R^P \leq 1 \tag{10}$$

On the other hand, the purpose of the overfitting rule is to detect models with an excess of bad molecular descriptors. This rule stipulates that, if $R^N < t^N$ (ε), the model is rejected. The t^N (ε) values are calculated by the Equation (11).

$$t^N(\varepsilon) = \frac{p \cdot \varepsilon - R}{p \cdot R} \tag{11}$$

where values range from 0.01 to 0.1 and p is the number of variables in the model. R^N is defined by Equation (12).

$$R^N = \sum_{j=1}^{P^-} M_j; \; M_j < 0 \;\; and \;\; -1 \leq R^N \leq 0 \tag{12}$$

where M_j is defined by Equation (13).

$$M_j = \frac{R_{jY}}{R} - \frac{1}{P}; \;\; -\frac{1}{P} \leq M_j \leq \frac{p-1}{p} \tag{13}$$

R_{jY} is the absolute value of the regression coefficient between the jth descriptors and the response Y.

Moreover, we evaluated the predictive ability of our model by the Leave-One-Out (Q^2_{LOO}) method, in which one compound is removed from the data set and the activity (Y_{exp}) is correlated using the rest of the data set. The Equation (14) was employed to calculate Q^2_{LOO}.

$$Q^2_{LOO} = 1 - \frac{\sum_{i=1}^{n}\left(y_i - \hat{y}_i\right)^2}{\sum_{i=1}^{n}\left(y_i - \bar{y}\right)^2} \tag{14}$$

where $\hat{y}_{i/i}$ is the predicted value of the activity (Y_{pred}).

Applicability domain evaluation was carried out by means of William plot construction, which depends on the leverage values and the standardized error in the calculation. The leverage values (h) are obtained from the leverage matrix H, which contains information about the descriptors on which the model is built. The leverage matrix H is defined as Equation (15).

$$H = X \cdot (X^T \cdot X)^{-1} \cdot X^T \tag{15}$$

where X is the selected descriptor matrix; X^T is the transpose matrix of X; and $(X^T \cdot X)^{-1}$ is the inverse of matrix $(X^T \cdot X)$. The leverage values are the diagonal elements of the H matrix. The warning leverage (h^*) is calculated as $h = 3\,p/n$, where n is the number of molecules and p is the number of descriptors in the model plus one. If one of the compounds has a leverage value higher than the h^*, it will be considered an outlier, this is, out of the applicability domain of the model.

4. Conclusions

In this study, Geniposide and its aglycone Genipin were tested against different cervical cancer cell lines (CaLo, CaSki, and INBL) from different FIGO stagings and with the most high-risk HPV types. Geniposide did not exert cytotoxic activity, and Genipin was more active against CaLo (IIB, HPV18) and CaSki (metastatic, HPV16) than against INBL (IVB, HPV18).

Derived from the structure–activity relationship and the molecular similarity analysis, we found that the dipole moment is relevant to the cytotoxic activity against the HeLa cell line. Moreover, we observed that the presence of different functional groups, such as an aldehyde or a carboxylic acid, the hydroxyls in C1 and C8, and the lack of the double bond in C7–C8 influenced the biological activity of the iridoids.

Derived from the QSAR study, we obtained a model with a good prediction of the biological activity against HeLa, that reveals the dipole moment as a principal descriptor that impacts on the activity of the iridoids. The designed iridoids incorporated the most relevant structural characteristics of simple iridoids based on the Genipin structure. Therefore, we propose ten of the designed iridoids (D9, D10, D35, D36, D55, D56, D58, D60, D61, and D62), since their predicted activity was lower (0.002–0.146 µM) than the activity of the most cytotoxic iridoid reported in the literature (0.2 µM), according to our QSAR model.

Supplementary Materials: The following supporting information can be downloaded at: https://www.mdpi.com/article/10.3390/ph16121647/s1, Figure S1: Structure of iridoid skeleton. Principal substituents in R_2 and R_6 are specified.; Figure S2: The 2D structures of iridoids with reported cytotoxic activity against the HeLa cell line.; Figure S3: The 3D structures of iridoid glycosides evaluated against the HeLa cell line, including the vector dipole (gold arrow). (A) Geniposidic acid, (B) 10-*O*-(E)-*p*-coumaroylgeniposidic acid, (C) Catalpol, (D) Geniposide, (D) Lamiide, (F) Pulchelloside I, (G) 5-deoxypulchelloside I, (H) Spinomannoside. Figure S4: Molecular electrostatic potential iso-surface of -10 kcal/mol of iridoid glycosides. (A) Pulchelloside I, (B) Catalpol, (C) Lamiide, (D) Spinomannoside, (E) 5-deoxypulchelloside I, (F) Geniposidic acid, (G) 10-*O*-(E)-*p*-coumaroylgeniposidic acid, (H) Geniposide. Figure S5: Molecular electrostatic potential map of iridoid glycosides. (A) Pulchelloside I, (B) Catalpol, (C) Lamiide, (D) Spinomannoside, (E) 5-deoxypulchelloside I, (F) Geniposidic acid, (G) 10-*O*-(E)-*p*-coumaroylgeniposidic acid, (H) Geniposide. Figure S6: Alignment of Genipin with Geniposide. (A) Common similarity centers by CFDs of Genipin (purple circles represent the CFDs selected for the alignment). (B) Dipole vector represented by gold arrows of both iridoids aligned is shown (a: Genipin, b: Geniposide). Figure S7: The 3D structures of the best designed iridoids based on Genipin. Gold arrows represent dipole vector in each iridoid. (A) D9, (B) D10, (C) D35, (D) D36, (E) D55, (F) D56, (G) D58, (H) D60, (I) D61, (J) D62. Figure S8: Molecular electrostatic potential iso-surface of -10 kcal/mol of the best designed iridoids (A) D9, (B) D10, (C) D35, (D) D36, (E) D55, (F) D56, (G) D58, (H) D60, (I) D61, (J) D62. Figure S9: Molecular electrostatic potential map of the best designed iridoids. (A) D9, (B) D10, (C) D35, (D) D36, (E) D55, (F) D56, (G) D58, (H) D60, (I) D61, (J) D62. Figure S10: Independent correlations between the biological activity and the descriptors of the QSAR model. (A) $-\text{Log IC}_{50}$ vs Dipole moment,

(B) $-$Log IC$_{50}$ vs ΔPSA, (C) $-$Log IC$_{50}$ vs LogS, (D) $-$Log IC$_{50}$ vs ΔPolarizability^2. Table S1: Pearson correlation matrix. Table S2: The pKa values of the acid iridoids. Table S3: Molecular descriptors of designed iridoids.

Author Contributions: Conceptualization, D.L.-L., R.S.R.-H. and V.R.-L.; methodology, D.L.-L. and J.N.S.-C.; software, R.S.R.-H. and M.A.L.-P.; validation, D.L.-L., R.S.R.-H. and V.R.-L.; formal analysis, D.L.-L.; investigation, D.L.-L.; resources, V.R.-L.; data curation, D.L.-L.; writing—original draft preparation, D.L.-L.; writing—review and editing, R.S.R.-H., V.R.-L., C.M.-P., J.N.S.-C., O.A.P.-M. and M.A.L.-P.; visualization, C.M.-P. and O.A.P.-M.; supervision, R.S.R.-H. and V.R.-L.; project administration, R.S.R.-H. and V.R.-L.; funding acquisition, V.R.-L. All authors have read and agreed to the published version of the manuscript.

Funding: Research was funded by CONAHCyT, grant number 667926.

Institutional Review Board Statement: Not applicable.

Informed Consent Statement: Not applicable.

Data Availability Statement: Data are contained within the article and Supplementary Materials.

Acknowledgments: The authors are thankful for the financial support from CONAHCyT (Projects No. 319550, No. 320243 and Grant 667926). We also thank María de Lourdes Gutiérrez Xicoténcatl for her donation of the CaLo and INBL cell lines.

Conflicts of Interest: The authors declare no conflict of interest.

References

1. World Health Organization (WHO). Available online: https://www.who.int/news-room/fact-sheets/detail/cancer (accessed on 5 July 2023).
2. GLOBOCAN-Global Cancer Observatory. Available online: https://gco.iarc.fr/ (accessed on 10 July 2023).
3. Okunade, K.S. Human papillomavirus and cervical cancer. *J. Obstet. Gynaecol.* **2020**, *40*, 602–608. [CrossRef]
4. Anand, U.; Dey, A.; Chandel, A.K.S.; Sanyal, R.; Mishra, A.; Pandey, D.K.; De Falco, V.; Upadhyay, A.; Kandimalla, R.; Chaudhary, A.; et al. Cancer chemotherapy and beyond: Current status, drug candidates, associated risks and progress in targeted therapeutics. *Genes Dis.* **2022**, *10*, 1367–1401. [CrossRef]
5. Çakır, C.; Kılıç, F.; Dur, R.; Yüksel, D.; Ünsal, M.; Korkmaz, V.; Kılıç, Ç.; Kimyon Cömert, G.; Boran, N.; Türkmen, O.; et al. Neoadjuvant chemotherapy for locally advanced stage (IB2-IIA2-IIB) cervical carcinoma: Experience of a tertiary center and comprehensive review of the literature. *Turk. J. Obstet. Gynecol.* **2021**, *18*, 190–202. [CrossRef] [PubMed]
6. Xiong, Y.; Liang, L.Z.; Cao, L.P.; Min, Z.; Liu, J.H. Clinical effects of irinotecan hydrochloride in combination with cisplatin as neoadjuvant chemotherapy in locally advanced cervical cancer. *Gynecol Oncol.* **2011**, *123*, 99–104. [CrossRef]
7. Zhang, H.; Zhang, Y. Application of vincristine and cisplatin combined with intensity-modulated radiation therapy in the treatment of patients with advanced cervical cancer. *Am. J. Transl. Res.* **2021**, *13*, 13894–13901. [PubMed]
8. Bajaj, A.; Gopalakrishnan, M.; Harkenrider, M.M.; Lurain, J.R.; Small, W., Jr. Advanced small cell carcinoma of the cervix-Successful treatment with concurrent etoposide and cisplatin chemotherapy and extended field radiation: A case report and discussion. *Gynecol. Oncol. Rep.* **2017**, *23*, 4–6. [CrossRef]
9. Park, S.H.; Kim, M.; Lee, S.; Jung, W.; Kim, B. Therapeutic Potential of Natural Products in Treatment of Cervical Cancer: A Review. *Nutrients* **2021**, *13*, 154. [CrossRef] [PubMed]
10. Huang, M.; Lu, J.J.; Ding, J. Natural Products in Cancer Therapy: Past, Present and Future. *Nat. Prod. Bioprospect.* **2021**, *11*, 5–13. [CrossRef]
11. Naeem, A.; Hu, P.; Yang, M.; Zhang, J.; Liu, Y.; Zhu, W.; Zheng, Q. Natural Products as Anticancer Agents: Current Status and Future Perspectives. *Molecules* **2022**, *27*, 8367. [CrossRef]
12. Wang, C.; Gong, X.; Bo, A.; Zhang, L.; Zhang, M.; Zang, E.; Zhang, C.; Li, M. Iridoids: Research Advances in Their Phytochemistry, Biological Activities, and Pharmacokinetics. *Molecules* **2020**, *25*, 287. [CrossRef]
13. Hussain, H.; Green, I.R.; Saleem, M.; Raza, M.L.; Nazir, M. Therapeutic Potential of Iridoid Derivatives: Patent Review. *Inventions* **2019**, *4*, 29. [CrossRef]
14. Bianco, A. Recent developments in iridoids chemistry. *Pure Appl. Chem.* **1994**, *86*, 2335–2338. [CrossRef]
15. Ornano, L.; Feroci, M.; Guarcini, L.; Venditti, A.; Bianco, A. Anti-HIV agents from nature: Natural compounds from *Hypericum hircinum* and carbocyclic nucleosides from iridoids. *Stud. Nat. Prod. Chem.* **2018**, *56*, 173–228. [CrossRef]
16. Kim, C.W.; Choi, K.C. Potential roles of iridoid glycosides and their underlying mechanisms against diverse cancer growth and metastasis: Do they have an inhibitory effect on cancer progression? *Nutrients* **2021**, *13*, 2974. [CrossRef]
17. Ndongwe, T.; Witika, B.A.; Mncwangi, N.P.; Poka, M.S.; Skosana, P.P.; Demana, P.H.; Summers, B.; Siwe-Noundou, X. Iridoid Derivatives as Anticancer Agents: An Updated Review from 1970–2022. *Cancers* **2023**, *15*, 770. [CrossRef]

18. Chen, Z.; Xu, H.; Wang, X.; Liu, Z. Lactobacillus raises in vitro anticancer effect of Geniposide in HSC-3 human oral squamous cell carcinoma cells. *Exp. Ther. Med.* **2017**, *14*, 4586–4594. [CrossRef]

19. Bai, G.; Chen, B.; Xiao, X.; Li, Y.; Liu, X.; Zhao, D.; Zhang, L.; Zhao, D. Geniposide inhibits cell proliferation and migration in human squamous carcinoma cells via AMPK and JNK signaling pathways. *Exp. Ther. Med.* **2022**, *24*, 706. [CrossRef] [PubMed]

20. Habtemariam, S.; Lentini, G. Plant-derived anticancer agents: Lessons from the pharmacology of Geniposide and its aglycone, Genipin. *Biomedicines* **2018**, *6*, 39. [CrossRef] [PubMed]

21. Feng, Q.; Cao, H.L.; Xu, W.; Li, X.R.; Ren, Y.Q.; Du, L.F. Apoptosis induced by Genipin in human leukemia K562 cells: Involvement of c-Jun N-terminal kinase in G2/M arrest. *Acta Pharmacol. Sin.* **2011**, *31*, 519–527. [CrossRef]

22. Kim, E.S.; Jeong, C.S.; Moon, A. Genipin, a constituent of Gardenia jasminoides Ellis, induces apoptosis and inhibits invasion in MDA-MB-231 breast cancer cells. *Oncol. Rep.* **2012**, *27*, 567–572. [CrossRef]

23. Ko, H.; Kim, J.M.; Kim, S.J.; Shim, S.H.; Ha, C.H.; Chang, H.I. Induction of apoptosis by Genipin inhibits cell proliferation in AGS human gastric cancer cells via Egr1/p21 signaling pathway. *Bioorganic Med. Chem. Lett.* **2015**, *25*, 4191–4196. [CrossRef]

24. Li, Z.; Zhang, T.B.; Jia, D.H.; Sun, W.Q.; Wang, C.L.; Gu, A.Z.; Yang, X.M. Genipin inhibits the growth of human bladder cancer cells via inactivation of PI3K/Akt signaling. *Oncol. Lett.* **2018**, *15*, 2619–2624. [CrossRef]

25. Shanmugam, M.K.; Shen, H.; Tang, F.R.; Arfuso, F.; Rajesh, M.; Wang, L.; Kumar, A.P.; Bian, J.; Goh, B.C.; Bishayee, A.; et al. Potential role of Genipin in cancer therapy. *Pharmacol. Res.* **2018**, *133*, 195–200. [CrossRef]

26. Maggiora, G.; Vogt, M.; Stumpge, D.; Bajorath, J. Molecular Similarity in Medicinal Chemistry. *J. Med. Chem.* **2014**, *57*, 3186–3204. [CrossRef]

27. Daina, A.; Röhrig, U.F.; Zoete, V. Computer-aided drug design for cancer therapy. In *Systems Medicine: Integrative, Qualitative and Computation Approaches*, 1st ed.; Wolkenhauer, O., Ed.; Elsevier: Amsterdam, The Netherlands, 2021; pp. 386–401. [CrossRef]

28. Zuñiga Martinez, M.D.L.; López Mendoza, C.M.; Tenorio Salazar, J.; García Carrancá, A.M.; Cerbón Cervantes, M.A.; Alcántara-Quintana, L.E. Establishment, authenticity, and characterization of cervical cancer cell lines. *Mol. Cell. Oncol.* **2022**, *9*, 2078628. [CrossRef]

29. Neri-Numa, I.A.; Pessôa, M.G.; Arruda, H.S.; Pereira, G.A.; Paulino, B.N.; Angolini, C.F.F.; Ruiz, A.L.T.G.; Pastore, G.M. Genipap (*Genipa americana* L.) fruit extract as a source of antioxidant and antiproliferative iridoids. *Food Res. Int.* **2020**, *134*, 109252. [CrossRef]

30. Hwang, H.; Kim, C.; Kim, S.M.; Kim, W.S.; Choi, S.H.; Chang, I.M.; Ahn, K.S. The hydrolyzed products of iridoid glycoside with β-glucosidase treatment exert anti-proliferative effects through suppression of STAT3 activation and STAT3-regulated gene products in several human cancer cells. *Pharm. Biol.* **2012**, *50*, 8–17. [CrossRef]

31. Marcotullio, M.C.; Loizzo, M.R.; Messina, F.; Temperini, A.; Tundis, R.; Menichini, F.; Curini, M. Bioassay-guided fractionation of *Euphrasia pectinata* Ten. and isolation of iridoids with antiproliferative activity. *Phytochem. Lett.* **2015**, *12*, 252–256. [CrossRef]

32. Feng, S.X.; Yi, B.; Zhang, M.; Xu, J.; Lin, H.; Xu, W.T. Iridoid glycosides from *Callicarpa nudiflora* Hook. *Nat. Prod. Res.* **2017**, *31*, 181–189. [CrossRef]

33. Wang, C.; Xin, P.; Wang, Y.; Zhou, X.; Wei, D.; Deng, C.; Sun, S. Iridoids and sfingolipids from *Hedyotis diffusa*. *Fitoterapia* **2018**, *124*, 152–159. [CrossRef]

34. Cao, H.; Feng, Q.; Xu, W.; Li, X.; Kang, Z.; Ren, Y.; Du, L. Genipin induced apoptosis associated with activation of the c-Jun NH2-terminal kinase and p53 protein in HeLa cells. *Biol. Pharm. Bull.* **2010**, *33*, 1343–1348. [CrossRef] [PubMed]

35. Li, N.; Di, L.; Gao, W.C.; Wang, K.J.; Zu, L.B. Cytotoxic iridoids from the roots of *Patrinia scabra*. *J. Nat. Prod.* **2012**, *72*, 1723–1728. [CrossRef] [PubMed]

36. Krohn, K.; Gehle, D.; Dey, S.K.; Nahar, N.; Mosihuzzaman, M.; Sutana, N.; Sohrab, M.H.; Stephens, P.J.; Pan, J.J.; Sasse, F. Prismatomerin, a new iridoid from *Prismatomeris tetranda*. Structure elucidation, determination of absolute configuration, and cytotoxicity. *J. Nat. Prod.* **2007**, *70*, 1339–1343. [CrossRef]

37. Kırmızıbekmez, H.; Kúsz, N.; Bérdi, P.; Zupkó, I.; Hohmann, J. New iridoids from the roots of *Valeriana dioscoridis* Sm. *Fitoterapia* **2018**, *130*, 73–78. [CrossRef]

38. Sheng, L.; Yang, Y.; Zhang, Y.; Li, N. Chemical constituents of *Patrinia heterophylla* Bunge and selective cytotoxicity against six human tumor cells. *J. Ethnopharmacol.* **2019**, *236*, 129–135. [CrossRef]

39. Saidi, I.; Baccari, W.; Marchal, A.; Waffo-Téguo, W.; Harrath, A.H.; Mansour, L.; Jannet, H.B. Iridoid glycosides from the Tunisian *Citharexylum spinosum* L.: Isolation, structure elucidation, biological evaluation, molecular docking and SAR analysis. *Ind. Crops Prod.* **2020**, *151*, 112440. [CrossRef]

40. Saidi, I.; Nimbarte, V.D.; Schwalbe, H.; Wafoo-Téguo, P.; Harrath, A.H.; Mansour, L.; Alwasel, S.; Jannet, H.B. Anti-tyrosinase, anti-cholinesterase and cytotoxic activities of extracts and phytochemicals from the Tunisian *Citharexylum spinosum* L.: Molecular docking and SAR analysis. *Bioorganic Chem.* **2020**, *102*, 104093. [CrossRef] [PubMed]

41. Hu, Z.; Wang, H.; Fu, Y.; Ma, K.; Ma, X.; Wang, J. Gentiopicroside inhibits cell growth and migration on cervical cancer via the recriprocal MAPK/Akt signaling pathways. *Nutr. Cancer* **2021**, *73*, 1459–1470. [CrossRef] [PubMed]

42. Qu, Z.; Ma, L.; Zhang, Q.; Yang, R.; Hou, G.; Wang, Y.; Zhao, F. Characterization, crystal structure and cytotoxic activity of a rare iridoid glycoside from *Lonicera saccata*. *Acta Crystallogr. Sect. C Struct. Chem.* **2020**, *C76*, 269–275. [CrossRef]

43. Fukuyama, Y.; Minoshima, Y.; Kishimoto, Y.; Chen, I.S.; Takahashi, H.; Esumi, T. Iridoid glucosides and *p*-coumaroyl iridoids from *Viburnum luzonicum* and their cytotoxicity. *J. Nat. Prod.* **2004**, *67*, 1833–1838. [CrossRef]

44. Discovery Studio 2021. Available online: https://discover.3ds.com/discovery-studio-visualizer-download (accessed on 5 August 2023).
45. Yang, Y.; Yang, Y.; Hou, J.; Ding, Y.; Zhang, T.; Zhang, Y.; Wang, J.; Shi, C.; Fu, W.; Cai, Z. The hydroxyl at position C1 of Genipin is the active inhibitory group that affects mitochondrial uncoupling protein 2 in Panc-1 cells. *PLoS ONE* **2016**, *11*, e0147026. [CrossRef]
46. Brown, S.; Clastre, M.; Courdavault, V.; O'Connor, S.E. De novo production of the plant-derived alkaloid strictosidine in yeast. *Proc. Natl. Acad. Sci. USA* **2015**, *112*, 3205–3210. [CrossRef] [PubMed]
47. Nagatoshi, M.; Terasaka, K.; Nagatsu, A.; Mizukami, H. Iridoid-specific glucosyltransferase from *Gardenia jasminoides*. *J. Biol. Chem.* **2011**, *286*, 32866–32874. [CrossRef] [PubMed]
48. Pungitore, C.R.; García, C.; Sotero Martín, V.; Tonn, C.E. Inhibition of Taq DNA polymerase by iridoid aglycone derivates. *Cell. Mol. Biol.* **2012**, *58*, 1786–1790. [CrossRef]
49. Skehan, P.; Storeng, R.; Scudiero, D.; Monks, A.; McMahon, J.; Vistica, D.; Warren, J.T.; Bokesch, H.; Kenney, S.; Boyd, M.R. New colorimetric cytotoxic assay for anticancer-drug screening. *J. Natl. Cancer Inst.* **1990**, *82*, 1107–1112. [CrossRef]
50. Vichai, V.; Kirtikara, K. Sulforhodamine B colorimetric assay for cytotoxicity screening. *Nat. Protoc.* **2006**, *1*, 1112–1116. [CrossRef]
51. Peña-Morán, O.A.; Villarreal, M.L.; Álvarez-Berber, L.; Meneses-Acosta, A.; Rodríguez-López, V. Cytotoxicity, Post-Treatment Recovery, and Selectivity Analysis of Naturally Occurring Podophyllotoxins from *Bursera fagaroides* var. *fagaroides* on Breast Cancer Cell Lines. *Molecules* **2016**, *21*, 1013. [CrossRef]
52. Sanchez-Carranza, J.N.; González-Maya, L.; Razo-Hernández, R.S.; Salas-Vidal, E.; Nolasco-Quintana, N.Y.; Clemente-Soto, A.F.; García-Arizmendi, L.; Sánchez-Ramos, M.; Marquina, S.; Alvarez, L. Achillin Increases Chemosensitivity to Paclitaxel, Overcoming Resistance and Enhancing Apoptosis in Human Hepatocellular Carcinoma Cell Line Resistant to Paclitaxel (Hep3B/PTX). *Pharmaceutics* **2019**, *11*, 512. [CrossRef]
53. Halgren, T.A. Merck Molecular Force Field. I. Basis, form, scope, parameterization and performance of MMFF94. *J. Comput. Chem.* **1996**, *17*, 490–519. [CrossRef]
54. Stewart, J.P.J. Optimization of parameters for semiempirical methods I. Method. *J. Comput. Chem.* **1989**, *10*, 209–220. [CrossRef]
55. Stephens, P.J.; Devlin, F.; Chabalowski, C.F.; Frisch, M.J. Ab Initio calculation of vibrational absorption and circular dichroism spectra using density functional force fields: A comparison of local, nonlocal, and hybrid density functionals. *J. Phys. Chem.* **1994**, *45*, 11623–11627. [CrossRef]
56. Hay, P.J.; Wadt, W.R. Ab initio effective core potentials for molecular calculations. Potentials for main group elements Na to Bi. *J. Chem. Phys.* **1985**, *82*, 284–298. [CrossRef]
57. Chambers, C.C.; Hawkins, G.D.; Cramer, C.J.; Truhlar, D.G. Model for aqueous solvation based on class IV atomic charges and first solvation shell effects. *J. Chem. Phys.* **1996**, *100*, 16385–16398. [CrossRef]
58. Petersson, G.A.; Tensfeldt, T.G.; Montgomery, J.A. A complete basis set model chemistry. III. The complete basis set-quadratic configuration interaction family of methods. *J. Chem. Phys.* **1991**, *94*, 6091–6101. [CrossRef]
59. Wavefunction, Inc. Spartan'20. Available online: https://www.wavefun.com (accessed on 30 July 2023).
60. Virtual Computational Chemistry Laboratory. Available online: https://vcclab.org/lab/alogps/ (accessed on 25 August 2023).
61. Razo-Hernández, R.S.; Pineda-Urbina, K.; Velazco-Medel, M.A.; Villanueva-García, M.; Sumaya-Martínez, M.T.; Martínez-Martínez, F.J.; Gómez-Sandoval, Z. QSAR study of the DPPH· radical scavenging activity of coumarin derivatives and xanthine oxidase inhibition by molecular docking. *Cent. Eur. J. Chem.* **2014**, *12*, 1067–1080. [CrossRef]
62. Marquina, S.; Maldonado-Santiago, M.; Sánchez-Carranza, J.N.; Antúnez-Mojica, M.; González-Maya, L.; Razo-Hernández, R.S.; Alvarez, L. Design, synthesis and QSAR study of 2′-hydroxy-4′-alkoxy chalcone derivatives that exert cytotoxic activity by the mitochondrial apoptotic pathway. *Bioorganic Med. Chem.* **2019**, *27*, 43–54. [CrossRef]

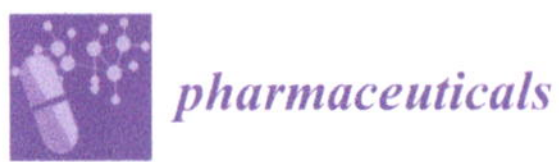 *pharmaceuticals*

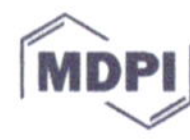

Article

Analgesic Activity of 5-Acetamido-2-Hydroxy Benzoic Acid Derivatives and an In-Vivo and In-Silico Analysis of Their Target Interactions

Cleydson B. R. Santos [1,2,*], Cleison C. Lobato [1,2], Sirlene S. B. Ota [2], Rai C. Silva [1,2], Renata C. V. S. Bittencourt [1], Jofre J. S. Freitas [3], Elenilze F. B. Ferreira [4], Marília B. Ferreira [1,3], Renata C. Silva [3], Anderson B. De Lima [3], Joaquín M. Campos [5,6], Rosivaldo S. Borges [2] and José A. H. M. Bittencourt [1,*]

[1] Laboratory of Modeling and Computational Chemistry, Department of Biological and Health Sciences, Federal University of Amapá, Macapá 68902-280, AP, Brazil; cleyson.cl@gmail.com (C.C.L.); camposchemistry@gmail.com (R.C.S.); recrisvale@hotmail.com (R.C.V.S.B.); maribrazaof@gmail.com (M.B.F.)
[2] Graduate Program on Medicinal Chemistry and Molecular Modeling, Institute of Health Science, Federal University of Pará, Belém 66075-110, PA, Brazil; sayuriota@gmail.com (S.S.B.O.); rosborg@ufpa.br (R.S.B.)
[3] Laboratory of Morphophysiology Applied to Health, State University of Pará, Belém 66095-662, PA, Brazil; jofre.freitas@uepa.br (J.J.S.F.); renatacs690@gmail.com (R.C.S.); andersonbentes@uepa.br (A.B.D.L.)
[4] Laboratory of Organic Chemistry and Biochemistry, University of the State of Amapá, Macapá 68900-070, AP, Brazil; elenilze.batista@ueap.edu.br
[5] Department of Pharmaceutical and Organic Chemistry, Faculty of Pharmacy, Campus of Cartuja, University of Granada, 18071 Granada, Spain; jmcampos@ugr.es
[6] Biosanitary Institute of Granada (ibs.GRANADA), University of Granada, 18071 Granada, Spain
[*] Correspondence: breno@unifap.br (C.B.R.S.); joseadolfo@unifap.br (J.A.H.M.B.)

Citation: Santos, C.B.R.; Lobato, C.C.; Ota, S.S.B.; Silva, R.C.; Bittencourt, R.C.V.S.; Freitas, J.J.S.; Ferreira, E.F.B.; Ferreira, M.B.; Silva, R.C.; De Lima, A.B.; et al. Analgesic Activity of 5-Acetamido-2-Hydroxy Benzoic Acid Derivatives and an In-Vivo and In-Silico Analysis of Their Target Interactions. *Pharmaceuticals* **2023**, *16*, 1584. https://doi.org/10.3390/ph16111584

Academic Editors: Halil İbrahim Ciftci, Belgin Sever and Hasan Demirci

Received: 4 June 2023
Revised: 4 October 2023
Accepted: 27 October 2023
Published: 9 November 2023

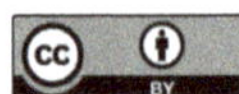

Abstract: The design, synthesis, and evaluation of novel non-steroidal anti-inflammatory drugs (NSAIDs) with better activity and lower side effects are big challenges today. In this work, two 5-acetamido-2-hydroxy benzoic acid derivatives were proposed, increasing the alkyl position (methyl) in an acetamide moiety, and synthesized, and their structural elucidation was performed using ^{1}H NMR and ^{13}C NMR. The changes in methyl in larger groups such as phenyl and benzyl aim to increase their selectivity over cyclooxygenase 2 (COX-2). These 5-acetamido-2-hydroxy benzoic acid derivatives were prepared using classic methods of acylation reactions with anhydride or acyl chloride. Pharmacokinetics and toxicological properties were predicted using computational tools, and their binding affinity (kcal/mol) with COX-2 receptors (*Mus musculus* and *Homo sapiens*) was analyzed using docking studies (PDB ID 4PH9, 5KIR, 1PXX and 5F1A). An in-silico study showed that 5-acetamido-2-hydroxy benzoic acid derivates have a better bioavailability and binding affinity with the COX-2 receptor, and in-vivo anti-nociceptive activity was investigated by means of a writhing test induced by acetic acid and a hot plate. PS3, at doses of 20 and 50 mg/kg, reduced painful activity by 74% and 75%, respectively, when compared to the control group (20 mg/kg). Regarding the anti-nociceptive activity, the benzyl showed reductions in painful activity when compared to acetaminophen and 5-acetamido-2-hydroxy benzoic acid. However, the proposed derivatives are potentially more active than 5-acetamido-2-hydroxy benzoic acid and they support the design of novel and safer derivative candidates. Consequently, more studies need to be conducted to evaluate the different pharmacological actions, the toxicity of possible metabolites that can be generated, and their potential use in inflammation and pain therapy.

Keywords: analgesic; 5-acetamido-2-hydroxy benzoic acid; molecular docking; ADME; toxicity

1. Introduction

The inflammatory process has a great impact on several pathophysiological functions in living organisms. However, some events, especially those promoted by the uncontrolled immune system, have a negative effect on the body, such as inflammation, pain, aggression, and loss of function. One way to alleviate the symptoms resulting from this process is using non-steroidal anti-inflammatory drugs. However, these medications may have adverse effects such as gastric irritation, hepatotoxicity, nephrotoxicity, and other side effects [1,2]. The undesirable side effects promoted by these therapeutic agents have directed the search for new compounds for which the anti-inflammatory potential is accompanied by greater selectivity, greater specificity, minimal side effects and a low cost of production [3,4].

Moreover, 5-acetamido-2-hydroxy benzoic acid (PS1) was developed through rational drug design and molecular modeling using the molecular association between paracetamol (PAR) or acetaminophen and salicylic acid (SAC) at the Nucleus of Studies and Selection of Bioactive Molecules (NESBio) at the Federal University of Pará (UFPA, Brazil), in partnership with the research group Applied Computational Chemistry at the Federal University of Amapá (UNIFAP, Brazil—http://dgp.cnpq.br/dgp/espelhogrupo/10685, accessed on 10 March 2021) (see Figure 1). It showed a superior capacity when compared to other salicylates used in anti-inflammatory therapy and could represent an important strategy in the development of aspirin derivatives when applied to patients with a risk of resistance to the preventive treatment of cerebral vascular accident [5,6]. After that, a study to evaluate its acute oral toxicity, anti-nociceptive and anti-inflammatory properties was conducted by the pharmacology group at the College of Pharmacy at UFPA, Brazil [7,8].

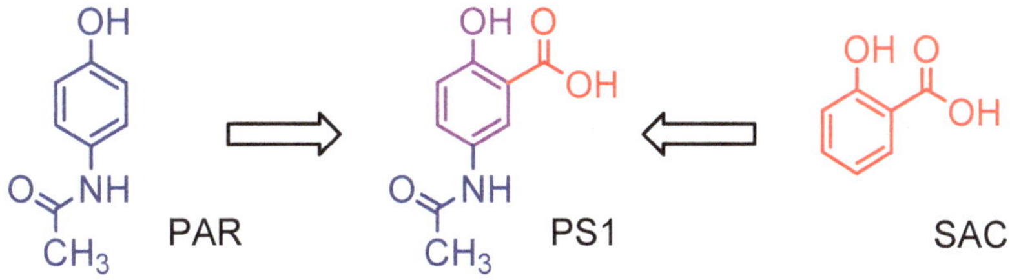

Figure 1. Chemical structure of 5-acetamido-2-hydroxy benzoic acid (PS1).

Acute toxicity was based on OECD guideline 423, where no death was observed due to the administration of 5-acetamido-2-hydroxy benzoic acid at doses of 2000 and 5000 mg/kg. When comparing with their relatives, we emphasize a value of 1500 mg/kg for the acute toxicity (LD_{50}) of acetylsalicylic acid (ASA) and 1944 mg/kg for acetaminophen (ACP) [6]. Next, the anti-nociceptive properties of 5-acetamido-2-hydroxy benzoic acid were investigated using the contortion, hot-plate and formalin tests in Swiss mice. The anti-edematogenic properties were evaluated using the carrageenan-induced paw edema model and croton oil-induced dermatitis in Wistar rats, and 5-acetamido-2-hydroxy benzoic acid did not promote behavioral changes or animal deaths during the acute evaluation of oral toxicity [6].

The 5-acetamido-2-hydroxy benzoic acid exhibited peripheric anti-nociceptive activity, evidenced by the reduction in the behavior of abdominal writhing induced by acetic acid, presenting an ED_{50} value of 4.95 mg/kg, as well as an anti-inflammatory effect in the formalin test in the inflammatory phase but not in the neurogenic phase [6]. When comparing this analgesic effect with its AAS relatives, which present values of 67.5 mg/kg and 125 mg/kg for the ACP, it shows a superior activity 10 to 25 times more potent than its precursors. In addition, 5-acetamido-2-hydroxy benzoic acid induced central anti-nociceptive activity in the hot-plate test both in the neurogenic phase and in the inflammatory phase of the formalin test, being effective in reducing edema formation induced by carrageenan or croton oil [6,7].

The main problem with its possible therapeutic application was its low plasma bioavailability; the compound shows a peak in the first two hours and then begins to fall rapidly [7–10]. However, the changes in methyl red (PS1) in larger groups such as phenyl (PS2) and benzyl (PS3) aim to increase their selectivity over cyclooxygenase 2 (COX-2), also increasing the bioavailability parameters (see Figure 2).

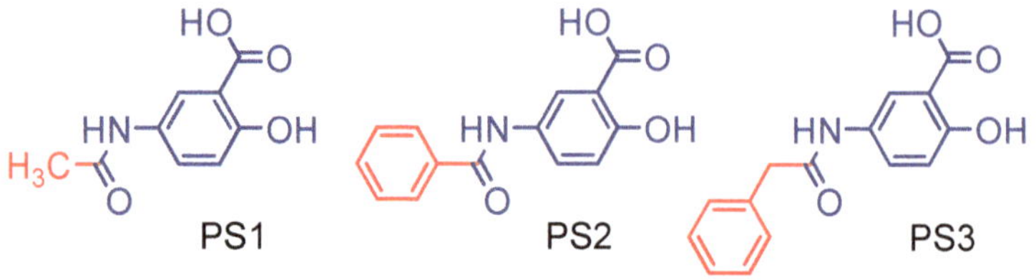

Figure 2. The 5-acetamido-2-hydroxy benzoic acid (PS1) and derivatives (PS2 and PS3).

In this study, the main objective was to evaluate the pharmacokinetic, toxicity, biological activity, and analgesia properties of the new 5-acetamido-2-hydroxy benzoic acid derivatives through the association of computational techniques and in-vivo experimental studies.

2. Results

2.1. Synthesis of 5-Acetamido-2-Hydroxy Benzoic Acid and Derivatives

The 5-amino-2-hydroxy benzoic acid (A) was used as the starting reagent to obtain 5-acetamido-2-hydroxy benzoic acid and its derivatives by acetylation (PS1) and *N*-acylation reactions with benzoyl chloride (PS2) or phenylacetyl chloride (PS3), using water or ethyl acetate as solvents and potassium carbonate as a catalyst (see Figure 3).

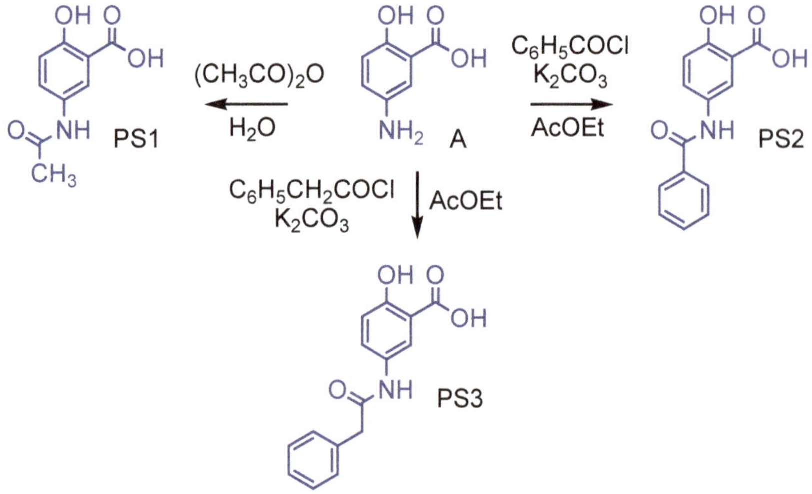

Figure 3. Synthetic methodology for the preparation of 5-acetamido-2-hydroxy benzoic acid and derivatives.

The salicylamide (5-acetamido-2-hydroxy benzoic acid, PS1) was obtained by a reaction between 5-amino salicylic acid and acetic anhydride using water as a solvent. It was cold-soluble in ethanol, methanol, dimethylsulfoxide (DMSO), acetonitrile, acetic acid and acetone, and hot-soluble in ethyl acetate and water. The 5-benzamidosalicylic acid compound (PS2) was obtained by a reaction between 5-amino-salicylic acid and benzoyl chloride using ethyl acetate as a solvent and potassium carbonate as a catalyst. It was cold-soluble in methanol and DMSO and hot-soluble in ethyl acetate, acetonitrile, acetone, acetic acid and ethanol. The 5-phenylacetamidosalicylic acid compound (PS3) was obtained by a reaction between 5-amino-salicylic acid and phenylacetoyl chloride using ethyl acetate as a solvent and potassium carbonate as a catalyst. It was cold-soluble in methanol, DMSO, ethyl acetate, acetonitrile, acetone, acetic acid and ethanol.

2.2. In-Silico Study of Oral Bioavailability, Bioactivity, ADME and Toxicity Risk Assessment

Molecular weight is an important aspect of therapeutic drug action; if it increases beyond a certain limit, the bulkiness of the compounds also increases correspondingly, which in turn affects the drug action [11–13].

Even some drug molecules with a molecular weight higher than that established by Lipinski's five rule (<500 Da) violate this principle and may have a good liposolubility profile. Druglikeness molecular descriptors of 5-acetamido-2-hydroxy benzoic acid derivatives are given in Table 1 and were tested against Lipinski's rule of five. Compounds PS1, PS2 and PS3 have a molecular weight that varied from 208.21 to 271.27 Da, respectively. Thus, drug molecules that present MW < 500 are easily transported, diffused and absorbed as compared to heavy molecules [12] (see Table 1).

Table 1. Oral bioavailability properties for 5-acetamido-2-hydroxy benzoic acid derivatives.

Compounds	MW [1] (<500 Da)	HBA [2] ($\leq$10)	HBD [3] ($\leq$5)	LogP ($\leq$5) [4]	MPSA (Å^2) [5]	MV (Å^3) [6]	NRB [7]
Ibuprofen	206.28	2	1	3.46	37.30	211.19	4
Diclofenac	296.15	3	2	4.57	49.33	238.73	4
Acetaminophen	151.16	3	2	0.68	49.33	140.01	1
Salicylic acid	137.11	3	1	−1.81	60.36	116.32	1
Rofecoxib	314.36	4	0	0.71	60.45	264.79	3
PS1	208.21	5	3	1.06	86.62	167.01	2
PS2	210.19	5	3	2.74	86.62	221.86	3
PS3	271.27	5	3	2.83	86.62	238.66	4

[1] Molecular weight, [2] Hydrogen bond acceptor, [3] Hydrogen bond donor, [4] Logarithm of the partition between of n-octanol and water phases, [5] MPSA (molecular polar surface area), [6] MV (molecular volume) and [7] NRB (number of rotatable bonds) were obtained.

The activity of 5-acetamido-2-hydroxy benzoic acid derivatives against the GPCR ligand, ion channel modulator, kinase inhibitor, nuclear receptor ligand, protease inhibitor and enzyme inhibitory activity were predicted via the Molinspiration server (https://www.molinspiration.com, accessed on 21 November 2021.) and are summarized in Table 2. The molecules with a bioactivity score of more than 0.00 are likely to possess considerable biological activities, according to Roy et al. (2015) [13]. The values from −0.50 to 0.00 are expected to be moderately active, and if the score is less than −0.50, it is presumed to be inactive.

Table 2. Bioactivity of the 5-acetamido-2-hydroxy benzoic acid derivatives and commercial drug [1].

Compounds	GPCR	Ion Channel Modulator	Kinase Inhibitor	Nuclear Receptor Ligand	Protease Inhibitor	Enzyme Inhibitor
Ibuprofen	−0.17	−0.01	−0.72	0.05	−0.21	0.12
Diclofenac	0.14	0.20	0.17	0.09	−0.10	0.25
Acetaminophen	−1.05	−0.54	−1.04	−1.21	−1.20	−0.68
Rofecoxib	0.20	−0.18	−0.18	0.12	0.26	0.61
Salicylic Acid	−1.00	−0.41	−1.26	−1.26	−1.13	−0.48
PS1	−0.67	−0.38	−0.70	−0.64	−0.76	−0.33
PS2	−0.20	−0.21	−0.13	−0.15	−0.25	−0.04
PS3	−0.10	−0.19	−0.15	−0.04	−0.14	−0.02

[1] Score Values > 0.00 = considerable biological activities; Score Values −0.50 to 0.00 = moderately active; score values < −0.50 = considerable inactive.

The prediction of Absorption, Distribution, Metabolism and Excretion (ADME) proprieties for 5-acetamido-2-hydroxy benzoic acid derivatives are shown in Table 3. Such ADME predictions were based on literature studies [14–18].

Table 3. Absorption and distribution properties in percentages of PPB and penetration of the blood–brain barrier for 5-acetamido-2-hydroxy benzoic acid derivatives and commercial drug.

Compounds	Absorption			Distribuition	
	HIA [1]	P_{caco-2} [2]	P_{MDCK} [3]	PPB (%) [4]	C_{Brain}/C_{Blood} [5]
Ibuprofen	98.38	21.20	136.48	88.24	1.26
Diclofenac	95.95	24.53	51.46	91.95	1.39
Acetaminophen	88.23	18.78	15.43	0.00	0.61
Salicylic Acid	86.59	20.43	25.36	7.31	0.43
Rofecoxib	98.22	2.72	11.27	0.00	0.61
PS1	75.97	19.93	5.17	14.34	0.35
PS2	91.29	18.29	51.99	69.05	0.50
PS3	91.95	20.70	31.04	66.41	0.15

[1] Percentage of human intestinal absorption; [2] cell permeability (Caco-2 in nm/s); [3] cell permeability Maden Darby Canine Kidney in nm/s; [4] percentage of plasma protein binding; [5] penetration of the blood–brain barrier.

Table 4 shows the results of toxicity predictions using the identification of toxicophoric groups of 5-acetamido-2-hydroxy benzoic acid derivatives. This evaluation was conducted using the Deductive Estimation of Risk from Existing Knowledge (DEREK) 10.0.2 program [19–21]. We have considered DEREK alerts of toxicity involving the human species that are classified as plausible in mammals.

Table 4. Toxicity prediction by the identification of toxicophoric groups and LD_{50} for 5-acetamido-2-hydroxy benzoic acid and derivatives.

Compounds	Toxicity Prediction Alert (Lhasa Prediction)	Toxicophoric Group	Toxicity Alert	LD_{50} Toxic [1]	Toxicity Class [2]
Ibuprofen	Hepatotoxicity in human, mouse and rat	2-arylacetic or 3-arylpropionic acid	PLAUSIBLE	299	III
		Alpha-substituted propionic acid or ester			
Diclofenac	Hepatotoxicity in human	2-arylacetic or 3-arylpropionic acid	CERTAIN	53	III
	Nephrotoxicity in human, mouse and rat	Aryl or fulvenyl acetic or 2-propionic acid derivative	PLAUSIBLE		
Acetaminophen	Chromosome damage in vitro in human	Phenol	CERTAIN	338	III
		Phenol	PROBABLE		
	Hepatotoxicity in human, mouse and rat	Para-aminophenol or derivative	CERTAIN		
Rofecoxib	-	-	NO ALERTS	4500	V
Salicylic Acid	-	-	NO ALERTS	480	IV
PS1	Hepatotoxicity in human, mouse and rat	Salicylic acid or analog	PLAUSIBLE	2800	V
		Para-Aminophenol or derivative			
PS2	Carcinogenicity in mouse and rat	Alkylaryl or bisaryl carboxylic acid or precursor	PLAUSIBLE	2400	V
	Hepatotoxicity in human, mouse and rat	Salicylic acid or analog			
	Peroxisome proliferation in mouse and rat	Para-aminophenol or derivative			
PS3	Hepatotoxicity in human, mouse and rat	Salicylic acid or analog	PLAUSIBLE	2175	V
		Para-aminophenol or derivative			

[1] Values in mg/kg body weight. [2] Class I: fatal if swallowed ($LD_{50} \leq 5$); Class II: fatal if swallowed ($5 < LD_{50} \leq 50$); Class III: toxic if swallowed ($50 < LD_{50} \leq 300$); Class IV: harmful if swallowed ($300 < LD_{50} \leq 2000$); Class V: may be harmful if swallowed ($2000 < LD_{50} \leq 5000$); Class VI: non-toxic ($LD_{50} > 5000$) [12].

2.3. Molecular Docking Simulations

The comparison between crystallographic ligands ibuprofen, rofecoxib, diclofenac and salicylic acid (red color) and the best conformation predicted by molecular docking (green color) can be seen in Figure 4, and the comparisons between experimental and predicted binding affinities are shown in Table 5.

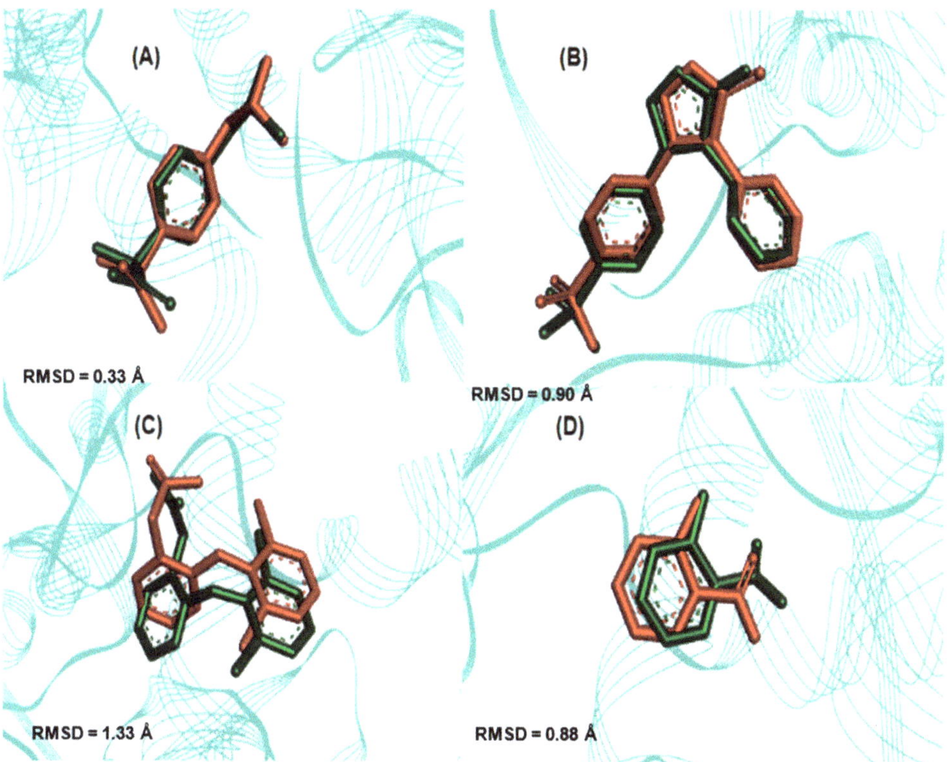

Figure 4. Superpositions of crystallographic ligands poses (in red) with the calculated poses (in green): (**A**) COX-2 (*Mus musculus*, PDB ID 4PH9–RMSD 0.33 Å), (**B**) COX-2 (*Homo sapiens*, PDB ID 5KIR–RMSD 0.90 Å), (**C**) COX-2 (*Mus musculus*, PDB ID 1PXX–RMSD 1.34 Å) and (**D**) COX-2 (*Homo sapiens*, PDB ID 5F1A–RMSD 0.88 Å) with respective crystallographic ligands.

Table 5. Comparison between experimental and theoretical binding affinities.

Enzyme COX2	Ligand	Experimental Binding Affinity * (kcal/mol)	Ki (nM)	Docking Predicted Binding Affinity (kcal/mol)	Resolution (Å)
(PDB ID 4PH9)	Ibuprofen	−7.3	$7.2.10^3$ [22]	−7.6	1.81
(PDB ID 5KIR)	Rofecoxib	−9.2	310 [23]	−10.0	2.69
(PDB ID 1PXX)	Diclofenac	−11.3	1.10^4 [24]	−8.6	2.90
(PDB ID 5F1A)	salicylic acid	−6.7	1.10^4 [25]	−6.1	2.38
(PDB ID 4PH9)	Ibuprofen	−7.3	$7.2.10^3$ [22]	−7.6	1.81

* Values calculated from experimentally determined inhibition constants (Ki), found in the PDBs, according to Equation: $\Delta G = R.T.\ln Ki$ [26,27], were R (constant of gas) = $1.987 \cdot 10^{-3}$ kcal/(mol K) and T (temperature) = 310 K.

The validation was accepted despite the minor deviation observed between the poses because the two crystallographic poses are possible. This was in order to evaluate whether the changes made would lead to a higher binding affinity than the respective inhibitor to each target. After validation, molecular docking was used to predict the modes of interaction and binding affinity of the PS1, PS2 and PS3 ligands. Figure 5 shows the best binding affinity values, in kcal/mol, of the ligands with COX-2 (PDB ID 4PH9).

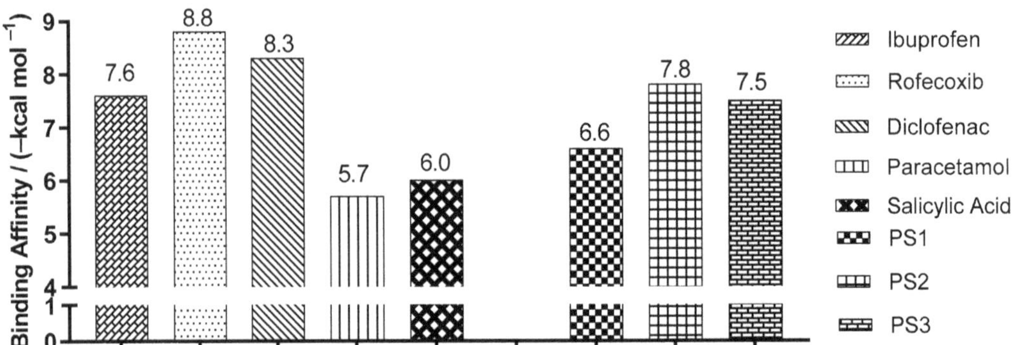

Figure 5. Binding affinity values of the ligands with COX-2 (*Mus musculus*) PDB ID 4PH9, by molecular docking.

Figure 6 shows the best binding affinity values, in kcal/mol, of the ligands with COX-2 (PDB ID 5KIR) of *Homo sapiens*. The control structure of rofecoxib exhibited a binding affinity of -10.0 kcal/mol, lower than PS1, PS2 and PS3, which presented values of -7.2, -8.5, -9.1 kcal/mol, with a variation of ±2.8, ±1.5 and ±0.9 kcal/mol, respectively.

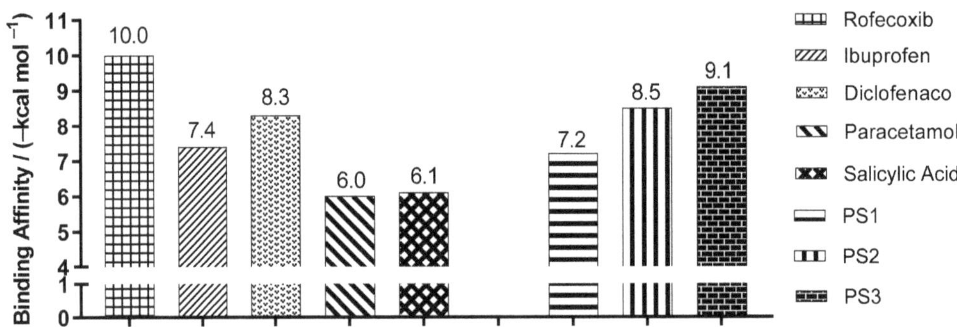

Figure 6. Binding affinity values of the ligands with COX-2 (*Homo sapiens*) PDB ID 5KIR, obtained by molecular docking.

Figure 7 shows the best binding affinity values, in kcal/mol, of the ligands with COX-2 (PDB ID 1PXX) of *Mus musculus*. The control structure of diclofenac exhibited a binding affinity of -8.6 kcal/mol, smaller than PS1, varying by ±2.2 kcal/mol. When compared to the PS2 and PS3 structures, the affinity values were the same.

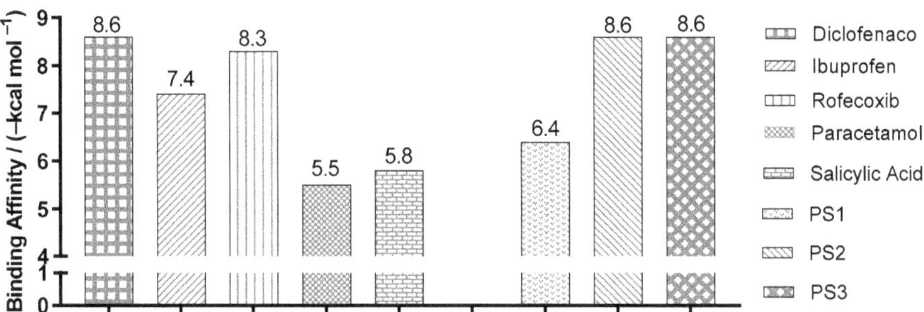

Figure 7. Binding affinity values of the ligands with COX-2 (*Mus musculus*) PDB ID 1PXX, obtained by molecular docking.

Figure 8 shows the best binding affinity values, in kcal/mol, of the ligands with COX-2 (PDB ID 5F1A) of *Homo sapiens*. The control structure of salicylic acid exhibited a binding affinity of -6.1 kcal/mol. Compared with salicylic acid, PS1, PS2 and PS3 showed better bond affinity values of -6.7, -7.2 and -7.8 kcal/mol, with a variation of ±0.6, ±1.1 and ±1.7 kcal/mol, respectively.

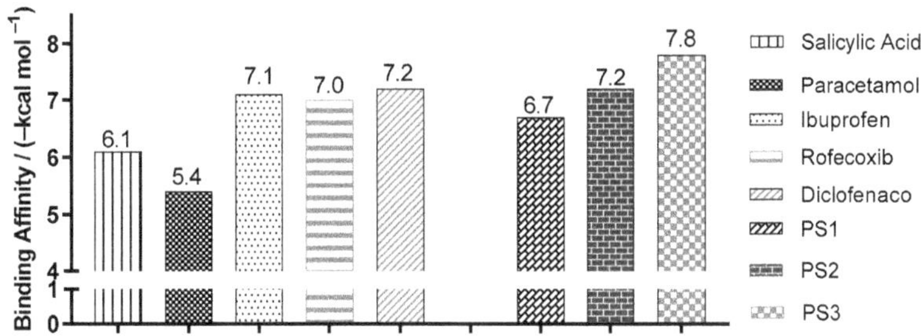

Figure 8. Binding affinity values of the ligands with COX-2 (Homo sapiens) PDB ID 5F1A, obtained by molecular docking.

Crystallographic structures of the COX-2 enzyme with carboxylic acid-containing non-steroidal anti-inflammatory drugs show that the inhibitors are positioned in a similar manner with their coordinated carboxylates for Arg120 and their aromatic functionality protruding into the active site of cyclooxygenase toward Tyr385 [24] (see Figure 9).

2.4. Anti-Nociceptive Activity

2.4.1. Central Analgesic Activity

PS1 at a dose of 20 mg/kg prolonged the increase in latency (the time that the animals needed to manifest a stereotyped reaction to the heat stimulus) in a significant way in 30 min, and PS2 had a high variation in the same time period. PS3 and acetaminophen did not show central analgesic activity when compared to the control group. However, morphine (an opioid drug) significantly prolonged the latency at 30, 60 and 90 min in the hot-plate test (see Figure 10).

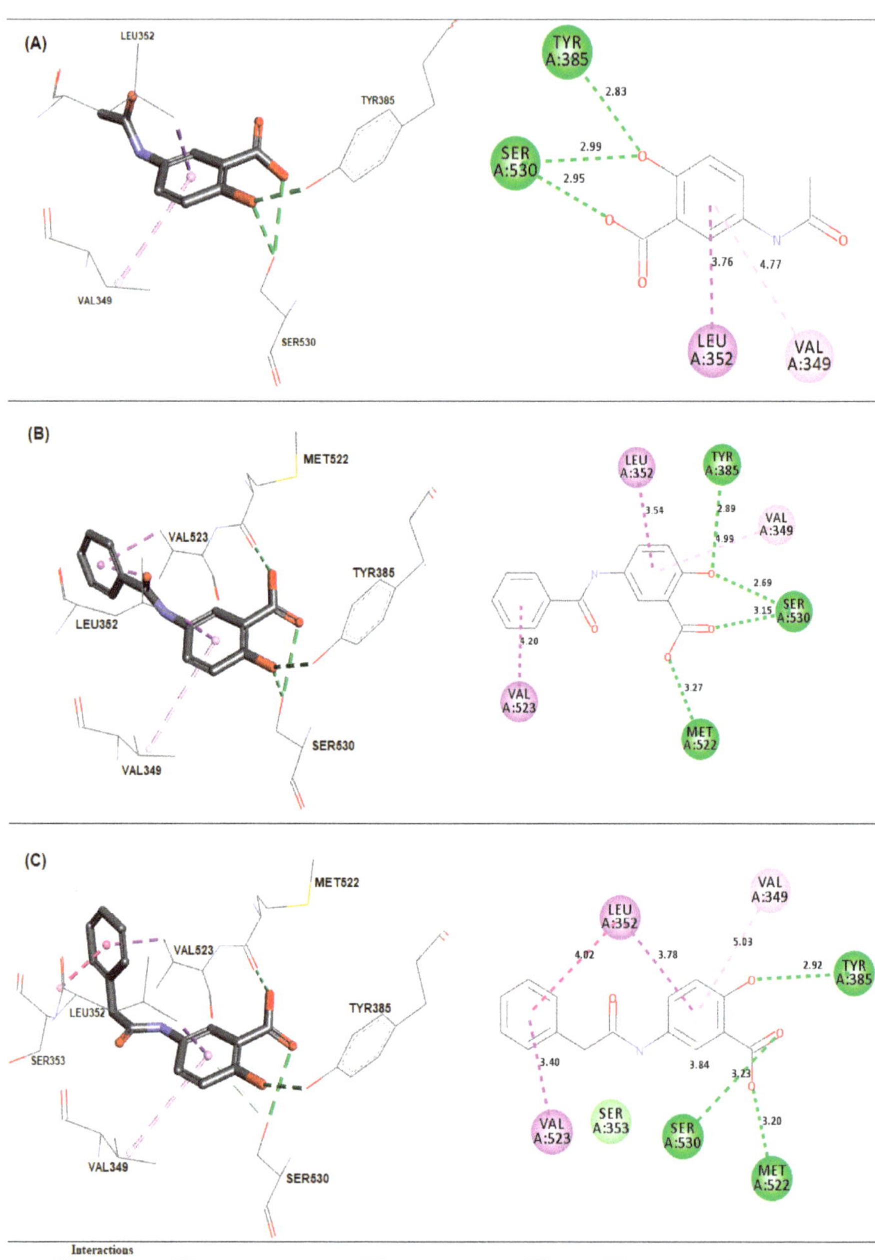

Figure 9. Interactions and distances (Å) predicted between the active site of COX-2 and compound PS1 (**A**), PS2 (**B**) and PS3 (**C**).

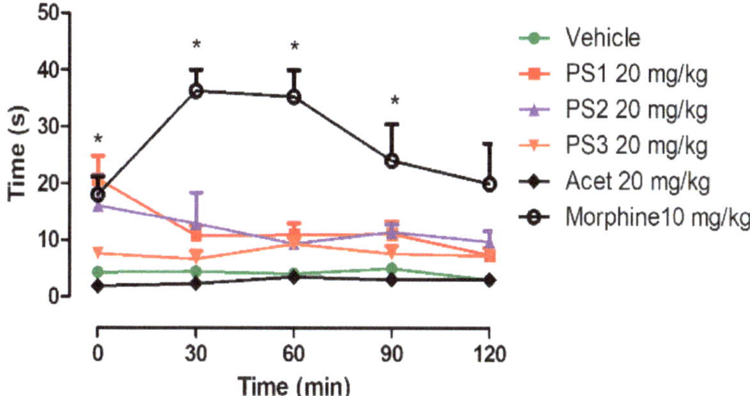

Figure 10. Effect of PS1, PS2, PS3 and Acetaminophen (Acet) at a dose of 20 mg/kg and morphine at a dose of 10 mg/kg on the nociceptive heat stimulus (55 ± 0.1 °C) induced in mice. Each point represents mean ± e.p.m. of five animals. * $p < 0.05$, when compared to the control group; ANOVA, Dunn's method.

2.4.2. Peripheral Analgesic Activity

In this model, acetic acid releases endogenous mediators (histamine, serotonin, bradykinin, substance P, and prostaglandins, especially PGI2, as well as some cytokines such as interleukin 1β (IL-1β), tumor necrosis factor (TNF-α) and interleukin 8) that are involved in the development of inflammatory pain. Acetaminophen is an analgesic drug used as the standard drug in this study (control group) (see Figure 11).

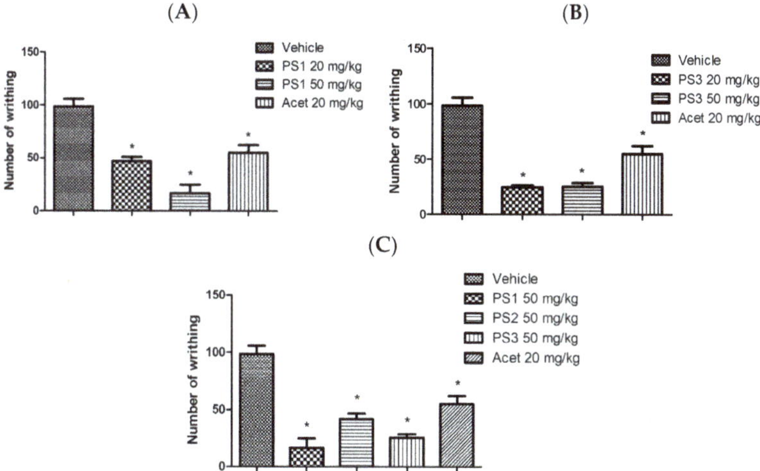

Figure 11. (**A**) Effect of PS1 and Acetaminophen (Acet) on the nociceptive stimulus induced by intraperitoneal injection of 0.6% acetic acid in mice. (**B**) Effect of PS3 and Acet on the nociceptive stimulus induced by the intraperitoneal injection of 0.6% acetic acid in mice. (**C**) Comparison of compounds (PS1, PS2 and PS3 at a dose of 50 mg/kg) with Acet at a dose of 20 mg/kg on the nociceptive stimulus induced by the intraperitoneal injection of 0.6% acetic acid in mice. Each column represents mean ± e.p.m. of five animals. * $p < 0.05$, when compared to the control group; ANOVA, Student-Newman–Keuls test.

3. Discussion

3.1. Synthesis of 5-Acetamido-2-Hydroxy Benzoic Acid and Derivatives

Compound PS1 is insoluble in dichloromethane, chloroform and hexane. It is a colorless crystalline solid and has a melting point between 228.0 and 230.0 °C [28]. ^{1}H NMR (300 MHz, DMSO-d6) δ (ppm) 6.89 (1H, d, J = 9.0 Hz, H-3), 7.64 (1H, dd, 9.3 and 2.7 Hz, H-4), 8.08 (1H, d, J = 2.7 Hz, H6), 2.00 (3H, s, CH_3, C-8), 9.87 (1H, s, NH). ^{13}C NMR (75 MHz; DMSO-d6) δ (ppm) 112.52 (C-1), 157.16 (C-2), 117.30 (C-3), 120.54 (C-4), 131.28 (C-5), 127.54 (C-6), 171.97 (COOH, C-7), 168.22 (CONH, C-8), 23.94 (CH_3, C-9).

The 5-benzamidosalicylic acid compound, PS2, is insoluble in dichloromethane, chloroform and hexane. It is a crystalline solid of slightly white coloration and has a melting point between 278.4 and 279.8 °C [28]. ^{1}H-NMR (300 MHz; DMSO-d6) δ (ppm) 6.97 (1H, d, 9.0 Hz, H-3), 7.89 (1H, dd, 8.7 and 2.7 Hz, H-4), 8.29 (1H, d, 2.7 Hz, H-6), 10.24 (1H, NH), 7.96 (2H, dd, 6.9 and 1.2 Hz, H-2$'$ and H-6$'$), 7.53 (3H, m, H-3$'$, H-4$'$ and H-5$'$). ^{13}C NMR (75 MHz; DMSO-d6) δ (ppm) 112.54 (C-1), 157.56 (C-2), 117.21 (C-3), 130.99 (C-4), 131.66 (C-5), 128.80 (C-6), 171.92 (COOH, C-7), 165.39 (CONH, C-8), 121.97 (C-1$'$), 127.71 (C-2$'$ and C-6$'$), 128.52 (C-3$'$ and C-5$'$), 134.87 (C-4$'$). All compounds and the numeration studied here are shown in Figure 12.

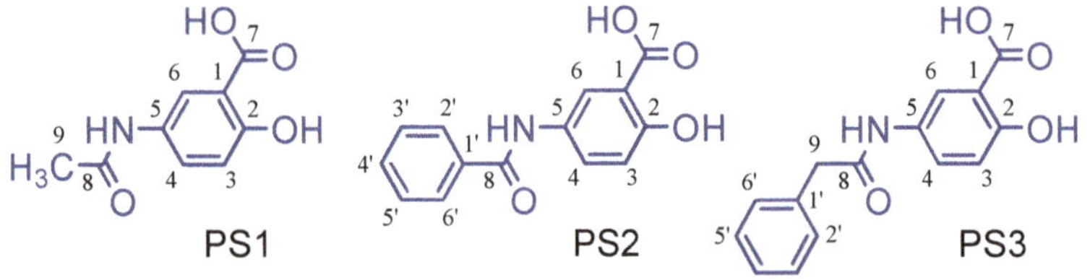

Figure 12. Structure and numeration of all derivatives studied here (PS1, PS2 and PS3).

The 5-phenylacetamidosalicylic acid compound, PS3, is insoluble in dichloromethane, chloroform and hexane. It is a crystalline solid of white coloration with a melting point between 296.4 and 298.8 °C. ^{1}H-NMR (300 MHz; CD_3COCD_3) δ (ppm) 6.90 (1H, d, 9.0 Hz, H-3), 7.75 (1H, dd, 8.7 and 2.7 Hz, H-4), 8.27 (1H, d, 2.7 Hz, H-6), 9.27 (1H, sb, NH), 3.68 (2H, s, CH_2, C-9), 7.33 (2H, dd, 6.9 and 1.2 Hz, H-2$'$ and H-6$'$), 7.40 (2H, m, H-3$'$ and H-5$'$), 7.26 (1H, m, H-4$'$). 13C NMR (75 MHz; CD_3COCD_3) δ (ppm) 117.11 (C-1), 158.06 (C-2), 111.72 (C-3), 131.16 (C-4), 135.99 (C-5), 129.32 (C-6), 171.44 (COOH, C-7), 168.69 (CONH, C-8), 39.40 (CH_2, C-9), 128.25 (C-1$'$), 126.55 (C-2$'$ and C-6$'$), 127.88 (C-3$'$ and C-5$'$), 120.76 (C-4$'$). The compound was compared with previously published results [28].

3.2. In-Silico Study of Oral Bioavailability, Bioactivity, ADME and Toxicity Risk Assessment

In the process of the discovery and development of new drugs, the success rate of new candidates selected for clinical development is approximately 20% [29], with most of the difficulties attributed to nonviable pharmacokinetic properties. Properties include low absorption rate, high liver extraction, and hepatic clearance, which cause low and variable bioavailability. In-vitro metabolic studies provide guidance for subsequent clinical studies [11].

PS1 showed moderate activity as an ion-channel modulator and enzyme inhibitor. Otherwise, PS2 and PS3 showed moderate activity as GPCR ligands, ion-channel modulators, kinase inhibitors, nuclear receptor ligands, protease inhibitors and enzyme inhibitors, also presenting a better profile of biological activity than salicylate and acetaminophen.

Since the G-protein coupled receptors (GPCRs) represent the largest family of cell surface molecules involved in signal transduction [30], some ligands can bind and activate GPCRs, including light-sensitive compounds, odors, pheromones, hormones, neurotransmitters, and peptides or proteins [31–34].

Also, several GPCRs have been reported to be involved in the activation and regulation of the NLRP3 inflammasome by sensing multiple ions, metabolites, neurotransmitters [35] and other therapeutic applications [36,37], including cancer, on similar molecules related to analgesic and anti-inflammatory drugs [38].

Otherwise, these properties can be related to promiscuity molecular prediction. In fact, drug promiscuity is defined as the property of a drug to act with multiple molecular targets and exhibit distinct pharmacological effects [39]. These properties are little explored but can be used in the discovery of new compounds by exploring molecular patterns and multi-target activity spaces [40].

However, no experimental evidence was observed for rofecoxib and diclofenac on GPCRs. Finally, similar compound predictions can be performed on the Molinspiration server and other online programs using druglikeness property determination [39].

Additionally, it is known that GPCRs play important roles in inflammation due to inflammatory cells (polymorphonuclear leukocytes (PMN), monocytes and macrophages) being able to express GPCRs. NSAIDS are effective anti-inflammatory and pain-relieving agents primarily because they block the synthesis of prostaglandins, which are lipid-derived autacoids that can interact with about nine prostanoid receptors that couple to several GPCR proteins [40–42].

In addition to the well-known activity in cyclooxygenase (COX) receptors, there is additional evidence that diclofenac probably activates GPCRs. Prostaglandins (PGs) collectively interact with prostanoid receptors that associate with a variety of G proteins and are responsible for several features of inflammation, including pain and edema [40,41]. Among the various arachidonic acid metabolites, PGE2 interacts with several GPCRs.

Evidence suggests that ATP-sensitive K+ channels are important in the anti-nociceptive action of non-steroidal anti-inflammatory drugs (NSAIDs) [43–45]. This result demonstrates the probable participation of the G+ channels coupled to the G protein in the internal rectifier and in the anti-nociceptive effect of diclofenac [43–45].

Thus, the prediction of the bioactivity of new drug candidates is critical for describing the possible mechanisms of action. In addition, it may assist in the selection of experimental tests to evaluate their pharmacological effects [46–48].

The prediction of human intestinal absorption is a major objective in the optimization and selection of candidates for the development of oral medications. The focus on the discovery of modern drugs is not simply on the pharmacological activity but is also on the search for more favorable pharmacokinetic properties [15].

The results of human intestinal absorption are the sum of absorption and bioavailability, evaluated from the proportion of excretion or cumulative excretion in urine, bile and feces [15,16]. The investigated compounds PS2 and PS3 showed, through prediction, good human intestinal absorption, with values of HIA >90%; this was not the case for PS1, which showed the lowest absorption of 75.9775%.

P_{Caco-2} (nm/s) and P_{MDCK} (nm/s) cell models have been used as reliable in-vitro models for the prediction of oral drug absorption, with the Caco-2 cells being derived from human colon adenocarcinoma, and they have various routes of drug transport through the intestinal epithelium [15,16].

The compounds in Table 3 show a mean permeability of 19.6422, as proposed by Yazdanian et al. (1998) [17]. PS2 showed the lowest value of cell permeability with 18.293 nm/s. According to Irvine et al. (1999) [18], an MDCK cell system can be used as a tool for the rapid screening of permeability. Only PS2 and PS3 showed high permeability in the cell system MDCK (>25). PS1 had the lowest permeability values of MDCK of 5.172 when compared to the controls, PS2 and PS3. The distribution of a drug depends on its plasma protein binding (PPB) and partition in adipose tissue and other tissues. In plasma, the drug may be in an unbound or a bound form, which depends on the affinity that the drug presents by the plasmatic protein (drug target). If the protein binding is reversible, then a chemical equilibrium will exist between bound and unbound states. The protein binding can influence the biological half-life in the body. The bound portion may act as a reservoir or deposit to which the drug is slowly released in the unbound form. As the non-bound form is metabolized and/or excreted from the body, the fraction it is bound to will be released in order to maintain that balance [49,50].

Table 3 shows the results of the distribution properties (PPB% and C_{Brain}/C_{blood}) for the investigated compounds. The salicylamide derivatives PS2 and PS3 showed moderate plasma protein binding with a PPB of 69.05416% and 66.41028%, respectively.

The penetration of the blood–brain barrier is critical in the pharmaceutical field because compounds that act on the central nervous system (CNS) should go through it and inactive compounds in the CNS should not, in order to avoid collateral effects of the CNS [51]. The investigated compounds (PS1, PS2 and PS3) do not show an absorption value in the CNS greater than 1, and this agrees with the classification proposed by Ma et al. (2005) [52]. Compounds that showed a value greater than 1 ($C_{Brain}/C_{Blood} > 1$) were classified as active in the CNS and may cause collateral effects. Compounds that showed values below 1 ($C_{Brain}/C_{Blood} < 1$) were classified as inactive in the CNS, as seen in Table 3.

The DEREK program makes the prediction of the toxicity of the compounds in a qualitative way; it is a specialist system that focuses attention on the toxic action of chemical compounds. The system performs this analysis based on implemented rules and depicts the relationship between a structural feature and toxicophoric groups present in the compounds, which are possible inducers of certain types of toxicity. It is considered that in addition to toxicity, DEREK can identify aspects related to carcinogenicity, mutagenicity, skin sensitization, irritation, teratogenicity and neurotoxicity [19–21].

The anti-inflammatory drugs derived from 2-arylacetic and 3-arylpropionic acids, such as ibuprofen and diclofenac, may cause hepatotoxicity and the irritation of the gastric mucosa. The hepatotoxicity is due to an idiosyncratic metabolic and/or immune reaction, not associated with the fact that mice treated with benoxaprofen developed this problem [53]. In studies carried out by Geneve et al. (1987) [53], high doses of pirprofen and ibuprofen were shown to significantly inhibit the mitochondrial beta-oxidation of fatty acids in mice, leading to the microvesicular steatosis of the liver. This may lead to less serious events such as mild elevations in serum transaminases to severe hepatocellular and/or cholestatic injury, which are relatively rare but important due to the potential for progression to fulminant hepatic failure. Jaundice, centrilobular necrosis, microvesicular steatosis, fibrosis, and symptoms suggestive of a hypersensitivity syndrome are clinical findings associated with the use of these agents [54,55].

The derivation of modified protein adducts is thought to be essential to the hepatotoxicity induced by these agents. Two alternative metabolic pathways may play a causative role: hepatic acyl glucuronidation catalyzed by the uridine diphospho-glucurosyl transferase (UGT) system and acyl-coenzyme A (acyl-CoA) formation. It is well established that acyl glucuronides are reactive electrophiles that can undergo covalent u with plasma or tissue proteins via a transacylation or glycation mechanism [53,55].

In the former, protein adducts are formed by the nucleophilic displacement of the glucuronic acid moiety. In the latter, intramolecular migration of the acyl residue allows for the opening of the glucuronic acid ring to create an aldehyde intermediate susceptible to nucleophilic attacks [53,55]. However, the gastric mucosal irritation of the nonsteroidal anti-inflammatory propionic acid (NSAIDs are mainly a consequence of the physicochemical disruption of the gastric mucosal barrier, resulting from alpha-substituted propionic acids or esters) causes a loss in protection resulting from the inhibition of the cyclo-oxygenase activity of the gastrointestinal mucosa [21]. Cyclo-oxygenase inhibition is also the mechanism by which propionic acids, and other NSAIDs, exert their anti-inflammatory action [56].

Diclofenac can cause distinct forms of nephrotoxicity in man and other mammals because of the presence of aryl or fulvenyl acetic or 2-propionic acid derivative, which have all been associated with a high incidence of dose-independent idiosyncratic acute renal failure (ARF) secondary to acute interstitial nephritis (AIN) in man, with or without nephrotic syndrome typically characterized by (membranous) glomerulonephritis or minimal change disease [53–59].

The presence of phenols substituted in acetaminophen in the para-position by nitrogen or oxygen gives a positive response in the in-vitro chromosome aberration test in human lymphocytes, as well as in the L5178Y TK+/− assay [58–60]. Activity is generally observed in both the presence and absence of the S9 mix. Since such compounds are not associated with significant activity in the Ames test, this suggests that the response in the L5178Y TK+/− assay is most likely due to a chromosomal rather than a mutagenic effect. Possible mechanisms for the observed activity include the generation of reactive oxygen species (ROS), metabolism to quinone-type intermediates or the inhibition of the enzyme ribonucleotide reductase [58–60] (see Table 4).

Acetaminophen and salicylamide derivatives (PS1, PS2 and PS3) showed toxicity alerts for hepatotoxicity, probably due to the presence of the toxicophoric group p-aminophenol and has been proven to require metabolic activation mediated by the cytochrome P450 system. The reactive metabolite is thought to be *N*-acetylbenzoquinone imine (NAPQI). After a toxic dose of the compound and subsequent glutathione depletion, NAPQI can covalently bind to a number of intracellular target proteins, resulting, in particular, in mitochondrial damage and ATP depletion. Other factors such as inflammatory cytokines, oxidative stress, tyrosine nitration, and mitochondrial permeability transition are also thought to play a causative role [61–65]. PS2 showed alerts for carcinogenicity in mice and rats and peroxisome proliferation in mice and rats, but these effects are not seen in higher mammals, including in man.

Depending on the toxicity, classes are defined according to the globally harmonized system of classification of labelling chemicals (GHS) [15]. Table 4 shows clearly that the LD_{50} prediction values were 2800 (PS1), 2400 (PS2) and 2175 (PS3) mg/kg. Thus, the compounds of the present study have an advantage over the commercial compound. This shows that such compounds may have greater safety in use, since they may be used in a higher concentration than the commercial compound. From the results, it was clear that the commercial compounds should be given with more caution under experimental study to avoid any loss of animals due to toxicity, which may, in turn, affect the statistical analysis of the experiment.

3.3. Molecular Docking Simulations

The comparison between crystallographic ligands ibuprofen, rofecoxib, diclofenac and salicylic acid and the best conformation predicted by molecular docking is seen in Figure 4, which shows the poses with RMSD values of 0.33, 0.90, 1.34 and 0.88 Å for ibuprofen, rofecoxib, diclofenac and salicylic acid, respectively. The docking had the ability to reproduce the experimental binding affinities, and according to the literature, the mode of connection prediction using docking should present an RMSD value <2.0 Å in the crystallographic pose of the binder [66–70]. So, the search parameters are suitable for the docking step. We have emphasized similar results in our previous work using molecular docking tools to search for new potential leads or hits [21,71–74].

We identified the sites of interaction described for rofecoxib (PDB ID 5KIR) around the alpha-helix located between the amino acid residues Thr118-Ser121, Tyr348-Leu352 and Met522-Gly526, as well as around the beta-sheet located between the amino acid residues Ser353-Phe357. For the binder, it is possible to observe common hydrogen bonds with residues Tyr355 and Arg120. There are also hydrophobic interactions with the residues Val349, Ser353, Leu352, Val523 and Ala527, according to studies in the literature [23].

In molecular docking, the theoretical binding affinity for ibuprofen was −7.6 kcal/mol, and a variation of ±0.3 kcal/mol was observed when compared with the experimental value of −7.3 kcal/mol [22]. For rofecoxib, the theoretical binding affinity was −10.0 kcal/mol, and a variation of ±0.8 kcal/mol was found when compared with the experimental value of −9.2 kcal/mol [23]. For diclofenac, the variation was ±2.9 kcal/mol, which was between the experimental bond affinity value of −11.3 kcal/mol [75] and the theoretical bond affinity for the docking of −6.1 kcal/mol. For salicylate, the binding affinity was −6.1 kcal/mol, varying by ±0.9 kcal/mol, when compared to the experimental value of

-6.7 kcal/mol [25]. Thus, the molecular docking methodology was able to accurately reproduce the experimental binding modes for ibuprofen, rofecoxib and salicylic acid. However, the values obtained for diclofenac may be due to the low resolution of PDB 1PXX when compared to the other PDBs (see Table 5).

Using the docking methodology selected here, we identified a potential binding mode for the compound capable of interacting with the active site of COX-2, similar to the observed crystallographic pose for ibuprofen (PDB ID 4PH9) around the alpha-helix located between the amino acid residues Asn86-Thr93, Lys114-Ser121, Val349-Ser353, Met522-Lys532 as well as around the beta-sheet located between the amino acid residues Gly354-Phe357, Leu384-Trp387, Ala516-Gly519. For the binder, it is possible to observe common hydrogen bonds formed with residues Arg120 and Tyr355. There are also hydrophobic interactions with residues Val116, Val349, Trp387, Met522, Val523, Gly526, Ala527, Leu531 and Ser530, according to a study found in the literature [22].

For diclofenac (PDB ID 1PXX), the sites of interactions observed were around the alpha-helix located between the amino acid residues Met197-Phe205, Lys342-Ser353 and Val523-Met535, as well as around the beta-sheet located between the residues of amino acids Tyr385-His388. For the ligand, hydrogen bonds are observed with residues Tyr385 and Ser530, according to previously reported results [24].

The interactions observed for salicylic acid (PDB ID 5F1A) were around the alpha-helix located between the amino acid residues Tyr348-Leu352 and Met522-Ser530, as well as around the beta-sheet located between the amino acid residues Tyr385-His388. For the binder, a hydrogen bond with the Ser530 residue is observed, according to previous studies [25].

The control structure of ibuprofen showed a binding affinity of -7.6 kcal/mol, a close value when compared to PS1 and PS3, which presented values of -6.6 and -7.5 kcal/mol with variation of ± 1.0 and ± 0.1 kcal/mol, respectively. Compound PS2 presented a binding affinity value of -7.8 kcal/mol, a better value when compared to ibuprofen, with a variation of ± 0.2 kcal/mol. When comparing the PS2 compounds with rofecoxib, a variation of ± 1.0 kcal/mol was observed (see Figure 5).

The active site of the COX-2 enzyme has three important regions. First, there is the hydrophobic pocket, which is coated with the amino acid residues Tyr385, Trp387, Phe518, Ala201, Tyr248 and Leu352. The second region is located at the site entrance and contains the hydrophilic amino acid residues Arg120, Glu524 and Tyr355, while the third is a side pouch with the amino acid residues His90, Arg513 and Val523 [76]. Some amino acid residues (Arg120, Tyr355, His90, Arg513, Val523, Ser353 and Glu124) are believed to play a significant role in the entry of the ligand into the active site, as shown in the analysis of the crystal structure of various selective COX-2 inhibitors [77].

The individually observed interactions between PS1 and the active site are located around the alpha-helix between the amino acid residues Val349-Leu352 and Met522-Ser530, as well as around the beta-sheet located between the amino acid residues Tyr385-His388; they were similar to those described in the literature [22,24,76], as can be seen in Figure 9A. For PS1, hydrogen bonds formed with residues Ser530 and Tyr385 are observed. The latter residue participates in the catalytic process exerted by COX-2 [24,77] and hydrophobic interactions with Leu352 and Val349 residues. In the interactions observed between PS2 and PS3 compounds and the active site, both ligands exhibited the same hydrogen interactions with amino acid residues Ser530 and Tyr385 and hydrophobic interactions with residues Val349, Leu352, Met522 and Val523 (Figure 9B,C). Analyses in a crystallographic complex of COX-2 and arachidonic acid revealed a unique conformation of the substrate in which the substrate was inverted with its coordinated carboxylate for Ser530 and Tyr385 [23]. Studies by Rowlinson et al. (2003) [24] suggest that Tyr385/Ser530 chelation is critical for the inhibition of COX-2 by clinically used NSAIDs such as diclofenac, piroxicam and nimesulide.

3.4. Anti-Nociceptive Activity

The results presented in Figure 11A show the dose-dependent effect of PS1 on the number of abdominal writhes induced by 0.6% acetic acid. PS1 at doses of 20 and 50 mg/kg reduced the amount of abdominal writhing by 52% and 83%, respectively, when compared to the control group. In Figure 11B, the PS3, at doses of 20 and 50 mg/kg, reduced painful activity by 74% and 75%, respectively, when compared to the control group (20 mg/kg). PS2 in the dose of 50 mg/kg did not show good results when compared to the compounds (PS1 and PS3), and this can be seen in Figure 11C.

The anti-nociceptive potential of these salicylamide derivatives was evaluated using two different methodologies. The writhing test was used to evaluate the peripheral nociceptive activity in order to characterize the nature of the pain and indirectly verify the anti-inflammatory potential of the evaluated compounds. The hot-plate test was used to evaluate the involvement of the opioid system in the central nervous system.

4. Materials and Methods

4.1. Chemicals and Equipment

Varian Spectrometer, Gemini model: ^{1}H-NMR (300 MHz) and ^{13}C-NMR (75 MHz); Digital Fusion Point, model MQAPF–302 Microquímica (Campinas, Brazil). Analytical balance–Sartorios (Göttingen, Germany); Heating plate with magnetic stirrer–Quimis (Aguaí, Brazil); Becker (Carnegie, PA, USA) 100 mL and 250 mL; 125 mL Erlenmeyer, 250 mL and 500 mL; Petri dish; 25 mL, 50 mL and 100 mL beakers; 1 mL and 5 mL pipettes; 250 mL separation funnel; test tubes; watch glass; ice cube; glass rod; filter paper; chromatographic plate; magnetic bar; capillaries; Ethyl acetate–Synth (San Francisco, CA, USA); 5-Amino-salicylic acid–Fluka (Buchs, Switzerland); benzoyl chloride–Merck; phenylacetyl chloride–Aldrich (St. Louis, MO, USA); acetic acid–Nuclear (Diadema, Brazil); sulfuric acid–Synth; nitric acid–Synth; sodium chloride–New Chemistry (Campinas, Brazil); distilled water; acetonitrile–Merck (Rahway, NJ, USA); ethyl acetate; Nuclear; chloroform–Merck; dichloromethane-Synth; dimethylsulfoxide–Riedel-de-Haen (Berlin, Germany); ethanol Synth; hexane-Synth; methanol-Synth; toluene-Synth.

4.2. Synthetic Methodology

The acylation reactions were performed in temperature-controlled (60 to 80 °C) environments using an amine and anhydride or acyl chloride using a nucleophilic addition reaction of the amine group on acyl carbon followed by acetic anhydride or hydrochloride elimination. Under these reaction conditions, only the amine acylation occurs [11]. All derivatives were identified by means of physicochemical characterizations, such as melting points, solubility tests and H^1 and C^{13} nuclear magnetic resonance (NMR) spectra [78–81].

4.3. In-Silico Study of Oral Bioavailability, Bioactivity, ADME and Toxicity Risk Assessment

The compounds used in this study were: ibuprofen, rofecoxib, diclofenac, acetaminophen, salicilate, PS1, PS2 and PS3. The molecular descriptors and druglikeliness (oral bioavailability) properties of the compounds were analyzed via the Molinspiration server (see site http://www.molinspiration.com, accessed on 21 November 2021) based on the Lipinski rule of five [82,83].

The rule states that most "druglike" compounds have a molecular weight (MW $\leq$ 500 Da), a number of hydrogen bond acceptors (HBA $\leq$ 10), a number of hydrogen bond donors (HBD $\leq$ 5), and an octanol/water partition coefficient (log P $\leq$ 5); compounds violating more than one of these rules can have problems with oral bioavailability. Molinspiration supports the calculation of important molecular properties such as MW, LogP, polar surface area, and the number of hydrogen bond donors and acceptors, as well as the prediction of the bioactivity score for the most important drug targets (GPCR ligands, kinase inhibitors, ion channel modulators, enzymes and nuclear receptors were predicted in this study [13]).

To identify any undesirable toxic properties of salicylamide derivates, the toxicity prediction server Protox [84] (see site http://tox.charite.de/tox, accessed on 11 January

2022) was used in this study. The prediction was based on the functional group similarity for the query compounds with the in-vitro and in-vivo validated compounds present in this database. The toxic properties such as toxicity class, toxic fragment generation, LD_{50} values in mg/kg, toxicity targets, drug-relevant properties [c Log P, Log S (Solubility)], molecular weight and overall drug score were calculated [84]. This approach was based on studies by Roy et al. (2015) [13].

The toxicity profile of the synthesized compounds was also evaluated using the Deductive Estimation of Risk from Existing Knowledge (DEREK) 10.0.2 program. We have considered DEREK alerts of toxicity involving the human species, mice and rats. The DEREK program conducts the prediction of the toxicity of the structures in a qualitative way and is a specialist system that focuses attention on the toxic action of chemical compounds. The system performs this analysis based on implemented rules and depicts the relationships between structural features and toxicophore groups present in the compounds as possible inducers of certain types of toxicity. It is considered that in addition to toxicity, DEREK can identify aspects related to carcinogenicity, mutagenicity, skin sensitization, irritation, teratogenicity and neurotoxicity [72,85,86].

4.4. Molecular Docking Simulations

The molecular docking study was performed with the aid of the AutoDock Vina 1.1.2 program [87] and its graphical interface PyRx 0.8 [88]. One of the most valuable features of docking methods is their ability to reproduce experimentally observed binding modes, even functioning as a form of validation. To perform a test of this level, a binder is extracted from its crystallographic complex and subjected to simulations with the binding site of the protein. Thus, the binding modes obtained in the simulations are compared with the respective binding modes obtained experimentally [87].

In this work, re-docking was performed to evaluate the accuracy of the docking program. The crystallographic models of cyclooxygenase-2 (COX-2) were selected from the Protein Data Bank (COX-2) and complexed with ibuprofen (PDB ID 4PH9) [22]; COX-2 (*Homo sapiens*) was complexed with rofecoxib (PDB ID 5KIR) [23]; COX-2 (*Mus musculus*) was complexed with diclofenac (PDB ID 1PXX) [24]; and COX-2 (*Homo sapiens*) was complexed with salicylic acid (PDB ID 5F1A) [25], with resolutions of 1.81, 2.69, 2.90 and 2.38 Å, respectively.

The crystallographic structure obtained in the PDB was edited in the program Discovery Studio Visualizer v.17.2 [89] to separate the protein from the ligand, and then the two molecules were submitted to molecular docking in the program AutoDock Vina 1.1.2 [87]. The search space was defined using experimentally solved protein–ligand complex structures (PDBs) [22–25]. First, an initial docking box was constructed to enclose the bound ligand, and then the box size was increased until it included the entire region of the active site to allow for the rotation and translation of the ligand in this region.

Molecular docking was performed to obtain a population of possible conformations and orientations for the ligand at the binding site. The protein was loaded in PyRx, creating a PDBQT file that contains a protein structure with hydrogens in all polar residues. All calculations for protein-fixed ligand-flexible docking were performed using the Lamarckian Genetic Algorithm (LGA) method, which presents the best results in the search for the global minimum [90].

The docking site on the protein target was defined by establishing a grid box with the dimensions shown in Table 6. Ten runs via AutoDock Vina, with an exhaustiveness default = 8 [87], were performed in all cases per each ligand structure, and for each run the best pose with the lowest binding free energy and lower RMSD was selected, saved, and analyzed. The RMSD was calculated in the Discovery Studio Visualizer v.17.2 program by comparing the crystallographic ligand pose and the docking predicted pose using all atoms.

Table 6. Protocols used in the study of molecular docking study.

Enzyme COX2	Inhibitor *	Coordinates of the Grid Center (Angstrom)	Grid Dimensions (Angstrom)
(PDB ID 4PH9)	Ibuprofen	X = 12.58 Y = 24.20 Z = 25.33	X = 17 Y = 17 Z = 16
(PDB ID 5KIR)	Rofecoxib	X = 23.63 Y = 1.30 Z = 34.07	X = 18 Y = 19 Z = 18
(PDB ID 1PXX)	Diclofenac	X = 27.16 Y = 24.45 Z = 15.30	X = 18 Y = 19 Z = 18
(PDB ID 5F1A)	Salicylic acid	X = 41.72 Y = 24.24 Z = 240.03	X = 18 Y = 17 Z = 17

* Acetaminophen (Acet) and the crystallographic structures of ibuprofen, rofecoxib, diclofenac and salicylic acid were used as a positive control.

The X-ray diffraction (PDB ID 4PH9, 5KIR, 1PXX and 5F1A) was overlaid with the lowest RMSD conformation obtained in the docking to visually evaluate the best obtained result of the validation. After the identification with the best search parameters, the study of molecular docking with the PS1, PS2 and PS3 structures was carried out.

The X, Y and Z spatial coordinates were determined in the active site region according to the observed interaction between the enzymes and their respective crystallographic binders, according to studies available in the literature [91–96].

The coordinates used for the center and the box size can be seen in Table 6. Visualizations as well as distance measures of the interactions between the ligands and enzymes were produced using the program Discovery Studio Visualizer v.17.2.

4.5. Anti-Nociceptive Activity

This project is characterized as an experimental, prospective, and interventional study aimed at evaluating the in-vivo therapeutic efficacy of salicylamide (PS1), (PS2) and (PS3) derivatives in nociception models. This experimental study was carried out in the city of Belém-Pará, at UEPA's Laboratory of Morphophysiology Applied to Health.

4.5.1. Animals

This project is characterized as an experimental, prospective, and interventional study aimed at evaluating the in-vivo therapeutic efficacy of salicylamide (PS1) derivatives (PS2) and (PS3) in nociception models. All experiments reported in this study were conducted in accordance with current guidelines for care of laboratory animals and ethical guidelines for investigation of experimental pain in conscious animals (CEUA-UEPA N° 14/2017).

Sixty-three Swiss mice belonging to the *Mus musculus* strain weighing between 30 g and 40 g were used. Adult males were used for each study group in vivo; they were from the Bioterio Evandro Chagas Institute (IEC) and were transferred and kept in the Luiz Carlos de Lima Silveira–UEPA/CCBS, where they were placed in appropriate acrylic cages with a bed of wood and kept at a temperature between 22 and 25 °C, receiving water ad libitum during the experiment period with a night light cycle/day of 12 h. The cleaning and the exchange of shavings and water were carried out on alternate days. The determination of the sample number was based on the central limit theory, once it was considered that the sample had a normal distribution.

4.5.2. Writhing Test Induced by Acetic Acid

The writhing tests were induced by the intraperitoneal administration of 0.6% acetic acid. In this concentration, the contraction of the abdominal muscles is generated [97].

The animals were subdivided into five groups: acetaminophen, saline, PS1, PS2 and PS3, totaling 25 animals, and they were pre-treated orally. After 60 min, the acetic acid administration was performed. The anti-nociceptive activity was expressed by the number of contortions in 30 min.

4.5.3. Hot Plate

The hot-plate test was used to measure the latency of response to the thermoceptive stimulus, according to the method described by Woolfe and Macdonald (1944) [98]. The mice were subdivided into six groups: vehicle, PS1, PS2, PS3, acetaminophen and morphine, totaling 30 animals. They were pre-treated orally with 20 mg/kg and only 10 mg/kg morphine. Each individual animal was placed on the hot plate (55 ± 0.5) °C. The time measurement was interrupted when the animal presented the instinctive behavior of jumping on the plate or licking or raising the legs, or after 35 s, to avoid tissue injury. The measurements to be analyzed were taken at the times of 30, 60, 90 and 120 min after the administration of the substance.

4.5.4. Ethical Aspects

All animals in the present research were cared for according to the national legislation for Procedures for the Scientific Use of Animals in force (Federal Law 11,794 of 8 October 2008), the rules of the Brazilian College of Animal Experimentation (COBEA) (CEPA) of the University of the State of Pará (UEPA) and the coordinator of the Laboratory of Applied Morphophysiology for Health of UEPA/CCBS, and the guidelines and responsibilities for veterinarians.

5. Conclusions

Two salicylamide derivates were designed and their chemical structures were spectrally confirmed. The in-silico properties of pharmacokinetics and the bioactivity, bioavailability and toxicity of the compounds were analyzed. The compounds showed a better bioavailability, and the molecular docking results obtained here indicate that compounds PS2 and PS3 have a superior potential capacity of COX-2 inhibition in human and mice enzymes, as they exhibited similar interactions to those observed for the templates or control compounds (ibuprofen, diclofenac, acetaminophen, rofecoxib, and salicylate). In the anti-nociceptive activity, the compounds reduced the painful activity in different concentrations. However, the proposed derivatives are potentially more active than salicylamide and they support the design of novel and safer derivative candidates. Consequently, more studies need to be conducted to evaluate the different pharmacological actions, the toxicity of possible metabolites that can be generated, and potential uses in inflammation and pain therapy.

Author Contributions: Conceptualization, C.B.R.S., M.B.F., R.C.S. (Renata C. Silva), A.B.D.L., R.S.B. and J.A.H.M.B.; Methodology, C.B.R.S., C.C.L., R.C.S. (Rai C. Silva), R.C.V.S.B., J.J.S.F., R.C.S. (Renata C. Silva), A.B.D.L., J.M.C., R.S.B. and J.A.H.M.B.; Software, C.C.L. and E.F.B.F.; Validation, A.B.D.L.; Formal analysis, C.C.L., S.S.B.O., R.C.S. (Rai C. Silva), R.C.V.S.B., J.J.S.F., M.B.F., J.M.C., R.S.B. and J.A.H.M.B.; Investigation, S.S.B.O., R.C.V.S.B., J.J.S.F., R.C.S. (Renata C. Silva) and J.A.H.M.B.; Data curation, R.C.V.S.B., J.M.C. and J.A.H.M.B.; Writing—original draft, C.C.L., S.S.B.O., A.B.D.L., R.S.B. and J.A.H.M.B.; Writing—review & editing, C.B.R.S., E.F.B.F., M.B.F. and J.M.C.; Visualization, S.S.B.O., R.C.S. (Rai C. Silva), J.J.S.F., E.F.B.F., M.B.F. and R.C.S. (Renata C. Silva); Supervision, C.B.R.S. and R.S.B.; Funding acquisition, C.B.R.S. and J.M.C. All authors have read and agreed to the published version of the manuscript.

Funding: This research received no external funding.

Institutional Review Board Statement: The study was conducted according to the guidelines of the Declaration of Helsinki and approved by the Institutional Review Board of (CEPA) of the University of the State of Pará (UEPA) (protocol code n° 14/2017 and date of approval 12 December 2017).

Informed Consent Statement: Not applicable.

Data Availability Statement: Data is contained within the article.

Acknowledgments: We gratefully acknowledge the financial support provided by the Graduate Program in Medicinal Chemistry and Molecular Modeling—Federal University of Pará (UFPA-Belém-Brazil), PROPESP/UFPA, CNPq, Graduate Program in Pharmaceutical Innovation—Federal University of Amapá, Laboratory of Modeling and Computational Chemistry—Federal University of Amapá (UNIFAP-Macapá-Brazil), Laboratory of Molecular Modeling—State University of Feira de Santana (UEFS-Bahia-Brazil) and Department of Pharmaceutical and Organic Chemistry-Institute of Biosanitary Research ibs.GRANADA—University of Granada (UGR-Granada-Spain).

Conflicts of Interest: The authors declare no conflict of interest.

References

1. Mansouri, M.T.; Hemmati, A.A.; Naghizadeh, B.; Mard, S.A.; Rezaie, A.; Ghorbanzadeh, B. A study of the mechanisms underlying the anti-inflammatory effect of ellagic acid in carrageenan-induced paw edema in rats. *Indian J. Pharmacol.* **2015**, *47*, 292–298. [PubMed]
2. Richy, F.; Bruyere, O.; Ethgen, O.; Rabenda, V.; Bouvenot, G.; Audran, M.; Herrero-Beaumont, G.; Moore, A.; Eliakim, R.; Haim, M.; et al. Time dependent risk of gastrointestinal complications induced by non-steroidal anti-inflammatory drug use: A consensus statement using a meta-analytic approach. *Ann. Rheum. Dis.* **2004**, *63*, 759–766. [CrossRef]
3. Beck, P.L.; Xavier, R.; Lu, N.; Nanda, N.N.; Dinauer, M.; Podolsky, D.K.; Seed, B. Mechanisms of NSAID-induced gastrointestinal injury defined using mutant mice. *Gastroenterology* **2000**, *119*, 699–705. [CrossRef]
4. Chan, F.K.L.; Graham, D.Y. Prevention of non-steroidal anti-inflammatory druggastrointestinal complications—Review and recommendations basedon risk assessment. *Aliment. Pharmacol. Ther.* **2004**, *19*, 1051–1061. [CrossRef] [PubMed]
5. Borges, R.S. *Planejamento, Síntese e Avaliação Antioxidante de Inibidores Fenólicos da PGES Derivados da Associação p-Aminofenol e Salicilatos*; Tese de Doutorado em Neurociências e Biologia Celular, UFPA: Belém, Brazil, 2007.
6. Borges, R.S.; Alves, C.N.; Nascimento, J.L.M. Aplicação de Derivados da Associação Molecular como Antiagregantes Plaquetários e Inibidores de Radicais Livres. PI1001434-9, 20 January 2010.
7. Borges, R.S.; Pereira, G.A.N.; Vale, J.K.L.; França, L.C.S.; Monteiro, M.C.; Alves, C.N.; Silva, A.B.F.d. Design and evaluation of 4-aminophenol and salicylate derivatives as free-radical scavenger. *Chem. Biol. Drug Des.* **2013**, *81*, 414–419. [CrossRef]
8. Borges, R.S.; Castle, S.L. The antioxidant properties of salicylate derivatives: A possible new mechanism of anti-inflammatory activity. *Bioorganic Med. Chem. Lett.* **2015**, *25*, 4808–4811. [CrossRef] [PubMed]
9. Guedes, K.M.M.; Borges, R.S.; Fontes-Júnior, E.A.; Silva, A.S.B.; Fernandes, L.M.P.; Cartágenes, S.C.; Pinto, A.C.G.; Silva, M.L.; Queiroz, L.M.D.; Vieira, J.L.F.; et al. Salicytamide: A New Anti-inflammatory Designed Drug Candidate. *Inflammation* **2018**, *41*, 1349–1360. [CrossRef] [PubMed]
10. Hawkey, C.J. COX-1 and COX-2 inhibitors. *Best Pract. Res. Clin. Gastroenterol.* **2001**, *15*, 801–820. [CrossRef]
11. Tanhehco, E.J. Potassium channel modulators as anti-inflammatory agents. *Expert. Opin. Ther. Pat.* **2001**, *11*, 1137–1145. [CrossRef]
12. Van De Waterbeemd, H.; Gifford, E. ADMET in silico modelling: Towards prediction paradise? *Nat. Rev. Drug Discov.* **2003**, *2*, 192–204. [CrossRef]
13. Roy, S.; Samant, L.; Chowdhary, A. In silico pharmacokinetics analysis and ADMET of phytochemicals of Datura metel Linn. and Cynodon dactylon Linn. *J. Chem. Pharm. Res.* **2015**, *7*, 385–388.
14. Cunha, E.L.; Santos, C.F.; Braga, F.S.; Costa, J.S.; Silva, R.C.; Favacho, H.A.; Hage-Melim, L.I.; Carvalho, J.C.; Silva, C.H.; Santos, C.B. Computational Investigation of Antifungal Compounds Using Molecular Modeling and Prediction of ADME/Tox Properties. *J. Comput. Theor. Nanosci.* **2015**, *12*, 3682–3691. [CrossRef]
15. Yee, S. In vitro permeability across caco-2 cells (colonic) can predict in vivo (small intestinal) absorption in man-fact or myth. *Pharm. Res.* **1997**, *14*, 763–766. [CrossRef]
16. Zhao, Y.H.; Le, J.; Abraham, M.H.; Hersey, A.; Eddershaw, P.J.; Luscombe, C.N.; Platts, J.A. Evaluation of human intestinal absorption data and subsequent derivation of a quantitative structure activity relationship (QSAR) with the Abraham descriptors. *J. Pharm. Sci.* **2001**, *90*, 749–784. [CrossRef] [PubMed]
17. Yazdanian, M.; Glynn, S.L.; Wright, J.L.; Hawi, A. Correlating Partitioning and Caco-2 Cell Permeability of Structurally Diverse Small Molecular Weight Compounds. *Pharm. Res.* **1998**, *15*, 1490–1494. [CrossRef]
18. Irvine, J.D.; Takahashi, L.; Lockhart, K.; Cheong, J.; Tolan, J.W.; Selick, H.E.; Grove, J.R. MDCK (Madin–Darby canine kidney) cells: A tool for membrane permeability screening. *J. Pharm. Sci.* **1999**, *88*, 28–33. [CrossRef] [PubMed]
19. Costa, J.S.; Costa, K.S.L.; Cruz, J.V.; Ramos, R.S.; Silva, L.B.; Brasil, D.S.B.; Silva, C.H.T.P.; Santos, C.B.R.; Macêdo, W.J.C. Virtual screening and statistical analysis in the design of new caffeine analogues molecules with potential epithelial anticancer activity. *Curr. Pharm. Des.* **2018**, *24*, 576–594. [CrossRef]
20. Cruz, J.V.; Neto, M.F.A.; Silva, L.B.; Ramos, R.; Costa, J.; Brasil, D.S.B.; Lobato, C.C.; Costa, G.V.; Bittencourt, J.A.H.M.; Silva, C.H.T.P.; et al. Identification of novel protein kinase receptor type 2 inhibitors using pharmacophore and structure-based virtual screening. *Molecules* **2018**, *23*, 453. [CrossRef]
21. Alberga, D.; Trisciuzzi, D.; Mansouri, K.; Mangiatordi, G.F.; Nicolotti, O. Prediction of Acute Oral Systemic Toxicity Using a Multifingerprint Similarity Approach. *Toxicol. Sci.* **2018**, *167*, 484–495. [CrossRef]

22. Orlando, B.J.; Lucido, M.J.; Malkowski, M.G. The structure of ibuprofen bound to cyclooxygenase-2. *J. Struct. Biol.* **2015**, *189*, 62–66. [CrossRef]

23. Orlando, B.J.; Malkowski, M.G. Crystal structure of rofecoxib bound to human cyclooxygenase-2. *Acta Crystallogr. Sect. F Struct. Biol. Commun.* **2016**, *72*, 772–776. [CrossRef] [PubMed]

24. Rowlinson, S.W.; Kiefer, J.R.; Prusakiewicz, J.J.; Pawlitz, J.L.; Kozak, K.R.; Kalgutkar, A.S.; Stallings, W.C.; Kurumbail, R.G.; Marnett, L.J. A novel mechanism of cyclooxygenase-2 inhibition involving interactions with Ser-530 and Tyr-385. *J. Biol. Chem.* **2003**, *278*, 45763–45769. [CrossRef] [PubMed]

25. Lucido, M.J.; Orlando, B.J.; Vecchio, A.J.; Malkowski, M.G. Crystal structure of aspirin-acetylated human cyclooxygenase-2: Insight into the formation of products with reversed stereochemistry. *Biochemistry* **2016**, *55*, 1226–1238. [CrossRef] [PubMed]

26. Cera, E.D. *Thermodynamic Theory of Site-Specific Binding Processes in Biological Macromolecules*; Cambridge University Press: Cambridge, UK; Washington University: St Louis, MO, USA, 1995.

27. Gohlke, H.; Klebe, G. Approaches to the description and prediction of the binding affinity of small-molecule ligands to macromolecular receptors. *Angew. Chem. Int. Ed.* **2002**, *41*, 2644–2676. [CrossRef]

28. Sportoletti, G.; Testi, V. Amino-Salicylic Acid Derivatives and Pharmaceutical Compositions. WO 86/03199 A1, 26 November 1985.

29. Serhan, C.N. Resolution phase of inflammation: Novel endogenous anti-inflammatory and proresolving lipid mediators and pathways. *Annu. Rev Immunol.* **2007**, *25*, 101–137. [CrossRef]

30. Cherezov, V.; Rosenbaum, D.M.; Hanson, M.A.; Rasmussen, S.G.; Thian, F.S.; Kobilka, T.S.; Choi, H.J.; Kuhn, P.; Weis, W.I.; Kobilka, B.K.; et al. High-resolution crystal structure of an engineered human beta2-adrenergic G protein-coupled receptor. *Science* **2007**, *318*, 1258–1265. [CrossRef]

31. Gurevich, V.V.; Gurevich, E.V. Molecular Mechanisms of GPCR Signaling:A Structural Perspective. *Int. J. Mol. Sci.* **2017**, *18*, 2519 [CrossRef]

32. Filmore, D. It's a GPCR world. *Mod. Drug Discov.* **2004**, *28*, 24–26.

33. Overington, J.P.; Al-Lazikani, B.; Hopkins, A.L. How many drug targets are there? *Nat. Rev. Drug Discov.* **2006**, *5*, 993–996 [CrossRef]

34. Hauser, A.S.; Attwood, M.M.; Rask-Andersen, M.; Schiöth, H.B.; Gloriam, D.E. Trends in GPCR drug discovery: New agents, targets and indications. *Nat. Rev. Drug Discov.* **2017**, *16*, 829–842. [CrossRef]

35. Tang, T.; Gong, T.; Jiang, W.; Zhou, R. GPCRs in NLRP3 Inflammasome Activation, Regulation, and Therapeutics. *Trends Pharmacol. Sci.* **2018**, *39*, 798–811. [CrossRef]

36. Bermudez, M.; Nguyen, T.N.; Omieczynski, C.; Wolber, G. Strategies for the discovery of biased GPCR ligands. *Drug Discov. Today* **2019**, *24*, 1031–1037. [CrossRef]

37. Muratspahić, E.; Freissmuth, M.; Gruber, C.W. Nature-Derived Peptides: A Growing Niche for GPCR Ligand Discovery. *Trends Pharmacol. Sci.* **2019**, *40*, 309–316. [CrossRef]

38. Ashok, S.R.; Shivananda, M.K.; Manikandan, A.; Chandrasekaran, R. Discovery and synthesis of 2-amino-1-methyl-1H-imidazol-4(5H)-ones as GPCR ligands; an approach to develop breast cancer drugs via GPCR associated PAR1 and PI3Kinase inhibition mechanism. *Bioorg. Chem.* **2019**, *86*, 641–651. [CrossRef] [PubMed]

39. Bantscheff, M.; Scholten, A.; Heck, A.J.R. Revealing promiscuous drug-target interactions by chemical proteomics. *Drug Discov. Today* **2009**, *14*, 1021–1029. [CrossRef]

40. Hu, Y.; Gupta-Ostermann, D.; Bajoratha, J. Exploring Compound Promiscuity Patterns and Multi-Target Activity Spaces. *Comput. Struct. Biotechnol. J.* **2014**, *9*, e201401003. [CrossRef] [PubMed]

41. Sun, L.; Ye, R.D. Role of G protein-coupled receptors in inflammation. *Acta Pharmacol. Sin.* **2012**, *33*, 342–350. [CrossRef] [PubMed]

42. Vane, J.R. Inhibition of Prostaglandin Synthesis as a Mechanism of Action for Aspirin-like Drugs. *Nat. New Biol.* **1971**, *231*, 232–235. [CrossRef]

43. Vane, J.R.; Botting, R.M. Mechanism of action of aspirin-like drugs. *Semin. Arthritis Rheum.* **1997**, *26*, 2–10. [CrossRef]

44. Ortiz, M.; Granados, S.V.; Castañeda, H.G. Possible Activation of Inward Rectifier-and G Protein-Coupled K^+ Channels in the Antinociception Induced by Non-steroidal Anti-inflammatory Drugs. *Proc. West. Pharmacol.* **2006**, *49*, 141–144.

45. Wulff, H.; Palle, C. Recent developments in ion channel pharmacology. *Channels* **2015**, *9*, 335. [CrossRef] [PubMed]

46. Gfeller, D.; Michielin, O.; Zoete, V. Shaping the interaction landscape of bioactive molecules. *Bioinformatics* **2013**, *29*, 3073–3079 [CrossRef] [PubMed]

47. Wang, L.; Ma, C.; Wipf, P.; Liu, H.; Su, W.; Xie, X.-Q. TargetHunter: An in silico target identification tool for predicting therapeutic potential of small organic molecules based on chemogenomic database. *AAPS J.* **2013**, *15*, 395–406. [CrossRef] [PubMed]

48. Ramirez, G.; Coletto, L.; Sciorati, C.; Bozzolo, E.; Manunta, P.; Rovere-Querini, P.; Manfredi, A. Ion Channels and Transporters in Inflammation: Special Focus on TRP Channels and TRPC6. *Cells* **2018**, *7*, 70. [CrossRef]

49. Roberts, M.S. *Dermal Absorption and Toxicity Assessment*, 2nd ed.; CRC Press: Boca Raton, FL, USA, 2007.

50. Pratt, W.B. The entry, distribution, and elimination of drugs. In *Principles of Drug Action: The Basis of Pharmacology*, 3rd ed.; Pratt W.B., Taylor, P., Eds.; Churchill Livingstone: New York, NY, USA, 1990.

51. Ajay, A.; Bemis, G.W.; Murcko, M.A. Designing libraries with CNS activity. *J. Med. Chem.* **1999**, *42*, 4942–4951. [CrossRef]

52. Ma, X.L.; Chen, C.; Yang, J. Predictive model of blood-brain barrier penetration of organic compounds. *Acta Pharmacol. Sin.* **2005**, *26*, 500–512. [CrossRef]

53. Geneve, J.E.A.N.; Hayat-Bonan, B.; Labbe, G.; Degott, C.; Letteron, P.; Freneaux, E.; Pessayre, D. Inhibition of mitochondrial beta-oxidation of fatty acids by pirprofen. Role in microvesicular steatosis due to this nonsteroidal anti-inflammatory drug. *J. Pharmacol. Exp. Ther.* **1987**, *242*, 1133–1137.

54. Dahl, S.L.; Ward, J.R. Pharmacology, clinical efficacy, and adverse effects of the nonsteroidal anti-inflammatory agent benoxaprofen. *Pharmacother. J. Hum. Pharmacol. Drug Ther.* **1982**, *2*, 354–365. [CrossRef]

55. Zimmerman, H.J. *Hepatotoxicity: The Adverse Effects of Drugs and Other Chemicals on the Liver*, 2nd ed.; Lippincott Williams & Wilkins: Dallas, TX, USA, 1999.

56. Li, C.; Grillo, M.P.; Benet, L.Z. In vivo mechanistic studies on the metabolic activation of 2-phenylpropionic acid in rat. *J. Pharmacol. Exp. Ther.* **2003**, *305*, 250–256. [CrossRef]

57. Boelsterli, U.A. Diclofenac-induced liver injury: A paradigm of idiosyncratic drug toxicity. *Toxicol. Appl. Pharmacol.* **2003**, *192*, 307–322. [CrossRef]

58. Dong, J.Q.; Liu, J.; Smith, P.C. Role of benoxaprofen and flunox-aprofen acyl glucuronides in covalent binding to rat plasma and liver proteins in vivo. *Biochem. Pharmacol.* **2005**, *70*, 937–948. [CrossRef] [PubMed]

59. Tsutsui, T.; Hayashi, N.; Maizumi, H.; Huff, J.; Barrett, J.C. Benzene-,catechol-, hydroquinone- and phenol-induced cell transformation, gene mutations, chromosome aberrations, aneuploidy, sister chro-matid exchanges and unscheduled DNA synthesis in Syrian hamster embryo cells. *Mutat. Res. Fundam. Mol. Mech. Mutagen.* **1997**, *373*, 113–123. [CrossRef] [PubMed]

60. Bolton, J.L.; Trush, M.A.; Penning, T.M.; Dryhurst, G.; Monks, T.J. Role of quinones in toxicology. *Chem. Res. Toxicol.* **2000**, *13*, 135–160. [CrossRef] [PubMed]

61. Rannug, U.; Holme, J.A.; Hongslo, J.K.; Šrám, R.J. An evalution of the genetic toxicityof paracetamol. *Mutat. Res. Fundam. Mol. Mech. Mutagen.* **1995**, *327*, 179–200. [CrossRef] [PubMed]

62. Gujral, J.S.; Knight, T.R.; Farhood, A.; Bajt, M.L.; Jaeschke, H. Mode of cell death after acetaminophen overdose in mice: Apoptosis or oncotic necrosis? *Toxicol. Sci.* **2002**, *67*, 322–328. [CrossRef]

63. Calder, I.C.; Hart, S.J.; Smail, M.C.; Tange, J.D. Hepatotoxicity of phenacetin and paracetamol in the Gunn rat. *Pathology* **1981**, *13*, 757–762. [CrossRef]

64. Kalgutkar, A.S.; Gardner, I.; Obach, R.S.; Shaffer, C.L.; Callegari, E.; Henne, K.R.; O'Donnell, J.P. A comprehensive listing of bioactivation pathways of organic functional groups. *Curr. Drug Metab.* **2005**, *6*, 161–225. [CrossRef]

65. Nelson, S.D.; Forte, A.J.; McMurtry, R.J. Decreased toxicity of the N-methyl analogs of acetaminophen and phenacetin. *Res. Commun. Chem. Pathol. Pharmacol.* **1978**, *22*, 61–71.

66. Bursulaya, B.D.; Totrov, M.; Abagyan, R.; Brooks, C.L. Comparative study of several algorithms for flexible ligand docking. *J. Comput. Aided. Mol. Des.* **2003**, *17*, 755–763. [CrossRef]

67. Cole, J.C.; Murray, C.W.; Nissink, J.W.M.; Taylor, R.D.; Taylor, R. Comparing protein–ligand docking programs is difficult. *Proteins Struct. Funct. Bioinf.* **2005**, *60*, 325–332. [CrossRef]

68. Hevener, K.E.; Zhao, W.; Ball, D.M.; Babaoglu, K.; Qi, J.; White, S.W.; Lee, R.E. Validation of molecular docking programs for virtual screening against dihydropteroate synthase. *J. Chem. Inf. Model.* **2009**, *49*, 444–460. [CrossRef] [PubMed]

69. Kontoyianni, M.; McClellan, L.M.; Sokol, G.S. Evaluation of Docking Performance: Comparative Data on Docking Algorithms. *J. Med. Chem.* **2004**, *47*, 558–565. [CrossRef]

70. Nissink, J.W.M.; Murray, C.; Hartshorn, M.; Verdonk, M.L.; Cole, J.C.; Taylor, R. A new test set for validating predictions of protein-ligand interaction. *Proteins Struct. Funct. Bioinf.* **2002**, *49*, 457–471. [CrossRef] [PubMed]

71. Barcellos, M.P.; Santos, C.B.R.; Federico, L.B.; Almeida, P.F.D.; Silva, C.H.D.P.; Taft, C.A. Pharmacophore and structure-based drug design, molecular dynamics and admet/tox studies to design novel potential pad4 inhibitors. *J. Biomol. Struct. Dyn.* **2019**, *37*, 966–981. [CrossRef] [PubMed]

72. Borges, R.S.; Palheta, I.C.; Ota, S.S.B.; Morais, R.B.; Barros, V.A.; Ramos, R.S.; Silva, R.C.; Costa, J.S.; Silva, C.H.T.P.; Campos, J.M.; et al. Toward of Safer Phenylbutazone Derivatives by Exploration of Toxicity Mechanism. *Molecules* **2019**, *24*, 143. [CrossRef]

73. Costa, J.S.; Ramos, R.S.; Costa, K.S.L.; Brasil, D.S.B.; Silva, C.H.T.P.; Ferreira, E.F.B.; Borges, R.S.; Campos, J.M.; Macêdo, W.J.C.; Santos, C.B.R. An in silico study of the antioxidant ability for two caffeine analogs using molecular docking and quantum chemical methods. *Molecules* **2018**, *23*, 2801. [CrossRef] [PubMed]

74. Ramos, R.D.S.; Costa, J.D.S.; Silva, R.C.; Costa, G.V.; Rodrigues, A.B.L.; Rabelo, É.D.M.; Santos, C.B.R.D. Identification of Potential Inhibitors from Pyriproxyfen with Insecticidal Activity by Virtual Screening. *Pharmaceuticals* **2019**, *12*, 20. [CrossRef]

75. Esser, R.; Berry, C.; Du, Z.; Dawson, J.; Fox, A.; Fujimoto, R.A.; Haston, W.; Kimble, E.F.; Koehler, J.; Peppard, J.; et al. Preclinical Pharmacology of Lumiracoxib: A Novel Selective Inhibitor of Cyclooxygenase-2. *Br. J. Pharmacol.* **2005**, *144*, 538–550. [CrossRef] [PubMed]

76. Kurumbail, R.G.; Stevens, A.M.; Gierse, J.K.; McDonald, J.J.; Stegeman, R.A.; Pak, J.Y.; Gildehaus, D.; Miyashiro, J.M.; Penning, T.D.; Seibert, K.; et al. Structural basis for selective inhibition of cyclooxygenase-2 by anti-inflammatory agents. *Nature* **1996**, *384*, 644–648. [CrossRef] [PubMed]

77. Marnett, L.J. Cyclooxygenase mechanisms. *Curr. Opin. Chem. Biol.* **2000**, *4*, 545–552. [CrossRef]

78. House, H.O. *Modern Organic Reactions*; The Benjamin Publishing Co.: Amsterdam, The Netherlands, 1972.

79. Patani, G.A.; LaVoie, E.J. Bioisosterism: A Rational Approach in Drug Design. *Chem. Rev.* **1996**, *96*, 3147–3176. [CrossRef]

80. Biagi, G.; Giorgi, I.; Livi, O.; Nardi, A.; Calderone, V.; Martelli, A.; Martinotti, E.; LeRoy, S.O. Synthesis and biological activity of novel substituted benzanilides as potassium channel activators. V. *Eur. J. Med. Chem.* **2004**, *39*, 491–498. [CrossRef] [PubMed]

81. Silverstein, R.M.; Bassler, G.C.; Morril, T.C. *Indentificação Espectrometria de Compostos Orgânicos*; Guanabara Dois: Rio de Janeiro, Brazil, 1994.
82. Lipinski, C.A. Drug-like properties and the causes of poor solubility and poor permeability. *J. Pharmacol. Toxicol. Methods* **2000**, *44*, 235–249. [CrossRef]
83. Lipinski, C.A.; Lombardo, F.; Dominy, B.W.; Feeney, P.J. Experimental and computational approaches to estimatesolubility and permeability in drug discovery and developmentqsettings. *Adv. Drug Deliv. Rev.* **2001**, *46*, 3–26. [CrossRef] [PubMed]
84. Drwal, M.N.; Banerjee, P.; Dunkel, M.; Wettig, M.R.; Preissner, R. ProTox: A web server for the in silico prediction of rodent oral toxicity. *Nucleic Acids Res.* **2014**, *42*, W53–W58. [CrossRef]
85. Santos, C.B.R.; Ramos, R.S.; Ortiza, B.L.S.; Silva, G.M.; Giuliatti, S.; Navarrete, J.L.A.; Carvalho, J.C.T. Oil from the fruits of Pterodon emarginatus Vog.: A traditional anti-inflammatory. Study combining in vivo and in silico. *J. Ethnopharmacol.* **2018**, *222*, 107–120. [CrossRef] [PubMed]
86. *Derek for Windows*, version 10.0.2; User Guide. Lhasa Limited; Department of Chemistry, University of Leeds: Leeds, UK, 2007.
87. Trott, O.; Olson, A.J. AutoDock Vina: Improving the speed and accuracy of docking with a new scoring function, efficient optimization and multithreading. *J. Comput. Chem.* **2010**, *31*, 455–461. [CrossRef] [PubMed]
88. Dallakyan, S.; Olson, A.J. Small-molecule library screening by docking with PyRx. *Methods Mol. Biol.* **2015**, *1263*, 243–250.
89. BIOVIA Dassault Systèmes. *BIOVIA Discovery Studio Visualizer*, version 17.2; Dassault Systèmes: San Diego, CA, USA, 2017.
90. Turner, G.W.; Tedesco, E.; Harris, K.D.; Johnston, R.L.; Kariuki, B.M. Implementation of lamarckian concepts in a genetic algorithm for structure solution from powder diffraction data. *Chem. Phys. Lett.* **2000**, *321*, 183–190. [CrossRef]
91. Bittencourt, J.A.H.M.; Neto, M.F.A.; Lacerda, P.S.; Bittencourt, R.C.V.S.; Silva, R.C.; Lobato, C.C.; Silva, L.B.; Leite, F.A.; Zuliani, J.P.; Rosa, J.M.C.; et al. In silico evaluation of ibuprofen and two benzoylpropionic acid derivatives with potential anti-inflammatory activity. *Molecules* **2019**, *24*, 1476. [CrossRef]
92. dos Santos, K.L.B.; Cruz, J.N.; Silva, L.B.; Ramos, R.S.; Neto, M.F.A.; Lobato, C.C.; Ota, S.S.B.; Leite, F.H.A.; Borges, R.S.; da Silva, C.H.T.P.; et al. Identification of Novel Chemical Entities for Adenosine Receptor Type 2A Using Molecular Modeling Approaches. *Molecules* **2020**, *25*, 1245. [CrossRef]
93. Santos, C.B.R.; Santos, K.L.B.; Cruz, J.N.; Leite, F.H.A.; Borges, R.S.; Taft, C.A.; Campos, J.M.; Silva, C.H.T.P. Molecular modeling approaches of selective adenosine receptor type 2A agonists as potential anti-inflammatory drugs. *J. Biomol. Struct. Dyn.* **2020**, *38*, 3115–3127. [CrossRef]
94. Leão, R.P.; Cruz, J.V.; da Costa, G.V.; Cruz, J.N.; Ferreira, E.F.B.; Silva, R.C.; de Lima, L.R.; Borges, R.S.; dos Santos, G.B.; Santos, C.B.R. Identification of New Rofecoxib-Based Cyclooxygenase-2 Inhibitors: A Bioinformatics Approach. *Pharmaceuticals* **2020**, *13*, 209. [CrossRef]
95. Araújo, P.H.F.; Ramos, R.S.; da Cruz, J.N.; Silva, S.G.; Ferreira, E.F.B.; de Lima, L.R.; Macêdo, W.J.C.; Espejo-Román, J.M.; Campos, J.M.; Santos, C.B.R. Identification of Potential COX-2 Inhibitors for the Treatment of Inflammatory Diseases Using Molecular Modeling Approaches. *Molecules* **2020**, *25*, 4183. [CrossRef]
96. Cruz, J.V.; Giuliatti, S.; Alves, L.B.; Silva, R.C.; Ferreira, E.F.B.; Kimani, N.M.; Silva, C.H.T.P.; de Souza, J.S.N.; Espejo-Román, J.M.; Santos, C.B.R. Identification of novel potential cyclooxygenase-2 inhibitors using ligand- and structure-based virtual screening approaches. *J. Biomol. Struct. Dyn.* **2021**, *39*, 5386–5408. [CrossRef]
97. Koster, R.; Anderson, M.; Ej, D.B. Acetic acid for analgesic screening. *Fed. Proc.* **1959**, *18*, 412.
98. Woolfe, G.; MacDonald, A.D. The evaluation of the analgesic action of pethidine hydrochloride (demerol). *J. Pharmacol. Exp. Ther.* **1944**, *80*, 300–307.

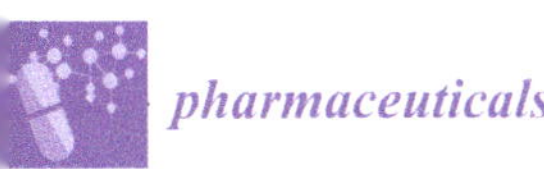

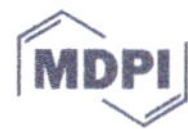

Article

Unraveling the Neuroprotective Effect of Natural Bioactive Compounds Involved in the Modulation of Ischemic Stroke by Network Pharmacology

Juan Carlos Gomez-Verjan [1,†], Emmanuel Alejandro Zepeda-Arzate [1,†], José Alberto Santiago-de-la-Cruz [1], Edgar Antonio Estrella-Parra [2] and Nadia Alejandra Rivero-Segura [1,*]

[1] Dirección de Investigación, Instituto Nacional de Geriatría (INGER), Blvd. Adolfo Ruiz Cortines 2767, Mexico City 10200, Mexico; jverjan@inger.gob.mx (J.C.G.-V.); bm.ezepeda@gmail.com (E.A.Z.-A.); alberto.santiago@alumnos.uacm.edu.mx (J.A.S.-d.-l.-C.)

[2] Laboratorio de Fitoquímica, UBIPRO, FES-Iztacala, Unidad Nacional Autónoma de México, Av. De los Barrios No.1, Los Reyes Iztacala, Tlalnepantla 54090, Mexico; estreparr@iztacala.unam.mx

* Correspondence: nrivero@inger.gob.mx; Tel.: +52-1-(55)-55738601

† These authors contributed equally to this work.

Abstract: Ischemic stroke (IS) is one of the leading causes of mortality worldwide. It is characterized by the partial or total occlusion of arteries that supply blood to the brain, leading to the death of brain cells. In recent years, natural bioactive compounds (NBCs) have shown properties that ameliorate the injury after IS and improve the patient's outcome, which has proven to be a potential therapeutic strategy due to their neuroprotective effects. Hence, in the present study, we use both systems pharmacology and chemoinformatic analyses to identify which NBCs have the most potential to be used against IS in clinics. Our results identify that flavonoids and terpenoids are the most studied NBCs, and, mainly, salidrosides, ginkgolides A, B, C, and K, cordycepin, curcumin, baicalin, resveratrol, fucose, and cannabidiol, target the main pathological processes occurring in IS. However, the medicinal chemistry properties of such compounds demonstrate that only six fulfill such criteria. However, only cordycepin and salidroside possess properties as leader molecules, suggesting that these compounds may be considered in developing novel drugs against IS.

Keywords: natural bioactive compounds; natural products; network pharmacology; neuroprotection; ischemic stroke; flavonoids; terpenoids

Citation: Gomez-Verjan, J.C.; Zepeda-Arzate, E.A.; Santiago-de-la-Cruz, J.A.; Estrella-Parra, E.A.; Rivero-Segura, N.A. Unraveling the Neuroprotective Effect of Natural Bioactive Compounds Involved in the Modulation of Ischemic Stroke by Network Pharmacology. *Pharmaceuticals* **2023**, *16*, 1376. https://doi.org/10.3390/ph16101376

Academic Editors: Halil Ibrahim Ciftci, Belgin Sever and Hasan Demirci

Received: 21 August 2023
Revised: 20 September 2023
Accepted: 25 September 2023
Published: 28 September 2023

1. Introduction

Ischemic stroke (IS) is one of the leading causes of mortality worldwide [1,2]. It is characterized by the partial or total occlusion of arteries that supply blood to the brain, leading to the massive death of brain cells [3]. Currently, canonical IS management relies on the revascularization and prevention of secondary neuronal injury by combining both thrombolytic (recombinant tissue plasminogen activator—rtPA) and surgical procedures, also known as endovascular therapies [4]. However, these therapies have many drawbacks. For instance, the rtPA administration has a narrow window of time (4.5 h of stroke onset), and a tiny proportion of individuals develop symptomatic hemorrhage, and it is recognized that rtPA has neurotoxic effects [5]. On the other hand, despite the newest mechanical devices to perform surgical procedures (mechanical thrombectomy) that are more effective (restoring the blood supply in almost 90% of the cases), these only focus on restoring blood supply to the brain (stopping the ischemia) but do not prevent the damage caused by the reperfusion [6]. In this sense, current research focuses on neuroprotective and neurorestorative therapies by identifying and developing novel compounds to overcome the current drugs' drawbacks. In this sense, natural products, a broad term encompassing either primary or secondary metabolites from plants, marine products, and microorganisms, represent a valuable source for developing and obtaining small molecules. In fact, from 1981 to 2019, about 36.3% of the clinically used drugs approved by the FDA (antimicrobial, antiparasitic, and anticancer treatments) were natural products or derivatives [7,8]. Particularly in the field of IS, natural bioactive compounds (NBCs), a subset of natural products that have biological activity [9–11], are recognized as a rich source of compounds with beneficial effects against the most common pathological effects induced by such conditions [12]. For instance, many authors report that different NBCs reduce infarct size by targeting oxidative stress. However, several NBCs also decrease neuroinflammation due to their immunomodulatory properties (reducing proinflammatory cytokines), inhibiting microglia activation, preventing excitotoxicity and apoptosis, and improving neuroplasticity and endothelial stiffness [13–18].

Moreover, network pharmacology has emerged as an exciting field that combines biology, bioinformatics, and network science to analyze the interaction among bioactive compounds, drugs, genes, proteins, or other biological molecules, leading to improved identification of new drug targets, the design of new drugs, and the prediction of their side effects [19,20]. In this sense, the IS research field has also benefited from network pharmacology since several studies aim to identify potential drug targets and molecular mechanisms induced by NBCs against IS [21–23]. Nevertheless, such studies focus only on a compound or plant extract. Only one published study summarizes the most commonly used NBCs in traditional Chinese medicine. It identifies the primary molecular targets of such NBCs [24] but does not perform cheminformatic analysis to rationally suggest which NBCs are more suitable to be used in therapeutics. Therefore, in the present article, we aim to identify which NBCs have potential to be used against IS in clinics through both systems pharmacology and chemoinformatic analyses. First, we perform a systematic review of the literature published in the last 12 years regarding NBCs used against IS, and then we retrieve the most relevant data for the network pharmacology analyses; these analyses lead us to identify the most connected NBCs in the network, and finally, such NBCs were subjected to chemoinformatic analyses to identify which NBCs are more suitable for success in the clinics. So, with this study, we provide a guide on trends in research towards the neuroprotective effects of NBCs.

2. Results

2.1. Twelve Chemical Classes of NBCs Target the Principal Pathological Processes Elicited by IS, but Only Flavonoids and Terpenoids Are the Most Studied

According to our research in the literature published between 2010 and 2022, there is a lack of studies that report which NBCs are the most studied against IS, compared to the vast number of narrative reviews describing the biological activities and molecular mechanisms elicited by such NBCs used against IS. In this context, our results from Figure 1A demonstrate that, even though twelve chemical classes of NBCs have been tested against IS, only flavonoids (27 studies) and terpenoids (13 studies) are the most studied chemical classes of NBCs. In contrast, the remaining NBCs had fewer studies in the period covered by our search; for instance, polyphenols (10 studies), alkaloids (9 studies), saponin and iridoid glycosides (8 studies each), glycosides (5 studies), phytocannabinoids (4 studies), adenosine analogues and N-linked glycans (3 studies each), anthraquinones (2 studies), and trans-cinnamaldehyde (1 study). Additionally, this result is validated by the results from Figure 1B, since according to the structural network analysis, flavonoids are the most connected nodes in the network (49 edges) in comparison with other NBCs such as terpenoids (23 edges), polyphenols (17 edges), and alkaloids (12 edges), meaning that flavonoids may interact with more targets associated with IS than other compounds.

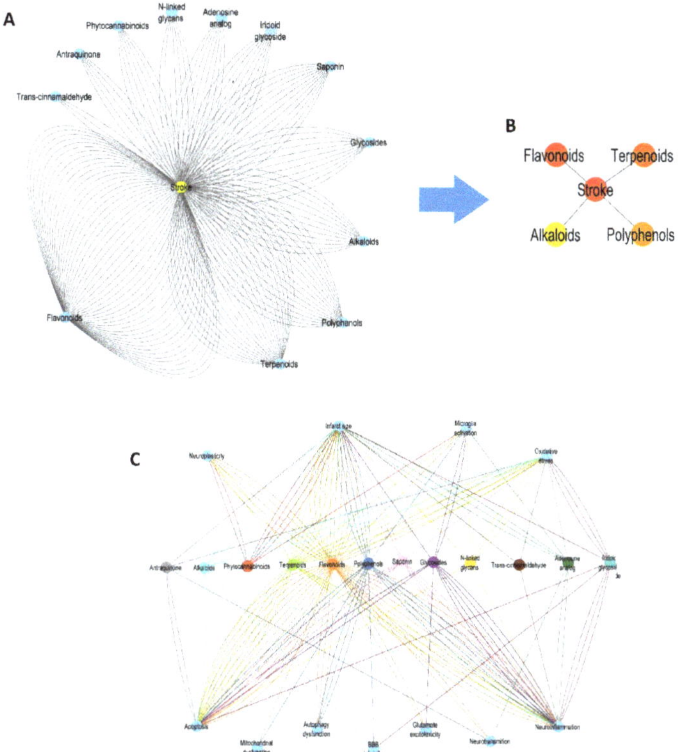

Figure 1. Chemical classes of the NBCs studied against IS. (**A**) Blue nodes represent the NBCs (flavonoids, terpenoids, polyphenols, alkaloids, glycosides, saponin, iridoid glycosides, phytocannabinoids, adenosine analogues, N-linked glycans, anthraquinones, and trans-cinnamaldehyde). Edges (black) represent a single pathological target for each node. Number of nodes: 15, number of edges: 166, network diameter: 1. (**B**) The structural network represents the top five of the most connected nodes in the network. The most connected nodes in the network are flavonoids and terpenoids. The most connected nodes are colored red, and the less connected nodes are colored yellow. (**C**) The structural network shows the chemical classes (central nodes) considered in this study (saponin (pink), iridoid glycoside (aqua), phytocannabinoids (red), N-linked glycans (yellow), flavonoids (orange), alkaloids (light blue), polyphenols (blue), terpenoids (light green), anthraquinone (grey), adenosine analogues (green), and trans-cinnamaldehyde (brown)). Edges connect these nodes (blue) to the main pathological processes that underlie IS. Each edge represents an individual NBC derived from their chemical class. The edges are colored according to the chemical class of each compound. Number of nodes: 23, number of edges: 163, network diameter: 1.

Once we had results from the first network, we built another network with NBCs and the pathological processes they target (Figure 1C). According to the results, the main targets of the NBCs against IS are infarct size, microglia activation, oxidative stress, neuroinflammation, neurotransmission, glutamate excitotoxicity, blood-brain barrier (BBB) integrity, autophagy, mitochondrial dysfunction, and apoptosis. Nevertheless, since the chemical classes of these NBCs include more than hundreds of compounds, we aim to identify which natural compounds target each process mentioned above.

2.2. Network of NBCs and the Most Common Pathological Pathways Associated with IS

As seen in the structural network from Figure 2A, there are 34 NBCs (astragaloside, *Panax notoginseng* saponin-TSPN, and ginsenoside Rg1, picroside II, catalpol, and geniposide, cannabidiol, fucose, baicalin, scutellarin, vitexin, apigenin, icariin, quercetin, calycosin, xanthohumol, carthamin yellow, and dihydromyricetin, berberine, ligustrazine, daurisoline, tetrahydropalmatine, neferine, curcumin, resveratrol, asiaticoside and salidroside, andrographolide, ginkgolides (A, B, C, K), borneol, and daidzein, emodin, cordycepin, and cinnamaldehyde) which target the most common pathological pathways associated with IS. According to the structural network from Figure 2B, the most connected nodes are ginkgolides (A, B, C, and K), curcumin, baicalin, fucose, cannabidiol, resveratrol, cordycepin, icariin, and salidroside. Additionally, we built another network showing the most connected NBCs and the molecular targets of such compounds (Figure 2C). As a result, the networks show that each NBC has its own molecular targets but also shares other molecular targets such as IL1-β, Bax, Bcl-2, SOD, TNF-α, Caspase-3, IL-8, IL-6, NF-κB, BDNF, GFAP, and Iba-1, suggesting that the development of novel drugs against IS may be directed towards these targets. Moreover, this network shows that the selected NBCs seem to decrease the expression or protein content of the molecular target since the number of green edges is higher than the number of red edges colored red.

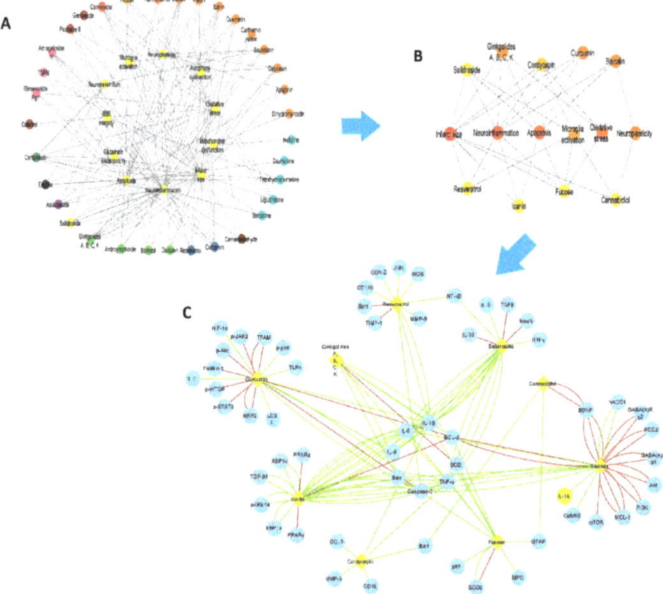

Figure 2. Nine NBCs are required to target the most common pathological processes that underlie IS. (**A**) The network shows the pathological processes that each NBC targets in IS. Number of nodes: 45; number of edges: 163; and network diameter: 1. (**B**) The structural network represents the top 15 of the most connected nodes in the network. Nine NBCs (ginkgolides (A, B, C, K) (terpenoid), curcumin (polyphenol), baicalin (flavonoid), fucose (N-linked glycans), cannabidiol (phytocannabinoids), resveratrol (polyphenol), cordycepin (adenosine analogue), icariin (flavonoid), and salidroside (glycoside) target the main pathological processes that underlie IS (infarct size, neuroinflammation, apoptosis, oxidative stress, neuroplasticity, and microglial activation). The most connected nodes are colored red, and the less connected nodes are colored yellow. (**C**) The network shows the molecular targets of the pathological pathways in IS (blue nodes) connected to the most connected compounds (yellow nodes). The edges represent the effect of the NBCs on each target; green lines represent decreased expression; and red lines represent increased expression. Each edge represents an independent report. In the network's center are the targets shared among the NBCs. Number of nodes: 64; number of edges: 141; and network diameter: 3.

2.3. Chemoinformatic Analysis of the NBCs

Once we identify the most connected NBCs that target the main pathological processes in IS, we perform a chemoinformatic analysis to identify which compounds are more suitable to become therapeutic agents against IS. According to our results (Table 1), cordycepin, curcumin, fucose, ginkgolide A, ginkgolide B, resveratrol, and salidroside meet Lipinski's rules. However, once we analyze the pharmacokinetic simulated properties, our results suggest that ginkgolides B, C, and K are not suitable for therapeutics since the gastrointestinal absorption is lower in contrast to other NBCs such as cannabidiol, cordycepin, curcumin, fucose, ginkgolide A, resveratrol, and salidroside. In addition, the medicinal chemistry properties suggest that ginkgolides A, B, C, and K are unsuitable for chemical synthesis.

Interestingly, only cordycepin and salidroside (Figure 3) possess remarkable pharmacokinetic properties and meet the lead-likeness criteria, suggesting they could be considered hits and leaders in developing novel drugs against IS.

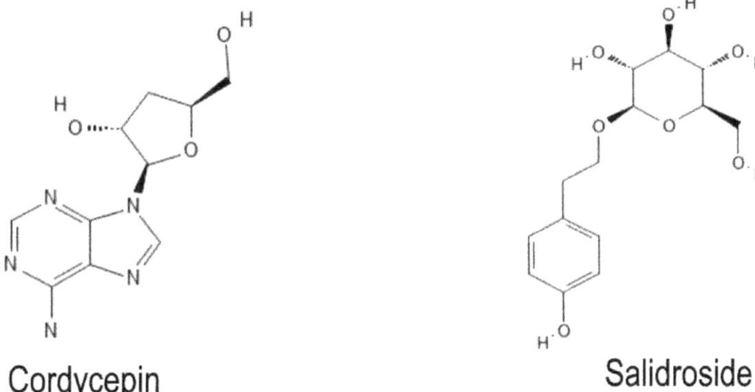

Figure 3. The chemical structure of both NBCs met the lead-likeness criteria.

Table 1. Molecular descriptors of the most connected natural compounds against IS.

		Baicalin	Cannabidiol	Cordycepin	Curcumin	Fucose	Ginkgolide A	Ginkgolide B	Ginkgolide C	Ginkgolide K	Icariin	Resveratrol	Salidroside
Physicochemical Properties	Log P	1.051	6.158	−2.195	1.945	−0.994	1.176	0.146	−1.095	0.914	1.092	2.048	−1.071
	Log S	−2.724	−4.493	−2.724	−3.622	−0.256	−2.526	−2.127	−1.728	−2.277	−4.133	−2.864	−1.016
	TPSA	183.21	40.46	116.03	93.06	90.15	128.59	148.82	169.05	128.59	234.29	60.69	119.61
	MW	446.08	314.46	251.1	368.38	164.16	408.4	424.4	440.13	406.38	676.24	228.24	300.3
	nRB	4	6	2	8	0	1	1	1	1	9	2	5
	HBD	6	2	3	2	4	2	3	4	2	8	3	5
	HBA	11	2	8	6	5	9	10	11	9	15	3	7
Pharmacokinetic Properties	GI absorption	Low	High	High	High	High	High	Low	Low	Low	Low	High	High
	BBB permeable	No	Yes	No	No	No	No	No	No	No	No	Yes	No
	P-gp substrate	Yes	No	No	No	Yes	Yes	Yes	Yes	Yes	Yes	No	No
	CYP1A2 inhibitor	No	No	No	No	No	No	No	No	No	No	Yes	No
	CYP2C19 inhibitor	No	Yes	No	No	No	No	No	No	No	No	No	No
	CYP2C9 inhibitor	No	Yes	No	Yes	No	No	No	No	No	No	Yes	No
	CYP2D6 Inhibitor	No	Yes	No	No	No	No	No	No	No	No	No	No
	CYP3A4 inhibitor	No	Yes	No	Yes	No	No	No	No	No	No	Yes	No
	Log Kp (Skin permeation)	−8.23	−3.59	−8.27	−6.28	−8.79	−8.37	−9.16	−9.95	−9.95	−9.25	−5.47	−8.88
Medicinal Chemistry Properties	Lipinski violations	2	1	0	0	0	0	0	1	1	3	0	0
	Ghose violations	0	1	1	0	2	0	1	1	1	3	0	1
	Veber violations	1	0	0	0	0	0	0	1	1	1	0	0
	Bioavailability Score	0.11	0.55	0.55	0.55	0.55	0.55	0.55	0.55	0.55	0.17	0.55	0.55
	Lead-likeness violations	1	1	0	2	1	1	1	1	1	2	1	0
	Synthetic accessibility	5.09	4.05	3.67	2.97	4.05	6.28	6.38	6.48	6.48	7.24	2.02	4.26
Toxicoinformatic Properties	Mutagenic	none	none	none	none	none	none	none	none	none	high	high	none
	Tumorigenic	none	none	none	none	none	none	none	none	none	none	none	none
	Irritant	none	none	none	none	none	none	none	none	none	none	none	none
	Reproductive effects	none	none	none	none	none	none	none	none	none	high	high	none

3. Discussion

IS represents a global health problem since it is the second cause of mortality and disability worldwide. Hence, current research in the field seeks novel protocols that improve IS diagnosis and treatment to overcome adverse outcomes [25,26]. As a result of this concern, several approaches have been developed; one of them relies on identifying natural products that target the main pathological processes underlying IS [27,28]. However, despite the significant number of original articles or reviews that seek to highlight the relevance of considering the use of natural products against IS, they limit themselves to adding more evidence of the effectiveness of the natural compounds or summarizing the results from other studies without suggesting the next step in the development of novel drugs or their application in clinical practice. Hence, to fill the gaps in the knowledge mentioned above, in the present study, we aim to identify which NBCs are the most studied against IS and then suggest which of them have the potential to formulate and design more effective pharmacological treatments against the pathological processes elicited by IS.

Accordingly, we perform a network pharmacology analysis based on a systematic review, demonstrating that flavonoids are the most studied compounds against IS; this result may be because flavonoids are enriched in many herbal products and, concomitantly, since their chemical structure (the hydroxy groups) influences their bioavailability and pharmacological activity [29]. For instance, flavonoids are associated with several beneficial biological properties such as anti-inflammatory, anticancer, anti-aging, cardio-protective, neuroprotective, immunomodulatory, antidiabetic, antibacterial, antiparasitic, and antiviral [30–32]. On the other hand, the same network identifies terpenoids as the second most studied NBCs against IS. Terpenoids, a class of terpenes with different functional groups and oxidized methyl groups, are the second most widespread NBCs that show antiviral, antibacterial, antimalarial, anti-inflammatory, anticancer, and hypoglycemic activities, and such compounds are found in plants, fungi, and some animals [33–35]. Additionally, these results also suggest that studying a plant or marine product rich in flavonoids or terpenoids is more likely to have neuroprotective effects against IS. Nevertheless, it is essential to note that clinical trials in humans are necessary to confirm their effects in real-world scenarios. Further studies may be conducted to develop a library of compounds derived or inspired by flavonoids and terpenoids to treat IS efficiently.

Since the chemical classes of NBCs include more than hundreds of compounds, we performed another network pharmacology analysis to identify which NBCs target each pathological process. Such a network identified nine compounds (ginkgolides (A, B, C, K), curcumin, baicalin, fucose, cannabidiol, resveratrol, cordycepin, icariin, and salidroside) as the most connected nodes in the network since they target six out of eleven of the most common pathological processes induced by IS (infarct size, neuroinflammation, apoptosis, oxidative stress, neuroplasticity, and microglia activation). Interestingly, many of these compounds are found in herbal medicines. For instance, ginkgolides (A, B, C, and K), a group of terpene trilactones, are isolated from the *Ginkgo biloba* tree and have shown a beneficial role in health and wellbeing since it is well described that ginkgo extract induces antiparasitic, antifungal, antibacterial, and antiviral activities [36]. Interestingly, it has been reported that the bioavailability of ginkgolides is low; however, the preparation method of ginkgol extracts influences the bioavailability [37].

On the other hand, curcumin (1,7-bis-(4-hydroxy-3-methoxyphenyl)-hepta-1,6-diene-3,5-dione) isolated from *Curcuma longa* belongs to the polyphenol group [38–40]. It has been reported that curcumin has enormous therapeutic potential since it exhibits anti-inflammatory, antioxidant, antiviral, proapoptotic, chemo-preventive, chemotherapeutic, antinociceptive, antiproliferative, antiparasitic, and antimalarial effects [41]. However, poor absorption, rapid metabolism, and systemic elimination, leading to poor bioavailability, are curcumin's main limitations in reaching therapeutics [42]. Moreover, baicalin (5,6-dihydroxy-7-O-glucuronide flavone) is the main active compound of the medicinal plants *Scutellaria baicalensis* and *Oroxylum indicum* [43]; such NBC is a flavonoid that has antibacterial, antiviral, anticancer, anticonvulsant, antioxidant, hepatoprotective, and neuroprotective effects in experimental models; however, its use is limited in clinical trials due to poor bioavailability [44,45]. Conversely, fucose is a monosaccharide that induces biological activities such as anticancer, anti-allergic, anti-coagulant, and anti-aging. Nevertheless, despite the great potential that fucose represents for the food, cosmetics, and pharmaceutical industries, its main limitation is the complexity and high cost of performing its chemical synthesis [46,47]. Likewise, cannabidiol represents the most abundant and therapeutically relevant component in *Cannabis sativa*, *Cannabis indica*, and *Cannabis ruderalis*. According to the literature, cannabidiol induces neuroprotective, antiepileptic, anxiolytic, antipsychotic, and anti-inflammatory effects. However, this NBC has bioavailability and solubility issues, and current studies have focused on developing a novel series of CBD analogues to overcome such drawbacks [48,49]. Similarly, resveratrol (3,5,4'-Trihydroxystilbene) is a polyphenol with a stilbene structure isolated from *Veratrum grandiflorum*. Resveratrol has antioxidant, anti-inflammatory, cardioprotective, antimicrobial, and anti-tumorigenic properties [50]. However, resveratrol also shows poor solubility in water, leading to low oral bioavailability; also, resveratrol has a shorter half-life when administered intravenously [51,52]. Finally, icariin is an isoprenoid flavonoid that represents the active compound of *Epimedii herba* [53,54]; this NBC induces anti-inflammatory, antioxidant, antidepressant, and aphrodisiac effects [55,56]; however, a Phase I trial demonstrated that icariin has low bioavailability of the oral formulation [57]. So, this growing body of evidence suggests that the main limitation of the NBCs we identified by our network analysis is their low bioavailability and the complexity and high cost of performing their chemical synthesis. Our chemoinformatic analysis strengthens such results, as discussed in the following paragraphs.

Since several drugs failed in clinical trials due to their pharmacokinetic properties, we performed a chemoinformatic analysis of the medicinal chemistry properties of the nine NBCs described above so we may identify which NBC may have more potential to be used to alleviate the most common pathological processes in IS. Such analysis shows that only cordycepin, curcumin, fucose, ginkgolide A, ginkgolide B, resveratrol, and salidroside fulfill Lipinski's rule of five. However, only cordycepin and salidroside fulfill lead-likeness rules since neither contains any toxicoinformatics properties. Interestingly, neither of the NBCs are flavonoids, suggesting that despite flavonoids being the more studied NBC against IS, salidroside (phenolic glycoside) and cordycepin (adenosine analogue) may be easier to incorporate as therapeutic drugs against IS. Moreover, these results suggest that both NBCs could be considered in developing novel strategies to develop drugs against IS or to search for natural products with a high content of these compounds. In this sense, cordycepin is an alkaloid and the primary bioactive molecule derived from *Cordyceps*, a well-known fungus used in Chinese traditional medicine for the last 300 years to treat fatigue, sickness, kidney disease, and low sex drive [58]. Various IS-related activities have been described for this NBC, such as anti-inflammatory, inhibition of platelet aggregation, and immunomodulatory effects [58,59]. On the other hand, salidroside is the main bioactive component in *Rhodiola* species; it is a phenylpropanoid glycoside that has also been associated with IS-related pathways, such as suppressing oxidative stress, inflammation, and enhancing cell survival [60].

Finally, pure compounds alone may be helpful; however, a cocktail of NBCs could represent a viable alternative in searching for IS treatments with a novel increase in phytomedicine. In this context, it is pretty interesting that there is a renewed interest in developing this type of product due to the success of NeuroAID [61], recently approved in China, Singapur, South Korea, Indonesia, and Vietnam to be used on IS and composed of nine herbal components. Thus, expectations are great for these types of products.

4. Materials and Methods

4.1. Data Collection

Following the PRISMA statement [62], we systematically reviewed the literature published between January 2010 and January 2022 (Figure 4). MESH terms, including *'cerebral ischemia'*, '*natural medicine*', '*stroke*', '*neuroprotection mechanism*', '*natural products*', '*therapeutic applications*', and '*natural extracts*', were submitted to the Pubmed database (https://pubmed.ncbi.nlm.nih.gov/, accessed on 30 March to 30 April 2023). Two independent reviewers curated the selected articles according to the following criteria:

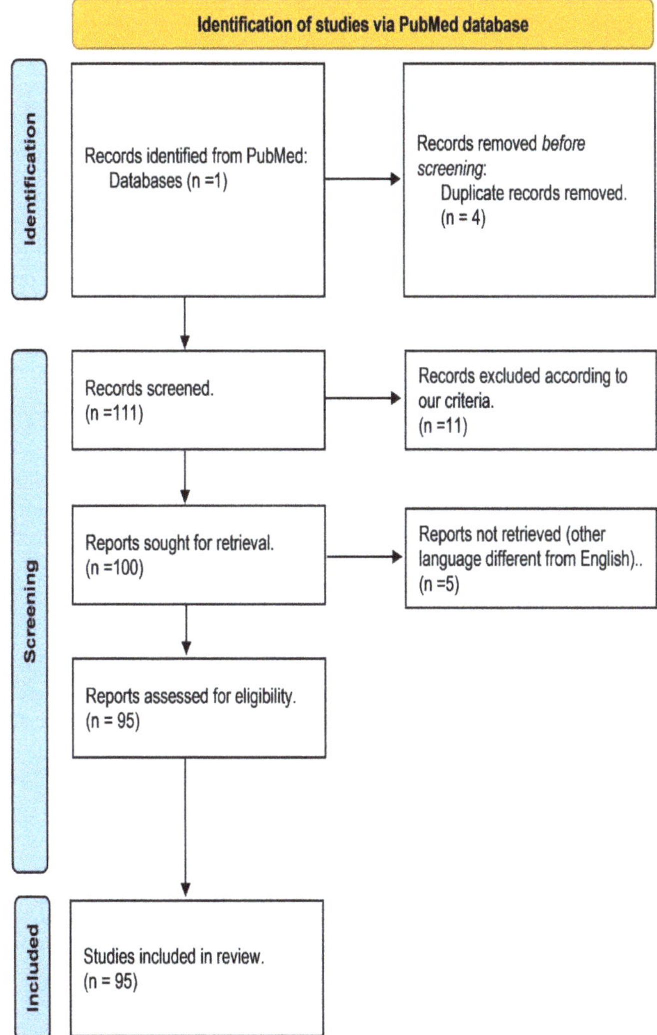

Figure 4. PRISMA flow diagram of the article selection for the systematic review of NBCs against IS. According to our selection criteria for this study, we selected 95 articles, from which we retrieved the following information: chemical class, chemical compound name, experimental model (in vivo or in vitro), molecular target, treatment (doses), biological activity, and reference (Table S1–Supplementary Materials). (http://prisma-statement.org/prismastatement/FlowDiagram.aspx, accessed on 1 January 2022) [62].

Inclusion criteria: Studies published between January 2010 and January 2022 (12 years of research window), original research articles, studies focused on neuroprotection induced by NBCs in IS models, and studies performed on in vitro or in vivo models using NBCs against IS.

Exclusion criteria: Studies that have not met the inclusion criteria, studies published in languages excluding English, articles that were narrative reviews, intervention studies, letters to editors or non-original articles, preprints or studies with incomplete datasets, studies without available data, studies without controls, studies focused on neuroprotection for neurodegenerative diseases (e.g., Huntington's disease, Alzheimer's disease, Parkinson's disease, among others), and articles not available in the PubMed database.

We retrieved all the relevant information from each selected study, as depicted in Table S1 in the Supplementary Materials.

4.2. Network Pharmacology Analysis

Pharmacological networks were built using Cytoscape (v 3.9.1) [63,64]. Networks were built with the data retrieved from the selected articles (Table S1 from the Supplementary Materials). Additionally, we identify the most connected nodes in the networks using the Cytohubba plugin available on the Cytoscape webpage [65].

4.3. Cheminformatic Analyses

Molecular descriptors (1-3D) were calculated for each NBC using three software and web tools: DruLiTo v.1.0 (Nagar, India) is open-source software that can calculate different molecular properties and screen molecules based on pharmacological property rules such as the Lipinski rule, MDDR rule, Veber rule, Ghose filter, BBB rule, CMC-50 rule, and quantitative estimation of pharmacological properties (QED) [66]; DataWarrior v.5.5.0 (Allschwil, Switzerland) [67], an open-source program for visualization and data analysis with chemical intelligence following the methodology of [67]; SwissADME (http://www.swissadme.ch/, Lausanne, Switzerland), a website that allows calculating physicochemical descriptors as well as predicting ADME parameters, pharmacokinetic properties, pharmacological nature, and medical chemical compatibility of single or multiple small molecules to support drug discovery. Such analysis was based on Lipinski's rules: molecular weight (MW) equal to or less than 500 Da, octanol-water partition coefficient equal to or less than 5 (cLogP), the total number of hydrogen acceptors equal to or less than 10 (HBA), and the total number of hydrogen donors equal to or less than 5 (HBD) [68–70] and pharmacokinetics [71].

5. Conclusions

In the present article, we resume most of the studies performed on natural products and IS through 12 years of research to guide trends in research towards the neuroprotective effects of NBCs against IS. In this sense, we found that flavonoids are the most studied NBCs tested against IS to date (2023). We also identify that of the nine NBCs that target the most common pathological process in IS, only cordycepin (adenosine analogue) and salidroside (phenolic glycoside) may be considered leaders to be used in developing chemical libraries and novel molecules against such a pathology. Finally, our study highlights the importance of searching for plant extracts that contain these compounds, which could represent the source for phytomedicine development.

Supplementary Materials: The following supporting information can be downloaded at https://www.mdpi.com/article/10.3390/ph16101376/s1. Table S1: Database of natural products against IS.

Author Contributions: N.A.R.-S.: Conceptualization, Investigation, Writing—Original Draft, Writing Review and Editing; Supervision and Project administration. E.A.Z.-A.: Conceptualization, Investigation, Data Curation, Methodology, Validation; Formal analysis, Software, Writing—Original Draft and Editing and Visualization. J.C.G.-V.: Validation; Formal analysis, Writing—Review and Editing and Visualization. J.A.S.-d.-l.-C.: Software, Formal Analysis, Writing-Original Draft, Writing-Review and Editing. E.A.E.-P.: Investigation, Data Curation, Formal Analysis and Writing-Original Draft. All authors have read and agreed to the published version of the manuscript.

Funding: This study was supported by the Consejo Nacional de Humanidades, Ciencias y Tecnologías, México; Project 319706. The publication of this paper was conducted by the Instituto Nacional de Geriatría, México, and financially supported by the Consejo Nacional de Humanidades

Ciencias y Tecnologías, México; Project 319706. E.A.Z.-A. received a scholarship from the Consejo Nacional de Humanidades Ciencias y Tecnologías (CONAHCYT), México project 319706, "¿Se pueden revertir el envejecimiento con fármacos?"

Institutional Review Board Statement: Not applicable.

Informed Consent Statement: Not applicable.

Data Availability Statement: Data is contained within the article.

Acknowledgments: This study was part of a registered project at the Instituto Nacional de Geriatría DI-PI-002-2020 (NARS). The publication of this paper was supported by the Instituto Nacional de Geriatría, México.

Conflicts of Interest: The authors declare no conflict of interest.

References

1.   CDC Stroke Facts. Available online: https://www.cdc.gov/stroke/facts.htm (accessed on 17 August 2023).
2.   Saini, V.; Guada, L.; Yavagal, D.R. Global Epidemiology of Stroke and Access to Acute Ischemic Stroke Interventions. *Neurology* **2021**, *97*, S6–S16. [CrossRef]
3.   Campbell, B.C.V.; De Silva, D.A.; Macleod, M.R.; Coutts, S.B.; Schwamm, L.H.; Davis, S.M.; Donnan, G.A. Ischaemic Stroke. *Nat. Rev. Dis. Primers* **2019**, *5*, 70. [CrossRef]
4.   Herpich, F.; Rincon, F. Management of Acute Ischemic Stroke. *Crit. Care Med.* **2020**, *48*, 1654–1663. [CrossRef]
5.   O'Carroll, C.B.; Aguilar, M.I. Management of Postthrombolysis Hemorrhagic and Orolingual Angioedema Complications. *Neurohospitalist* **2015**, *5*, 133–141. [CrossRef]
6.   Hurd, M.D.; Goel, I.; Sakai, Y.; Teramura, Y. Current Status of Ischemic Stroke Treatment: From Thrombolysis to Potential Regenerative Medicine. *Regen. Ther.* **2021**, *18*, 408–417. [CrossRef]
7.   Rivero-Segura, N.A.; Gomez-Verjan, J.C. In Silico Screening of Natural Products Isolated from Mexican Herbal Medicines against COVID-19. *Biomolecules* **2021**, *11*, 216. [CrossRef]
8.   Calixto, J.B. The Role of Natural Products in Modern Drug Discovery. *An. Acad. Bras. Cienc.* **2019**, *91* (Suppl. S3), e20190105. [CrossRef]
9.   *Natural Bioactive Compounds: Technological Advancements*; Sinha, R.P.; Häder, h.c.D.-P. (Eds.) Academic Press: San Diego, CA, USA, 2020; ISBN 9780128206553.
10. Sytar, O.; Smetanska, I. Special Issue "Bioactive Compounds from Natural Sources (2020, 2021)". *Molecules* **2022**, *27*, 1929. [CrossRef]
11. Mohd Sairazi, N.S.; Sirajudeen, K.N.S. Natural Products and Their Bioactive Compounds: Neuroprotective Potentials against Neurodegenerative Diseases. *Evid. Based Complement. Alternat. Med.* **2020**, *2020*, 6565396. [CrossRef]
12. George, P.M.; Steinberg, G.K. Novel Stroke Therapeutics: Unraveling Stroke Pathophysiology and Its Impact on Clinical Treatments. *Neuron* **2015**, *87*, 297–309. [CrossRef]
13. Putteeraj, M.; Lim, W.L.; Teoh, S.L.; Yahaya, M.F. Flavonoids and Its Neuroprotective Effects on Brain Ischemia and Neurodegenerative Diseases. *Curr. Drug Targets* **2018**, *19*, 1710–1720. [CrossRef] [PubMed]
14. Xie, Q.; Li, H.; Lu, D.; Yuan, J.; Ma, R.; Li, J.; Ren, M.; Li, Y.; Chen, H.; Wang, J.; et al. Neuroprotective Effect for Cerebral Ischemia by Natural Products: A Review. *Front. Pharmacol.* **2021**, *12*, 607412. [CrossRef] [PubMed]
15. She, Y.; Shao, L.; Zhang, Y.; Hao, Y.; Cai, Y.; Cheng, Z.; Deng, C.; Liu, X. Neuroprotective Effect of Glycosides in Buyang Huanwu Decoction on Pyroptosis Following Cerebral Ischemia-Reperfusion Injury in Rats. *J. Ethnopharmacol.* **2019**, *242*, 112051. [CrossRef] [PubMed]
16. Lin, B. Polyphenols and Neuroprotection against Ischemia and Neurodegeneration. *Mini Rev. Med. Chem.* **2011**, *11*, 1222–1238.
17. Zhang, Q.; Zhao, Y.-H. Therapeutic Angiogenesis after Ischemic Stroke: Chinese Medicines, Bone Marrow Stromal Cells (BMSCs) and Their Combinational Treatment. *Am. J. Chin. Med.* **2014**, *42*, 61–77. [CrossRef] [PubMed]
18. Ismailoglu, U.B.; Saracoglu, I.; Harput, U.S.; Sahin-Erdemli, I. Effects of Phenylpropanoid and Iridoid Glycosides on Free Radical-Induced Impairment of Endothelium-Dependent Relaxation in Rat Aortic Rings. *J. Ethnopharmacol.* **2002**, *79*, 193–197. [CrossRef]
19. Noor, F.; Tahir Ul Qamar, M.; Ashfaq, U.A.; Albutti, A.; Alwashmi, A.S.S.; Aljasir, M.A. Network Pharmacology Approach for Medicinal Plants: Review and Assessment. *Pharmaceuticals* **2022**, *15*, 572. [CrossRef]
20. Hopkins, A.L. Network Pharmacology: The next Paradigm in Drug Discovery. *Nat. Chem. Biol.* **2008**, *4*, 682–690. [CrossRef]
21. Liu, F.; Li, L.; Chen, J.; Wu, Y.; Cao, Y.; Zhong, P. A Network Pharmacology to Explore the Mechanism of in the Treatment of Ischemic Stroke. *Biomed Res. Int.* **2021**, *2021*, 6611018.
22. Yang, T.; Chen, X.; Mei, Z.; Liu, X.; Feng, Z.; Liao, J.; Deng, Y.; Ge, J. An Integrated Analysis of Network Pharmacology and Experimental Validation to Reveal the Mechanism of Chinese Medicine Formula Naotaifang in Treating Cerebral Ischemia-Reperfusion Injury. *Drug Des. Devel. Ther.* **2021**, *15*, 3783–3808. [CrossRef]

23. Zhang, W.; Zhang, L.; Wang, W.J.; Ma, S.; Wang, M.; Yao, M.; Li, R.; Li, W.W.; Zhao, X.; Hu, D.; et al. Network Pharmacology and Experimental Verification to Explore the Mechanism of Sanhua Decoction in the Treatment of Ischaemic Stroke. *Pharm. Biol.* **2022**, *60*, 119–130. [CrossRef]

24. Zhu, T.; Wang, L.; Wang, L.-P.; Wan, Q. Therapeutic Targets of Neuroprotection and Neurorestoration in Ischemic Stroke: Applications for Natural Compounds from Medicinal Herbs. *Biomed. Pharmacother.* **2022**, *148*, 112719. [CrossRef] [PubMed]

25. Lanas, F.; Seron, P. Facing the Stroke Burden Worldwide. *Lancet Glob Health* **2021**, *9*, e235–e236. [CrossRef] [PubMed]

26. Feigin, V.L.; Norrving, B.; Mensah, G.A. Global Burden of Stroke. *Circ. Res.* **2017**, *120*, 439–448. [CrossRef] [PubMed]

27. Fang, C.; Xu, H.; Yuan, L.; Zhu, Z.; Wang, X.; Liu, Y.; Zhang, A.; Shao, A.; Lou, M. Natural Compounds for SIRT1-Mediated Oxidative Stress and Neuroinflammation in Stroke: A Potential Therapeutic Target in the Future. *Oxid. Med. Cell. Longev.* **2022**, *2022*, 1949718. [CrossRef]

28. Li, X.-H.; Yin, F.-T.; Zhou, X.-H.; Zhang, A.-H.; Sun, H.; Yan, G.-L.; Wang, X.-J. The Signaling Pathways and Targets of Natural Compounds from Traditional Chinese Medicine in Treating Ischemic Stroke. *Molecules* **2022**, *27*, 3099. [CrossRef]

29. Câmara, J.S.; Albuquerque, B.R.; Aguiar, J.; Corrêa, R.C.G.; Gonçalves, J.L.; Granato, D.; Pereira, J.A.M.; Barros, L.; Ferreira, I.C.F.R. Food Bioactive Compounds and Emerging Techniques for Their Extraction: Polyphenols as a Case Study. *Foods* **2021**, *10*, 37. [CrossRef]

30. Jucá, M.M.; Cysne Filho, F.M.S.; de Almeida, J.C.; Mesquita, D.d.S.; Barriga, J.R.d.M.; Dias, K.C.F.; Barbosa, T.M.; Vasconcelos, L.C.; Leal, L.K.A.M.; Ribeiro, J.E.; et al. Flavonoids: Biological Activities and Therapeutic Potential. *Nat. Prod. Res.* **2020**, *34*, 692–705. [CrossRef]

31. Di Ferdinando, M.; Brunetti, C.; Fini, A.; Tattini, M. Flavonoids as Antioxidants in Plants Under Abiotic Stresses. In *Abiotic Stress Responses in Plants*; Springer: New York, NY, USA, 2012; pp. 159–179. ISBN 9781461406334.

32. Maleki, S.J.; Crespo, J.F.; Cabanillas, B. Anti-Inflammatory Effects of Flavonoids. *Food Chem.* **2019**, *299*, 125124. [CrossRef]

33. Perveen, S.; Al-Taweel, A. *Terpenes and Terpenoids*; BoD—Books on Demand: Norderstedt, Germany, 2018; ISBN 9781789847765.

34. Yang, W.; Chen, X.; Li, Y.; Guo, S.; Wang, Z.; Yu, X. Advances in Pharmacological Activities of Terpenoids. *Nat. Prod. Commun.* **2020**, *15*, 1934578X2090355. [CrossRef]

35. Martin-Smith, M.; Khatoon, T. Biological Activity of The Terpenoids and Their Derivatives. *Fortschr. Arzneimittelforsch.* **1963**, *5*, 279–346. [PubMed]

36. Boonkaew, T.; Camper, N.D. Biological Activities of Ginkgo Extracts. *Phytomedicine* **2005**, *12*, 318–323. [CrossRef] [PubMed]

37. Li, C.L.; Wong, Y.Y. The Bioavailability of Ginkgolides in Ginkgo Biloba Extracts. *Planta Med.* **1997**, *63*, 563–565. [CrossRef] [PubMed]

38. Den Hartogh, D.J.; Gabriel, A.; Tsiani, E. Antidiabetic Properties of Curcumin II: Evidence from In Vivo Studies. *Nutrients* **2019**, *12*, 58. [CrossRef]

39. Hosseini, A.; Hosseinzadeh, H. Antidotal or Protective Effects of Curcuma Longa (turmeric) and Its Active Ingredient, Curcumin, against Natural and Chemical Toxicities: A Review. *Biomed. Pharmacother.* **2018**, *99*, 411–421. [CrossRef]

40. Vaiserman, A.M.; Lushchak, O.V.; Zayachkivska, A.; Koliada, A. Curcumin. In *Anti-Aging Pharmacology*; Elsevier: Amsterdam, The Netherlands, 2023; pp. 153–176. ISBN 9780128236796.

41. Kunnumakkara, A.B.; Bordoloi, D.; Padmavathi, G.; Monisha, J.; Roy, N.K.; Prasad, S.; Aggarwal, B.B. Curcumin, the Golden Nutraceutical: Multitargeting for Multiple Chronic Diseases. *Br. J. Pharmacol.* **2017**, *174*, 1325–1348. [CrossRef]

42. Urošević, M.; Nikolić, L.; Gajić, I.; Nikolić, V.; Dinić, A.; Miljković, V. Curcumin: Biological Activities and Modern Pharmaceutical Forms. *Antibiotics* **2022**, *11*, 135. [CrossRef]

43. Ezzat, S.M.; Salama, M.M.; Salem, M.A. Bioactive Lead Compounds and Molecular Targets for the Treatment of Heart Diseases. In *Phytochemicals as Lead Compounds for New Drug Discovery*; Elsevier: Amsterdam, The Netherlands, 2020; pp. 67–94. ISBN 9780128178904.

44. Huang, T.; Liu, Y.; Zhang, C. Pharmacokinetics and Bioavailability Enhancement of Baicalin: A Review. *Eur. J. Drug Metab. Pharmacokinet.* **2019**, *44*, 159–168. [CrossRef]

45. Hu, Z.; Guan, Y.; Hu, W.; Xu, Z.; Ishfaq, M. An Overview of Pharmacological Activities of Baicalin and Its Aglycone Baicalein: New Insights into Molecular Mechanisms and Signaling Pathways. *Iran. J. Basic Med. Sci.* **2022**, *25*, 14–26.

46. Xiao, M.; Ren, X.; Yu, Y.; Gao, W.; Zhu, C.; Sun, H.; Kong, Q.; Fu, X.; Mou, H. Fucose-Containing Bacterial Exopolysaccharides: Sources, Biological Activities, and Food Applications. *Food Chem. X* **2022**, *13*, 100233. [CrossRef]

47. Hong, S.-B.; Choi, J.-H.; Chang, Y.K.; Mun, S. Production of High-Purity Fucose from the Seaweed of Undaria Pinnatifida through Acid-Hydrolysis and Simulated-Moving Bed Purification. *Sep. Purif. Technol.* **2019**, *213*, 133–141. [CrossRef]

48. Morales, P.; Reggio, P.H.; Jagerovic, N. An Overview on Medicinal Chemistry of Synthetic and Natural Derivatives of Cannabidiol. *Front. Pharmacol.* **2017**, *8*, 422. [CrossRef] [PubMed]

49. Kinney, W.A.; McDonnell, M.E.; Zhong, H.M.; Liu, C.; Yang, L.; Ling, W.; Qian, T.; Chen, Y.; Cai, Z.; Petkanas, D.; et al. Discovery of KLS-13019, a Cannabidiol-Derived Neuroprotective Agent, with Improved Potency, Safety, and Permeability. *ACS Med. Chem. Lett.* **2016**, *7*, 424–428. [CrossRef] [PubMed]

50. Meng, Q.; Li, J.; Wang, C.; Shan, A. Biological Function of Resveratrol and Its Application in Animal Production: A Review. *J. Anim. Sci. Biotechnol.* **2023**, *14*, 25. [CrossRef] [PubMed]

51. Das, S.; Lin, H.-S.; Ho, P.C.; Ng, K.-Y. The Impact of Aqueous Solubility and Dose on the Pharmacokinetic Profiles of Resveratrol. *Pharm. Res.* **2008**, *25*, 2593–2600. [CrossRef]

52. Wang, L.-X.; Heredia, A.; Song, H.; Zhang, Z.; Yu, B.; Davis, C.; Redfield, R. Resveratrol Glucuronides as the Metabolites of Resveratrol in Humans: Characterization, Synthesis, and Anti-HIV Activity. *J. Pharm. Sci.* **2004**, *93*, 2448–2457. [CrossRef]
53. He, C.; Wang, Z.; Shi, J. Pharmacological Effects of Icariin. *Adv. Pharmacol.* **2020**, *87*, 179–203.
54. Liu, F.-Y.; Ding, D.-N.; Wang, Y.-R.; Liu, S.-X.; Peng, C.; Shen, F.; Zhu, X.-Y.; Li, C.; Tang, L.-P.; Han, F.-J. Icariin as a Potential Anticancer Agent: A Review of Its Biological Effects on Various Cancers. *Front. Pharmacol.* **2023**, *14*, 1216363. [CrossRef]
55. Wang, S.; Ma, J.; Zeng, Y.; Zhou, G.; Wang, Y.; Zhou, W.; Sun, X.; Wu, M. Icariin, an Up-and-Coming Bioactive Compound Against Neurological Diseases: Network Pharmacology-Based Study and Literature Review. *Drug Des. Devel. Ther.* **2021**, *15*, 3619–3641. [CrossRef]
56. Szabó, R.; Rácz, C.P.; Dulf, F.V. Bioavailability Improvement Strategies for Icariin and Its Derivates: A Review. *Int. J. Mol. Sci.* **2022**, *23*, 7519. [CrossRef]
57. Brown, E.S.; Bice, C.; Putnam, W.C.; Leff, R.; Kulikova, A.; Nakamura, A.; Ivleva, E.I.; Van Enkevort, E.; Holmes, T.; Miingi, N. Human Safety and Pharmacokinetics Study of Orally Administered Icariin: Randomized, Double-Blind, Placebo-Controlled Trial. *Nat. Prod. Commun.* **2019**, *14*, 1934578X1985678. [CrossRef]
58. Ashraf, S.A.; Elkhalifa, A.E.O.; Siddiqui, A.J.; Patel, M.; Awadelkareem, A.M.; Snoussi, M.; Ashraf, M.S.; Adnan, M.; Hadi, S. Cordycepin for Health and Wellbeing: A Potent Bioactive Metabolite of an Entomopathogenic Medicinal Fungus and Its Nutraceutical and Therapeutic Potential. *Molecules* **2020**, *25*, 2735. [CrossRef]
59. Wang, D.; Zhang, Y.; Lu, J.; Wang, Y.; Wang, J.; Meng, Q.; Lee, R.J.; Wang, D.; Teng, L. Cordycepin, a Natural Antineoplastic Agent, Induces Apoptosis of Breast Cancer Cells via Caspase-Dependent Pathways. *Nat. Prod. Commun.* **2016**, *11*, 63–68. [CrossRef] [PubMed]
60. Han, J.; Luo, L.; Wang, Y.; Wu, S.; Kasim, V. Therapeutic Potential and Molecular Mechanisms of Salidroside in Ischemic Diseases. *Front. Pharmacol.* **2022**, *13*, 974775. [CrossRef] [PubMed]
61. Venketasubramanian, N.; Kumar, R.; Soertidewi, L.; Abu Bakar, A.; Laik, C.; Gan, R. The NeuroAiD Safe Treatment (NeST) Registry: A Protocol. *BMJ Open* **2015**, *5*, e009866. [CrossRef]
62. Page, M.J.; McKenzie, J.E.; Bossuyt, P.M.; Boutron, I.; Hoffmann, T.C.; Mulrow, C.D.; Shamseer, L.; Tetzlaff, J.M.; Akl, E.A.; Brennan, S.E.; et al. The PRISMA 2020 Statement: An Updated Guideline for Reporting Systematic Reviews. *BMJ* **2021**, *372*, n71. [CrossRef]
63. Shannon, P.; Markiel, A.; Ozier, O.; Baliga, N.S.; Wang, J.T.; Ramage, D.; Amin, N.; Schwikowski, B.; Ideker, T. Cytoscape: A Software Environment for Integrated Models of Biomolecular Interaction Networks. *Genome Res.* **2003**, *13*, 2498–2504. [CrossRef]
64. Barrera-Vázquez, O.S.; Gomez-Verjan, J.C.; Ramírez-Aldana, R.; Torre, P.G.-D.; Rivero-Segura, N.A. Structural and Pharmacological Network Analysis of miRNAs Involved in Acute Ischemic Stroke: A Systematic Review. *Int. J. Mol. Sci.* **2022**, *23*, 4663. [CrossRef]
65. Chin, C.-H.; Chen, S.-H.; Wu, H.-H.; Ho, C.-W.; Ko, M.-T.; Lin, C.-Y. cytoHubba: Identifying Hub Objects and Sub-Networks from Complex Interactome. *BMC Syst. Biol.* **2014**, *8* (Suppl. S4), S11. [CrossRef]
66. Kumar, T.D.A. *Elementary Pharmacoinformatics*; Pharmamed Press: London, UK, 2015; ISBN 9789385433665.
67. Sander, T.; Freyss, J.; von Korff, M.; Rufener, C. DataWarrior: An Open-Source Program for Chemistry Aware Data Visualization and Analysis. *J. Chem. Inf. Model.* **2015**, *55*, 460–473. [CrossRef]
68. Daina, A.; Michielin, O.; Zoete, V. SwissADME: A Free Web Tool to Evaluate Pharmacokinetics, Drug-Likeness and Medicinal Chemistry Friendliness of Small Molecules. *Sci. Rep.* **2017**, *7*, 42717. [CrossRef] [PubMed]
69. Lipinski, C.A. Lead- and Drug-like Compounds: The Rule-of-Five Revolution. *Drug Discov. Today Technol.* **2004**, *1*, 337–341. [CrossRef] [PubMed]
70. Castillo-Arellano, J.I.; Gómez-Verjan, J.C.; Rojano-Vilchis, N.A.; Mendoza-Cruz, M.; Jiménez-Estrada, M.; López-Valdés, H.E.; Martínez-Coria, H.; Gutiérrez-Juárez, R.; González-Espinosa, C.; Reyes-Chilpa, R.; et al. Chemoinformatic Analysis of Selected Cacalolides from (A. Gray) H. Rob. & Brettell and (Kunth) Cass. and Their Effects on FcεRI-Dependent Degranulation in Mast Cells. *Molecules* **2018**, *23*, 3367. [CrossRef] [PubMed]
71. Bertram-Ralph, E.; Amare, M. Factors Affecting Drug Absorption and Distribution. *Anaesth. Intensive Care Med.* **2023**, *24*, 221–227. [CrossRef]

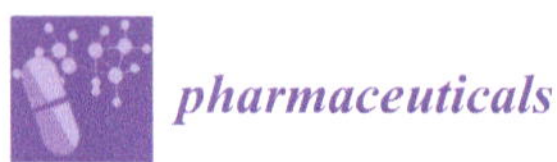 *pharmaceuticals* 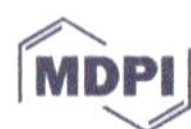

Article

Design of β-Keto Esters with Antibacterial Activity: Synthesis, In Vitro Evaluation, and Theoretical Assessment of Their Reactivity and Quorum-Sensing Inhibition Capacity

Maximiliano Martínez-Cifuentes [1,*], Emmanuel Soto-Tapia [1], Camila Linares-Pipón [1], Ben Bradshaw [2], Paulina Valenzuela-Hormazabal [3], David Ramírez [3], Patricio Muñoz-Torres [4,*] and Claudio Parra [1,*]

[1] Departamento de Química Orgánica, Facultad de Ciencias Químicas, Universidad de Concepción, Edmundo Larenas 129, Concepción 4070371, Chile; emsoto2019@udec.cl (E.S.-T.); clinares@udec.cl (C.L.-P.)
[2] Laboratori de Química Orgánica, Facultat de Farmàcia, IBUB, Universitat de Barcelona, Av. Joan XXIII, s/n, 08028 Barcelona, Spain; benbradshaw@ub.edu
[3] Departamento de Farmacología, Facultad de Ciencias Biológicas, Universidad de Concepción, Concepción 4030000, Chile; paulinvalenzuela@udec.cl (P.V.-H.); dramirezs@udec.cl (D.R.)
[4] Laboratorio de Patología Vegetal y Bioproductos, Facultad de Ciencias Agronómicas, Universidad de Tarapacá, Av. General Velásquez 1775, Arica 1000000, Chile
[*] Correspondence: maxmartinez@udec.cl (M.M.-C.); pmunozt@academicos.uta.cl (P.M.-T.); cparra@udec.cl (C.P.)

Citation: Martínez-Cifuentes, M.; Soto-Tapia, E.; Linares-Pipón, C.; Bradshaw, B.; Valenzuela-Hormazabal, P.; Ramírez, D.; Muñoz-Torres, P.; Parra, C. Design of β-Keto Esters with Antibacterial Activity: Synthesis, In Vitro Evaluation, and Theoretical Assessment of Their Reactivity and Quorum-Sensing Inhibition Capacity. *Pharmaceuticals* **2023**, *16*, 1339. https://doi.org/10.3390/ph16101339

Academic Editors: Halil İbrahim Ciftci, Belgin Sever and Hasan Demirci

Received: 25 August 2023
Revised: 15 September 2023
Accepted: 18 September 2023
Published: 22 September 2023

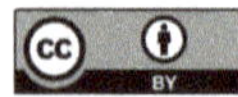

Abstract: This work proposes the design of β-keto esters as antibacterial compounds. The design was based on the structure of the autoinducer of bacterial quorum sensing, *N*-(3-oxo-hexanoyl)-l-homoserine lactone (3-oxo-C6-HSL). Eight β-keto ester analogues were synthesised with good yields and were spectroscopically characterised, showing that the compounds were only present in their β-keto ester tautomer form. We carried out a computational analysis of the reactivity and ADME (absorption, distribution, metabolism, and excretion) properties of the compounds as well as molecular docking and molecular dynamics calculations with the LasR and LuxS quorum-sensing (QS) proteins, which are involved in bacterial resistance to antibiotics. The results show that all the compounds exhibit reliable ADME properties and that only compound **7** can present electrophile toxicity. The theoretical reactivity study shows that compounds **6** and **8** present a differential local reactivity regarding the rest of the series. Compound **8** presents the most promising potential in terms of its ability to interact with the LasR and LuxS QS proteins efficiently according to its molecular docking and molecular dynamics calculations. An initial in vitro antimicrobial screening was performed against the human pathogenic bacteria *Pseudomonas aeruginosa* and *Staphylococcus aureus* as well as the phytopathogenic bacteria *Pseudomonas syringae* and *Agrobacterium tumefaciens* Compounds **6** and **8** exhibit the most promising results in the in vitro antimicrobial screening against the panel of bacteria studied.

Keywords: β-keto esters; DFT; docking; LasR and LuxS; quorum sensing

1. Introduction

In the last few decades, the emergence of antibiotic-resistant bacteria has become a significant concern for developing economies and global health. The World Health Organization (WHO) has published reports showing an increasing worry about this problem, which is predicted to worsen in the coming years [1]. The primary cause behind this development is the excessive use of antibiotics in both human and animal treatment and their widespread application in the commercial industry [2,3]. Although many countries have implemented strict regulations on antibiotic consumption, these measures have yet to halt antibiotic resistance's continuous development effectively. As a result, cases of multidrug resistant strains of common bacteria, such as *Escherichia coli*, *Streptococcus pneumoniae*, and nontyphoidal *Salmonella*, have been documented worldwide [1]. It is essential to address this issue through research, developing new and more robust therapeutic strategies and implementing methods for bacterial control in industry and agriculture. This will ensure access to food and health resources for future generations [1,3].

One promising avenue of research is interfering with bacterial cell communication, known as quorum sensing (QS), which synchronises the behaviours of the individual cells within a multicellular community [4,5]. This process relies on producing, releasing, and detecting small diffusible signalling molecules called autoinducers. In Gram-negative bacteria, QS is regulated by a two-component system, including synthesizing the autoinducer with LuxI homologs and the autoinducer-dependent transcriptional activator, a LuxR homolog [6]. Many pathogenic bacteria use QS to facilitate pathogenesis, producing the virulence factors necessary for host infection or evading the immune system by coordinating swarming behaviour and forming biofilms [7,8]. Therefore, interfering with bacterial communication has become an attractive target for developing new therapies in medicine and the agricultural and aquacultural industries.

Figure 1 shows the chemical structure of the autoinducer (3-oxo-C6-HSL) discovered in the 1980s in the *Vibrio fischeri* lux genes of the QS system, which is responsible for bioluminescence [9]. Since many Gram-negative bacteria use *N*-acyl-homoserine lactones (AHLs) as autoinducers, these natural ligands are important starting points and inspiration for discovering new QS modulators. Numerous synthetic ligands have been designed, synthesised, and evaluated in this field, mimicking natural AHLs' biological activity. The backbone of AHLs consists of three fundamental parts: a lactone ring, their amide function, and an acyl chain. It has been demonstrated that incorporating aryl functionality with electron-withdrawing groups in the acyl side chain converts many small molecules of AHL mimics into potent quorum-sensing inhibitors [10,11]. The central amide-connecting function of AHLs can be replaced with various nonnatural moieties, and these derivatives still retain their activity as synthetic LuxR-based quorum-sensing modulators [12,13]. On the other hand, the hydrolysis of the lactone present in AHLs by mammalian lactonases limits their potential as antivirulence drugs [14]. Several groups have identified nonnatural quorum-sensing modulators inspired by AHLs in which the native homoserine lactone group has been replaced by an aromatic group or carbocyclic rings [15,16].

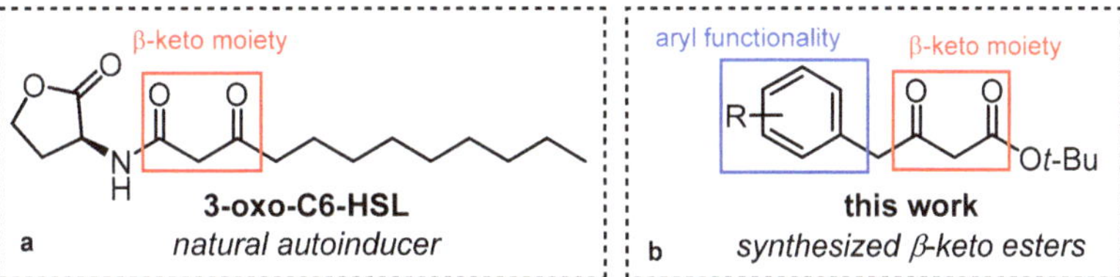

Figure 1. (**a**) Natural autoinducer employed by *V. fischeri*. (**b**) Our proposed QS inhibitor chemotype.

Additionally, other QS systems important to several types of bacteria correspond to LuxS/AI-2 (S-ribosylhomocysteine lyase/autoinducer-2) and LasI-LasR with 3-oxo-C6-HSL as an autoinducer. The first system is implicated in biofilm formation in bacteria such as *Staphylococcus aureus* [17–19]. In contrast, the second is implicated in several characteristics related to bacteria's pathogenicity, such as those of *Pseudomonas aeruginosa* and *S. aureus* [18,20,21].

Various commercial β-keto esters, the simplest structures with potential anti-QS activity, have also been analysed [22]. It has been observed that these compounds, incorporating an aryl substituent, interact with Lux-R-type proteins, thereby inhibiting quorum-sensing (QS) communication. Evaluating more β-keto esters will provide crucial information about the structure–activity relationships necessary for developing antivirulence agents. Therefore, this study designed and synthesised eight β-keto ester analogues of AHL natural autoinducers as potential quorum-sensing inhibitors (Figure 1). The compounds were chemically characterized, and a computational analysis of the reactivity and ADME (absorption, distribution, metabolism, and excretion) properties of the compounds as well as molecular docking and molecular dynamics calculations with the LasR and LuxS quorum-sensing (QS) proteins were carried out. An initial in vitro antimicrobial screening was carried out against human pathogenic and phytopathogenic bacteria.

2. Results and Discussion

2.1. Synthesis and Spectroscopic Characterisation of β-Keto Esters

β-keto esters were synthesised from eight easily accessible commercial carboxylic acids, yielding between 65% and 96%. The choice of carboxylic acid was based on their substituents, with a primary focus on studying the impact of the *ortho* substitution of the phenyl group and its interaction with the active site of the LasR and LuxS QS proteins. We examined the interactions of the resonance-activating groups (**3**) or induction-activating groups (**2**, **5**, **6**, **7**, and **8**) and the deactivating groups (**4**) concerning this model compound (**1**). As shown in Scheme 1, target compounds **1–8** were synthesised. First of all, the commercially available phenylacetic acid derivatives were activated with 4-dimethylaminopyridine (DMAP) and *N,N′*-Dicyclohexylcarbodiimide (DCC) at 0 °C in dichloromethane solutions. Subsequently, condensation with Meldrum's acid at room temperature overnight afforded the proper intermediates. Finally, the β-keto esters were efficiently obtained by refluxing the intermediates in *tert*-butanol.

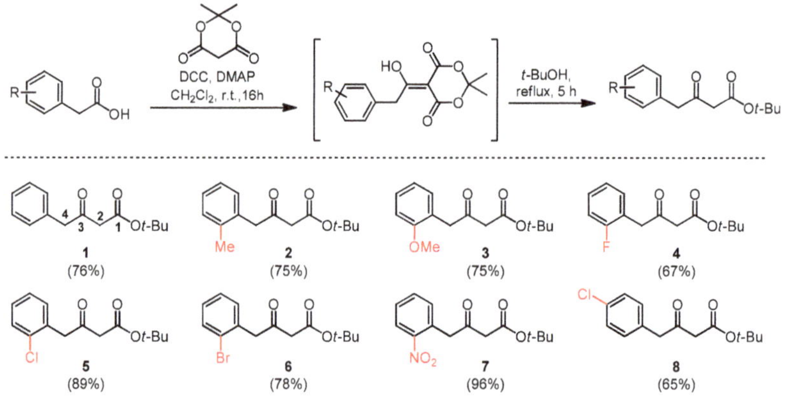

Scheme 1. Synthesis of β-keto esters.

To analyse these structures, we conducted NMR experiments using $CDCl_3$ as the solvent. In all the compounds, we observed three singlet signals at 1.46–1.50 ppm, 3.37–3.55 ppm, and 3.82–4.25 ppm, which were assigned to the protons of the methyl group ($-CH_3$) and the methylene groups ($-CH_2$) of carbons 2 and 4, respectively. These signals confirmed that all the synthesised compounds existed in their keto form rather than their enolic form. However, the signals of the phenyl group varied depending on the type of substituent they had (see supporting information). Overall, all these analyses supported both the proposed structures and the purity of the β-keto esters, making these compounds suitable for bioassays.

2.2. Computational Analysis of the Reactivity and ADME Properties

It has been described that the quantitative relationship between the bioactivity/toxicity and the chemical structure of any compound can be established based on three aspects: [23] the compound's hydrophobic, electronic, and steric characteristics. The weight of these three factors vary depending on the specific biological mechanism in which the compound is involved; particularly, the steric aspects can be relevant, for example, in specific interactions within the active site of the enzyme, which can be aborded through docking and molecular dynamics modelling [24]. Lipophilicity (hydrophobicity) has been the main focus in this area. However, electronic characteristics related to electrophile–nucleophile reactivity have also emerged as effective parameters to preliminarily assess the biological and toxicological activities of compounds of pharmacological interest [25–27].

2.2.1. ADME Properties of the β-Keto Esters

We obtained the lipophilicity and other structural parameters, which allowed us to estimate the pharmacokinetic properties (ADME: absorption, distribution, metabolism, and excretion) of the compounds using the SwissADME server [28]. The descriptors predicted by the SwissADME server are presented in Table 1.

Table 1. Physicochemical and pharmacokinetic descriptors calculated with SwissADME.

ID	Physicochemical Properties					Lipophilicity	Water Solubility	Pharmacokinetics		
	MW [1]	Rot. Bond [2]	HB-A [3]	HB-D [4]	TPSA [5]	Consensus Log $P_{o/w}$ [6]	Solubility (mol/L)	GI Abs [7]	BBB [8]	log K_p (cm/s) [9]
1	234.29	6	3	0	43.37	2.6	8.67×10^{-5}	High	Yes	−5.92
2	248.32	6	3	0	43.37	2.97	3.56×10^{-5}	High	Yes	−5.75
3	264.32	7	4	0	52.6	2.63	6.53×10^{-5}	High	Yes	−6.12
4	252.28	6	4	0	43.37	2.96	4.58×10^{-5}	High	Yes	−5.96
5	268.74	6	3	0	43.37	3.18	2.13×10^{-5}	High	Yes	−5.68
6	313.19	6	3	0	43.37	3.24	1.29×10^{-5}	High	Yes	−5.91
7	279.29	7	5	0	89.19	1.93	3.69×10^{-4}	High	No	−6.31
8	268.74	6	3	0	43.37	3.19	2.13×10^{-5}	High	Yes	−5.68

[1] Molecular weight (g/mol); [2] number of rotatable bonds; [3] number of hydrogen-bond acceptors; [4] number of hydrogen-bond donors; [5] topological polar surface area [29]; [6] average of iLOGP, XLOGP, WLOGP, MLOGP, and SILICOS-IT predictions [28]; [7] gastrointestinal absorption; [8] blood–brain barrier permeation; and [9] skin permeation: QSPR model [30].

All the compounds presented acceptable parameters, meeting the drug-likeness criteria (Table 2) according to Lipinski's rule of five [31,32]. It is worth noting that seven of the eight compounds should be able to permeate the blood–brain barrier, except for compound **7** (which contains a para-nitro group in the aromatic ring).

Table 2. Drug-likeness properties of the compounds calculated with SwissADME.

ID	Lipinski # Violations [1]	Ghose # Violations [2]	Veber # Violations [3]	Egan # Violations [4]	Muegge # Violations [5]
1	0	0	0	0	0
2	0	0	0	0	0
3	0	0	0	0	0
4	0	0	0	0	0
5	0	0	0	0	0
6	0	0	0	0	0
7	0	0	0	0	0
8	0	0	0	0	0

[1] Lipinski (Pfizer) filter [32]: MW ≤ 500; MLOGP ≤ 4.15; N or O ≤ 10; and NH or OH ≤ 5. [2] Ghose filter [33]: 160 ≤ MW ≤ 480; −0.4 ≤ WLOGP ≤ 5.6; 40 ≤ MR ≤ 130; and 20 ≤ atoms ≤ 70. [3] Veber (GSK) filter [34]: rotatable bonds ≤ 10, and TPSA ≤ 140. [4] Egan (Pharmacia) filter [35]: WLOGP ≤ 5.88, and TPSA ≤ 131.6. [5] Muegge (Bayer) filter [36]: 200 ≤ MW ≤ 600; −2 ≤ XLOGP ≤ 5; TPSA ≤ 150; number of rings ≤ 7; number of carbon atoms > 4; number of heteroatoms > 1; and number of rotatable bonds ≤ 15.

2.2.2. Reactivity Indices Based on Electronic Structure

The description of the electronic aspect of the compounds is critical, for example, in aqueous toxicity mechanisms where nucleophile–electrophile interactions are the driving force [27]. It has been described that strong electrophiles can exert toxicity by covalently bonding with biological nucleophiles such as the cysteine or lysine amino-acid residues in enzymes, among others [37]. We focused mainly on the tendency of these compounds to react with potential biological nucleophiles by analysing their global electrophilicity and the local electrophilic sites within the compound.

The previous experimental spectroscopic evidence shows that the compounds were in their keto form; therefore, we calculated the compounds considering only this tautomer. β-keto esters **1–8** were optimised at the DFT M062x/6-311+G(d,p) level. We conducted a conformational analysis on compound **1** to find the minimal energy conformation, identifying three stable conformations. The minimal energy conformation is presented in Figure 2.

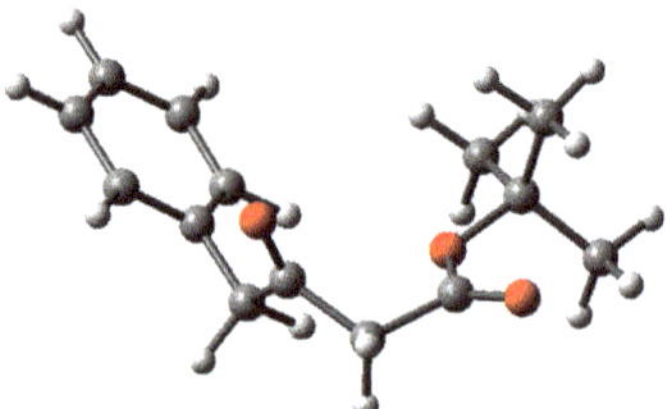

Figure 2. Molecular structure for the minimal energy conformation of compound **1**.

To study the susceptibility of β-keto esters **1–8** to suffering a reaction with biological nucleophiles, we employed reactivity descriptors from conceptual DFT [27,38,39], which are presented in Table 3.

Table 3. Vertical ionisation potential (*IPv*), vertical electron affinity (*EAv*), hardness (η), electronic chemical potential (μ), and global electrophilicity (ω) calculated at DFT M062x/6-311+G(d,p) level (all values in eV).

Compound	IP_v	EA_v	η	μ	ω
1	8.98	−0.77	9.75	−4.11	0.86
2	8.76	−0.79	9.55	−3.98	0.83
3	8.27	−0.89	9.17	−3.69	0.74
4	9.12	−0.76	9.88	−4.18	0.88
5	9.05	−0.73	9.78	−4.16	0.88
6	8.99	−0.72	9.72	−4.14	0.88
7	9.58	0.63	8.95	−5.10	1.46
8	8.91	−0.62	9.53	−4.15	0.90

The results for the electronic chemical potential (μ) show that compound **3** presented the highest escaping tendency of its electrons from equilibrium, while compound **7** presents the lowest tendency. These results reflect the effect of the strongest electron-donating and electron-accepting substituents on the aromatic ring. The molecular hardness, a measure of the resistance of a compound to a charge transfer, shows that compound **4** presented the highest resistance, while compound **7** presented the lowest resistance to a charge transfer. This descriptor can be combined to produce a new descriptor, global electrophilicity (ω), which accounts for energy stabilisation due to the maximum electron flow from a donor environment. Compound **7** presented a remarkably high electrophilicity, indicating the highest tendency towards undergoing a nucleophilic attack from a potential biological nucleophile and, therefore, potential electrophilic toxicity [37]. Interestingly, there is also the comparison between isomers **5** and **8** (ortho- and para-Cl), where the last one presented the highest tendency towards undergoing a nucleophilic attack.

In order to analyse the local reactivity of the β-keto esters at more reactive positions, C-carbonyl atoms 1 and 3, we calculated the condensed Fukui functions for an electrophilic (f_k^-) and nucleophilic (f_k^+) attack and the condensed dual descriptor (f_k^2). We condensed the local hypersoftness ($s_k^{(2)}$) at these positions (Table 4). f_k^- and f_k^+ give us information about susceptibility to undergoing an electrophilic and nucleophilic attack separately, while the condensed dual descriptor (f_k^2) considers both reactivities simultaneously [38]. A positive value of f_k^2 indicates an atom that tends to react with nucleophiles, while a negative value indicates an atom that tends to react with electrophiles. These descriptors, very useful for analysing the reactivity inside a molecule, do not allow a comparison among different molecules. To overcome this drawback, another local reactivity descriptor has been developed, local hypersoftness ($s_k^{(2)}$), which allows us to compare the local reactivity site among different molecules.

Table 4. Condensed Fukui functions for an electrophilic (f_k^-) and nucleophilic (f_k^+) attack, condensed dual descriptor f_k^2, and condensed local hypersoftness $s_k^{(2)}$ over the C-carbonyl atoms of compounds **1–8** (all values in eV).

Compound	Atom	f_k^+	f_k^-	f_k^2	$s_k^{(2)}$
1	C1	0.53	−0.18	0.71	5.56
	C3	0.84	0.21	0.63	4.90
2	C1	0.61	−0.17	0.78	6.33
	C3	0.25	0.16	0.09	0.77
3	C1	0.44	−0.16	0.60	5.25
	C3	−0.15	0.11	−0.25	−2.23
4	C1	0.34	−0.18	0.51	3.90
	C3	−0.11	0.25	−0.36	−2.71
5	C1	0.17	−0.16	0.33	2.54
	C3	0.16	0.16	0.00	0.03
6	C1	0.07	−0.17	0.24	1.86
	C3	0.35	0.09	0.26	2.02
7	C1	−0.14	−0.28	0.14	1.30
	C3	0.26	0.83	−0.57	−5.27
8	C1	0.33	−0.16	0.49	4.01
	C3	0.76	0.16	0.60	4.89

Experimentally, β-keto esters tend to react with nucleophiles at the esters' C-carbonyl atom, for example, in the transesterification reaction [40]. The presence of *tert*-butyl can be a factor that alters this tendency through steric hindrance; however, it has been described that transesterification occurs without a problem in β-keto esters with a *tert*-butyl attached to their ester [40,41]. Our results for $s_k^{(2)}$ show that C1 was more susceptible to a nucleophilic attack in β-keto esters **1**, **2**, **3**, **4**, **5**, and **7**. On the other hand, for β-keto esters **6** and **8**, we found that their C3 was more electrophilic than their C1. These results suggest that compounds **6** and **8** could react differently than the rest of the series.

2.3. In Silico Analysis of Quorum-Sensing Activity

2.3.1. Molecular Docking

To study how the compounds interact with the key targets involved in bacterial quorum sensing, we docked them in LasR and LuxS, and then we rescored the docking solutions using MM-GBSA. The results of these evaluations are presented in Table 5. This table details the docking score and binding-free-energy values for each of the eight compounds in their interaction with the proteins above. Lower binding-score values suggest a higher binding affinity between a compound and the corresponding protein. On the other hand, the MM-GBSA ΔGBind values provide a more accurate estimate of the binding free energy when considering the mechanistic and solvation terms. These values reflect the strength and stability of compound–protein interactions. Compounds with shallow docking scores and MM-GBSA ΔGBind values were identified in the analysis of the results, as is the case for compound 8. These values highlight a high affinity and stability in the interaction of **8** with both proteins. β-Keto ester **8** shows a promising potential in efficiently interacting with these key proteins in bacterial communication.

Table 5. Docking and binding free energy of compounds **1–8**.

Compound	LuxS		LasR	
	Docking Score (kcal/mol)	MMGBSA ΔG Bind (kcal/mol)	Docking Score (kcal/mol)	MMGBSA ΔG Bind (kcal/mol)
1	−3.781	−22.82	−6.405	−69.71
2	−3.475	−29.17	−2.742	−75.95
3	−4.052	−28.77	−5.253	−71.19
4	−4.265	−28.34	−7.291	−73.54
5	−3.981	−28.55	−7.439	−80.07
6	−4.011	−28.35	−4.335	−77.37
7	−1.188	−31.69	−3.555	−73.08
8	−4.085	−31.38	−4.649	−77.67

2.3.2. Molecular Dynamics

Molecular dynamics simulations were carried out to explore the interactions between compound **8** and both the LuxS and LasR proteins. Using simulations of a 500 ns duration for each system, the time evolution of the complexes was analysed in detail. In this context, the behaviour of compound **8** at the binding site of both proteins was examined, evaluating its stability and conformation throughout the simulations. The results provide fundamental information on the dynamics of these interactions and allow a more complete understanding of the interaction between compound **8** and the LuxS and LasR proteins. Specifically, remarkable stability was observed in the LuxS–compound **8** and LasR–compound **8** complexes over the 500 ns of the trajectories. This stability is evidenced by the root mean square deviation (RMSD) values of the protein backbones as shown in Figure 3A,B. The constancy in the structural conformation over this period suggests a robust interaction between compound **8** and both targets, reinforcing the validity of these interactions in the context of their long-lived molecular dynamics. In the case of LuxS, the RMSD of compound **8** remained consistently below 6 Å for the first 450 ns of the simulation. However, beyond this point, a significant increase in the RMSD of the ligand was observed, reaching approximately 40 Å. This change indicates an alteration in the interaction between the compound and LuxS. On the other hand, in the case of LasR, the RMSD of compound **8** remained relatively constant, in the range of 6 to 7 Å, throughout the entire 500 ns simulation. This points to a sustained and well-tuned ligand position at the LasR binding site, indicating a more persistent and stable interaction.

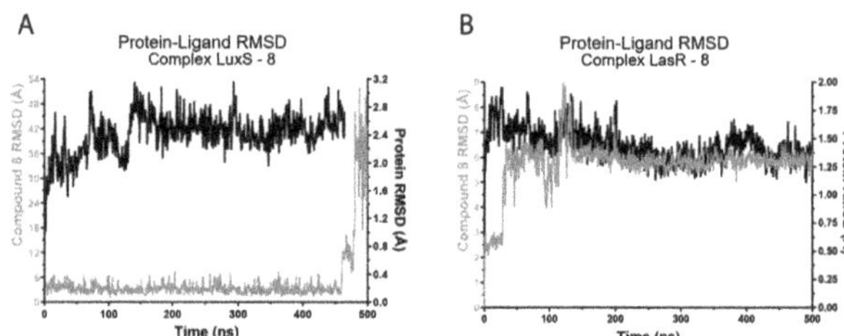

Figure 3. Root mean square deviation (RMSD) of the MD trajectories for compound **8**. (**A**) Complex of LuxS–**8** and (**B**) complex of LasR–**8**.

During the 500 ns MD, we analysed the interaction frequencies within the complexes. We focused mainly on the residues that exhibited interactions with a frequency higher than 20% during the trajectory. In the case of the LuxS–**8** complex (Figure 4A), different interactions were detected. These included π–π interactions involving His54; hydrophobic interactions with Ala60 and Ala120; and ionic interactions with His54, His58, and Cys126. In the LasR–**8** complex (Figure 4B), the residues Tyr64, Leu36, and Ala127 presented interactions with a significant frequency. In addition, π–π interactions were identified with Tyr64 and Trp60, whereas hydrogen-bonding interactions were established with Trp60.

Notably, water-bridge interactions were observed with Tyr47 and Asp65. These interaction profiles contribute significantly to the stability of the LuxS–**8** and LasR–**8** complexes.

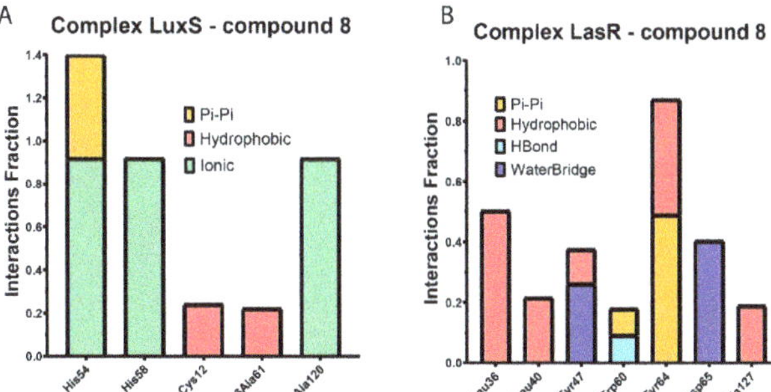

Figure 4. Interaction fractions over 500 ns of molecular dynamics simulations. Only residues that presented an interaction percentage higher than 20% over 500 ns of molecular dynamics simulations. (**A**) Complex of LuxS with **8** and (**B**) complex of LasR with **8**. The interactions of the protein with the ligand could be controlled throughout the simulation. Protein–ligand interactions are classified into four types: hydrogen bonds, hydrophobic interactions, ionic interactions, and water bridges. Each type of interaction contains more specific subtypes.

Additionally, interaction modes corresponding to each complex are presented in Figure 5 where we also compare how the cocrystalised ligands interacted with the key proteins (Figure 5A,C). Compound **8** interacted with LuxS (Figure 5B) and LasR (Figure 5D) similar to the cocrystalised ligands; this suggests a possible shared affinity toward these residues regarding their ligand–protein interactions.

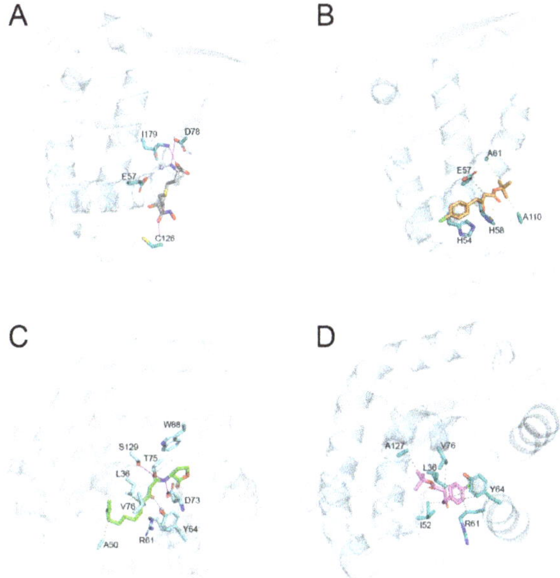

Figure 5. Representation of interactions. (**A**) LuxS–cocrystalised ligand complex (PDB code: 2FQO), (**B**) LuxS–**8** complex, (**C**) LasR–cocrystalised ligand complex (PDB code: 3IX3), and (**D**) LasR–**8** complex. Dashed black lines correspond to hydrophobic interactions; dashed yellow lines correspond to salt bridges; magenta lines correspond to hydrogen bonds; and grey lines correspond to water bridges.

2.4. Antibacterial Activity

Following the theoretical assessment of the reactivity of the β-keto esters, an initial exploration was conducted to ascertain the antibacterial efficacy of these compounds against both pathogenic and phytopathogenic strains. Previous works have described various compounds' antibacterial properties, potentially possessing antiquorum-sensing attributes [42,43]. Notably, several synthesised compounds could inhibit the activities of *P. aeruginosa*, *S. aureus*, *P. syringae*, and *A. tumefaciens*.

Figure 6 illustrates the inhibitory diameters of the β-keto ester compounds against two common foodborne pathogens and two phytopathogenic bacteria. This technique is widely acknowledged as a useful semiquantitative method for assessing the sensitivity of microorganisms to specific compounds. Negative controls were employed using disks impregnated with acetone. To prevent any antimicrobial effects from acetone, these disks were dried under the flow of a biosafety chamber. Among the tested compounds, **2**, **3**, **6**, and **8** demonstrated inhibitory activity against these pathogens, with diameters ranging from 8 to 15 mm, classified as moderate/mild inhibitory activity compared to the values reported by other authors [44]. The minimum inhibitory concentration (MIC) and minimum bactericidal concentration (MBC) were determined only for the compounds that showed inhibition.

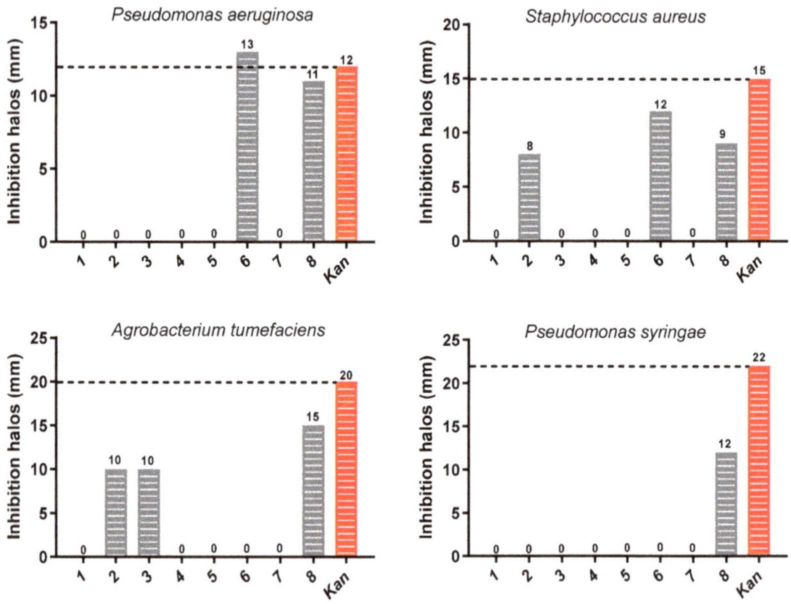

Figure 6. Inhibitory activity (mm) of β-keto ester compounds against pathogens and phytopathogenic bacteria. (■) β-keto ester compounds and (■) kanamycin, positive control.

Table 6 reveals that the selected microorganisms exhibited susceptibility to the action of these compounds, with MIC values ranging from 0.08 mg/mL to 0.63 mg/mL and MBC values from 1.25 mg/mL to 5.00 mg/mL. Notably, β-keto ester **3** demonstrated higher resistance to antimicrobial activity against most of the strains, except for *A. tumefaciens*. Kanamycin (50 µg) served as the positive control for bacterial inhibition. Among the phytopathogenic bacteria, *P. syringae* (1.25 mg/mL MIC and 5.00 mg/mL MCB) and *A. tumefaciens* (0.08 mg/mL MIC and 1.25 mg/mL MCB) exhibited the highest susceptibility to compound **8**, requiring lower concentrations to inhibit bacterial growth. On the other hand, the bacteria of clinical importance, *S. aureus* (0.32 mg/mL MIC and 2.50 mg/mL MCB), were most susceptible to β-keto ester **8**.

Table 6. Antibacterial activity of β-keto ester compounds.

Bacteria	MIC [1] (mg/mL)				Kan [3] (µg/mL)	MBC [2] (mg/mL)				Kan [3] (µg/mL)
	2	**3**	**6**	**8**		**2**	**3**	**6**	**8**	
Pathogenic										
Pseudomonas aeruginosa (ATCC 19429)	ND	ND	0.32	0.63	5.00	ND	ND	2.50	5.00	10.00
Staphylococcus aureus (ATCC 29737)	0.63	ND	0.63	0.32	2.50	5.00	ND	5.00	2.50	10.00
Phytopathogenic										
Pseudomonas syringae (MF547632)	ND	ND	ND	1.25	1.25	ND	ND	ND	5.00	2.50
Agrobacterium tumefaciens (ATCC 19358)	0.16	0.16	ND	0.08	1.25	2.50	2.50	ND	1.25	5.00

[1] Minimum inhibitory concentration. [2] Minimum bactericidal concentration. ND: inhibition not detected. ATCC: American Type Culture Collection (USA). MF547632 is the accession number to the Genbank of the respective bacteria. [3] Minimum bactericidal concentration (positive control).

3. Materials and Methods

3.1. Synthesis of β-Keto Esters

Synthesis of the β-keto esters used our group's previously described method (see supporting information) [45].

***tert*-Butyl 3-oxo-4-(o-tolyl)butanoate (2).** This compound was prepared according to the general procedure described in the supporting information using 2-methylphenylacetic acid (0.30 g, 2.00 mmol), Meldrum's acid (0.29 g, 2.00 mmol), DCC (0.45 g, 2.20 mmol), and DMAP (0.27 g, 2.20 mmol). Purification by column chromatography (0→1→2.5→5% EtOAc/hexane) gave β-keto ester **2** (0.37 g, 75%) as a yellow oil. ^{1}H NMR (CDCl$_3$, 400 MHz): δ 1.49 (s, 9H, CH$_3$), 2.28 (s, 3H, CH$_3$), 3.39 (s, 2H, H-2), 3.87 (s, 2H, H-4), and 7.15–7.22 (m, 4H, Ph). ^{13}C NMR (CDCl$_3$, 100 MHz): δ 19.7 (CH3), 28.0 (CH$_3$), 48.3 (C-4), 49.7 (C-2), 82.1 (CCH$_3$), 126.4, 127.7, 130.6, 132.4 (Ph), 166.4 (C-1), and 200.9 (C-3). HRMS calculated for C$_{15}$H$_{20}$O$_3$ [M-H]$^-$ was 247.1329; we found 247.1337.

***tert*-Butyl 4-(2-methoxyphenyl)-3-oxobutanoate (3).** This compound was prepared according to the general procedure described in the supporting information using 2-methoxyphenylacetic acid (0.30 g, 2.00 mmol), Meldrum's acid (0.29 g, 2.00 mmol), DCC (0.45 g, 2.20 mmol), and DMAP (0.27 g, 2.20 mmol). Purification by column chromatography (0→2.5→5→10% EtOAc/hexane) gave β-keto ester **3** (0.37 g, 75%) as a yellow oil. ^{1}H NMR (CDCl$_3$, 400 MHz): δ 1.48 (s, 9H, CH$_3$), 3.39 (s, 2H, H-2), 3.79 (s, 3H, CH$_3$), 3.83 (s, 2H, H-4), 6.99–6.86 (q, 2H, Ph), 7.16 (d, J = 7.3 Hz, 1H, Ph), and 7.28 (t, J = 7.8 Hz, 1H, Ph). ^{13}C NMR (CDCl$_3$, 100 MHz): δ 28.1 (CH$_3$), 44.8 (C-4), 49.8 (C-2), 55.5 (OCH$_3$), 81.8 (CCH$_3$), 110.7, 120.9, 128.9, 131.5 (Ph), 166.7 (C-1), and 201.5 (C-3). HRMS calculated for C$_{15}$H$_{20}$O$_4$ [M-H]$^-$ was 263.1278; we found 263.1295.

***tert*-Butyl 4-(2-Bromophenyl)-3-oxobutanoate (6).** This compound was prepared according to the general procedure described in the supporting information using 2-bromophenylacetic acid (0.59 g, 3.47 mmol), Meldrum's acid (0.50 g, 3.47 mmol), DCC (0.79 g, 3.82 mmol), and DMAP (0.47 g, 3.82 mmol). Purification by column chromatography (0→1→2.5→5% EtOAc/hexane) gave β-keto ester **6** (1.09 g, 78%) as a yellow oil. ^{1}H NMR (CDCl$_3$, 400 MHz): δ 1.49 (s, 9H, CH$_3$), 3.46 (s, 2H, H-2), 4.02 (s, 2H, H-4), 7.15–7.33 (m, 3H, Ph), and 7.60 (d, J = 8.0 Hz, 1H, Ph). ^{13}C NMR (CDCl$_3$, 100 MHz): δ 28.1 (CH$_3$), 50.1 (C-4), 50.3 (C-2), 82.3 (C), 125.2, 127.8, 129.2, 132.0, 133.0, 134.1 (Ph), 166,4 (C-1), and 199.8 (C-3). HRMS calculated for C$_{14}$H$_{17}$BrO$_3$ [M-H]$^-$ was 311.0277; we found 311.0257.

3.2. ADME Properties' Evaluation

The pharmacokinetic properties (ADME: absorption, distribution, metabolism, and excretion), physicochemical descriptors, and drug-likeness of the compounds were calculated using the SwissADME server [28]. Briefly, 42 descriptors were predicted for each compound, including physicochemical properties such as molecular weight, logP, solubility, and pharmacokinetic properties. Based on the descriptors obtained, the acceptability of the compounds based on bioavailability score (drug-likeness) could be assessed [28].

3.3. Quantum Chemical Calculation

β-keto esters were calculated using the Gaussian 09 [46] program package (Revision a.01; Gaussian, Inc.: Wallingford, CT, USA). No symmetry constraints were imposed on the optimisations performed at the DFT M06-2x/6-311+G(d,p) level. No imaginary vibrational frequencies were found at the optimised geometries, indicating true minima of the potential energy surfaces. Reactivity descriptors from Conceptual Density Functional Theory were obtained using the finite difference approximation (FDA) to analyse and compare the reactivity of β-keto esters.

Global reactivity descriptors were calculated as follows [27]:

$$\text{Electronic Chemical Potential} \quad \mu = -0.5\left(IP_v + EA_v\right) \tag{1}$$

$$\text{Chemical Hardness} \quad \eta = IP_v - EA_v \tag{2}$$

$$\text{Electrophilicity} \quad \omega = \frac{\mu^2}{\eta} \tag{3}$$

where IP_v and EA_v correspond to the vertical ionisation potential and vertical electron affinity, respectively.

Local reactivity descriptors were calculated as follows [38]:

$$\text{Fukui Function for Nucleophilic Attack} \quad f_k^+ = N_k(N) - N_k(N+1) \tag{4}$$

$$\text{Fukui Function for Electrophilic Attack} \quad f_k^- = N_k(N-1) - N_k(N) \tag{5}$$

$$\text{Dual Descript} \quad f_k^{(2)} = f_k^+ - f_k^- \tag{6}$$

$$\text{Local Hypersoftness} \quad s_k^{(2)} = \frac{f_k^{(2)}}{\eta^2} \tag{7}$$

where $N_k(N)$, $N_k(N+1)$, and $N_k(N-1)$ correspond to the electronic populations on atom k in neutral, radical anion, and radical cation species obtained through natural population analysis [39].

3.4. Docking and DM Calculations

To study the antibacterial potential of the β-keto esters, we selected the LasR and LuxS targets. These targets are involved in the pathogenicity of several bacteria, such as *P. aeruginosa* and *S. aureus* [14,18,20,21]. To determinate the binding site, we used the structure of LasR-OC1 cocrystalised with *N*-3-oxo-dodecanoyl-l-homoserine lactone (PDB code: 3IX3) [47] and LuxS cocrystalised with (2*S*)-2-amino-4-[(2*R*,3*R*)-2,3-dihydroxy-3-*N*-hydroxycarbamoyl-propylmercapto]butyric acid (PDB code: 2FQO) [48]. Prior to molecular docking calculations, proteins were prepared using the Protein Preparation Wizard tool included in Maestro. The ligands, waters (beyond 5 Å), and metals were removed from the structure; then, hydrogens were added, and ionisation states were calculated at pH 7.4 [49]. The proteins were energy-minimised with the OPLS4 force field. The centre of the grid boxes was located using the cocrystalised ligand in each structure. Molecular docking simulations were performed for LasR-OC1, with the outer edge of the grid set to 26 Å, and for LuxS, with the outer edge of the grid set to 22 Å. The standard precision function (SP) of Glide [50] was employed for docking simulations, and the best ten pose solutions per docked ligand were further subjected to postprocessing and rescoring by calculating binding free energy (ΔGbind) using the molecular-mechanics-generalised Born surface area (MM-GBSA) protocol in Prime [51]. The best complexes, according to ΔGbind, were subjected to 10 ns of equilibrium molecular dynamics (MD) simulations each using Desmond software [52] and the OPLS4 force field [53]. Then, 500 ns of production MD was performed for each complex. To prepare both systems, the complexes were solvated with pre-equilibrated single point charged (SPC) water molecules in a periodic-boundary-condition box. Neutralisation of the systems was done by adding Na^+ or Cl^- counterions, and then, to simulate physiological conditions, a final concentration of 0.15 M NaCl was set. Each system was relaxed using the default Desmond relaxation protocol and then was equilibrated for 10 ns using the NPT ensemble at 1 atm and 300 K. A spring constant of 10.0 kcal $\times$ mol^{-1} $\times$ Å^{-2} was applied to the ligand and the protein. The last frame of equilibration MD was employed to perform production MD of 500 ns using the same conditions as those described above.

3.5. Antibacterial Activity

3.5.1. Strain and Growth Conditions

β-keto esters were employed in assessing their antibacterial activity against several strains of bacteria, including the human pathogenic bacteria *Pseudomonas aeruginosa* (ATCC 19429) and *Staphylococcus aureus* (ATCC 29737) as well as the phytopathogenic bacteria *Pseudomonas syringae* (MF547632) and *Agrobacterium tumefaciens* (ATCC 19358). The bacteria were inoculated in nutrient broth containing 5.0 g/L of peptone and 3.0 g/L of meat extract followed by an incubation period of 18 h. Incubation temperatures were set to 25 °C for plant pathogens and to 35 °C for human pathogens. The incubation process was conducted with orbital shaking at 150 rpm utilising an incubator (MRC LOM-80).

3.5.2. Paper-Disk Diffusion Method

The antibacterial properties of β-keto ester compounds were assessed following a method originally outlined by Parra et al. with modifications [34]. Initially, a stock solution of β-keto esters at a 20 mg/mL concentration was prepared using acetone as the solvent. Subsequently, 15 µL of this stock solution was applied to 5 mm sterile cellulose filter paper disks. In parallel, control disks impregnated with acetone were prepared to serve as negative controls. The impregnated disks were then dried within a biosafety chamber.

Disks containing 50 µg of kanamycin were employed as positive controls assessing bacterial inhibition. Fresh bacterial inoculum for each bacterial species was prepared as previously described, was diluted to a 0.5 McFarland standard (representing a bacterial concentration of 1.5×10^8 CFU/mL), and was uniformly spread onto plates containing nutrient broth supplemented with 12 g/L of agar. The dried, impregnated disks were positioned equidistant from each other on the agar plates. Subsequently, the plates were incubated for 24 h at either 25 °C or 35 °C at the appropriate temperature. Following the incubation period, the diameter of bacterial-growth inhibition was measured, characterised by a transparent halo surrounding each disk where no bacterial growth was observed. To ensure precision and reproducibility, these tests were conducted in triplicate.

3.5.3. Minimum Inhibitory Concentration (MIC)

The determination of the minimum concentration of β-keto esters required to inhibit bacterial growth followed the methodology detailed by Parra et al. [34]. The β-keto esters were evaluated using a concentration range from 0 to 10 mg/mL. Each concentration was prepared in a final working volume of 200 µL and was inoculated with the respective bacteria to be tested. These inoculated samples were then incubated in 96-well plates at either 25 °C or 35 °C at the appropriate temperature.

To serve as a control, nutrient broth without the compound was inoculated with each bacterium to monitor normal growth (growth control). Additionally, nutrient broth containing β-keto esters at concentrations ranging from 0 to 10 mg/mL, without bacterial inoculation, was employed to assess the compounds' growth and sterility (negative control). To estimate the minimum inhibitory concentration (MIC) of acetone for each bacterium, an assay was conducted using acetone concentrations spanning from 0 to 90%. It was observed that acetone did not exhibit inhibitory effects on any of the four bacteria tested. After a 24 h incubation period, the lowest concentration of the compound at which no bacterial growth was detected was identified as the MIC for each bacterium.

3.5.4. Minimum Bactericidal Concentration (MCB)

The bactericidal capacity of β-keto esters was assessed based on a method detailed by Parra et al. [34], focusing on the last three wells in the MIC assay that exhibited no bacterial growth. To determine the minimum concentration of β-keto esters where no growth was observed (MCB) for each microorganism, 100 μL of the bacterial cultures was plated on nutrient-broth plates supplemented with 15 g/L of agar. A culture that exhibited microbial growth in the MIC test was employed to serve as a growth control. Subsequently, the plates were incubated for 24 h at the appropriate temperature. Following incubation, the concentration of β-keto esters at which no growth was detected was recorded as the MCB for each microorganism.

4. Conclusions

We modelled and synthesised β-keto esters as antibacterial compounds in this work. The design was based on the structure of autoinducers of quorum-sensing Gram-negative bacteria. Eight β-keto ester analogues were synthesised with good yields, and they were spectroscopically characterised, showing that the compounds were only in their β-keto ester tautomer form. We carried out a computational analysis of the reactivity and ADME (absorption, distribution, metabolism, and excretion) properties of the compounds as well as molecular docking and molecular dynamics calculations with the LasR and LuxS quorum-sensing (QS) proteins, which are involved in bacterial resistance to antibiotics. The results show that all the compounds exhibited reliable ADME properties; none violated Lipinski's rule. Based on the reactivity parameters obtained from the conceptual DFT calculations, only compound **7** could potentially present electrophile toxicity. The theoretical local reactivity study shows that compounds **6** and **8** reacted with nucleophiles at the keto C-carbonyl, unlike the rest of the series, which reacted with nucleophiles at the ester C-carbonyl. The molecular docking calculations show that compound **8** presented a better profile of affinity and stability in its interaction with the LasR and LuxS QS proteins. The molecular dynamics calculations allowed us to study the stability of the interaction between compound **8** and both proteins, being remarkable in both cases, particularly with LasR. An initial in vitro antimicrobial screening was performed against the human pathogenic bacteria *Pseudomonas aeruginosa* and *Staphylococcus aureus* as well as the phytopathogenic bacteria *Pseudomonas syringae* and *Agrobacterium tumefaciens*. Compounds 6 and 8 exhibited the most promising results in the in vitro antimicrobial screening against the panel of bacteria studied.

Supplementary Materials: The following supporting information can be downloaded at: https://www.mdpi.com/article/10.3390/ph16101339/s1, Experimental and NMR data of compounds, optimized geometries of compounds, and Docking and Molecular Dynamics data of compounds.

Author Contributions: Conceptualisation, M.M.-C. and C.P.; data curation, M.M.-C., P.M.-T. and C.P.; funding acquisition, M.M.-C., P.M.-T. and C.P.; investigation, M.M.-C., E.S.-T., C.L.-P., P.V.-H., D.R., P.M.-T. and C.P.; methodology, M.M.-C., D.R., P.M.-T. and C.P.; project administration, M.M.-C. and C.P.; supervision, M.M.-C. and C.P.; validation, M.M.-C. and C.P.; writing—original draft, M.M.-C., B.B., D.R., P.M.-T. and C.P.; writing—review and editing, M.M.-C., B.B. and C.P. All authors have read and agreed to the published version of the manuscript.

Funding: This study was funded by Fondecyt 11190698. D.R. acknowledges Fondecyt 1220656. M.M-C. acknowledges 2023000771INV. P.M.-T. acknowledges FIC-CORFO Project 13CEI2-21852 and the execution of the project coexecution agreement between the Universidad de Tarapacá and the University of California, Davis, Chile. Powered@NLHPC: this research was partially supported by the supercomputing infrastructure of the NLHPC (ECM-02).

Institutional Review Board Statement: Not applicable.

Informed Consent Statement: Not applicable.

Data Availability Statement: Data is contained within the article and Supplementary Material.

Acknowledgments: The authors wish to express their gratitude to the Rectoría of Universidad de Tarapacá for their financial and administrative support.

Conflicts of Interest: The authors declare that there are no conflict of interest.

References

1. Antimicrobial Resistance Division; WHO. *Antimicrobial Resistance: Global Report on Surveillance*; WHO: Geneva, Switzerland, 2014; p. 256.
2. Neu, H.C. The crisis in antibiotic-resistance. *Science* **1992**, *257*, 1064–1073. [CrossRef] [PubMed]
3. Brown, E.D.; Wright, G.D. Antibacterial drug discovery in the resistance era. *Nature* **2016**, *529*, 336–343. [CrossRef] [PubMed]
4. Waters, C.M.; Bassler, B.L. Quorum sensing: Cell-to-cell communication in bacteria. *Annu. Rev. Cell Dev. Biol.* **2005**, *21*, 319–346. [CrossRef] [PubMed]
5. Hall-Stoodley, L.; Costerton, J.W.; Stoodley, P. Bacterial biofilms: From the natural environment to infectious diseases. *Nat. Rev. Microbiol.* **2004**, *2*, 95–108. [CrossRef] [PubMed]
6. Papenfort, K.; Bassler, B.L. Quorum sensing signal-response systems in Gram-negative bacteria. *Nat. Rev. Microbiol.* **2016**, *14*, 576–588. [CrossRef] [PubMed]
7. Huigens, R.W.; Richards, J.J.; Parise, G.; Ballard, T.E.; Zeng, W.; Deora, R.; Melander, C. Inhibition of Pseudomonas aeruginosa biofilm formation with bromoageliferin analogues. *J. Am. Chem. Soc.* **2007**, *129*, 6966–6967. [CrossRef] [PubMed]
8. Rasamiravaka, T.; Labtani, Q.; Duez, P.; El Jaziri, M. The Formation of Biofilms by Pseudomonas aeruginosa: A Review of the Natural and Synthetic Compounds Interfering with Control Mechanisms. *Biomed. Res. Int.* **2015**, *2015*, 759348. [CrossRef]
9. Engebrecht, J.; Nealson, K.; Silverman, M. Bacterial Bioluminescence—Isolation and Genetic-Analysis of Functions from *Vibrio fischeri*. *Cell* **1983**, *32*, 773–781. [CrossRef]
10. Geske, G.D.; Oneill, J.C.; Miller, D.M.; Wezeman, R.J.; Mattmann, M.E.; Lin, Q.; Blackwell, H.E. Comparative analyses of N-acylated homoserine Lactones reveal unique structural features that dictate their ability to activate or inhibit quorum sensing. *Chembiochem* **2008**, *9*, 389–400. [CrossRef]
11. Wei, Z.Y.; Li, T.; Gu, Y.; Zhang, Q.; Wang, E.H.; Li, W.B.; Wang, X.; Li, Y.; Li, H.Y. Design, Synthesis, and Biological Evaluation of N-Acyl-Homoserine Lactone Analogs of Quorum Sensing in Pseudomonas aeruginosa. *Front. Chem.* **2022**, *10*, 948687. [CrossRef]
12. Qiang, Z.; Li, S.Z.; Queneau, Y.; Soulere, L. Synthesis of new 1,4-and 1,5-disubstituted N-ethyl acetate and N-alpha-butyro-gamma-lactone alkylimidazole derivatives as N-acylhomoserine lactone analogs. *J. Heterocycl. Chem.* **2021**, *58*, 2298–2303. [CrossRef]
13. Frezza, M.; Soulere, L.; Reverchon, S.; Guiliani, N.; Jerez, C.; Queneau, Y.; Doutheau, A. Synthetic homoserine lactone-derived sulfonylureas as inhibitors of Vibrio fischeri quorum sensing regulator. *Bioorg. Med. Chem.* **2008**, *16*, 3550–3556. [CrossRef] [PubMed]
14. Manson, D.E.; O'Reilly, M.C.; Nyffeler, K.E.; Blackwell, H.E. Design, Synthesis, and Biochemical Characterization of Non-Native Antagonists of the Pseudomonas aeruginosa Quorum Sensing Receptor LasR with Nanomolar IC50 Values. *ACS Infect. Dis.* **2020**, *6*, 649–661. [CrossRef]
15. Marsden, D.M.; Nicholson, R.L.; Skindersoe, M.E.; Galloway, W.; Sore, H.F.; Givskov, M.; Salmond, G.P.C.; Ladlow, M.; Welchd, M.; Spring, D.R. Discovery of a quorum sensing modulator pharmacophore by 3D small-molecule microarray screening. *Org. Biomol. Chem.* **2010**, *8*, 5313–5323. [CrossRef] [PubMed]
16. Boursier, M.E.; Combs, J.B.; Blackwell, H.E. N-Acyl L-Homocysteine Thiolactones Are Potent and Stable Synthetic Modulators of the RhlR Quorum Sensing Receptor in Pseudomonas aeruginosa. *ACS Chem. Biol.* **2019**, *14*, 186–191. [CrossRef]
17. Guo, N.; Bai, X.; Shen, Y.; Zhang, T.H. Target-based screening for natural products against *Staphylococcus aureus* biofilms. *Crit. Rev. Food Sci. Nutr.* **2023**, *63*, 2216–2230. [CrossRef]
18. Wang, Y.; Liu, B.B.; Grenier, D.; Yi, L. Regulatory Mechanisms of the LuxS/AI-2 System and Bacterial Resistance. *Antimicrob. Agents Chemother.* **2019**, *63*, 12. [CrossRef]
19. Xavier, K.B.; Bassler, B.L. LuxS quorum sensing: More than just a numbers game. *Curr. Opin. Microbiol.* **2003**, *6*, 191–197. [CrossRef]
20. Zhang, B.Z.; Ku, X.G.; Zhang, X.Q.; Zhang, Y.; Chen, G.; Chen, F.Z.; Zeng, W.; Li, J.; Zhu, L.; He, Q.G. The AI-2/luxS Quorum Sensing System Affects the Growth Characteristics, Biofilm Formation, and Virulence of *Haemophilus parasuis*. *Front. Cell. Infect. Microbiol.* **2019**, *9*, 15. [CrossRef]
21. Murray, E.J.; Crowley, R.C.; Truman, A.; Clarke, S.R.; Cottam, J.A.; Jadhav, G.P.; Steele, V.R.; O'Shea, P.; Lindholm, C.; Cockayne, A.; et al. Targeting *Staphylococcus aureus* Quorum Sensing with Nonpeptidic Small Molecule Inhibitors. *J. Med. Chem.* **2014**, *57*, 2813–2819. [CrossRef]
22. Forschner-Dancause, S.; Poulin, E.; Meschwitz, S. Quorum Sensing Inhibition and Structure-Activity Relationships of beta-Keto Esters. *Molecules* **2016**, *21*, 971. [CrossRef] [PubMed]
23. Hansch, C.; Fujita, T. P-σ-π Analysis: A method for the correlation of biological activity and chemical structure. *J. Am. Chem. Soc.* **1964**, *86*, 1616–1626. [CrossRef]
24. Issa, N.T.; Wathieu, H.; Ojo, A.; Byers, S.W.; Dakshanamurthy, S. Drug Metabolism in Preclinical Drug Development: A Survey of the Discovery Process, Toxicology, and Computational Tools. *Curr. Drug Metab.* **2017**, *18*, 556–565. [CrossRef] [PubMed]

25. Parthasarathi, R.; Subramanian, V.; Roy, D.R.; Chattaraj, P.K. Electrophillicity index as a possible descriptor of biological activity. *Bioorg. Med. Chem.* **2004**, *12*, 5533–5543. [CrossRef] [PubMed]
26. Padmanabhan, J.; Parthasarathi, R.; Subramanian, V.; Chattaraj, P.K. Group philicity and electrophilicity as possible descriptors for modeling ecotoxicity applied to chlorophenols. *Chem. Res. Toxicol.* **2006**, *19*, 356–364. [CrossRef] [PubMed]
27. Pal, R.; Patra, S.G.; Chattaraj, P.K. Quantitative Structure-Toxicity Relationship in Bioactive Molecules from a Conceptual DFT Perspective. *Pharmaceuticals* **2022**, *15*, 1383. [CrossRef] [PubMed]
28. Daina, A.; Michielin, O.; Zoete, V. SwissADME: A free web tool to evaluate pharmacokinetics, drug-likeness and medicinal chemistry friendliness of small molecules. *Sci. Rep.* **2017**, *7*, 42717. [CrossRef]
29. Ertl, P.; Rohde, B.; Selzer, P. Fast calculation of molecular polar surface area as a sum of fragment-based contributions and its application to the prediction of drug transport properties. *J. Med. Chem.* **2000**, *43*, 3714–3717. [CrossRef]
30. Potts, R.O.; Guy, R.H. Predicting skin permeability. *Pharm. Res.* **1992**, *9*, 663–669. [CrossRef]
31. Lipinski, C.A. Drug-like properties and the causes of poor solubility and poor permeability. *J. Pharmacol. Toxicol. Methods* **2000**, *44*, 235–249. [CrossRef]
32. Lipinski, C.A.; Lombardo, F.; Dominy, B.W.; Feeney, P.J. Experimental and computational approaches to estimate solubility and permeability in drug discovery and development settings. *Adv. Drug Deliv. Rev.* **1997**, *23*, 3–25. [CrossRef]
33. Ghose, A.K.; Viswanadhan, V.N.; Wendoloski, J.J. A knowledge-based approach in designing combinatorial or medicinal chemistry libraries for drug discovery. 1. A qualitative and quantitative characterization of known drug databases. *J. Comb. Chem.* **1999**, *1*, 55–68. [CrossRef] [PubMed]
34. Veber, D.F.; Johnson, S.R.; Cheng, H.Y.; Smith, B.R.; Ward, K.W.; Kopple, K.D. Molecular properties that influence the oral bioavailability of drug candidates. *J. Med. Chem.* **2002**, *45*, 2615–2623. [CrossRef] [PubMed]
35. Egan, W.J.; Merz, K.M.; Baldwin, J.J. Prediction of drug absorption using multivariate statistics. *J. Med. Chem.* **2000**, *43*, 3867–3877. [CrossRef] [PubMed]
36. Muegge, I.; Heald, S.L.; Brittelli, D. Simple selection criteria for drug-like chemical matter. *J. Med. Chem.* **2001**, *44*, 1841–1846. [CrossRef] [PubMed]
37. LoPachin, R.M.; Geohagen, B.C.; Nordstroem, L.U. Mechanisms of soft and hard electrophile toxicities. *Toxicology* **2019**, *418*, 62–69. [CrossRef] [PubMed]
38. Gacitua, M.; Carreno, A.; Morales-Guevara, R.; Paez-Hernandez, D.; Martinez-Araya, J.I.; Araya, E.; Preite, M.; Otero, C.; Rivera-Zaldivar, M.M.; Silva, A.; et al. Physicochemical and Theoretical Characterization of a New Small Non-Metal Schiff Base with a Differential Antimicrobial Effect against Gram-Positive Bacteria. *Int. J. Mol. Sci.* **2022**, *23*, 16. [CrossRef] [PubMed]
39. Zamora, P.P.; Bieger, K.; Cuchillo, A.; Tello, A.; Muena, J.P. Theoretical determination of a reaction intermediate: Fukui function analysis, dual reactivity descriptor and activation energy. *J. Mol. Struct.* **2021**, *1227*, 129369. [CrossRef]
40. Hennessy, M.C.; O'Sullivan, T.P. Recent advances in the transesterification of beta-keto esters. *RSC Adv.* **2021**, *11*, 22859–22920. [CrossRef]
41. Rao, G.B.D.; Anjaneyulu, B.; Kaushik, M.P. Greener and expeditious one-pot synthesis of dihydropyrimidinone derivatives using non-commercial beta-ketoesters via the Biginelli reaction. *RSC Adv.* **2014**, *4*, 43321–43325. [CrossRef]
42. Bacha, K.; Tariku, Y.; Gebreyesus, F.; Zerihun, S.; Mohammed, A.; Weiland-Brauer, N.; Schmitz, R.A.; Mulat, M. Antimicrobial and anti-Quorum Sensing activities of selected medicinal plants of Ethiopia: Implication for development of potent antimicrobial agents. *BMC Microbiol.* **2016**, *16*, 139. [CrossRef] [PubMed]
43. Wang, W.T.; Huang, X.Q.; Yang, H.X.; Niu, X.Q.; Li, D.X.; Yang, C.; Li, L.; Zou, L.T.; Qiu, Z.W.; Wu, S.H.; et al. Antibacterial Activity and Anti-Quorum Sensing Mediated Phenotype in Response to Essential Oil from Melaleuca bracteata Leaves. *Int. J. Mol. Sci.* **2019**, *20*, 5696. [CrossRef] [PubMed]
44. Simirgiotis, M.J.; Burton, D.; Parra, F.; López, J.; Muñoz, P.; Escobar, H.; Parra, C. Antioxidant and Antibacterial Capacities of Origanum vulgare L. Essential Oil from the Arid Andean Region of Chile and its Chemical Characterization by GC-MS. *Metabolites* **2020**, *10*, 414. [CrossRef] [PubMed]
45. Bradshaw, B.; Parra, C.; Bonjoch, J. Organocatalyzed Asymmetric Synthesis of Morphans. *Org. Lett.* **2013**, *15*, 2458–2461. [CrossRef] [PubMed]
46. Frisch, M.J.; Trucks, G.W.; Schlegel, H.B.; Scuseria, G.E.; Robb, M.A.; Cheeseman, J.R.; Scalmani, G.; Barone, V.; Petersson, G.A.; Nakatsuji, H.; et al. *Gaussian 09*; Gaussian, Inc.: Wallingford, CT, USA, 2009.
47. Zou, Y.; Nair, S.K. LasR-OC12 HSL Complex. PDB ID: 3IX3 2009. Available online: https://www.wwpdb.org/pdb?id=pdb_0000 3ix3 (accessed on 14 September 2023).
48. Shen, G.; Rajan, R.; Zhu, J.G.; Bell, C.E.; Pei, D.H. Design and synthesis of substrate and intermediate analogue inhibitors of S-ribosylhomocysteinase. *J. Med. Chem.* **2006**, *49*, 3003–3011. [CrossRef] [PubMed]
49. Sastry, G.M.; Adzhigirey, M.; Day, T.; Annabhimoju, R.; Sherman, W. Protein and ligand preparation: Parameters, protocols, and influence on virtual screening enrichments. *J. Comput.-Aided Mol. Des.* **2013**, *27*, 221–234. [CrossRef] [PubMed]
50. Friesner, R.A.; Murphy, R.B.; Repasky, M.P.; Frye, L.L.; Greenwood, J.R.; Halgren, T.A.; Sanschagrin, P.C.; Mainz, D.T. Extra precision glide: Docking and scoring incorporating a model of hydrophobic enclosure for protein-ligand complexes. *J. Med. Chem.* **2006**, *49*, 6177–6196. [CrossRef]
51. Jacobson, M.P.; Pincus, D.L.; Rapp, C.S.; Day, T.J.F.; Honig, B.; Shaw, D.E.; Friesner, R.A. A hierarchical approach to all-atom protein loop prediction. *Proteins-Struct. Funct. Bioinform.* **2004**, *55*, 351–367. [CrossRef]

52. Bowers, K.J.; Chow, E.; Xu, H.; Dror, R.O.; Eastwood, M.P.; Gregersen, B.A.; Klepeis, J.L.; Kolossvary, I.; Moraes, M.A.; Sacerdoti; et al. Scalable algorithms for molecular dynamics simulations on commodity clusters. In Proceedings of the 2006 ACM/IEEE Conference on Supercomputing, Tampa, FL, USA, 11–17 November 2006; IEEE: Manhattan, NY, USA, 2006; p. 43.
53. Lu, C.; Wu, C.J.; Ghoreishi, D.; Chen, W.; Wang, L.L.; Damm, W.; Ross, G.A.; Dahlgren, M.K.; Russell, E.; Von Bargen, C.D.; et al. OPLS4: Improving Force Field Accuracy on Challenging Regimes of Chemical Space. *J. Chem. Theory Comput.* **2021**, *17*, 4291–4300. [CrossRef]

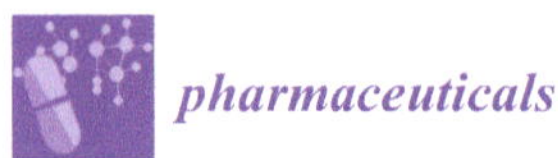 *pharmaceuticals*

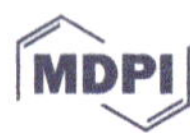

Review

An Innovative Approach to Address Neurodegenerative Diseases through Kinase-Targeted Therapies: Potential for Designing Covalent Inhibitors

Swapnil P. Bhujbal [1] and Jung-Mi Hah [2,*]

[1]   College of Pharmacy, Hanyang University, Ansan 426-791, Republic of Korea; swapnil18@hanyang.ac.kr
[2]   Institute of Pharmaceutical Science and Technology, Hanyang University, Ansan 426-791, Republic of Korea
*   Correspondence: jhah@hanyang.ac.kr; Tel.: +82-31-400-5803

Abstract: Owing to the dysregulation of protein kinase activity in various diseases such as cancer and autoimmune, cardiovascular, neurodegenerative, and inflammatory conditions, the protein kinase family has emerged as a crucial drug target in the 21st century. Notably, many kinases have been targeted to address cancer and neurodegenerative diseases using conventional ATP-mimicking kinase inhibitors. Likewise, irreversible covalent inhibitors have also been developed for different types of cancer. The application of covalent modification to target proteins has led to significant advancements in the treatment of cancer. However, while covalent drugs have significantly impacted medical treatment, their potential for neurodegenerative diseases remains largely unexplored. Neurodegenerative diseases present significant risks to brain function, leading to progressive deterioration in sensory, motor, and cognitive abilities. Alzheimer's disease (AD), Huntington's disease (HD), Parkinson's disease (PD), and multiple sclerosis (MS) are among the various examples of such disorders. Numerous research groups have already reported insights through reviews and research articles on FDA-approved covalent inhibitors, revealing their mechanisms and the specific covalent warheads that preferentially interact with particular amino acid residues in intricate detail. Hence, in this review, we aim to provide a concise summary of these critical topics. This summary endeavors to guide medicinal chemists in their quest to design covalent inhibitors for protein kinases, specifically targeting neurodegenerative diseases.

Keywords: protein kinase; cancer; neurodegenerative diseases; covalent inhibitors

---

Citation: Bhujbal, S.P.; Hah, J.-M. An Innovative Approach to Address Neurodegenerative Diseases through Kinase-Targeted Therapies: Potential for Designing Covalent Inhibitors. *Pharmaceuticals* **2023**, *16*, 1295. https://doi.org/10.3390/ph16091295

Academic Editors: Anna Artese, Alessandra Ammazzalorso, Halil İbrahim Ciftci, Belgin Sever and Hasan Demirci

Received: 28 July 2023
Revised: 7 September 2023
Accepted: 12 September 2023
Published: 13 September 2023

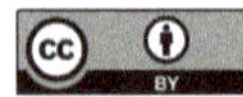

1. Introduction

Kinases are a class of enzymes responsible for catalyzing the transfer of a phosphate group from a high-energy donor molecule (usually ATP) to a substrate molecule [1]. These enzymes are categorized based on the type of substrate they phosphorylate, leading to two main groups: metabolic kinases and protein kinases. The protein kinases are further divided into three subcategories: tyrosine-specific kinases, serine/threonine-specific kinases, and mixed-specificity kinases [1–3]. They play a crucial role in regulating the intracellular signaling pathways that govern vital cellular processes, such as cell proliferation, survival, differentiation, and apoptosis. Both protein and metabolic kinases hold vital significance in numerous human diseases, encompassing immune disorders and cancers [3]. The dysregulation of kinase activity has been linked to over 400 diseases [4]. For example, mutations in genes encoding protein kinases can lead to excessive kinase activity. To address this, several clinically approved drugs, such as selective kinase inhibitors, have been designed to target and inhibit the enzymatic activity of specific protein kinases [1–5]. The FDA-approved kinase inhibitors encompass conventional acyclic, macrocyclic, and covalent inhibitors, all developed to enhance efficacy and selectivity against their respective kinase targets. This review specifically concentrates on exploring opportunities for designing covalent kinase inhibitors to treat neurodegenerative diseases.

1.1. Protein Kinases in Drug Discovery

Due to overexpression and genetic alterations, such as mutations and translocations, protein kinase activity becomes dysregulated. This contributes to the pathogenesis of numerous diseases, including autoimmune, cardiovascular, nervous, and inflammatory conditions, as well as various malignancies. Consequently, the kinase family has emerged as a crucial drug target in the 21st century [6,7], with approximately one-quarter of the world's drug discovery efforts focusing on protein kinases [8]. Remarkably, there are currently 62 FDA-approved therapeutic agents that target around two dozen distinct protein kinases [8]. The public domain hosts over five thousand protein kinase structures, serving as valuable resources for structure-based drug development. Additionally, the pharmaceutical industry holds a considerable number of proprietary structures utilized in the drug development process. The ongoing clinical trials worldwide involve about 175 different orally effective protein kinase antagonists [9], and a comprehensive listing of these drugs, regularly updated, can be accessed at www.icoa.fr/pkidb/ (accessed on 16 June 2023). Despite these impressive numbers, it is worth noting that the 62 FDA-approved therapeutic agents and the additional drugs in clinical trials only target a fraction of the vast 518-member protein kinase enzyme family [5,9].

1.1.1. Protein Kinases in Neurodegenerative Diseases

Neuroregeneration refers to the processes of regeneration within the nervous system, encompassing the generation of new neurons, axons, glia, and synapses [6,7,10]. It involves the progressive structural and functional recovery of the damaged nervous system over time. Damage to the central nervous system (CNS) can result from cell death, failure of axonal regeneration, demyelination, and overall deficits in neuronal structure and function [5]. These conditions, whether partial or complete, occurring individually or in combination, and whether arising from genetic factors or acquired, collectively give rise to specific neurological disorders known as neurodegenerative disorders. These neurodegenerative disorders pose significant threats to the normal functioning of the brain, leading to gradual deterioration or even total loss of sensory, motor, and cognitive function. Examples of such disorders include Alzheimer's disease (AD), Huntington's disease (HD), Parkinson's disease (PD), and multiple sclerosis (MS), among others [5].

Significantly, neurodegenerative diseases are characterized by the abnormal accumulation of proteins in the brain or tissue. For instance, Alzheimer's disease (AD) involves the buildup of β-amyloid, while Huntington's disease (HD) is associated with misfolded Huntington protein aggregation. In amyotrophic lateral sclerosis, there is an aggregation of ubiquitinated proteins [11]; multiple sclerosis (MS) plaques exhibit the accumulation of Tau and β-amyloid [8]; while Parkinson's disease (PD) is marked by α-synuclein accumulation. Additionally, traumatic brain injuries are linked to Tau neurofibrillary tangles [12]. Compelling evidence indicates that the spread of misfolded proteins from one cell to another contributes to the disease's progression [5,13]. Currently, there are no cures for neurodegenerative diseases, especially in their advanced stages. However, the development of therapeutic approaches remains of paramount importance to address physiological and cognitive deficits [5].

Neurodegenerative diseases impact distinct regions of the brain, exhibiting unique and evident characteristics at the phenotypic level, such as the progressive loss of sensory–motor and cognitive functions [14]. However, despite these differences, they share similar cellular and molecular etiologies [15]. Analyzing these commonalities offers the potential for therapeutic advancements that could simultaneously address multiple neurodegenerative disorders if we gain a clear understanding of their shared features [5,16]. Among these, Alzheimer's (AD), Parkinson's (PD), Huntington's disease (HD), and multiple sclerosis (MS) are the most prevalent forms. AD stands as the leading cause of dementia worldwide, severely impacting an individual's ability to perform everyday activities. In the United States alone, an estimated 5.4 million people are affected by AD, including approximately 200,000 individuals aged under 65, making up the younger-onset AD population [17]. The harmful etiological factors in AD involve the buildup of β-amyloid protein and intracellular aggregation of tau protein, which may trigger synaptopathies, glial inflammation, and eventual neuronal death in the cerebral cortex, sub-cortical regions, temporal and parietal lobes, and cingulate gyrus [5].

Both AD and PD are progressive diseases associated with the intracellular accumulation of toxic protein aggregates. Despite their distinct and evident phenotypic characteristics, they share a common etiology at the subcellular level [18,19]. However, the current treatment approaches for neurodegenerative diseases only target a small subset of the population and primarily focus on providing symptomatic relief, lacking the ability to alter the progression of the diseases [5,19]. Using a covalent kinase inhibitors (CKI) strategy in the design of new kinase inhibitors presents a compelling and innovative solution to address these challenges. CKI have been developed and reported as promising drug candidates for various diseases, with a particular emphasis on their therapeutic applications in the field of oncology [18,19]. Therefore, it is advisable to develop novel CKI-targeting kinases for which only anticancer inhibitors had been previously documented, for example, JNK3 (c-Jun N-terminal kinase 3).

1.1.2. JNK3 in Neurodegenerative Diseases

JNKs, part of the mitogen-activated protein kinases (MAPKs) family, are stress-activated serine-threonine protein kinases [20]. They play a crucial role in regulating various cellular activities, ranging from proliferation to cell death [21]. While JNK1 and JNK2 are widely expressed in all body tissues, JNK3 expression is restricted to the central nervous system (CNS), cardiovascular system, smooth muscle, and testis [21]. JNK3 primarily participates in neurodegenerative processes, including Alzheimer's disease (AD), Parkinson's disease (PD), cerebral ischemia, and other CNS disorders. Significantly, JNK3 has been detected in the cerebrospinal fluid (CSF) of AD patients, and its elevated levels have been statistically correlated with the rate of cognitive decline. This finding emphasizes JNK3's crucial role as a key player in AD, making it an attractive target for CNS drug development [20,21]. Moreover, JNK3 plays a pivotal role in the initial neurodegenerative event, known as synaptic dysfunction, which leads to the perturbation of physiological synapse structure and function. Excitingly, synaptic dysfunction and spine loss have been shown to be pharmacologically reversible, offering promising therapeutic directions for brain diseases. Additionally, JNK3 could serve as a valuable biomarker for disease detection, as its presence can be detected at the peripheral level, enabling early diagnosis of neurodegenerative diseases in their prodromal stages [20–22].

Given this information, it is worth considering JNK3 as an illustrative example since it has not been extensively studied as a target for the development of covalent inhibitors in the past. Targeting protein kinases like JNK3 could prove advantageous in the design and advancement of covalent inhibitors for the treatment of neurodegenerative disorders. With the wealth of existing 3D structures of JNK3 and comprehensive information on covalent inhibitors and their warheads, the enticing advantages and disadvantages have motivated us to embrace the challenge of designing covalent inhibitors for JNK3. Our aim is to target diseases like Alzheimer's while ensuring these inhibitors possess blood–brain barrier (BBB) permeability. Furthermore, aside from its involvement in neurodegenerative diseases (ND), JNK3's binding site contains a critical residue, cysteine154, which can form covalent bonds with most of the covalent warheads (as shown in Figure 1). This characteristic makes JNK3 an attractive target for the development of covalent inhibitors.

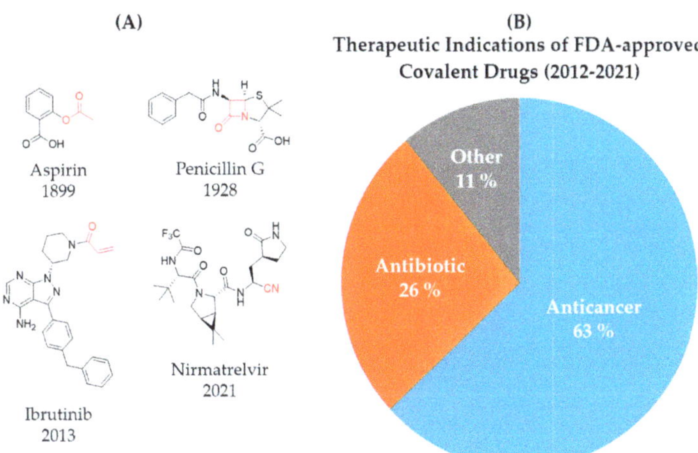

Figure 1. (**A**) Chemical structures of representative covalent inhibitors in early and recent years. (**B**) Therapeutic indications of covalent inhibitors [18].

1.2. Recent Studies on Neurodegenerative Diseases

Limited research endeavors have been commenced in the realm of neurodegenerative diseases, particularly those targeting diverse macromolecules. Instances of investigations focusing on kinases as targets are relatively scarce. Some of these studies are briefly outlined hereafter. Yun et al.'s study revealed the significant involvement of the NLRP3 inflammasome in innate immune-mediated inflammation, contributing to the development of various neurodegenerative diseases. Despite this, there is currently a lack of clinically available medications targeting the NLRP3 inflammasome. Although RRx-001, an anticancer agent under phase III clinical investigation, is known for its well-tolerated nature, its potential impact on inflammatory conditions remains unexplored. In light of this, Yun et al. demonstrated the remarkable potential of RRx-001 as a specific and potent NLRP3 inhibitor, yielding substantial benefits for NLRP3-driven inflammatory ailments. Mechanistically, RRx-001 forms a covalent bond with Cysteine409 of NLRP3 through its bromoacetyl group, effectively obstructing the crucial NLRP3-NEK7 interaction necessary for NLRP3 inflammasome assembly and activation [23].

Bratkowski et al. identified a significant revelation regarding the role of nicotinamide adenine dinucleotide (NAD) hydrolase SARM1, positioning it as a pivotal metabolic sensor and executor of axonal functions. This finding presents a captivating avenue for the creation of innovative neuroprotective treatments aimed at impeding or arresting the degenerative progression. They elucidated a category of SARM1 inhibitors reliant on NAD that act within the active site, effectively intercepting NAD hydrolysis and engaging in covalent bonding with the resulting product, adenosine diphosphate ribose (ADPR) [24]. Moreover, Huang et al. have documented that the phosphoinositide 3-kinase (PI3K)/protein kinase B (AKT)/mammalian target of rapamycin (mTOR) pathway holds significant importance as a therapeutic target for neurodegenerative disorders. Their examination encompassed recent advancements in ATP-competitive inhibitors, allosteric inhibitors, covalent inhibitors, and proteolysis-targeting chimeras within the context of the PI3K/AKT/mTOR pathway. They highlighted potential strategies to counteract the toxicities and acquired drug resistance associated with current treatments and put forth recommendations for the future formulation and development of promising agents targeting this pathway [25]. We have not discussed these studies extensively in our review because comprehensive outcomes and elucidations for these investigations are available within their respective referenced articles, mentioned earlier.

2. Covalent Inhibitors

Covalent inhibitors are extensively used as both biochemical tools and therapeutic agents, allowing for the targeting of proteins previously considered "undruggable" [18,26]. The advanced selectivity of modern covalent inhibitors has significantly alleviated concerns about potential toxicity arising from protein covalent modifications. Despite the remarkable clinical success achieved by current covalent inhibitors, there still remain unmet medical needs that require further attention. The application of covalent drugs has been instrumental in improving human lives by utilizing the covalent modification of target proteins [18,26]. Iconic examples of covalent drugs include aspirin, a well-known anti-inflammatory medication, and penicillin, one of the earliest antibiotics to be developed (Figure 1A) [27]. Historically, the discovery of covalent drugs has been largely serendipitous, providing only a limited window of opportunity for exploring the landscape of covalent inhibitors. However, in recent decades, advancements in crystallography, computer-aided drug design, and modern organic chemistry have made the rational design of covalent inhibitors more feasible and efficient [18,26].

The conventional mechanism of covalent inhibitors, from aspirin to nirmatrelvir (Figure 1A), has involved targeting the catalytic residues of pathological enzymes. However, when these traditional covalent inhibitors encounter highly conserved residues across protein family members, they may lack subtype selectivity. In 2011, Singh and colleagues introduced a novel strategy utilizing targeted covalent inhibitors (TCIs) [28]. This approach achieves subtype selectivity by focusing on poorly conserved and non-catalytic residues. A notable example of TCIs is Ibrutinib (Figure 1A), a first-in-class BTK inhibitor approved for the treatment of mantle cell lymphoma and chronic lymphocytic leukemia (CLL). The clinical success of Ibrutinib has propelled the utilization of TCIs as the preferred approach in the development of covalent drugs [18]. The majority of FDA-approved TCIs exhibit selective inhibition of kinases by targeting poorly conserved cysteine residues near ATP-binding pockets. However, it is essential to note that such targetable cysteine residues are not widespread in the human proteome [29]. Due to this limitation, lysine has gained attention as a promising target residue for covalent modification due to its prevalence in the human kinome [18].

Despite their promising therapeutic potential, covalent drugs currently constitute only 4.4% of the drugs approved by the U.S. Food and Drug Administration (FDA) in the past decade [30]. Among these covalent drugs, 90% function as anticancer or antibiotic agents (Figure 1B). FDA-approved covalent kinase inhibitors are listed in Table 1.

Table 1. FDA approved covalent kinase inhibitors.

Name/Structure	Targets	Therapeutic Indication	Warhead	Ref (Approval Date)
Wortmannin	Kinase (PI3K)	N/A	Furan	[24]
A5	Kinase (BCR-ABL)	Anticancer (chronic myeloid leukemia)	Aldehyde	[28]

Table 1. *Cont.*

Name/Structure	Targets	Therapeutic Indication	Warhead	Ref (Approval Date)
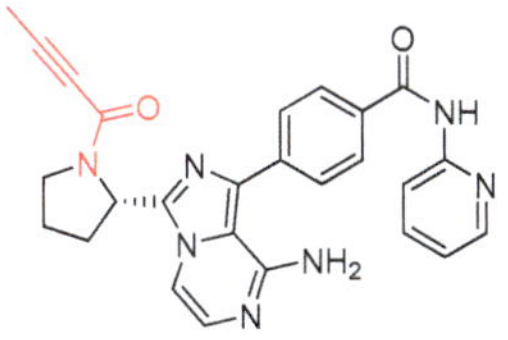 Acalabrutinib	Kinase (BTK)	Anticancer (mantle cell lymphoma	2-butyneamide	31 October 2017
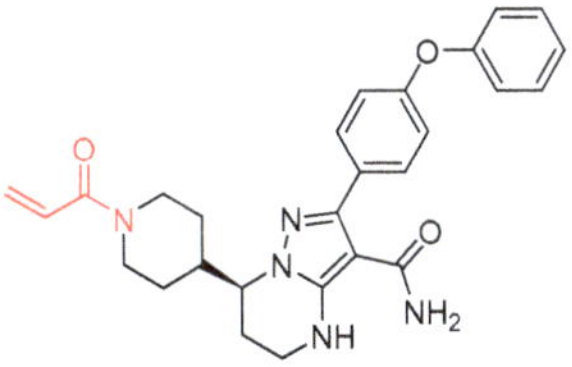 Zanubrutinib	Kinase (BTK)	Anticancer (mantle cell lymphoma	Acrylamide	14 November 2019
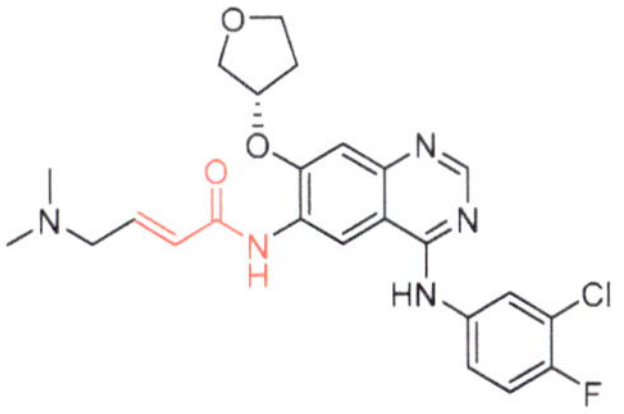 Afatinib	Kinase (EGFR T790M and pan-HER)	Anticancer (NSCLC)	Acrylamide	12 July 2013
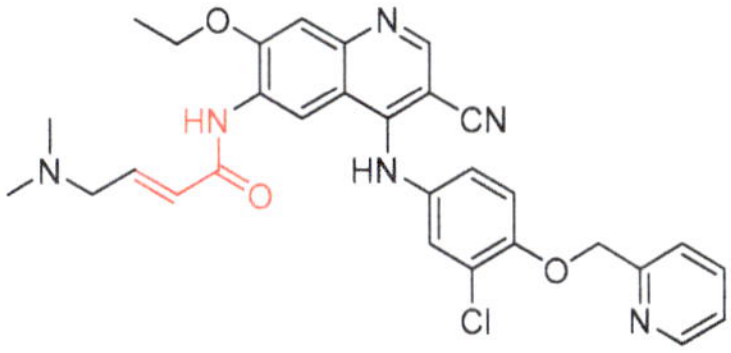 Neratinib	Kinase (pan-HER)	Anticancer (breast cancer)	Acrylamide	17 July 2017
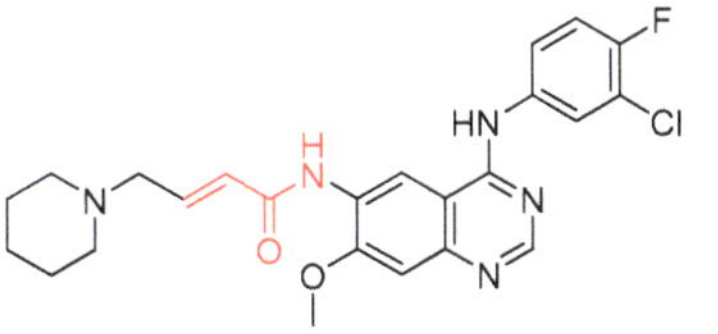 Dacomitinib	Kinase (pan-HER)	Anticancer (NSCLC)	Acrylamide	27 September 2018
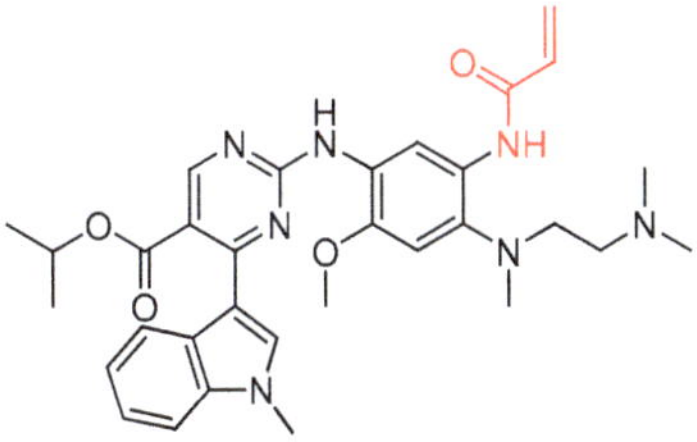 Mobocertinib	Kinase (EGFR ex20ins)	Anticancer (NSCLC)	Acrylamide	15 September 2021

Table 1. *Cont.*

Name/Structure	Targets	Therapeutic Indication	Warhead	Ref (Approval Date)
Lazertinib	Kinase (EGFR)	Anticancer (NSCLC)	Acrylamide	Accelerated approval, 21 May 2021, combination with amivantamab
Nazartinib	Kinase (EGFR)	Anticancer (NSCLC)	Acrylamide	[29]

3. Types of Covalent Inhibitors

In addition to categorizing covalent inhibitors based on reactive groups or modification sites, Alfred Tuley et al. [26] and Jesang Lee et al. [18] introduced a classification based on a mechanism depicted in Figure 2. This method emphasizes the common advantages and disadvantages inherent to each approach. The established categories for reversible and irreversible covalent inhibitors are briefly outlined below, along with representative examples for each class, including covalent reversible inhibitors, slow substrates, residue-specific reagents, affinity labels (classical, quiescent, and photoaffinity), and mechanism-based inactivators. For a more comprehensive understanding of these types of covalent inhibitors, interested readers are encouraged to refer to the detailed works by Lee et al. [18] and Tuley et al. [26].

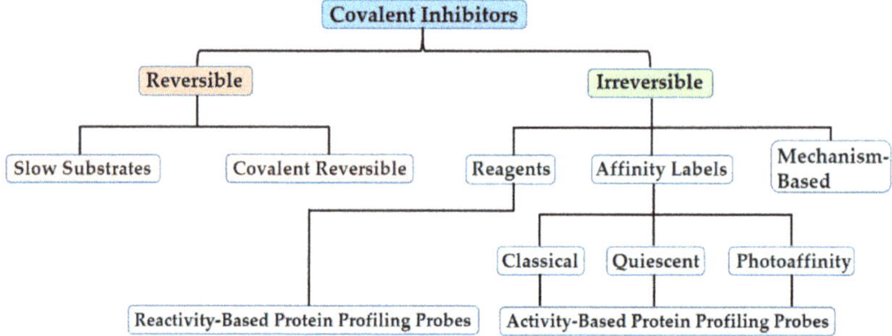

Figure 2. Taxonomy of covalent inhibitors. The classification of covalent enzyme inhibitors according to their mechanisms highlights diverse approaches aimed to balance reactivity and selectivity [26].

In general, covalent inhibitors can be broadly classified into two categories based on whether the inhibition is reversible or irreversible upon dialysis, competition with excess substrate, or extended incubation times. While different covalent inhibitors may exhibit the same reversibility or irreversibility of inhibition, each employs distinct strategies to selectively form and break bonds with the targeted enzyme. Identifying and categorizing these strategies helps to illuminate the inherent advantages and disadvantages associated with each mechanism [18–22,26].

3.1. Covalent Reversible Inhibitors

This class of inhibitors employs covalent bond formation with the enzyme to achieve inhibition, but enzyme activity is subsequently restored through the cleavage of this bond [2,3]. Covalent bond formation contributes to the overall affinity of the inhibitor, but the subsequent bond cleavage can decrease the duration of inhibition and lower the affinity [4]. This approach helps to mitigate some of the potential drawbacks associated with the formation of irreversible covalent adducts, but, at the same time, makes it more challenging to identify the proteins bound by these inhibitors. The most prevalent type of covalent inhibitor exhibiting reversible inhibition is named after this category because the term "reversible" accurately describes the underlying chemical mechanism [18].

3.2. Covalent Irreversible Inhibitors

The second major category of covalent inhibitors comprises those that induce irreversible inhibition (Figure 2). These inhibitors are also referred to as inactivators to underscore the irretrievable loss in enzyme activity they cause [26]. Since covalent modification by these inhibitors is not reversible, they cannot rely on thermodynamic equilibration to achieve selectivity. Instead, they employ different strategies to achieve selective modification. While forming an irreversible covalent adduct comes with some inherent disadvantages, this type of inhibitor offers the advantage of long-lasting inhibition that persists even as the inhibitor concentration in solution decreases. Additionally, irreversible inhibitors facilitate both target and off-target identification. Over time, the slow accumulation of inhibited enzymes, even in the presence of competing ligands, further contributes to the effectiveness of irreversible inhibitors [18,26].

In summary, it is important to highlight that, when dealing with this class of inhibitors, the use of IC_{50} values alone to guide structure–activity studies can be misleading due to the time-dependent nature of inhibition [31–33]. To accurately assess the inhibitory effects, parameters such as K_I, which describes the noncovalent binding affinity (denoted with a capital I to differentiate it from K_i values for reversible noncovalent inhibitors), and k_{inact}, which describes the kinetics of covalent modification, can be utilized. These parameters can be derived from fitting time-dependent inhibition studies through various methods described elsewhere [34,35]. Irreversible inhibitors are divided into three main categories: residue-specific reagents, affinity labels, and mechanism-based enzyme inactivators.

3.2.1. Residue-Specific Reagents

These are the least selective type of irreversible inhibitor, and they are primarily employed in vitro as biochemical tools [26]. These reactive compounds achieve selective modification by depending on chemoselectivity for specific nucleophiles, rather than noncovalent affinity to a particular binding site. The selectivity is also influenced by the relative nucleophilicity and steric availability of the reacting residues in the targeted proteins. Recently, many reagents used for residue-specific modification in proteins and peptides have been extensively reviewed [36]. Due to their limited noncovalent affinity for a specific protein site, these reagents typically exhibit second-order inactivation kinetics. A pertinent illustration of a residue-specific chemical modifying agent employed as a covalent inhibitor involves the use of methylmethanethiosulfonate to interact with cysteine residues in soluble guanylate cyclase. This process leads to the covalent attachment of methanethiol moieties through disulfide bonds to multiple cysteine residues located throughout the protein [37].

3.2.2. Affinity Labels

Rather than relying solely on chemoselectivity, affinity labels increase their site selectivity by coupling a reactive group, typically a poor electrophile, to a second moiety that provides noncovalent binding affinity to a specific binding site [38]. Each of the three different types of affinity labels within this class increases the effective molarity of the reactive group near the site of enzyme modification by using a moiety to provide noncovalent binding. However, the strategy used to attenuate reactivity varies by type and can impact selectivity [26]. In contrast to relying solely on chemoselectivity, affinity labels enhance their site selectivity by combining a reactive group, usually a poor electrophile, with a second moiety that provides noncovalent binding affinity to a specific binding site [38]. The three different types of affinity labels (classical, quiescent, and photoaffinity) within this class employ a moiety to provide noncovalent binding, thus increasing the effective molarity of the reactive group near the site of enzyme modification. However, the approach used to attenuate reactivity differs for each type, and this variation can influence the overall selectivity.

3.2.3. Covalent Mechanism-Based Enzyme Inactivators

Among all covalent enzyme inhibitors, those falling into the category of mechanism-based enzyme inactivators have the potential to be the most selective because they initially exist as unreactive molecules. These inhibitors bind to the active sites of enzymes and undergo normal catalytic processes, leading to the formation of a reactive species that results in covalent bond formation. The parameters K_I and k_{inact} represent a combination of individual rate constants, which, in certain cases (e.g., rapid equilibrium, $k_4 = 0$, k_2 is rate-limiting), can be simplified to represent the dissociation constant for the noncovalent complex and k_2, respectively [39].

4. Advantages and Disadvantages of Covalent Inhibitors

Basically, a covalent bond is formed when atoms equally share electron pairs. In the context of covalent kinase inhibitor (CKI) development, this usually involves a ligand electrophile (e.g., acrylamide) and a target nucleophile (e.g., a cysteine sulfhydryl). However, achieving selective kinase targeting poses challenges, and there is a risk of cytotoxicity due to extended or permanent off-target modifications [40]. In short, the following are some of the potential advantages associated with covalent inhibitors.

4.1. Potency

Within a covalent inhibitor, the covalent attachment plays a crucial role in contributing to the overall free energy of binding (GB), leading to significantly enhanced potency while maintaining a low molecular weight. Unlike non-covalent inhibitors, covalent therapeutics are less affected by competition with high concentrations of endogenous substrates (e.g., ATP). This advantage is due to their reliance on non-equilibrium binding kinetics [41].

4.2. Pharmacodynamics (PD)

When the target is appropriately chosen, covalent inhibitors can exhibit a prolonged duration of action compared to their non-covalent counterparts. This leads to a separation between pharmacodynamics (PD) and pharmacokinetics (PK), referred to as PK-PD decoupling. As a result, covalent inhibitors can maintain sustained efficacy beyond metabolic clearance [40].

4.3. Drug Dosing

Covalent binders offer a clinically relevant advantage due to their high potency, sustained action, and decoupled PK-PD effect. This advantage allows for the administration of smaller and less frequent doses as compared to non-covalent drugs. These relatively smaller doses often result in a significant reduction in negative side effects, particularly those arising from unpredictable idiosyncratic toxicities (IDTs). In contrast, many non-covalent drugs may require more frequent and larger doses to maintain therapeutically efficacious plasma concentrations [40,42].

4.4. Drug Resistance

The primary source of resistance typically arises from mutations within the ATP binding site. Recent studies on covalent inhibitors have confirmed their capacity to hinder and evade mutation events, enabling them to maintain potency against mutant targets [40,43]. These investigations have suggested that while active-site mutations may impede the initial reversible binding (i.e., K_i), subsequent covalent bond formation (i.e., k_{inact}) can still occur, assuming that the reactive residue remains unaltered. However, it is essential to consider the vulnerability of covalent kinase inhibitors (CKIs) to mutations of the nucleophilic residue. In such cases, the potency can be significantly reduced due to the critical role of covalent bond formation in the observed efficacy.

4.5. Target Scope

CKIs heavily depend on covalent interactions for their potency. In specific cases, due to their reduced reliance on non-covalent intermolecular interactions, covalent drugs may offer the advantage of targeting challenging active sites, such as those that are poorly defined, large, and solvent-exposed. The nature of a covalent inhibitor allows for high potency without requiring extensive binding surface contact, which can lead to a smaller-sized molecule. Moreover, target selectivity is a critical consideration in any drug discovery program, and covalent compounds can be deliberately designed to bind to poorly conserved target-specific nucleophilic residues [40,44].

5. Disadvantages

Despite their advantages, covalent inhibitors also come with potential drawbacks that need to be considered. These include the increased challenge of evaluating and achieving a balance between reactivity and selectivity. Covalent modification may extend to off-target proteins, nucleic acids, or small molecules due to nonselective reactions. Moreover, idiosyncratic adverse drug responses, inappropriate levels of enzyme inhibition when partial or short-duration inhibition is required, and limitations in achieving some of the benefits mentioned earlier are also among the concerns. Additionally, designing these inhibitors de novo may be perceived as challenging [26,40].

6. Need for Covalent Kinase Inhibitors

6.1. Importance of Cysteine Residue

Covalent compounds that react with cysteine have seen a resurgence as potent and selective tools for modifying protein function, serving both as chemical probes and clinically approved drugs [2]. The remarkable sensitivity of human immune cell signaling pathways to oxidative stress suggests that covalent probes hold significant potential for selective chemical immunomodulation, an area that is still relatively underexplored [45,46]. Recently, cysteine-reactive compounds have regained prominence as powerful tools for altering protein function, especially for challenging-to-target protein classes [2]. These compounds, often referred to as covalent compounds, contain electrophilic moieties that react either irreversibly or reversibly with the thiol side chain of specific cysteine residues. The preferential labeling of specific cysteine results from a combination of factors, including the intrinsic reactivity of the thiol, the nature and relative reactivity of the electrophile, and the molecular recognition of the binding portion of the molecule [47].

Cysteine presents an intriguing amino acid target for several compelling reasons. The unique chemistry of the cysteine thiol renders cysteine residues crucial for the structure and function of most human proteins [2]. Cysteines often serve as catalytic nucleophiles in enzymes, such as proteases. Additionally, cysteines are involved in coordinating metals, forming structural and redox-active disulfides, undergoing frequent post-translational modifications, and acting as sensors of oxidative stress [2]. Cysteine-reactive compounds can be skillfully designed to access small and less-defined binding sites, allowing them to efficiently block high-affinity interactions, such as protein–protein interactions, or compete with high concentrations of endogenous biomolecules like ATP [47]. There exists a wide array of examples of cysteine-reactive clinical candidates and drugs, including blockbuster covalent kinase inhibitors (CKIs); anti-cancer compounds like KPT3 [48], which reacts with a conserved cysteine in the nuclear export factor XPO1 [49]; and ARS-1620, which inhibits the Gly12Cys-mutated oncogenic form of the GTPase KRAS [50]. Remarkably, nearly all human proteins contain at least one cysteine (with an average of 13 cysteines per protein), and recent studies [2,47] indicate that a surprisingly significant portion of cysteines can react with cysteine-reactive compounds [2,47]. Commonly used cysteine-reactive electrophiles are depicted in Figure 3, below. In our review, we do not provide a detailed description of how each of the cysteine-reactive electrophiles reacts, as this information was already covered in a previously published article [2,47].

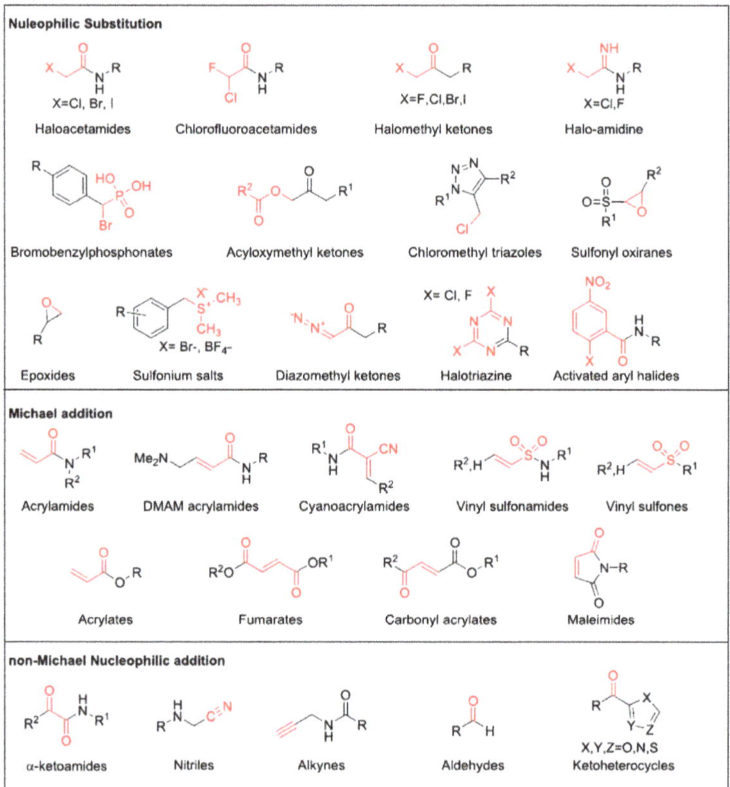

Figure 3. Commonly used cysteine-reactive electrophiles. Electrophilic groups, depicted in red, are categorized based on their specific mechanisms of covalent cysteine labeling.

6.2. Opportunities for Covalent Kinase Inhibitors (CKIs) by Targeting Kinases

Developing selective inhibitors for kinases poses a considerable challenge due to their high sequence and structural homology. Surprisingly, more than 200 members of the human protein kinase family have been found to harbor active site cysteines [51]. Targeting these residues with covalent kinase inhibitors (CKIs) offers an exciting strategy to create highly potent and selective ATP competitive kinase inhibitors, a topic covered extensively in recent comprehensive reviews [40]. CKIs have gained significant attention for their therapeutic efficacy in treating various cancers [2,40]. While many of the targeted kinases have clear immune-relevance, the full immunotherapeutic potential of CKIs is yet to be fully explored. To date, all identified CKIs primarily target protein kinases for cancer treatment; however, in this review, we focused on the opportunity to target kinases for neurodegenerative diseases. As some kinases exhibit higher degrees of promiscuous binding, an alternative strategy is to produce compounds targeting the inactive forms of kinases. However, complications arise, as some kinases can bind inhibitors more promiscuously when in their inactive conformation, making it challenging to generate selective inhibitors for inactive kinases, at least in certain cases.

Given this information, it is worth considering JNK3 as an illustrative example since it has not been extensively studied as a target for the development of covalent inhibitors in the past. Moreover, aside from its involvement in neurodegenerative diseases (ND), JNK3's binding site contains a critical residue, cysteine154, which can form covalent bonds with most of the covalent warheads. Targeting protein kinases like JNK3 could prove advantageous in the design and advancement of covalent inhibitors for the treatment of neurodegenerative disorders. Presently, our research group is actively engaged in designing and synthesizing covalent inhibitors specific to JNK3. However, we cannot disclose the chemical structures of these designed covalent inhibitors in this review. Instead, we intend to publish them as a separate research article in the near future.

7. Conclusions

Due to the dysregulation of protein kinase activity in various diseases, including cancer, autoimmune, neurodegenerative, and inflammatory conditions, the protein kinase family has emerged as a crucial drug target. In this review, we have extensively discussed previously approved covalent inhibitors, elucidating their mechanisms and the specific covalent warheads that typically react with particular amino acid residues, most of which were developed for cancer treatment. However, the potential of these inhibitors for neurodegenerative diseases remains largely unexplored. We have also highlighted the advantages and disadvantages of covalent kinase inhibitors (CKIs) over conventional kinase inhibitors. Moreover, our focus is on the importance of designing CKIs for specific protein kinases, such as JNK3, which plays a significant role in neurodegenerative diseases like Alzheimer's. We aim to help in the development of covalent inhibitors with high selectivity and improved blood–brain barrier (BBB) permeability. The concise summary provided in this review is intended to serve as a guide for the research community in their efforts to design covalent inhibitors for protein kinases, specifically targeting neurodegenerative diseases.

Author Contributions: Conceptualization, J.-M.H. and S.P.B.; methodology and formal analysis, S.P.B.; writing—original draft preparation, S.P.B.; writing—review and editing, J.-M.H. and S.P.B.; project administration, J.-M.H.; funding acquisition, J.-M.H. All authors have read and agreed to the published version of the manuscript.

Funding: This work was financially supported by a National Research Foundation of Korea grant (NRF-2020R1A6A1A03042854: Center for Proteinopathy), and Hanyang University (HY-2023).

Institutional Review Board Statement: Not applicable.

Informed Consent Statement: Not applicable.

Data Availability Statement: Data sharing is not applicable.

Conflicts of Interest: The authors declare no conflict of interest.

References

1. Guo, Y.; Liu, Y.; Hu, N.; Yu, D.; Zhou, C.; Shi, G.; Zhang, B.; Wei, M.; Liu, J.; Luo, L.; et al. Discovery of zanubrutinib (BGB-3111), a novel, potent, and selective covalent inhibitor of Bruton's tyrosine kinase. *J. Med. Chem.* **2019**, *62*, 7923–7940. [CrossRef] [PubMed]
2. Backus, K.M.; Cao, J.; Maddox, S.M. Opportunities and challenges for the development of covalent chemical immunomodulators. *Bioorg. Med. Chem.* **2019**, *27*, 3421–3439.
3. Cheng, H.; Nair, S.K.; Murray, B.W. Recent progress on third generation covalent EGFR inhibitors. *Bioorg. Med. Chem. Lett.* **2016**, *26*, 1861–1868. [CrossRef]
4. Fan, S.; Yue, L.; Wan, W.; Zhang, Y.; Zhang, B.; Otomo, C.; Li, Q.; Lin, T.; Hu, J.; Xu, P.; et al. Inhibition of autophagy by a small molecule through covalent modification of the LC3 protein. *Angew. Chem. Int. Ed.* **2021**, *60*, 26105–26114. [CrossRef]
5. Hussain, R.; Zubair, H.; Pursell, S.; Shahab, M. Neurodegenerative diseases: Regenerative mechanisms and novel therapeutic approaches. *Brain Sci.* **2018**, *8*, 177. [CrossRef] [PubMed]
6. Gage, F.H.; Temple, S. Neural stem cells: Generating and regenerating the brain. *Neuron* **2013**, *80*, 588–601. [CrossRef] [PubMed]
7. Malberg, J.E.; Eisch, A.J.; Nestler, E.J.; Duman, R.S. Chronic antidepressant treatment increases neurogenesis in adult rat hippocampus. *J. Neurosci.* **2000**, *20*, 9104–9110. [CrossRef]
8. David, M.A.; Tayebi, M.J. Detection of protein aggregates in brain and cerebrospinal fluid derived from multiple sclerosis patients. *Front. Neurol.* **2014**, *5*, 251. [CrossRef]

9. Altman, J. Are new neurons formed in the brains of adult mammals? *Science* **1962**, *135*, 1127–1128. [CrossRef]
10. Kuhn, H.G.; Dickinson-Anson, H.; Gage, F.H. Neurogenesis in the dentate gyrus of the adult rat: Age-related decrease of neuronal progenitor proliferation. *J. Neurosci.* **1996**, *16*, 2027–2033. [CrossRef]
11. Blokhuis, A.M.; Groen, E.J.; Koppers, M.; van den Berg, L.H.; Pasterkamp, R.J. Protein aggregation in amyotrophic lateral sclerosis *Acta Neuropathol.* **2013**, *125*, 777–794. [CrossRef] [PubMed]
12. Lucke-Wold, B.P.; Turner, R.C.; Logsdon, A.F.; Bailes, J.E.; Huber, J.D.; Rosen, C.L. Linking traumatic brain injury to chronic traumatic encephalopathy: Identification of potential mechanisms leading to neurofibrillary tangle development. *J. Neurotrauma* **2014**, *31*, 1129–1138. [CrossRef]
13. Hatters, D.M. Protein misfolding inside cells: The case of huntingtin and Huntington's disease. *IUBMB Life* **2008**, *60*, 724–728 [CrossRef]
14. Woolley, J.D.; Khan, B.K.; Murthy, N.K.; Miller, B.L.; Rankin, K.P. The diagnostic challenge of psychiatric symptoms in neurodegenerative disease: Rates of and risk factors for prior psychiatric diagnosis in patients with early neurodegenerative disease *J. Clin. Psychiatry* **2011**, *72*, 4437. [CrossRef]
15. Vadakkan, K.I. Neurodegenerative disorders share common features of "loss of function" states of a proposed mechanism of nervous system functions. *BioMedicine* **2016**, *83*, 412–430. [CrossRef]
16. Rubinsztein, D.C. The roles of intracellular protein-degradation pathways in neurodegeneration. *Nature* **2006**, *443*, 780–786 [CrossRef]
17. Alzheimer's Association. 2012 Alzheimer's disease facts and figures. *Alzheimer Dement.* **2012**, *8*, 131–168. [CrossRef]
18. Lee, J.; Park, S.B. Extended Applications of Small-Molecule Covalent Inhibitors toward Novel Therapeutic Targets. *Pharmaceuticals* **2022**, *15*, 1478. [CrossRef]
19. Roskoski, R., Jr. Properties of FDA-approved small molecule protein kinase inhibitors: A 2021 update. *Pharmacol. Res.* **2021**, *165*, 105463. [CrossRef] [PubMed]
20. Bhujbal, S.P.; Hah, J.-M. An Intriguing Purview on the Design of Macrocyclic Inhibitors for Unexplored Protein Kinases through Their Binding Site Comparison. *Pharmaceuticals* **2023**, *16*, 1009. [CrossRef] [PubMed]
21. Jun, J.; Yang, S.; Lee, J.; Moon, H.; Kim, J.; Jung, H.; Im, D.; Oh, Y.; Jang, M.; Cho, H.J. Discovery of novel imidazole chemotypes as isoform-selective JNK3 inhibitors for the treatment of Alzheimer's disease. *Eur. J. Med. Chem.* **2023**, *245*, 114894. [CrossRef] [PubMed]
22. Jun, J.; Moon, H.; Yang, S.; Lee, J.; Baek, J.; Kim, H.; Cho, H.; Hwang, K.; Ahn, S.; Kim, Y.J.; et al. Carbamate JNK3 Inhibitors Show Promise as Effective Treatments for Alzheimer's Disease: In Vivo Studies on Mouse Models. *J. Med. Chem.* **2023**, *66*, 6372–6390 [CrossRef]
23. Chen, Y.; He, H.; Lin, B.; Chen, Y.; Deng, X.; Jiang, W.; Zhou, R. RRx-001 ameliorates inflammatory diseases by acting as a potent covalent NLRP3 inhibitor. *Cell. Mol. Immunol.* **2021**, *18*, 1425–1436. [CrossRef] [PubMed]
24. Bratkowski, M.; Burdett, T.C.; Danao, J.; Wang, X.; Mathur, P.; Gu, W.; Beckstead, J.A.; Talreja, S.; Yang, Y.-S.; Danko, G.; et al Uncompetitive, adduct-forming SARM1 inhibitors are neuroprotective in preclinical models of nerve injury and disease. *Neuron* **2022**, *110*, 3711–3726.e3716. [CrossRef]
25. Huang, J.; Chen, L.; Wu, J.; Ai, D.; Zhang, J.-Q.; Chen, T.-G.; Wang, L. Targeting the PI3K/AKT/mTOR signaling pathway in the treatment of human diseases: Current status, trends, and solutions. *J. Med. Chem.* **2022**, *65*, 16033–16061. [CrossRef] [PubMed]
26. Tuley, A.; Fast, W. The taxonomy of covalent inhibitors. *Biochemistry* **2018**, *57*, 3326–3337. [CrossRef]
27. Bauer, R.A. Covalent inhibitors in drug discovery: From accidental discoveries to avoided liabilities and designed therapies. *Drug Discov. Today* **2015**, *20*, 1061–1073. [CrossRef]
28. Sutanto, F.; Konstantinidou, M.; Dömling, A.J. Covalent inhibitors: A rational approach to drug discovery. *RSC Med. Chem.* **2020** *11*, 876–884. [CrossRef]
29. Mukherjee, H.; Grimster, N.P. Beyond cysteine: Recent developments in the area of targeted covalent inhibition. *Curr. Opin. Chem Biol.* **2018**, *44*, 30–38. [CrossRef]
30. Singh, J. The ascension of targeted covalent inhibitors. *J. Med. Chem.* **2022**, *65*, 5886–5901. [CrossRef]
31. Chen, P.; Sun, J.; Zhu, C.; Tang, G.; Wang, W.; Xu, M.; Xiang, M.; Zhang, C.J.; Zhang, Z.M.; Gao, L.; et al. Cell-Active, Reversible and Irreversible Covalent Inhibitors That Selectively Target the Catalytic Lysine of BCR-ABL Kinase. *Angew. Chem. Int. Ed.* **2022** *61*, e202203878. [CrossRef] [PubMed]
32. Robichaux, J.P.; Le, X.; Vijayan, R.; Hicks, J.K.; Heeke, S.; Elamin, Y.Y.; Lin, H.Y.; Udagawa, H.; Skoulidis, F.; Tran, H.; et al Structure-based classification predicts drug response in EGFR-mutant NSCLC. *Nature* **2021**, *597*, 732–737.
33. Copeland, R. *Evaluation of Enzyme Inhibitors in Drug Discovery: A Guide to Chemists and Pharmacologists*; Wiley-Interscience Hoboken, NJ, USA, 2005.
34. Holdgate, G.A.; Meek, T.D.; Grimley, R.L. Mechanistic enzymology in drug discovery: A fresh perspective. *Nat. Rev. Drug Discov* **2018**, *17*, 115–132.
35. Silverman, R. Introduction in *"Mechanism-Based Enzyme Inactivation: Chemistry and Enzymology"*; CRC Press: Boca Raton, FL, USA 1988; Volume 1.
36. So, W.H.; Zhang, Y.; Kang, W.; Wong, C.T.; Sun, H.; Xia, J. Site-selective covalent reactions on proteinogenic amino acids. *Curr Opin. Biotechnol.* **2017**, *48*, 220–227. [PubMed]

37. Fernhoff, N.B.; Derbyshire, E.R.; Marletta, M.A. A nitric oxide/cysteine interaction mediates the activation of soluble guanylate cyclase. *Proc. Natl. Acad. Sci. USA* **2009**, *106*, 21602–21607. [CrossRef]
38. Plapp, B.V. Application of affinity labeling for studying structure and function of enzymes. In *Methods in Enzymology*; Elsevier: Amsterdam, The Netherlands, 1982; Volume 87, pp. 469–499.
39. Silverman, R.B. Mechanism-based enzyme inactivators. In *Methods in Enzymology*; Elsevier: Amsterdam, The Netherlands, 1995; Volume 249, pp. 240–283.
40. Abdeldayem, A.; Raouf, Y.S.; Constantinescu, S.N.; Moriggl, R.; Gunning, P.T. Advances in covalent kinase inhibitors. *Chem. Soc. Rev.* **2020**, *49*, 2617–2687. [PubMed]
41. Ward, R.A.; Colclough, N.; Challinor, M.; Debreczeni, J.E.; Eckersley, K.; Fairley, G.; Feron, L.; Flemington, V.; Graham, M.A.; Greenwood, R.; et al. Structure-guided design of highly selective and potent covalent inhibitors of ERK1/2. *J. Med. Chem.* **2015**, *58*, 4790–4801.
42. Smith, A.J.; Zhang, X.; Leach, A.G.; Houk, K. Beyond picomolar affinities: Quantitative aspects of noncovalent and covalent binding of drugs to proteins. *J. Med. Chem.* **2009**, *52*, 225–233.
43. Tan, L.; Wang, J.; Tanizaki, J.; Huang, Z.; Aref, A.R.; Rusan, M.; Zhu, S.-J.; Zhang, Y.; Ercan, D.; Liao, R.G.; et al. Development of covalent inhibitors that can overcome resistance to first-generation FGFR kinase inhibitors. *Proc. Natl. Acad. Sci. USA* **2014**, *111*, E4869–E4877.
44. Morgan, M.J.; Liu, Z.-G. Crosstalk of reactive oxygen species and NF-κB signaling. *Cell Res.* **2011**, *21*, 103–115.
45. Swaika, A.; Hammond, W.A.; Joseph, R.W. Current state of anti-PD-L1 and anti-PD-1 agents in cancer therapy. *Mol. Immunol.* **2015**, *67*, 4–17.
46. Van Kasteren, S.I.; Neefjes, J.; Ovaa, H. Creating molecules that modulate immune responses. *Nat. Rev. Chem.* **2018**, *2*, 184–193.
47. Backus, K.M.; Correia, B.E.; Lum, K.M.; Forli, S.; Horning, B.D.; González-Páez, G.E.; Chatterjee, S.; Lanning, B.R.; Teijaro, J.R.; Olson, A.; et al. Proteome-wide covalent ligand discovery in native biological systems. *Nature* **2016**, *534*, 570–574.
48. Hildeman, D.A.; Mitchell, T.; Kappler, J.; Marrack, P. T cell apoptosis and reactive oxygen species. *J. Clin. Investig.* **2003**, *111*, 575–581. [PubMed]
49. Lapalombella, R.; Sun, Q.; Williams, K.; Tangeman, L.; Jha, S.; Zhong, Y.; Goettl, V.; Mahoney, E.; Berglund, C.; Gupta, S.; et al. The Journal of the American Society of Hematology. Selective inhibitors of nuclear export show that CRM1/XPO1 is a target in chronic lymphocytic leukemia. *Blood J. Am. Soc. Hematol.* **2012**, *120*, 4621–4634.
50. Janes, M.R.; Zhang, J.; Li, L.-S.; Hansen, R.; Peters, U.; Guo, X.; Chen, Y.; Babbar, A.; Firdaus, S.J.; Darjania, L.; et al. Targeting KRAS mutant cancers with a covalent G12C-specific inhibitor. *Cell* **2018**, *172*, 578–589.e517.
51. Smith, G.A.; Uchida, K.; Weiss, A.; Taunton, J. Essential biphasic role for JAK3 catalytic activity in IL-2 receptor signaling. *Nat. Chem. Biol.* **2016**, *12*, 373–379. [PubMed]

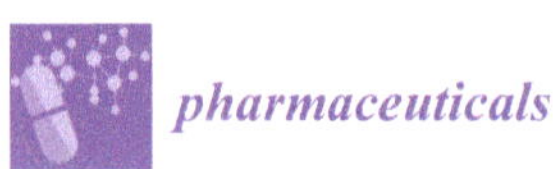 *pharmaceuticals*

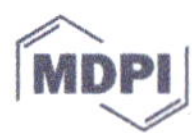

Article

Molecular Dynamics Simulations of Drug-Conjugated Cell-Penetrating Peptides

Márton Ivánczi [1], Balázs Balogh [1], Loretta Kis [1] and István Mándity [1,2,*]

[1] Institute of Organic Chemistry, Semmelweis University, Hőgyes Endre Utca 7., H-1092 Budapest, Hungary; kis.loretta97@gmail.com (L.K.)

[2] Artificial Transporters Research Group, Institute of Materials and Environmental Chemistry, Research Centre for Natural Sciences, Magyar Tudósok Körútja 2., H-1117 Budapest, Hungary

* Correspondence: mandity.istvan@semmelweis.hu or mandity.istvan@ttk.hu

Abstract: Cell-penetrating peptides (CPPs) are small peptides capable of translocating through biological membranes carrying various attached cargo into cells and even into the nucleus. They may also participate in transcellular transport. Our in silico study intends to model several peptides and their conjugates. We have selected three CPPs with a linear backbone, including penetratin, a naturally occurring oligopeptide; two of its modified sequence analogues (6,14-Phe-penetratin and dodeca-penetratin); and three natural CPPs with a cyclic backbone: Kalata B1, the Sunflower trypsin inhibitor 1 (SFT1), and Momordica cochinchinensis trypsin inhibitor II (MCoTI-II). We have also built conjugates with the small-molecule drug compounds doxorubicin, zidovudine, and rasagiline for each peptide. Molecular dynamics (MD) simulations were carried out with explicit membrane models. The analysis of the trajectories showed that the interaction of penetratin with the membrane led to spectacular rearrangements in the secondary structure of the peptide, while cyclic peptides remained unchanged due to their high conformational stability. Membrane–peptide and membrane–conjugate interactions have been identified and compared. Taking into account well-known examples from the literature, our simulations demonstrated the utility of computational methods for CPP complexes, and they may contribute to a better understanding of the mechanism of penetration, which could serve as the basis for delivering conjugated drug molecules to their intracellular targets.

Keywords: cell-penetrating peptides; molecular dynamics; drug conjugates; biological membrane; penetratin; cyclic peptides; explicit membrane model; intracellular target; Desmond; in silico simulation

Citation: Ivánczi, M.; Balogh, B.; Kis, L.; Mándity, I. Molecular Dynamics Simulations of Drug-Conjugated Cell-Penetrating Peptides. *Pharmaceuticals* **2023**, *16*, 1251. https://doi.org/10.3390/ph16091251

Academic Editors: Halil İbrahim Ciftci, Belgin Sever and Hasan Demirci

Received: 16 June 2023
Revised: 8 August 2023
Accepted: 11 August 2023
Published: 5 September 2023

1. Introduction

Membrane-active peptides are divided into two main categories: antimicrobial peptides (AMPs) and cell-penetrating peptides (CPPs). The AMPs (also known as host defense peptides or HDPs) are part of the innate immune response as potent, broad-spectrum antibiotics acting through the destabilization of membranes of the pathogens. Unlike AMPs, CPPs can translocate into living cells and their organelles without lasting damage under physiological conditions [1–3]. This peculiarity makes CPPs adequate to deliver drugs and other compounds to intracellular targets or across the blood–brain barrier [4,5].

Conjugated CPPs could improve various pharmacokinetic properties of drugs, including, for example, poor delivery and low bioavailability, and they may also decrease toxicity. Nearly all types of 'cargo' can be transported: small molecules, diagnostics, macromolecules (DNA, RNA, antibodies, peptides), or even nanoparticles [4]. The conjugation of penetratin with paclitaxel was one of the first applications. It not only increased the solubility of the compound but also helped to reach the nucleus, thereby improving the anticancer activity of the compound [6]. One of the most recent successful applications of CPPs is the development of orally active insulin with preclinical development in 2021 [7]. Penetratin also seems to be capable of delivering isoniazid into mycobacteria [8].

Different strategies were published in the literature for the conjugation of the cargo; for example, certain macromolecules could be attached in a non-covalent manner via charge-dependent complex formation with the CPP. However, small molecules were mostly bound covalently [4]. Conjugation can be formed by either the terminals of the peptide or through a side chain with the application of an appropriate functional group. A linker is frequently used in order to increase the distance between the peptide and the active ingredient or providing reversibility (capability of detachment under appropriate conditions) [9–13]. CPPs also can be the component of more complex drug delivery systems combined with polymers, dendrimers, or antibodies for targeting, especially in cancer therapy [14,15]. Homing peptides and targeting ligands are capable of combining with CPPs to improve cell specificity [16].

Several possible mechanisms of the penetration are described in the literature, with the two main types being energy-dependent or energy-independent [17,18]. The energy-dependent mechanism indicates that contribution by the cell is needed via nearly all ways of endocytosis: phagocytosis, macropinocytosis, clathrin-coated vesicles, caveola formation, and constitutive endocytosis (Figure 1A–E). Energy-independent penetrations may occur spontaneously through direct translocation, membrane thinning, pore formation, and inverted micelles (Figure 1F–J). According to the carpet model mechanism (Figure 1K), the peptides in high concentration are adsorbed on the surface of the membrane, then the lipids form toroid aggregates stabilized by the amphipathic peptides. This causes serious damage leading to cell death, unlike any other mechanisms belonging to this category [13,19]. Some peptides can penetrate and form pores even as oligomer complexes [20].

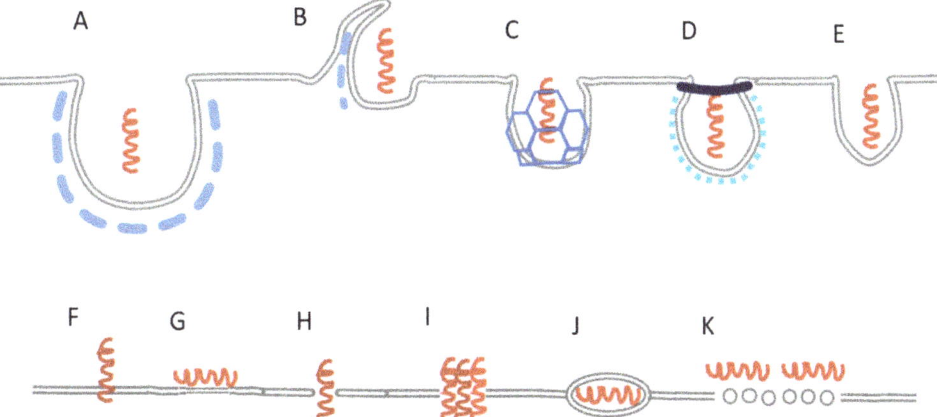

Figure 1. Active (**A–E**) and passive (**F–K**) mechanisms of the CPP penetration: (**A**) phagocytosis; (**B**) macropinocytosis; (**C**) clathrin-mediated endocytosis; (**D**) caveola; (**E**) constitutive endocytosis; (**F**) direct translocation; (**G**) membrane thinning; (**H**) toroidal pore; (**I**) barrel pore; (**J**) inverted micelle; (**K**) carpet model.

Our aim is to clarify the possible mechanisms with molecular dynamics simulations through a number of examples. The original aim was to model the internalization process, but it did not occur. Therefore, we focused on some aspects that might be involved in the penetration instead, such as the formation of intermolecular interactions, orientation, and conformational changes of the penetratin and analogues, and the influence of the conjugated small molecule on the process. In the literature, a wide range of computational chemistry techniques were used to investigate CPPs. Several attempts have been made to predict penetrating ability, including cheminformatic filters, artificial intelligence-based models, and quantitative structure–property relationships. In addition, a number of studies were aimed at the modeling of the mechanism of penetration, applying molecular dynamics [21–26].

The role of the membrane potential of living cells seems to be important in most mechanisms [27]. The correlation between CPPs and transmembrane potency may indicate that generating positive charges on the outer surface of the plasma membrane could decrease the free energy barrier associated with translocation. Additionally, it triggers pore formation [28]. It appears that the possibility, speed, and mechanism of penetration through asymmetric membranes may not be the same [29]. In the case of arginine-rich peptides, the penetrating capability may correlate with the backbone rigidity [30].

Lensink et al. carried out one of the first studies on simulating penetratin in 2005. The peptide did not translocate during the simulation utilizing Gromacs, but several interactions between the peptide and the membrane lipids were observed [31].

Herce and Garcia published an important study about MD simulations of CPPs in 2007. The HIV Tat peptide was found to translocate spontaneously, mainly via transient pores, while the positively charged side chains interacted with the phosphate groups of the membrane lipids [32]. Their next article in 2009 was about pore formation by arginine-rich peptides [33]. According to simulations and experiments, guanidium groups can lead the penetration not only in peptides, but in other similar macromolecules too [34]. The mentioned interactions between Tat and membranes were experimentally confirmed using X-ray diffraction [35,36].

In the following section, a few examples with respect to the topic of CPP penetration with MD will be addressed. The role of the membrane tension was confirmed in simulations with the coarse-grained MD method, with the finding that polyarginines in low concentrations were only adsorbed on the membrane surface, whereas translocation in higher concentration was completed in less than 100 ns [37].

In a study by Bennett in 2016, the CM15 antimicrobial peptide was shown not to translocate, but it only entered the membrane and reached its equilibrium point inside the lipid bilayer [38]. Further studies applying a similar setup makes the pore formation likely [29,39].

The direct translocation of pVEC (amphipathic CPP) was successfully simulated using the steered MD method. The penetration was led by the N-terminal amino acid of the peptide, while the cationic side chains were interacting with the phosphatide groups, enhancing the adsorption on the membrane [40]. The importance of transmembrane electric potential was also demonstrated in silico by the MARTINI coarse-grained MD and metadynamics simulations, in which the translocation of arginine-rich design peptides were successfully promoted by the introduction of the electrostatic gradient [41].

Ulmschneider, in 2017 and 2018, investigated the mechanism of antimicrobial peptides using molecular dynamics simulations [42,43]. Again, the importance of arginine was confirmed [44]. In the case of hydrophilic peptides, the computed free energy of membrane insertion does not depend on the MD method [45]. The energetic aspect of the transmembrane penetration of peptides was studied by Yao et al. in 2019 [46].

MD simulations were used to validate and prioritize the penetration of CPPs generated by artificial intelligence, and a novel CPP sequence named Pep-MD was de novo identified and then synthesized. Later, its penetration potential into living cells was demonstrated by in vitro experiments [47].

In simulations of CPPs containing unnatural amino acids, the mechanism of penetration may depend on the lipid composition of the membrane. In one study by Gimenez-Dejoz et al., the methyl groups of α-aminoisobutyric acid facilitated hydrophobic interactions inside the membrane, while side chains of lysines formed electrostatic interactions with the phosphatide groups in the outer layers. Other components of the membrane may also influence the penetration. In the same study, the addition of cholesterol into the bilayer decreased the efficiency of CPPs [48].

In some of the above-mentioned examples, coarse-grained models were used because of their cost-effectiveness in the case of limited computing capacity. However, the drastic improvement in computational capacities allowed for applying all-atom calculations instead of the simplified coarse-grained models when both explicit solvent and membrane models could be included [49]. Therefore, all-atom MD simulations have been applied in our study to investigate the CPP membrane contacts and clashes as well as their changes over time. We assume that this approach is suitable for the modeling of direct penetration, but its applicability might be limited for other energy-independent mechanisms [50,51].

In the current study, three linear and three cyclic CPPs were selected, representing two significantly different groups of CPPs. The linear ones were penetratin and its two known analogues (Table 1). Penetratin is one of the best known CPPs, and has been included in numerous studies; therefore, it is an ideal reference molecule. The two modified analogues (6,14-Phe-penetratin and Dodeca-penetratin) are lesser known, but their membrane translocation capabilities have been established in vitro. In the first analogue, the replacement of tryptophans with phenylalanines showed weaker penetration in vitro. In the dodeca analogue, in contrast, the removal of one cationic amino acid (together with three more) did not affect penetration. We intended to investigate whether these small differences would affect our simulations and learn if we would be able to differentiate between them. The three cyclic CPPs (Kalata B1, Sunflower trypsin inhibitor 1 (SFTI-1), and Momordica comhinchinensis trypsin inhibitor II (MCoTI-II)) (Table 1), although also known as CPPs, have been less examined. With the inclusion of these inhibitors, we intended to investigate whether the elimination of the charged N- and C-termini of the chain (as a result of the cyclization) and conjugation through the side chain (instead of the N-terminal) would affect the simulation. Furthermore, these peptides have various sizes, and consequently, we were able to analyze the penetration of peptides with small, medium, and large sizes.

Table 1. Amino acid sequences of the investigated peptides.

Peptide	PDB ID	Sequence	Reference
Penetratin	1KZ0	RQIKIWFQNRRMKWKK	[52]
6,14-Phe-penetratin	1KZ2	RQIKIFFQNRRMKFKK	[52]
Dodeca-penetratin	1KZ5	RQIKIWFRKWKK	[52]
Kalata B1	1NB1	[CGETCVGGTCNTPGCTCSWPVCTRNGLPV]	[53]
SFTI-1	1JBL	[GRCTKSIPPICFPD]	[54]
MCoTI-II	1HA9	[SGSDGGVCPKILKKCRRDSDCPGACICRGNGYCG]	[55]

Penetratin is a fragment of Antennapedia homeoprotein (helix III) isolated from Drosophila melanogaster and is one of the most frequently investigated CPPs. It consists of sixteen amino acids, including seven amino acids with cationic (three arginines, four lysines) and three with aromatic side chains (two triptofanes and a phenylalanine). The secondary structure of penetratin is roughly helical. However, depending on the conditions, it can be either α-helix or 3_{10}-helix (Figure 2A). Its capability of spontaneous translocation through cell membranes has been experimentally certified [56,57].

6,14-Phe-penetratin is an altered version of penetratin, in which both tryptophan units have been replaced with phenylalanines, resulting in a mostly α-helical and less flexible conformation compared to that of penetratin (Figure 2B). As a consequence, the biological activity was much lower than that of the original peptide, yet it was still a functional CPP [56,57].

Dodeca-penetratin is another modified version of penetratin, built of only 12 amino acids instead of 16 (Figure 2C). Even with this change, it has been shown to be effective because the critical cationic and aromatic residues have remained, despite its conformational instability [56].

Kalata B1 is a member of the cyclotide family isolated from the plant Oldenlandia affinis. Beyond its capability of membrane penetration, it has been characterized by high chemical and thermal stability together with pharmaceutical and insecticidal properties. Its 29 amino acids form a long cyclic backbone resulting from the formation of a peptide bond between the N- and C-terminals of the chain. This already hindered structure is further stabilized by three disulfide bonds formed within the peptide called knot motif, making it even more rigid and stable (Figure 2D) [53].

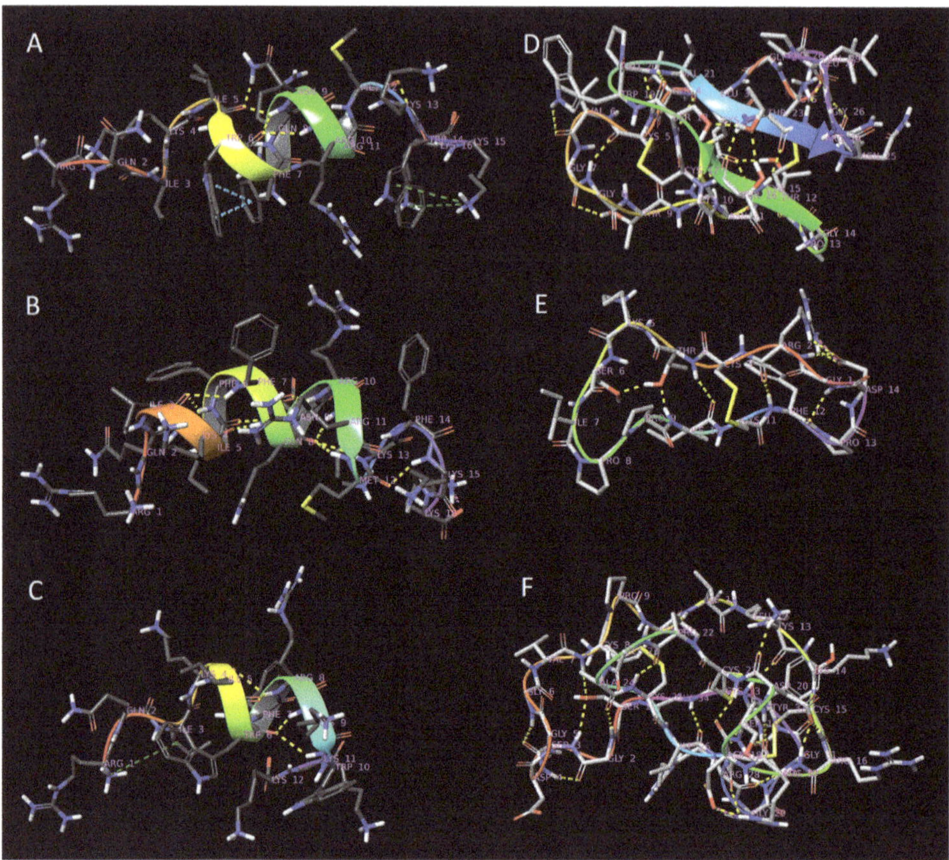

Figure 2. The 3D structures of the peptides determined by NMR from the Protein Database by the following PDB IDs: (**A**) 1KZ0—penetratin; (**B**) 1KZ2—6,14-Phe-penetratin; (**C**) 1KZ5—dodeca-penetratin; (**D**) 1NB1—Kalata B1; (**E**) 1JBL—SFTI-1; (**F**) 1HA9—MCoTI-II. Residue positions are colored from red to violet and intramolecular interactions are represented as dashed lines: hydrogen bond—yellow; π–π stacking—turquoise; π-cationic—dark green; salt bridge—purple.

SFTI-1 is another cyclic CPP of natural origin (isolated from Helianthus annuus), with the sunflower trypsin inhibitor indicating its enzymatic function. It is built of 14 amino acids, and its conformation is characterized by two anti-parallel β-strands stabilized by seven hydrogen bonding and a single disulfide bridge (Figure 2E) [54].

MCoTI-II (isolated from Momordica Cochinchinensis) is another example of a macro-cyclic knotin with a similar enzymatic function. The group it belongs to was named squash trypsin inhibitors. It is made of 34 amino acids, and its structure is stabilized by three disulfide bonds (Figure 2F) [55].

In the current study, three different types of drugs with known penetration-related difficulties were selected with different lipophylicity values (Table 2). All three were known for their peptide conjugates in the literature, but only one of these (rasagiline) was investigated before as a complex.

Doxorubicin is a topoisomerase-2 inhibitor anticancer drug. In animal tests, the peptide-conjugated form of doxorubicin has been excreted much more slowly, and, therefore, a much lower blood concentration was needed to have an equal therapeutic effect [11].

Rasagiline is a specific, irreversible MAO-B inhibitor used for the treatment of Parkinson's disease; that is, it has to get through the blood–brain barrier. It has been experimentally confirmed that the drug attached to the CPP was more effective than its unconjugated form [12,58].

Zidovudine, a reverse transcriptase inhibitor antiviral drug, has been developed to cure HIV infection. The peptide conjugation can increase its specificity towards the infected cells, thereby reducing the side effects [10].

Table 2. Partitioning of the investigated drugs.

Drug	Molar Weight (g/mol)	Experimental logP
Doxorubicin	543.52	0.32 [59]
Zidovudine	267.24	0.04 [60]
Rasagiline	171.24	2.462 [61]

Despite the high number of papers related to CPPs, no MD simulation studies of drug-conjugated CPPs have been published, and studies based on the comparison of more different peptides in conjugation with one or more small molecules are also rare.

2. Results

A complete structural rearrangement was observed with penetratin in the proximity of the surface of the POPC membrane model. At first, the helix uncoiled and ceased to exist entirely, and then slowly transformed into two-strand antiparallel β-sheets connected by a β-turn, laid to the surface of the membrane. The analysis of the last frame of the trajectory also revealed that four salt bridges and eleven hydrogen bonds were formed between the peptide and the membrane molecules, whereas no π-cation interactions were observed (see Figures 3A, 4 and 5 and summaries in numbers in Table 3 Entry 1). Both 6,14-Phe-penetratin and dodeca-penetratin preserved their helical structure until the end of the simulations, with their N-terminal partially sinking into the POPC membrane. The axis of the 6,14-Phe-penetratin closed at about a 60° angle with the plane of the membrane, while dodeca-penetratin was almost perpendicular (Figures 3B,C, 4 and 5). Despite the limited area of contact (compared to those of the penetration), 6,14-Phe-penetratin formed five salt bridges, seven hydrogen bonds, and a single π-cation interaction with membrane molecules (Table 3 Entry 5). Dodeca-penetratin connected even more loosely to the membrane surface with only one salt bridge and six hydrogen bonds (Table 3 Entry 9).

During 1000 ns simulations, the cargo molecules significantly affected the position of the conjugate relative to the membrane, and in the case of penetratin, they affected the conformation of the peptide as well. In contrast to native penetratin peptide, the unfolding mentioned above was not observed in the conjugated ones. In the case of the penetratin analogues, the helical structure remained intact similar to their unconjugated counterparts. We also observed that, unlike the unsubstituted penetratin and analogues, not all conjugated peptides positioned with their terminal towards the membrane with their longer axis perpendicular or at a closing angle, and they partially sank into the membrane. The three non-cyclic doxorubicin conjugates positioned differently. Penetratin-doxorubicin was one of the two conjugates that moved away from the membrane without forming any interaction (Figures 6A and 7; see the supplement for interaction diagrams that are not included in the text). The 6,14-Phe-penetratin-conjugate anchored to the membrane through its N-terminal with the doxorubicin tightly bound on the surface with three salt bridges and eight hydrogen bonds (Figure 6B, Table 3 Entry 6). The dodeca-penetratin conjugate anchored to the surface of the membrane with its C-terminal through a number of interactions with doxorubicin orientated into the opposing direction towards the water box (Figure 6C, Table 3 Entry 10). The rasagiline-conjugated penetratin and analogues always positioned with their N-terminals toward the membrane with the cargo compound sank into the bilayer. Their positions were stabilized by the formation of several hydrogen bonds and a few salt bridges between the peptide and membrane molecules (Figure 6D–F;

Table 3 Entries 3, 7, 10). The simulations with the zidovudine-linear peptide conjugates showed, among the three drugs, that this compound seemed to be the least likely to penetrate, and its conjugates had significantly less interaction with the membrane. The native penetratin zidovudine conjugate was positioned with its C-terminal towards the membrane connected with only a single hydrogen bond and the N-terminal with the cargo pointing towards the opposite direction (Figure 6G, Table 3 Entry 4). The 6,14-Phe-penetratin-zidovudine was the other example with the conjugate entirely moving away from the membrane without any possible bond formation (Figure 6H, Table 3 Entry 8). Only the dodeca-penetratin-zidovudine conjugate turned with its N-terminal towards the membrane with the formation of two salt bridges, with the cargo wedged between the peptide and the membrane (Figure 6I, Table 3 Entry 12).

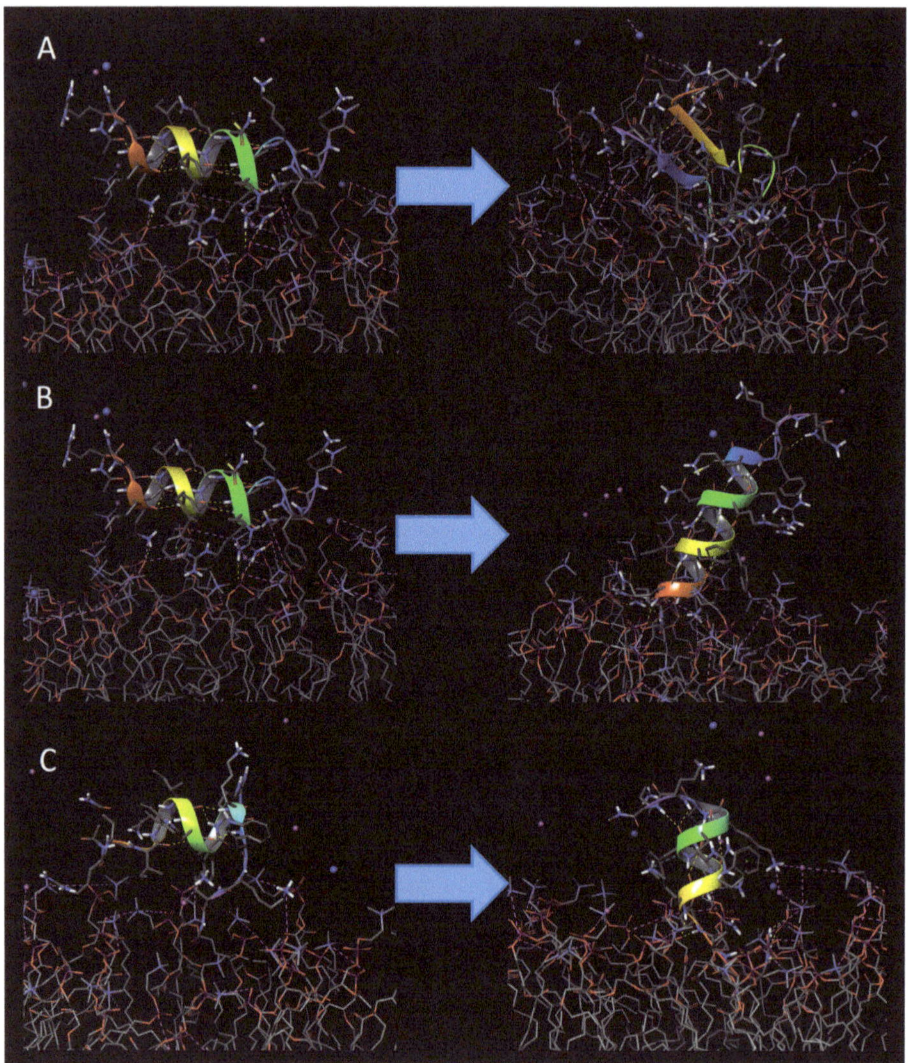

Figure 3. Comparison of the initial (**left**) and final (**right**) positions of unconjugated CCPs during the 1000 ns membrane simulations: (**A**) penetratin with POPC; (**B**) 6,14-Phe-penetratin with POPC; (**C**) dodeca-penetratin with POPC—all peptides starting from the surface of bilayer.

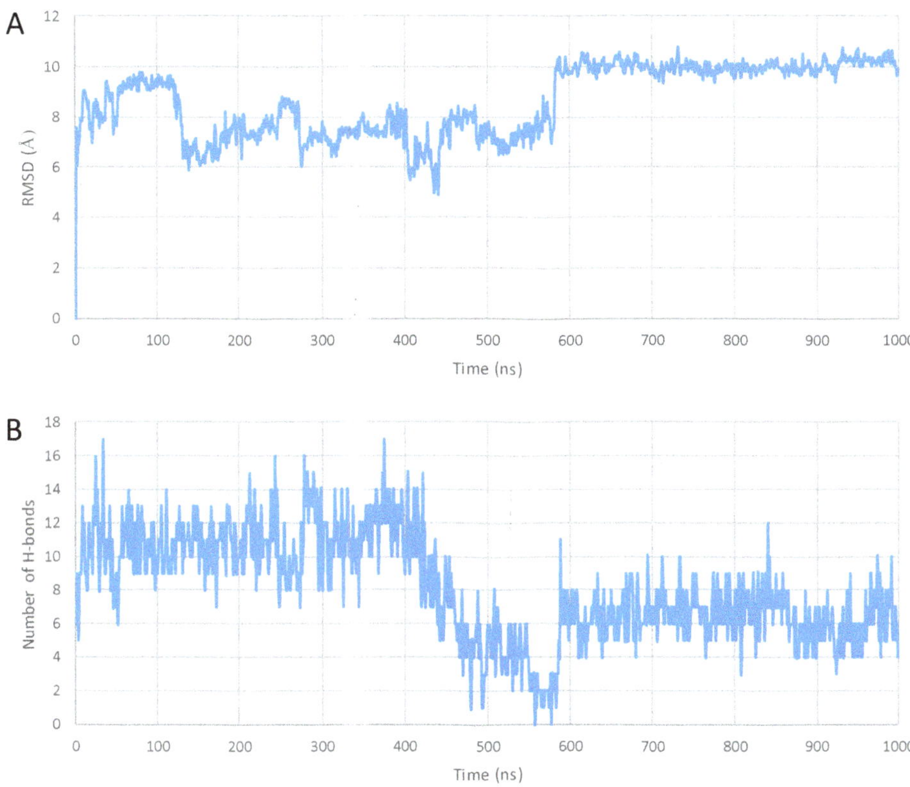

Figure 4. (**A**) RMSD diagram of the α-carbon atoms of the unconjugated penetratin peptide; (**B**) the total number of intramolecular hydrogen bonds plotted against simulation time during the 1000 ns MD simulation—starting from the top of the membrane bilayer.

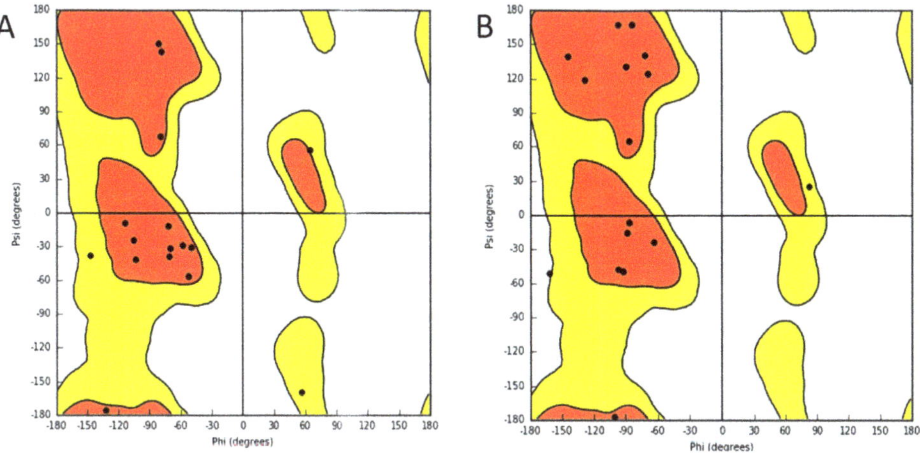

Figure 5. Comparison of the Ramachandran plots of the unconjugated penetratin peptide (**A**) at the beginning; (**B**) at the end of the 1000 ns simulation with the POPC membrane model—starting from the top of the membrane bilayer.

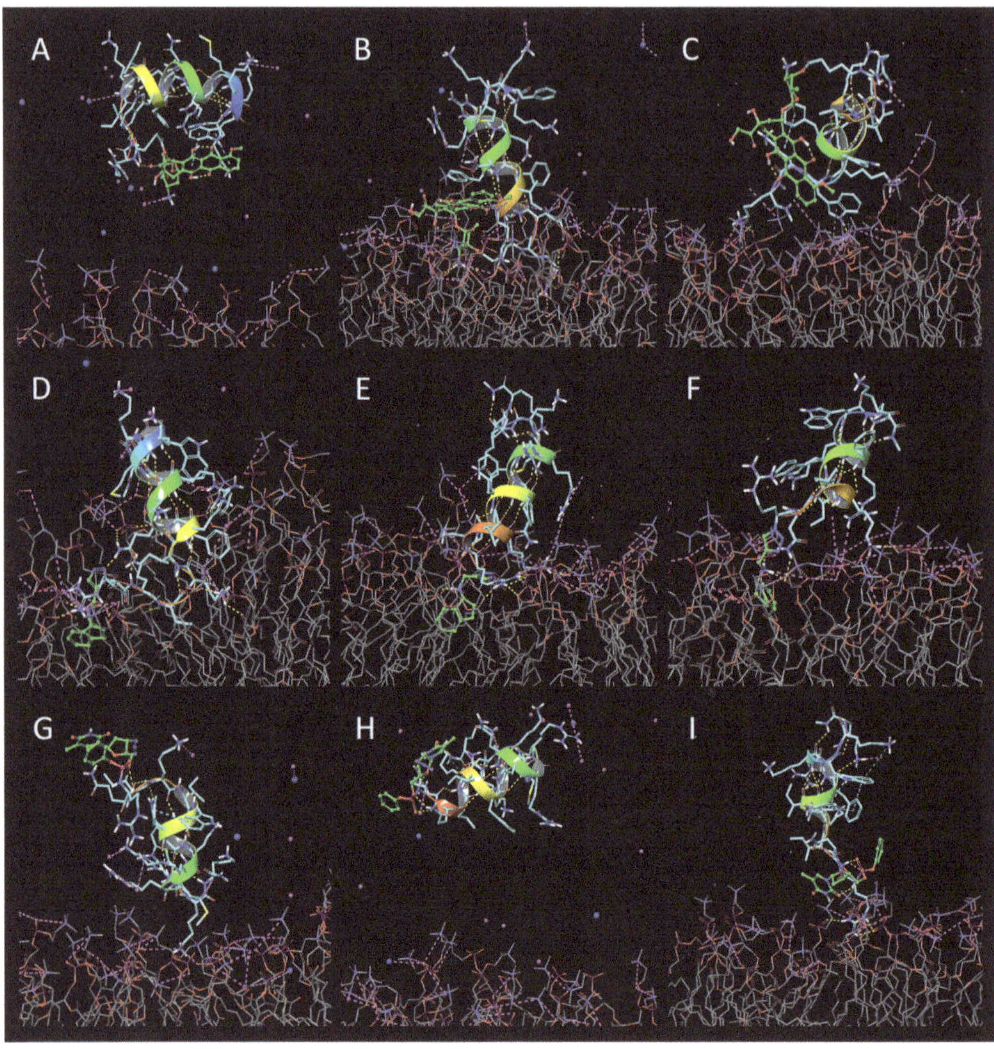

Figure 6. The final positions of the 1000 ns POPC membrane simulations with different CCP-conjugates: (**A**) penetratin–doxorubicin, (**B**) 6,14-Phe-penetratin–doxorubicin, (**C**) dodeca-penetratin–doxorubicin, (**D**) penetratin–rasagiline, (**E**) 6,14-Phe-penetratin–rasagiline, (**F**) dodeca-penetratin–rasagiline, (**G**) penetratin–zidovudine, (**H**) 6,14-Phe-penetratin–zidovudine, (**I**) dodeca-penetratin–zidovudine—all conjugates were started from the top of the membrane bilayer.

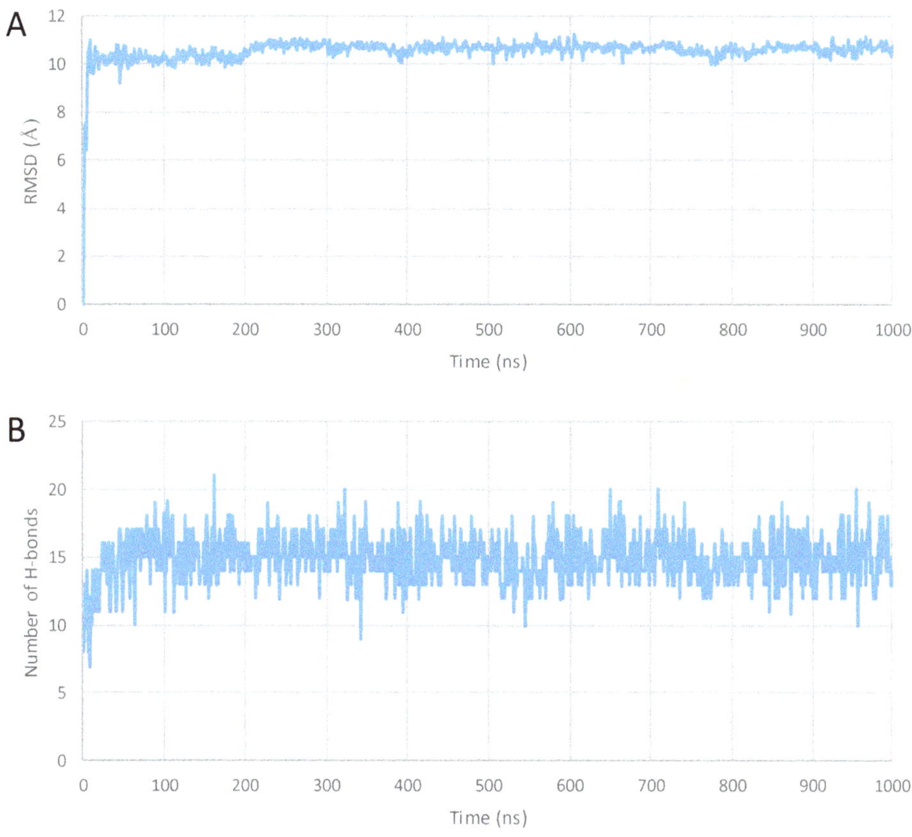

Figure 7. (**A**) The Root Mean Square Deviation (RMSD) diagram of the α-carbon atoms of the peptide; (**B**) the total number of intramolecular hydrogen bonds plotted against simulation time during the 1000 ns MD simulation of penetratin–doxorubicin conjugate—starting from the top of the membrane bilayer.

The structure of the unconjugated cyclic peptides did not show any significant change during the 1000 ns simulations (Figure 8). In the course of the runs, they all positioned toward the membrane and then tightly adhered to its surface with minimal sinking into the bilayer. Unlike penetratin, these cyclic peptides—with the exception of MCoTI-II—have only a few amino acids with polar side chains, which limits their capability to form ionic interactions. A high number of mostly uncharged hydrogen bonds were observed, where the peptide heteroatoms were the donors and the heteroatoms of the membrane were the acceptors. The lack of aromatic side chains also excluded the formation of π-cation interactions with the positively charged choline groups of the POPC membrane. The overall impact of conjugation in the case of the cyclic CPPs was much less significant than those of penetratin and its analogues. At the end of the simulation, the cyclic peptides had fewer interactions with the membrane compared to penetratin and its analogues. A possible explanation is that penetratins were mostly positioned outside the membrane where the polar phosphorous groups were available to form H-bonds and salt bridges. In contrast, the cyclic peptides sank into the hydrophobic interior of the membrane more deeply, further away from the polar surface. However, there were some exceptions, such as MCoTI-II-doxorubicin and MCoTI-II-zidovudine conjugates, both with a significant number of hydrogen bonds and salt bridges (Figure 9, Table 3 Entries 22 and 24).

At the end of the 1000 ns simulations, the positions of all cyclic conjugates compared to the POPC membrane model were very similar to their unconjugated forms, indicating that their capability for adherence was less hindered. All three cyclic doxorubicin conjugates sank into the membrane with the cargo positioned inside the medium. In the case of the SFTI-1-doxorubicin-conjugate, both the peptide and the cargo part positioned close to one surface (Figure 9D), while in the case of MCoTI-II- and Kalata-B1-doxorubicin-conjugates, the peptide parts were located in the proximity of one membrane surface while the cargos were translocated towards the opposing surface (Figure 9E,F). In the case of the rasagiline conjugates, all three peptides sank into the membrane, but the position of the cargo was very different. With SFTI-1, the rasagiline positioned close to the surface (Figure 9G); with Kalata B1, the rasagiline moved towards the center of the bilayer (Figure 9H); and when it was conjugated with MCoTI-II, it was closer to the opposite surface (Figure 9I). Similarly, the peptide part of all three zidovudine conjugates also sank deeply into the bilayer, and with both SFTI-1 and Kalata-B1, the cargo remained in the relative vicinity of the surface (Figure 9J,K). However, when conjugated with MCoTI-II, it positioned towards the direction of the opposing surface (Figure 9L). It is also important to point out that the simulation with MCoTI-II-zidovudine was the only example where a significant distortion of the membrane was observed, although neither full penetration nor perforation took place.

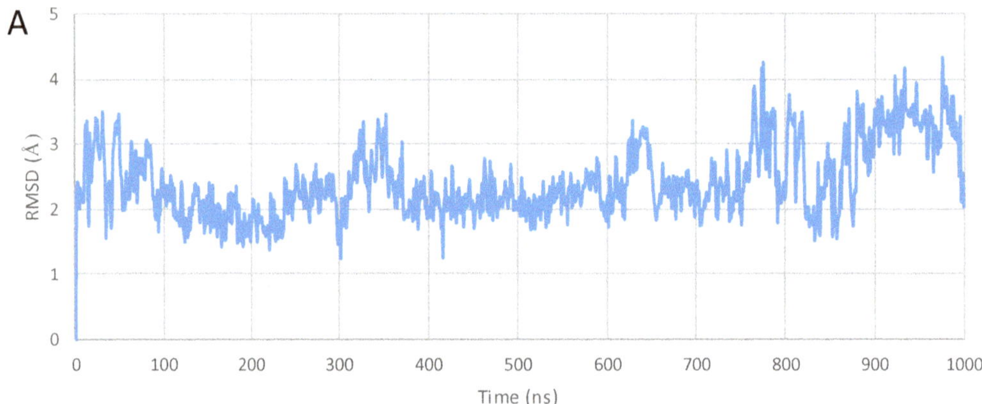

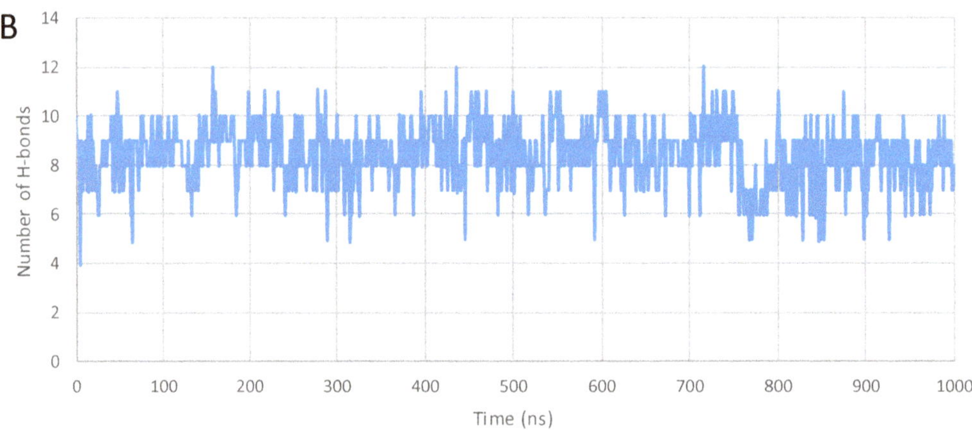

Figure 8. (**A**) The Root Mean Square Deviation (RMSD) diagram of the α-carbon atoms of the peptides; (**B**) the total number of intramolecular hydrogen bonds plotted against simulation time during the 1000 ns MD run of the unconjugated SFTI-1 peptide—starting from the top of the membrane bilayer.

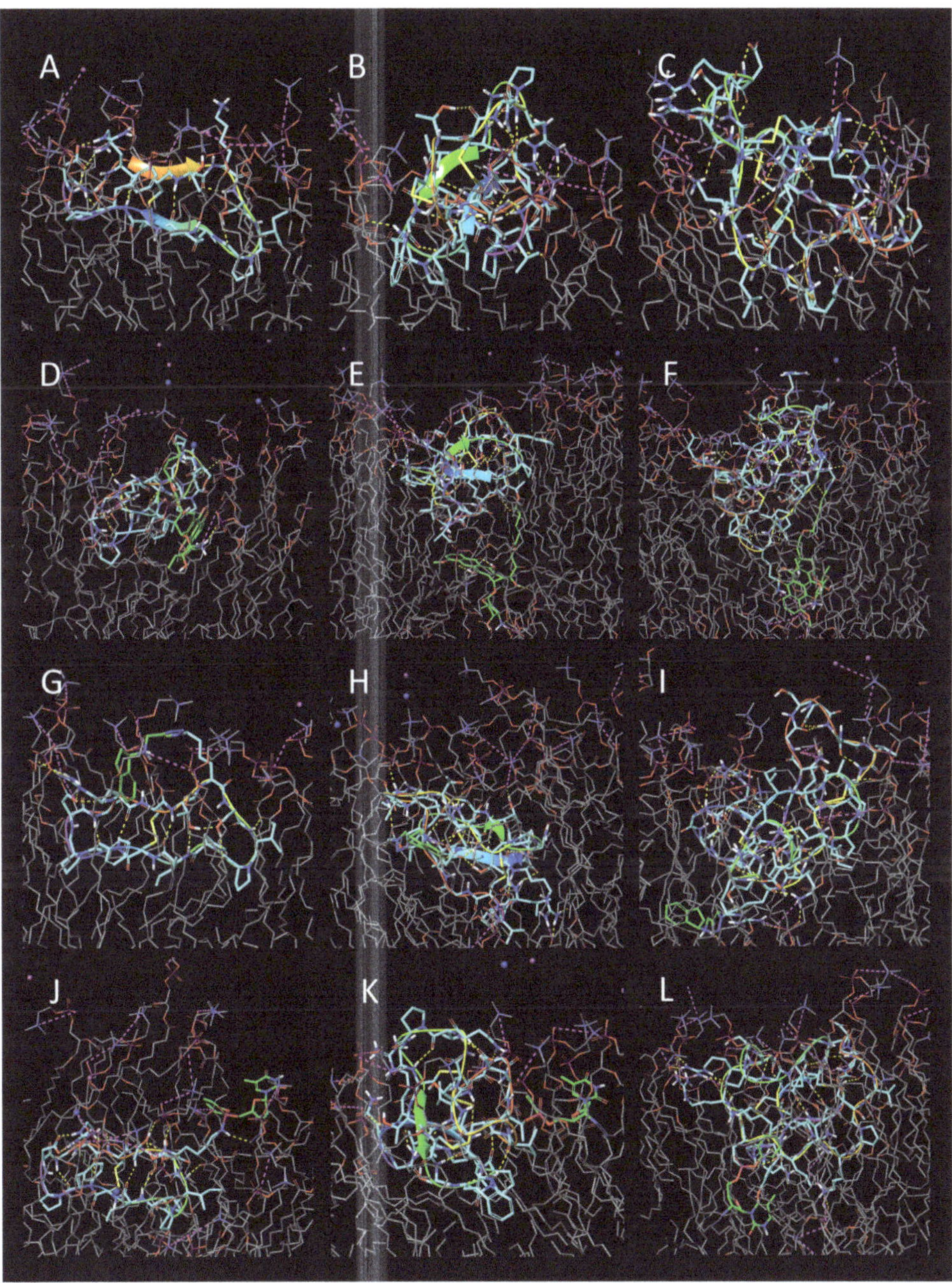

Figure 9. The final positions of the 1000 ns POPC membrane simulations with cyclic CCPs and their conjugates: (**A**) unconjugated SFTI-1, (**B**) unconjugated Kalata B1, (**C**) unconjugated MCoTI-II, (**D**) SFTI-1-doxorubicin, (**E**) Kalata B1-doxorubicin, (**F**) MCoTI-II-doxorubicin, (**G**) SFTI-1-rasagiline, (**H**) Kalata B1-rasagiline, (**I**) MCoTI-II-rasagiline, (**J**) SFTI-1-zidovudine, (**K**) Kalata B1-zidovudine, (**L**) MCoTI-II-zidovudine—all conjugates were started from the top of the membrane bilayer.

Table 3. The number of observed interactions between the peptides/conjugates and the POPC membrane molecules at the end of the 1000 ns simulations.

Entry	Peptide	Conjugate	H-Bond	π-Cation	Salt Bridge
1	penetratin (1KZ0)	unconjugated	11	0	4
2	penetratin (1KZ0)	doxorubicin	0	0	0
3	penetratin (1KZ0)	rasagiline	12	1	7
4	penetratin (1KZ0)	zidovudine	1	0	2
5	6,14-Phe-penetratin (1KZ2)	unconjugated	7	1	5
6	6,14-Phe-penetratin (1KZ2)	doxorubicin	8	0	3
7	6,14-Phe-penetratin (1KZ2)	rasagiline	10	0	4
8	6,14-Phe-penetratin (1KZ2)	zidovudine	0	0	0
9	dodeca-penetratin (1KZ5)	unconjugated	6	0	1
10	dodeca-penetratin (1KZ5)	doxorubicin	2	1	3
11	dodeca-penetratin (1KZ5)	rasagiline	5	0	4
12	dodeca-penetratin (1KZ5)	zidovudine	4	0	2
13	SFTI-1 (1NB1)	unconjugated	0	0	0
14	SFTI-1 (1NB1)	doxorubicin	10	0	2
15	SFTI-1 (1NB1)	rasagiline	6	0	2
16	SFTI-1 (1NB1)	zidovudine	2	0	2
17	Kalata B1 (1JBL)	unconjugated	2	0	0
18	Kalata B1 (1JBL)	doxorubicin	6	0	3
19	Kalata B1 (1JBL)	rasagiline	4	0	3
20	Kalata B1 (1JBL)	zidovudine	3	0	1
21	MCoTI-II (1HA9)	unconjugated	0	0	0
22	MCoTI-II (1HA9)	doxorubicin	8	0	11
23	MCoTI-II (1HA9)	rasagiline	6	0	8
24	MCoTI-II (1HA9)	zidovudine	16	0	6

3. Discussion

The original aim of this study was to simulate the penetration of the CPPs and conjugates throughout the POPC membrane bilayer.

A complete membrane penetration was not observed in 1000 ns for any of the molecules investigated. Only penetratin showed a significant structural rearrangement during the simulation, as the mostly helical structure uncoiled and a double-stranded β-sheet-like structure connected with a turn was formed. During the process, the peptide tightly adhered to the surface of the membrane with the formation of a number of hydrogen bonds and salt bridges. Ionic interactions were observed between the positively charged arginine side chains of the cationic peptides and the negatively charged head groups of the membrane phospholipids. Phe-modified penetratin and dodeca-penetratin derivative showed different behavior as they maintained their original helical structures. Instead of laying on the membrane, both peptides sank partially into it, with their N-terminal of the helix partially merging into the lipid bilayer, while the greater portion of the peptides remained above the membrane. Fewer H-bonds and salt bridges were formed compared to penetratin, but some additional π-cationic interactions were also observed.

The three cyclic peptides behaved in a completely different manner: they extruded the water between themselves and the membrane, and they were more tightly fitted to the lipid bilayer forming direct interactions. The attachment of the peptide to the membrane can be explained by entropic reasons, with water exclusion as the main cause.

In general, the conjugated molecules did not interact with the CPPs during the simulation. However, the conjugation of the drug molecule, in some cases, influenced interacting behavior between the membrane and the molecules.

Doxorubicin is an amphiphilic molecule possessing a hydrophobic anthraquinone ring substituted with a hydrophilic aminosugar derivative. When doxorubicin was attached to penetratin, the conjugate diverged from the membrane. In contrast, the Phe-derivative–doxorubicin conjugate behaved in a different way. Namely, the N-terminus equipped with the conjugate merged slightly into the membrane. The dodeca-penetratin derivative–doxorubicin conjugate merged slightly into the membrane with its C-terminal. The hydrophylic part of the molecule can form hydrogen bonds with phospholipids. These facts suggest that the amphipathic nature of doxorubicin influences the behavior of the conjugate.

The next drug investigated was zidovudine, which is a more hydrophilic molecule in comparison to doxorubicin. When it was attached to penetratins, no interaction was found between the two parts of the conjugates. The C-terminal of the penetratin conjugate slightly merged into the membrane, while the N-terminal with the zidovudine remained in the water. In the case of the Phe-derivative–zidovudine conjugate, the assembly diverged from the membrane and persisted between water molecules. In the case of the 12 AA-long dodeca-penetratin derivative conjugate, in turn, the N-terminus slightly merged into the membrane. The phosphate group of the zidovdine was able to form a salt bridge to the choline part of a POPC molecule.

Rasagiline, a hydrophobic compound, was also tested, and it conjugated to penetratins. All three compounds behaved in the same way, with the peptidic part retaining its helical conformation and merging slightly into the membrane with their N-terminal part. However, the rasagiline part merged deeply into the bilayer because of its highly nonpolar nature. The aromatic ring can form a π-cation interaction with the choline part of lecithine.

For the cyclic CPPs, the polarity of the small organic molecule had a dominant influence with respect to the behavior of the conjugate. In all cases, the peptide part was attached to the membrane, and water was extruded. Doxorubicin, as a conjugate, slightly merged into the membrane and formed a hydrogen bond, with the head part of the lipid oxygen atom bound to the phosphorous atom. Zidovudine diverged from the membrane because of its hydrophilic nature and formed hydrogen bonds with water molecules. The most hydrophobic rasagiline deeply merged into the membrane as long as its linker allowed.

4. Methods

4.1. Preparation of Peptides and Conjugates

The graphical user interface (GUI) Schrödinger molecular modeling package Maestro was used in the process of this study (Schrödinger Release 2022-3: Maestro, Schrödinger, LLC, New York, NY, USA, 2022). The peptide structures were downloaded from Research Collaboratory for Structural Bioinformatics Protein Database (RCSB PDB, http://rcsb.org accessed on 16 June 2023) based on the identifying code (PDB ID); see Table 1 [62]. All entries were derived from NMR spectroscopy, with multiple structures always working with the first member of the ensemble. Each structure was prepared using Schrödinger Protein Preparation Wizard, and the preprocess option was used to cap the termini of the linear peptides (the N-terminal was acetylated, and the C-terminal was transformed into an N-methyl-amide group) [63]. (Schrödinger Release 2022-3: Protein Preparation Wizard; Epik, Schrödinger, LLC, New York, NY, USA, 2022; Impact, Schrödinger, LLC, New York, NY, USA; Prime, Schrödinger, LLC, New York, NY, USA, 2022).

Drug molecules were drawn by the sketcher of the Maestro GUI, and they were minimized using the LigPrep module (Schrödinger Release 2022-3: LigPrep, Schrödinger, LLC, New York, NY, USA, 2022). The conjugates were made by merging the optimized small-molecule and selected peptide structures, and the linkers were added using the 3D Builder application within the interface: a glutaryl group for doxorubicin, a triazole ring for rasagiline, and phosphoric amide for zidovudine as indicated in the literature. In the case of the three linear peptides, the conjugations were formed through their N-terminal, while an appropriate amino acid side chain was utilized in the case of the cyclic peptides (Lys5 for SFTI-1, Lys14 for MCoTI-II, and Thr4 for Kalata B1; Table 4) [10–12]. That is, the simulations included the three unconjugated peptides together with all possible combinations of the three drugs and the six peptides, resulting in the building of 24 different peptides and conjugates.

Table 4. Schematic representation of conjugates investigated.

	Doxorubicin	Rasagiline	Zidovudine
penetratin and analogues	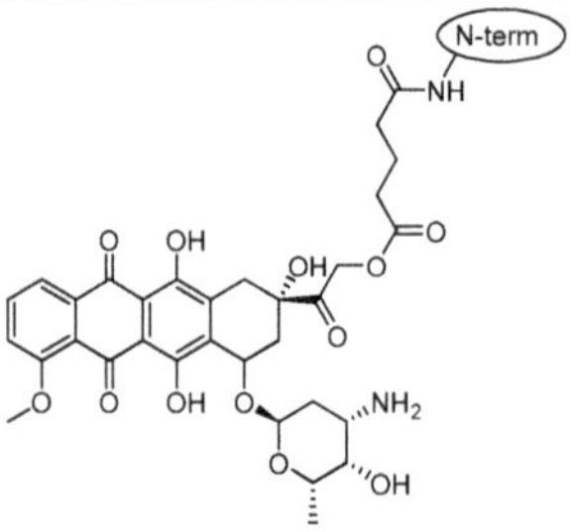 N-term	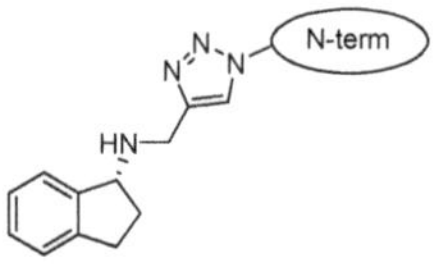 N-term	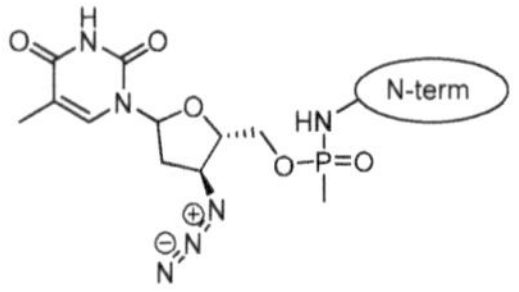 N-term
Kalata B1	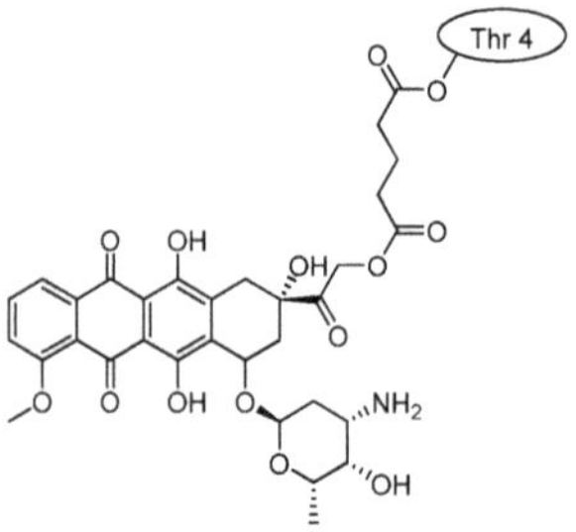 Thr 4	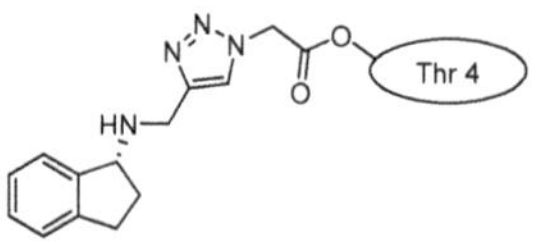 Thr 4	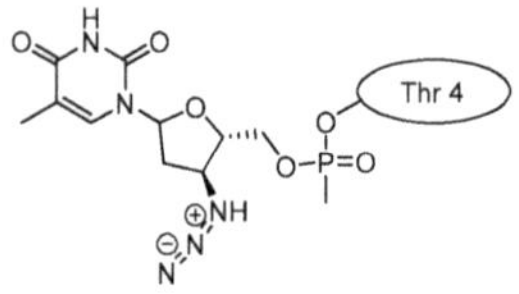 Thr 4
SFTI-1	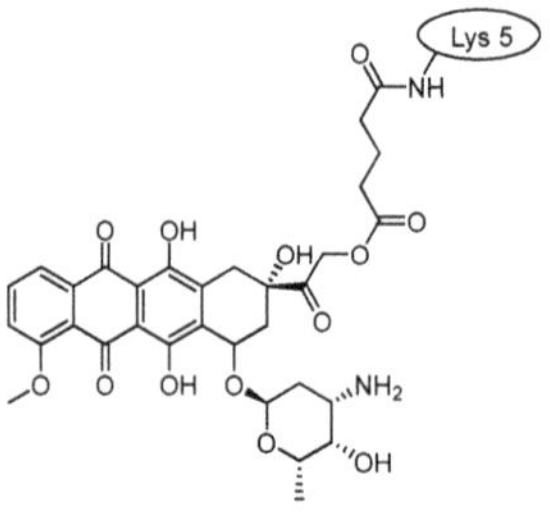 Lys 5	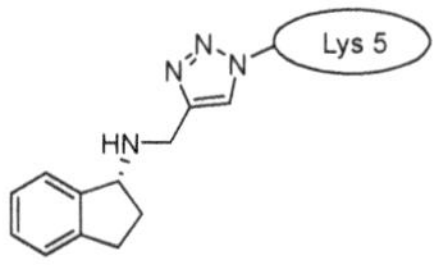 Lys 5	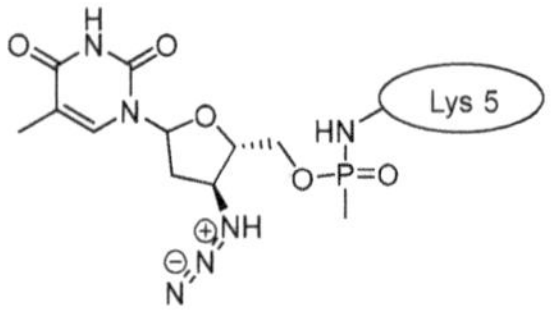 Lys 5
MCoTI-II	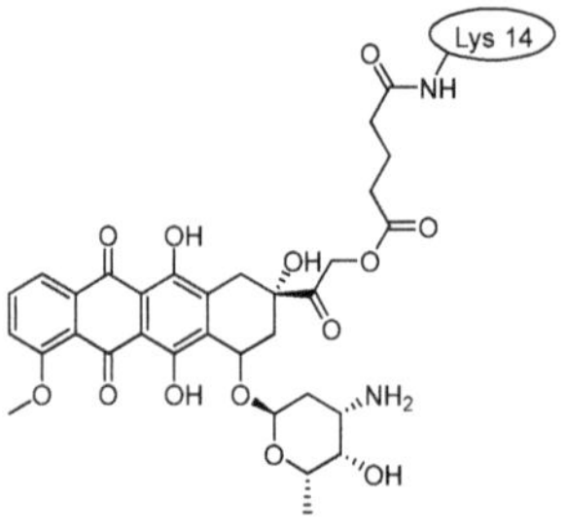 Lys 14	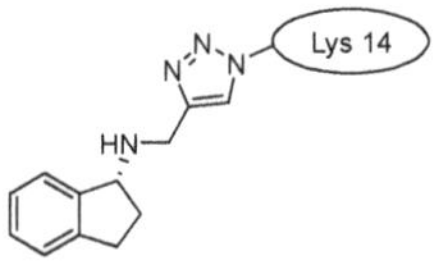 Lys 14	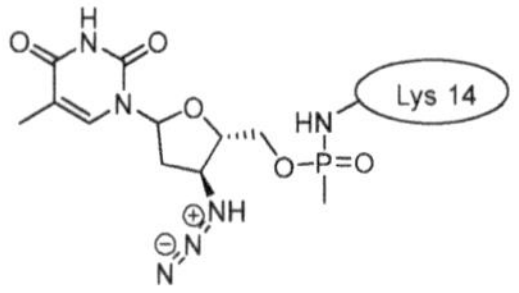 Lys 14

4.2. Setup and Building of the Systems

All MD simulations in this study were completed with the Desmond Molecular Dynamic software under Schrödinger (Schrödinger Release 2022-3: Desmond Molecular Dynamics System, D. E. Shaw Research, New York, NY, USA, 2022. Maestro–Desmond Interoperability Tools, Schrödinger, New York, NY, USA, 2022). Setups for the runs were assembled with Desmond System Builder application under Maestro. All simulations were run within an orthorhombic box full of explicit water molecules generated by the single-point charge (SPC) model [46]. This enclosed a unimolecular membrane bilayer made of palmitoyl-oleoyl-phosphatidylcholine (POPC) compounds added automatically. The peptides and conjugates were manually placed on the top of the membrane at a distance of approximately 10 Å from its surface. The size of the membrane was calculated by the software using the buffer method, with a medium spread of 10 Å in every direction from the peptide or conjugate [64]. The assembling was continued with water boxes on both the top and bottom of the membrane, also according to the buffer. The assembly was then completed with sodium and chloride ions to statistically reach the isotonic (0.15 M) concentration, and additional counter ions were added if needed in order to neutralize the charge of the peptide or conjugate so the net charge of the system was reduced to zero. Prior to the MD simulations, the assemblies were minimized with OPLS3e (optimized potential for liquid simulations) force field method for the final positioning of the molecules to avoid steric clashes. The OPLS-AA is an all-atom force field parameter for both proteins and many general classes of organic molecules; therefore, no further parametrization for the drug molecules is necessary [65–67]. According to the literature, this system is suitable for modeling peptides in the presence of POPC membrane [68].

All 24 peptides and peptide conjugates mentioned above were placed into the simulation box with POPC membrane; that is, altogether, 24 systems were included in the study.

4.3. MD Simulations

The completed setups were then loaded into Desmond's Molecular Dynamics interface, and simulations for 1000 ns runs were initialized [67]. All MD simulations began with the standard relaxation protocol, which also included equilibration utilizing the default settings: starting with 12 ps-long NVT (constant substance, volume, and temperature) ensemble simulation at 10 K temperature; followed by two 12 ps-long NPT (constant substance, temperature, and pressure) ensemble simulation at 10 K temperature and 1.01325 bar pressure; and, finally, a 24 ps-long NPT ensemble simulation at 300 K temperature and 1.01325 bar pressure [50].

Following the relaxation, all MD simulations were always carried out with NPT settings, where the pressure was 1.01325 bar, and the temperature was 300 K [69]. Additionally, the recording interval of the trajectory was set to 1000 ps (therefore, each trajectory contained 1000 frames).

Simulations were completed on hardware with nVidia® GeForce GTX 1070 Ti 1683 MHz x2432 graphics processing unit (GPU) under Linux Ubuntu. The 1000 ns simulations took a maximum of 70–80 h.

4.4. Analyzing the Structures

The Structure Analysis application of the Schrödinger was used to evaluate the trajectories (Schrödinger Release 2022-3: Prime, Schrödinger, LLC, New York, NY, USA, 2022). The most critical piece of data is the root mean square deviation (RMSD) of the alpha carbon atoms depending on the running time. All RMSD values were calculated compared to the 0 ns geometry of the trajectories (after relaxation/equilibration). If the RMSD does not change, the conformation is stable. In contrast, if the RMSD increases or decreases, the atoms are moving, and the system is not in equilibrium [70–72].

The evaluation also included monitoring the change of the number of intramolecular hydrogen bonds within the peptides over time, which correlates with the changes of the secondary structure. Fewer intramolecular hydrogen bonds may be indicative of irregular, less stable conformations, while a higher number usually means a more organized and energetically more stable folded structure.

The comparison of the Ramachandran plots of the peptides at different times of the simulation can also show structural differences. In the case of minor conformational movements during simulation, the Φ and Ψ dihedrals were quite similar at the initial and final frames. However, where significant changes were observed in the Φ and Ψ dihedrals on the Ramachandran plot, the coordinates of the dominant conformations changed.

Because of the limitations of the software, we were unable to track all interactions between the peptides, small molecules, and the membrane over the course of the simulations.

Therefore, we counted the hydrogen bonds, salt bridges, and π-cation interactions marked by the graphical interface manually in the final frame (at 1000 ns) within each trajectory. The entire modeling process has been summarized on a working flowchart (see Figure 10).

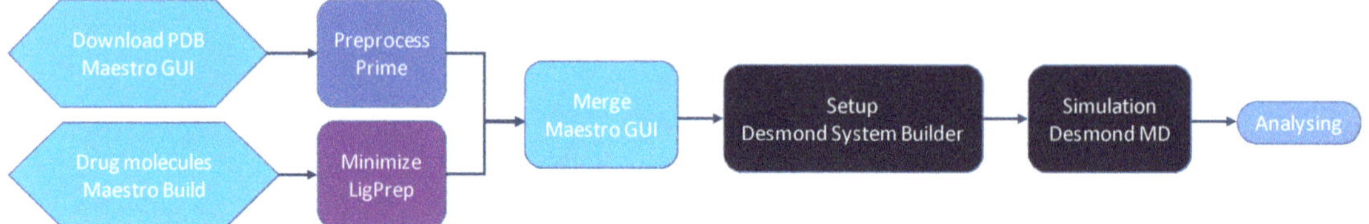

Figure 10. Schematic chart of the workflow.

5. Conclusions

In this study, we examined the behavior of CPPs with covalently conjugated drug molecules using all-atom MD simulations. Although a complete membrane penetration was not achieved, some interesting conformational and positional changes were observed during the 1000 ns simulation time.

We found that only the unconjugated penetratin underwent some major conformational rearrangement, while less flexible 6,14-Phe-penetratin and dodeca-penetratin retained their mostly helical structure. Penetratin and analogues thereof were more affected by the polarity of the conjugated small molecule. Namely, the hydrophilic zidovudine seemingly inhibited the interaction between the peptide and the membrane, the more hydrophobic rasagiline guided the entire conjugate in between the membrane bilayer, and the amphiphilic doxorubicin induced variable degrees of penetration for each peptide.

The three cyclic peptides (SFTI-1, Kalata B1, and MCoTI-II) behaved in a similar manner during the simulations. Due to their high structural stability, only minimal conformational changes were observed, and their position compared to the surface of the lipid bilayer was altered less. The influence of the conjugates for the penetration also seemed to be less significant, but the conjugated small molecules were oriented according to their polarity.

The lack of direct penetration might be the result of the relative simplicity of the model. Although we used all-atom MD, a simple monomolecular membrane model was applied, and neither the possible membrane components nor the membrane potential could be implemented properly. Our system contained only a single CPP peptide and, therefore, more complex multi-molecular mechanisms, such as complexation with other proteins or pore formation, could not be examined.

It is our sincere hope that we will be able to build a much larger simulation box, including more than just a single peptide in a sufficiently high concentration, and that, consequently, spontaneous penetration may be observed.

Supplementary Materials: The following supporting information can be downloaded at: https://www.mdpi.com/article/10.3390/ph16091251/s1, comprehensive list of the simulations, further rearrangement figures, RMSD and Ramachandran plots are added. Table S1. Comprehensive list of the simulations. All of the simulation boxes contained POPC membrane model, the peptide conjugates were placed in the water box above the membrane in parallel position. The simulation time always was 1000 ns and the temperature was 300 K. Figure S1. The arrangement of the MD simulation systems: starting from the top of the phosphatidylcholine (POPC) membrane bilayer. Figure S2. The 1000-ns MD simulation of the unconjugated penetratin (PDB ID: 1KZ0) in the POPC membrane model: the RMSD of α the carbon atoms plotted against the simulation time (a), the number of hydrogen bonds within the peptide plotted against the simulation time (b), the Ramachandran plot of the peptide at 0 ns (c) and at 1000 ns (d) starting from the top of the membrane. Figure S3. The 1000-ns MD simulation of the unconjugated 6,14-Phe-penetratin (PDB ID: 1KZ2) in the POPC membrane model: the RMSD of the α-carbon atoms plotted against the simulation time (a), the number of hydrogen bonds within the peptide plotted against the simulation time (b), the Ramachandran plot of the peptide at 0 ns (c) and at 1000 ns (d) starting from the top of the membrane. Figure S4. The 1000-ns MD simulation of the unconjugated dodeca-penetratin (PDB ID: 1KZ5) in the POPC membrane model: the RMSD of the α-carbon atoms plotted against the simulation time (a), the number of hydrogen bonds within the peptide plotted against the simulation time (b), the Ramachandran plot of the peptide at 0 ns (c) and at 1000 ns (d) starting from the top of the membrane. Figure S5. The 1000-ns MD simulation of the penetratin–doxorubicin conjugate in the POPC membrane model: the RMSD of the α-carbon atoms plotted against the simulation time (a), the number of hydrogen bonds within the peptide plotted against the simulation time (b), the Ramachandran plot of the peptide at 0 ns (c) and at 1000 ns (d) starting from the top of the membrane. Figure S6. The 1000-ns MD simulation of the of 6,14-Phe-penetratin–doxorubicin conjugate in the POPC membrane model: the RMSD of the α-carbon atoms plotted against the simulation time (a), the number of hydrogen bonds within the peptide plotted against the simulation time (b), the Ramachandran plot of the peptide at 0 ns (c) and at 1000 ns (d) starting from the top of the membrane. Figure S7. The 1000-ns MD simulation of the of dodeca-penetratin–doxorubicin conjugate in the POPC membrane model: the RMSD of the α-carbon atoms plotted against the simulation time (a), the number of hydrogen bonds within the peptide plotted against the simulation time (b), the Ramachandran plot of the peptide at 0 ns (c) and at 1000 ns (d) starting from the top of the membrane. Figure S8. The 1000 ns MD simulation of the penetratin–rasagiline conjugate in the POPC membrane model: the RMSD of the α-carbon atoms plotted against the simulation time (a), the number of hydrogen bonds within the peptide plotted against the simulation time (b), the Ramachandran plot of the peptide at 0 ns (c) and at 1000 ns (d) starting from the top of the membrane. Figure S9. The 1000-ns MD simulation of the of 6,14-Phe-penetratin–rasagiline conjugate in the POPC membrane model: the RMSD of the α-carbon atoms plotted against the simulation time (a), the number of hydrogen bonds within the peptide plotted against the simulation time (b), the Ramachandran plot of the peptide at 0 ns (c) and at 1000 ns (d) starting from the top of the membrane. Figure S10. The 1000-ns MD simulation of the of the dodeca-penetratin–rasagiline conjugate in the POPC membrane model: the RMSD of α the carbon atoms plotted against the simulation time (a), the number of hydrogen bonds within the peptide plotted against the simulation time (b), the Ramachandran plot of the peptide at 0 ns (c) and at 1000 ns (d) starting from the top of the membrane. Figure S11. The 1000-ns MD simulation of the penetratin–zidovudine conjugate in the POPC membrane model: the RMSD of the α-carbon atoms plotted against the simulation time (a), the number of hydrogen bonds within the peptide plotted against the simulation time (b), the Ramachandran plot of the peptide at 0 ns (c) and at 1000 ns (d) starting from the top of the membrane. Figure S12. The 1000-ns MD simulation of the 6,14-Phe-penetratin–zidovudine conjugate in the POPC membrane model: the RMSD of α the carbon atoms plotted against the simulation time (a), the number of hydrogen bonds within the peptide plotted against the simulation time (b), the Ramachandran plot of the peptide at 0 ns (c) and at 1000 ns (d) starting from the top of the membrane. Figure S13. The 1000-ns MD simulation of the dodeca-penetratin–zidovudine conjugate in the POPC membrane model: the RMSD of α the carbon atoms plotted against the simulation time (a), the number of hydrogen bonds within the peptide plotted against the simulation time (b), the Ramachandran plot of the peptide at 0 ns (c) and at 1000 ns (d) starting from the top of the membrane. Figure S14. The 1000-ns MD simulation of the unconjugated Kalata B1 (PDB ID: 1NB1) in the POPC membrane model: the RMSD of the α-carbon atoms plotted against the simulation time (a), the number of hydrogen bonds within the peptide plotted against the simulation time (b), the Ramachandran plot of the peptide at 0 ns (c) and at 1000 ns (d) starting from the top of the membrane. Figure S15. The 1000 ns MD simulation of the unconjugated SFTI-1 (PDB ID: 1JBL) in the POPC membrane model: the RMSD of the α-carbon atoms plotted against the simulation time (a), the number of hydrogen bonds within the peptide plotted against the simulation time (b), the Ramachandran plot of the peptide at 0 ns (c) and at 1000 ns (d) starting from the top of the membrane. Figure S16. The 1000-ns MD simulation of the unconjugated MCoTI-II (PDB ID: 1HA9) in the POPC membrane model: the RMSD of the α-carbon atoms plotted against the simulation time (a), the number of hydrogen bonds within the peptide plotted against the simulation time (b), the Ramachandran plot of the peptide at 0 ns (c) and at 1000 ns (d) starting from the top of the membrane. Figure S17. The 1000-ns MD simulation of the Kalata B1–doxorubicin conjugate in P the OPC membrane model: the RMSD of the α-carbon atoms plotted against the simulation time (a), the number of hydrogen bonds within the peptide plotted against the simulation time (b), the Ramachandran plot of the peptide at 0 ns (c) and at 1000 ns (d) starting from the top of the membrane. Figure S18. The 1000-ns MD simulation of the SFTI-1–doxorubicin conjugate in the POPC membrane model: the RMSD of the α-carbon atoms plotted against the simulation time (a), the number of hydrogen bonds within the peptide plotted against the simulation time (b), the Ramachandran plot of the peptide at 0 ns (c) and at 1000 ns (d) starting from the top of the membrane. Figure S19. The 1000-ns MD simulation of the MCo-TI-II–doxorubicin conjugate in the POPC membrane model: the RMSD the of α-carbon atoms plotted against the simulation time (a), the number of hydrogen bonds within the peptide plotted against the simulation time (b), the Ramachandran plot of the peptide at 0 ns (c) and at 1000 ns (d) starting from the top of the membrane. Figure S20. The 1000-ns MD simulation of the Kalata B1–rasagiline conjugate in the POPC membrane model: the RMSD of the α-carbon atoms plotted against the simulation time (a), the number of hydrogen bonds within the peptide plotted against the simulation time (b), the Ramachandran plot of the peptide at 0 ns (c) and at 1000 ns (d) starting from the top of the membrane. Figure S21. The 1000-ns MD simulation of the SFTI-1–rasagiline conjugate in the POPC membrane model: the RMSD of the α-carbon atoms plotted against the simulation time (a), the number of hydrogen bonds within the peptide plotted against the simulation time (b), the Ramachandran plot of the peptide at 0 ns (c) and at 1000 ns (d) starting from the top of the membrane. Figure S22. The 1000-ns MD simulation of the MCo-TI-II–rasagiline conjugate in the POPC membrane model: the RMSD of α the carbon atoms plotted against the simulation time (a), the number of hydrogen bonds within the peptide plotted against the simulation time (b), the Ramachandran plot of the peptide at 0 ns (c) and at 1000 ns (d) starting from the top of the membrane. Figure S23. The 1000-ns MD simulation of the Kalata B1–zidovudine conjugate in the POPC membrane model: the RMSD of the α-carbon atoms plotted against the simulation time (a), the number of hydrogen bonds within the peptide plotted against the simulation time (b), the Ramachandran plot of the peptide at 0 ns (c) and at 1000 ns (d) starting from the top of the membrane. Figure S24. The 1000-ns MD simulation of the SFTI-1–zidovudine conjugate in the POPC membrane model: the RMSD of the α-carbon atoms plotted against the simulation time (a), the number of hydrogen bonds within the peptide plotted against the simulation time (b), the Ramachandran plot of the peptide at 0 ns (c) and at 1000 ns (d) starting from the top of the membrane. Figure S25. The 1000-ns MD simulation of the MCoTI-II–zidovudine conjugate in the POPC membrane model: the RMSD of the α-carbon atoms plotted against the simulation time (a), the number of hydrogen bonds within the peptide plotted against the simulation time (b), the Ramachandran plot of the peptide at 0 ns (c) and at 1000 ns (d) starting from the top of the membrane

Author Contributions: Conceptualization, I.M.; Methodology, B.B. and I.M.; Software, B.B.; Investigation, M.I.; Data curation, B.B.; Writing—original draft, M.I. and L.K.; Writing—review & editing, I.M. All authors have read and agreed to the published version of the manuscript.

Funding: We are grateful to the Hungarian Scientific Research Fund (OTKA ANN 139484, OTKA 139216). The financial support of the National Research, Development, and Innovation Office (TKP2021-EGA-31) is acknowledged. Project no. RRF-2.3.1-21-2022-00015 has been implemented with the support provided by the European Union.

Institutional Review Board Statement: Not applicable.

Informed Consent Statement: Not applicable.

Data Availability Statement: Data is contained within the article and supplementary material.

Conflicts of Interest: The authors declare no conflict of interest.

References

1. Derossi, D.; Chassaing, G.; Prochiantz, A. Trojan peptides: The penetratin system for intracellular delivery. *Trends Cell Biol.* **1998**, *8*, 84–87. [CrossRef] [PubMed]
2. Bolhassani, A.; Jafarzade, B.S.; Mardani, G. In vitro and in vivo delivery of therapeutic proteins using cell penetrating peptides. *Peptides* **2017**, *87*, 50–63. [CrossRef]
3. Gautam, A.; Singh, H.; Tyagi, A.; Chaudhary, K.; Kumar, R.; Kapoor, P.; Raghava, G.P. CPPsite: A curated database of cell penetrating peptides. *Database* **2012**, *2012*, bas015. [CrossRef] [PubMed]
4. Bashyal, S.; Noh, G.; Keum, T.; Choi, Y.W.; Lee, S. Cell penetrating peptides as an innovative approach for drug delivery; then, present and the future. *J. Pharm. Investig.* **2016**, *46*, 205–220. [CrossRef]
5. Copolovici, D.M.; Langel, K.; Eriste, E.; Langel, U. Cell-Penetrating Peptides: Design, Synthesis, and Applications. *ACS Nano* **2014**, *8*, 1972–1994. [CrossRef]

6. Wang, S.; Zhelev, N.Z.; Duff, S.; Fischer, P.M. Synthesis and biological activity of conjugates between paclitaxel and the cell delivery vector penetratin. *Bioorg. Med. Chem. Lett.* **2006**, *16*, 2628–2631. [CrossRef]

7. Diedrichsen, R.G.; Harloff-Helleberg, S.; Werner, U.; Besenius, M.; Leberer, E.; Kristensen, M.; Nielsen, H.M. Revealing the importance of carrier-cargo association in delivery of insulin and lipidated insulin. *J. Control. Release* **2021**, *338*, 8–21. [CrossRef] [PubMed]

8. Pari, E.; Horvati, K.; Bosze, S.; Biri-Kovacs, B.; Szeder, B.; Zsila, F.; Kiss, E. Drug conjugation induced modulation of structural and membrane interaction features of cationic cell-permeable peptides. *Int. J. Mol. Sci.* **2020**, *21*, 2197. [CrossRef]

9. Balogh, B.; Ivanczi, M.; Nizami, B.; Beke-Somfai, T.; Mandity, I.M. ConjuPepDB: A database of peptide-drug conjugates. *Nucleic Acids Res.* **2021**, *49*, D1102–D1112. [CrossRef]

10. Liotard, J.F.; Mehiri, M.; Di Giorgio, A.; Boggetto, N.; Reboud-Ravaux, M.; Aubertin, A.M.; Condom, R.; Patino, N. AZT and AZT-monophosphate prodrugs incorporating HIV-protease substrate fragment: Synthesis and evaluation as specific drug delivery systems. *Antivir. Chem. Chemother.* **2006**, *17*, 193–213. [CrossRef]

11. Nasrolahi Shirazi, A.; Tiwari, R.; Chhikara, B.S.; Mandal, D.; Parang, K. Design and biological evaluation of cell-penetrating peptide-doxorubicin conjugates as prodrugs. *Mol. Pharm.* **2013**, *10*, 488–499. [CrossRef] [PubMed]

12. Vale, N.; Alves, C.; Sharma, V.; Lazaro, D.F.; Silva, S.; Gomes, P.; Outeiro, T.F. A new MAP-Rasagiline conjugate reduces alpha-synuclein inclusion formation in a cell model. *Pharmacol. Rep.* **2020**, *72*, 456–464. [CrossRef] [PubMed]

13. Dufourc, E.J.; Buchoux, S.; Toupe, J.; Sani, M.A.; Jean-Francois, F.; Khemtemourian, L.; Grelard, A.; Loudet-Courreges, C.; Laguerre, M.; Elezgaray, J.; et al. Membrane interacting peptides: From killers to helpers. *Curr. Protein Pept. Sci.* **2012**, *13*, 620–631. [CrossRef] [PubMed]

14. Asrorov, A.M.; Wang, H.; Zhang, M.; Wang, Y.; He, Y.; Sharipov, M.; Yili, A.; Huang, Y. Cell penetrating peptides: Highlighting points in cancer therapy. *Drug Dev. Res.* **2023**, *early view*. [CrossRef]

15. Mansur, A.A.P.; Carvalho, S.M.; Lobato, Z.I.P.; Leite, M.F.; Cunha, A.D.S., Jr.; Mansur, H.S. Design and Development of Polysaccharide-Doxorubicin-Peptide Bioconjugates for Dual Synergistic Effects of Integrin-Targeted and Cell-Penetrating Peptides for Cancer Chemotherapy. *Bioconj. Chem.* **2018**, *29*, 1973–2000. [CrossRef]

16. Borrelli, A.; Tornesello, A.L.; Tornesello, M.L.; Buonaguro, F.M. Cell Penetrating Peptides as Molecular Carriers for Anti-Cancer Agents. *Molecules* **2018**, *23*, 295. [CrossRef]

17. Kalafatovic, D.; Giralt, E. Cell-Penetrating Peptides: Design Strategies beyond Primary Structure and Amphipathicity. *Molecules* **2017**, *22*, 1929. [CrossRef]

18. Herce, H.D.; Garcia, A.E. Cell penetrating peptides: How do they do it? *J. Biol. Phys.* **2007**, *33*, 345–356. [CrossRef] [PubMed]

19. Durzynska, J.; Przysiecka, L.; Nawrot, R.; Barylski, J.; Nowicki, G.; Warowicka, A.; Musidlak, O.; Gondzicka-Jozefiak, A. Viral and other cell-penetrating peptides as vectors of therapeutic agents in medicine. *J. Pharmacol. Exp. Ther.* **2015**, *354*, 32–42. [CrossRef]

20. Strandberg, E.; Wadhwani, P.; Burck, J.; Anders, P.; Mink, C.; van den Berg, J.; Ciriello, R.A.M.; Melo, M.N.; Castanho, M.; Bardaji, E.; et al. Temperature-Dependent Re-alignment of the Short Multifunctional Peptide BP100 in Membranes Revealed by Solid-State NMR Spectroscopy and Molecular Dynamics Simulations. *ChemBioChem* **2023**, *24*, e202200602. [CrossRef] [PubMed]

21. de Oliveira, E.C.L.; da Costa, K.S.; Taube, P.S.; Lima, A.H.; Junior, C.d.S.d.S. Biological Membrane-Penetrating Peptides: Computational Prediction and Applications. *Front. Cell. Infect. Microbiol.* **2022**, *12*, 838259. [CrossRef]

22. Kabelka, I.; Brozek, R.; Vacha, R. Selecting Collective Variables and Free-Energy Methods for Peptide Translocation across Membranes. *J. Chem. Inf. Model.* **2021**, *61*, 819–830. [CrossRef] [PubMed]

23. Jobin, M.-L.; Vamparys, L.; Deniau, R.; Grelard, A.; Mackereth, C.D.; Fuchs, P.F.J.; Alves, I.D. Biophysical insight on the membrane insertion of an arginine-rich cell-penetrating peptide. *Int. J. Mol. Sci.* **2019**, *20*, 4441. [CrossRef] [PubMed]

24. Huang, K.; Garcia, A.E. Free energy of translocating an arginine-rich cell-penetrating peptide across a lipid bilayer suggests pore formation. *Biophys. J.* **2013**, *104*, 412–420. [CrossRef] [PubMed]

25. Walrant, A.; Vogel, A.; Correia, I.; Lequin, O.; Olausson, B.E.; Desbat, B.; Sagan, S.; Alves, I.D. Membrane interactions of two arginine-rich peptides with different cell internalization capacities. *Biochim. Biophys. Acta* **2012**, *1818*, 1755–1763. [CrossRef]

26. Reid, L.M.; Verma, C.S.; Essex, J.W. The role of molecular simulations in understanding the mechanisms of cell-penetrating peptides. *Drug Discov. Today* **2019**, *24*, 1821–1835. [CrossRef]

27. Gao, X.; Hong, S.; Liu, Z.; Yue, T.; Dobnikar, J.; Zhang, X. Membrane potential drives direct translocation of cell-penetrating peptides. *Nanoscale* **2019**, *11*, 1949–1958. [CrossRef]

28. Trofimenko, E.; Grasso, G.; Heulot, M.; Chevalier, N.; Deriu, M.A.; Dubuis, G.; Arribat, Y.; Serulla, M.; Michel, S.; Vantomme, G.; et al. Genetic, cellular, and structural characterization of the membrane potential-dependent cell-penetrating peptide translocation pore. *eLife* **2021**, *10*, e69832. [CrossRef] [PubMed]

29. Blumer, M.; Harris, S.; Li, M.; Martinez, L.; Untereiner, M.; Saeta, P.N.; Carpenter, T.S.; Ingolfsson, H.I.; Bennett, W.F.D. Simulations of Asymmetric Membranes Illustrate Cooperative Leaflet Coupling and Lipid Adaptability. *Front. Cell Dev. Biol.* **2020**, *8*, 575. [CrossRef]

30. Lattig-Tunnemann, G.; Prinz, M.; Hoffmann, D.; Behlke, J.; Palm-Apergi, C.; Morano, I.; Herce, H.D.; Cardoso, M.C. Backbone rigidity and static presentation of guanidinium groups increases cellular uptake of arginine-rich cell-penetrating peptides. *Nat. Commun.* **2011**, *2*, 453. [CrossRef] [PubMed]

31. Lensink, M.F.; Christiaens, B.; Vandekerckhove, J.; Prochiantz, A.; Rosseneu, M. Penetratin-membrane association: W48/R52/W56 shield the peptide from the aqueous phase. *Biophys. J.* **2005**, *88*, 939–952. [CrossRef] [PubMed]

32. Herce, H.D.; Garcia, A.E. Molecular dynamics simulations suggest a mechanism for translocation of the HIV-1 TAT peptide across lipid membranes. *Proc. Natl. Acad. Sci. USA* **2007**, *104*, 20805–20810. [CrossRef] [PubMed]
33. Herce, H.D.; Garcia, A.E.; Litt, J.; Kane, R.S.; Martin, P.; Enrique, N.; Rebolledo, A.; Milesi, V. Arginine-rich peptides destabilize the plasma membrane, consistent with a pore formation translocation mechanism of cell-penetrating peptides. *Biophys. J.* **2009**, *97*, 1917–1925. [CrossRef] [PubMed]
34. Herce, H.D.; Garcia, A.E.; Cardoso, M.C. Fundamental molecular mechanism for the cellular uptake of guanidinium-rich molecules. *J. Am. Chem. Soc.* **2014**, *136*, 17459–17467. [CrossRef] [PubMed]
35. Akabori, K.; Huang, K.; Treece, B.W.; Jablin, M.S.; Maranville, B.; Woll, A.; Nagle, J.F.; Garcia, A.E.; Tristram-Nagle, S. HIV-1 membrane interactions probed using X-ray and neutron scattering, CD spectroscopy and MD simulations. *Biochim. Biophys. Acta* **2014**, *1838*, 3078–3087. [CrossRef]
36. Neale, C.; Huang, K.; Garcia, A.E.; Tristram-Nagle, S. Penetration of HIV-1 Tat47-57 into PC/PE Bilayers Assessed by MD Simulation and X-ray Scattering. *Membranes* **2015**, *5*, 473–494. [CrossRef]
37. He, X.; Lin, M.; Sha, B.; Feng, S.; Shi, X.; Qu, Z.; Xu, F. Coarse-grained molecular dynamics studies of the translocation mechanism of polyarginines across asymmetric membrane under tension. *Sci. Rep.* **2015**, *5*, 12808. [CrossRef] [PubMed]
38. Bennett, W.F.; Hong, C.K.; Wang, Y.; Tieleman, D.P. Antimicrobial Peptide Simulations and the Influence of Force Field on the Free Energy for Pore Formation in Lipid Bilayers. *J. Chem. Theory Comput.* **2016**, *12*, 4524–4533. [CrossRef] [PubMed]
39. Bennett, W.F.; Sapay, N.; Tieleman, D.P. Atomistic simulations of pore formation and closure in lipid bilayers. *Biophys. J.* **2014**, *106*, 210–219. [CrossRef]
40. Alaybeyoglu, B.; Sariyar Akbulut, B.; Ozkirimli, E. Insights into membrane translocation of the cell-penetrating peptide pVEC from molecular dynamics calculations. *J. Biomol. Struct. Dyn.* **2016**, *34*, 2387–2398. [CrossRef]
41. Via, M.A.; Klug, J.; Wilke, N.; Mayorga, L.S.; Del Popolo, M.G. The interfacial electrostatic potential modulates the insertion of cell-penetrating peptides into lipid bilayers. *Phys. Chem. Chem. Phys.* **2018**, *20*, 5180–5189. [CrossRef]
42. Ulmschneider, J.P. Charged Antimicrobial Peptides Can Translocate across Membranes without Forming Channel-like Pores. *Biophys. J.* **2017**, *113*, 73–81. [CrossRef] [PubMed]
43. Ulmschneider, J.P.; Ulmschneider, M.B. Molecular Dynamics Simulations Are Redefining Our View of Peptides Interacting with Biological Membranes. *Acc. Chem. Res.* **2018**, *51*, 1106–1116. [CrossRef] [PubMed]
44. Ulmschneider, M.B.; Ulmschneider, J.P.; Freites, J.A.; von Heijne, G.; Tobias, D.J.; White, S.H. Transmembrane helices containing a charged arginine are thermodynamically stable. *Eur. Biophys. J.* **2017**, *46*, 627–637. [CrossRef] [PubMed]
45. Gumbart, J.C.; Ulmschneider, M.B.; Hazel, A.; White, S.H.; Ulmschneider, J.P. Computed Free Energies of Peptide Insertion into Bilayers are Independent of Computational Method. *J. Membr. Biol.* **2018**, *251*, 345–356, Erratum in *J. Membr. Biol.* **2018**, *251*, 357. [CrossRef] [PubMed]
46. Yao, C.; Kang, Z.; Yu, B.; Chen, Q.; Liu, Y.; Wang, Q. All-Factor Analysis and Correlations on the Transmembrane Process for Arginine-Rich Cell-Penetrating Peptides. *Langmuir* **2019**, *35*, 9286–9296. [CrossRef] [PubMed]
47. Tran, D.P.; Tada, S.; Yumoto, A.; Kitao, A.; Ito, Y.; Uzawa, T.; Tsuda, K. Using molecular dynamics simulations to prioritize and understand AI-generated cell penetrating peptides. *Sci. Rep.* **2021**, *11*, 10630. [CrossRef]
48. Gimenez-Dejoz, J.; Numata, K. Molecular dynamics study of the internalization of cell-penetrating peptides containing unnatural amino acids across membranes. *Nanoscale Adv.* **2022**, *4*, 397–407. [CrossRef]
49. Grasso, G.; Muscat, S.; Rebella, M.; Morbiducci, U.; Audenino, A.; Danani, A.; Deriu, M.A. Cell penetrating peptide modulation of membrane biomechanics by Molecular dynamics. *J. Biomech.* **2018**, *73*, 137–144. [CrossRef]
50. Bowers, K.J.; Chow, E.; Xu, H.; Dror, R.O.; Eastwood, M.P.; Gregersen, B.A.; Klepeis, J.L.; Kolossvary, I.; Moraes, M.A.; Sacerdoti, F.D.; et al. Scalable Algorithms for Molecular Dynamics Simulations on Commodity Clusters. In Proceedings of the ACM/IEEE Conference on Supercomputing (SC06), Tampa, FL, USA, 11–17 November 2006.
51. Bennett, W.F.; Tieleman, D.P. The importance of membrane defects-lessons from simulations. *Acc. Chem. Res.* **2014**, *47*, 2244–2251. [CrossRef] [PubMed]
52. Czajlik, A.; Mesko, E.; Penke, B.; Perczel, A. Investigation of penetratin peptides. Part 1. The environment dependent conformational properties of penetratin and two of its derivatives. *J. Pept. Sci.* **2002**, *8*, 151–171. [CrossRef]
53. Rosengren, K.J.; Daly, N.L.; Plan, M.R.; Waine, C.; Craik, D.J. Twists, knots, and rings in proteins. Structural definition of the cyclotide framework. *J. Biol. Chem.* **2003**, *278*, 8606–8616. [CrossRef] [PubMed]
54. Korsinczky, M.L.; Schirra, H.J.; Rosengren, K.J.; West, J.; Condie, B.A.; Otvos, L.; Anderson, M.A.; Craik, D.J. Solution structures by 1H NMR of the novel cyclic trypsin inhibitor SFTI-1 from sunflower seeds and an acyclic permutant. *J. Mol. Biol.* **2001**, *311*, 579–591. [CrossRef] [PubMed]
55. Heitz, A.; Hernandez, J.F.; Gagnon, J.; Hong, T.T.; Pham, T.T.; Nguyen, T.M.; Le-Nguyen, D.; Chiche, L. Solution structure of the squash trypsin inhibitor MCoTI-II. A new family for cyclic knottins. *Biochemistry* **2001**, *40*, 7973–7983. [CrossRef] [PubMed]
56. Letoha, T.; Gaal, S.; Somlai, C.; Venkei, Z.; Glavinas, H.; Kusz, E.; Duda, E.; Czajlik, A.; Petak, F.; Penke, B. Investigation of penetratin peptides. Part 2. In vitro uptake of penetratin and two of its derivatives. *J. Pept. Sci.* **2005**, *11*, 805–811. [CrossRef]
57. Dom, G.; Shaw-Jackson, C.; Matis, C.; Bouffioux, O.; Picard, J.J.; Prochiantz, A.; Mingeot-Leclercq, M.-P.; Brasseur, R.; Rezsohazy, R. Cellular uptake of Antennapedia penetratin peptides is a two-step process in which phase transfer precedes a tryptophan-dependent translocation. *Nucleic Acids Res.* **2003**, *31*, 556–561. [CrossRef] [PubMed]

58. Bera, S.; Kar, R.K.; Mondal, S.; Pahan, K.; Bhunia, A. Structural Elucidation of the Cell-Penetrating Penetratin Peptide in Model Membranes at the Atomic Level: Probing Hydrophobic Interactions in the Blood-Brain Barrier. *Biochemistry* **2016**, *55*, 4982–4996. [CrossRef] [PubMed]
59. Verma, R.P.; Hansch, C. Cytotoxicity of organic compounds against ovarian cancer cells: A quantitative structure-activity relationship study. *Mol. Pharm.* **2006**, *3*, 441–450. [CrossRef]
60. Machatha, S.G.; Bustamante, P.; Yalkowsky, S.H. Deviation from linearity of drug solubility in ethanol/water mixtures. *Int. J. Pharm.* **2004**, *283*, 83–88. [CrossRef]
61. Kong, Z.; Sun, D.; Jiang, Y.; Hu, Y. Design, synthesis, and evaluation of 1,4-benzodioxan-substituted chalcones as selective and reversible inhibitors of human monoamine oxidase B. *J. Enzyme Inhib. Med. Chem.* **2020**, *35*, 1513–1523. [CrossRef]
62. Berman, H.M.; Westbrook, J.; Feng, Z.; Gilliland, G.; Bhat, T.N.; Weissig, H.; Shindyalov, I.N.; Bourne, P.E. The Protein Data Bank. *Nucleic Acids Res.* **2000**, *28*, 235–242. [CrossRef]
63. Sastry, G.M.; Adzhigirey, M.; Day, T.; Annabhimoju, R.; Sherman, W. Protein and ligand preparation: Parameters, protocols, and influence on virtual screening enrichments. *J. Comput.-Aided Mol. Des.* **2013**, *27*, 221–234. [CrossRef] [PubMed]
64. Jorgensen, W.L.; Chandrasekhar, J.; Madura, J.D.; Impey, R.W.; Klein, M.L. Comparison of simple potential functions for simulating liquid water. *J. Chem. Phys.* **1983**, *79*, 926–935. [CrossRef]
65. Jorgensen, W.L.; Tirado-Rives, J. The OPLS [optimized potentials for liquid simulations] potential functions for proteins, energy minimizations for crystals of cyclic peptides and crambin. *J. Am. Chem. Soc.* **1988**, *110*, 1657–1666. [CrossRef] [PubMed]
66. Jorgensen, W.L.; Maxwell, D.S.; Tirado-Rives, J. Development and Testing of the OPLS All-Atom Force Field on Conformational Energetics and Properties of Organic Liquids. *J. Am. Chem. Soc.* **1996**, *118*, 11225–11236. [CrossRef]
67. Harder, E.; Damm, W.; Maple, J.; Wu, C.; Reboul, M.; Xiang, J.Y.; Wang, L.; Lupyan, D.; Dahlgren, M.K.; Knight, J.L.; et al. OPLS3: A Force Field Providing Broad Coverage of Drug-like Small Molecules and Proteins. *J. Chem. Theory Comput.* **2016**, *12*, 281–296. [CrossRef] [PubMed]
68. Kurki, M.; Poso, A.; Bartos, P.; Miettinen, M.S. Structure of POPC Lipid Bilayers in OPLS3e Force Field. *J. Chem. Inf. Model.* **2022**, *62*, 6462–6474. [CrossRef] [PubMed]
69. Ivanova, N.; Ivanova, A. Testing the limits of model membrane simulations-bilayer composition and pressure scaling. *J. Comput. Chem.* **2018**, *39*, 387–396. [CrossRef]
70. Jacobson, M.P.; Friesner, R.A.; Xiang, Z.; Honig, B. On the Role of the Crystal Environment in Determining Protein Side-chain Conformations. *J. Mol. Biol.* **2002**, *320*, 597–608. [CrossRef]
71. Jacobson, M.P.; Pincus, D.L.; Rapp, C.S.; Day, T.J.F.; Honig, B.; Shaw, D.E.; Friesner, R.A. A hierarchical approach to all-atom protein loop prediction. *Proteins Struct. Funct. Bioinform.* **2004**, *55*, 351–367. [CrossRef]
72. Ramachandran, B.; Muthupandian, S.; Jeyaraman, J.; Lopes, B.S. Computational exploration of molecular flexibility and interaction of meropenem analogs with the active site of oxacillinase-23 in *Acinetobacter baumannii*. *Front. Chem.* **2023**, *11*, 1090630. [CrossRef]

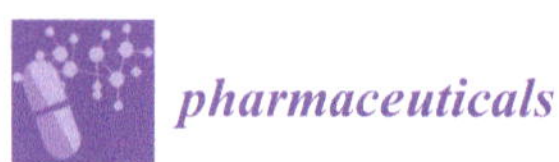

pharmaceuticals

MDPI

Article

Underlying Mechanisms of *Bergenia* spp. to Treat Hepatocellular Carcinoma Using an Integrated Network Pharmacology and Molecular Docking Approach

Shoukat Hussain [1], Ghulam Mustafa [1,*], Sibtain Ahmed [2,3] and Mohammed Fahad Albeshr [4]

[1] Department of Biochemistry, Government College University Faisalabad, Faisalabad 38000, Pakistan
[2] Scripps Institution of Oceanography, University of California San Diego, 9500 Gilman Drive, La Jolla, CA 92093, USA
[3] Department of Biochemistry, Bahauddin Zakariya University, Multan 60800, Pakistan
[4] Department of Zoology, College of Science, King Saud University, P.O. Box 2455, Riyadh 11451, Saudi Arabia
* Correspondence: drghulammustafa@gcuf.edu.pk

Abstract: Hepatocellular carcinoma (HCC) is the fifth most common and fatal cancer reported, representing 72.5% of malignancies around the world. The majority of HCC incidents have been associated with infections caused by hepatitis B and C viruses. Many first- and second-line conventional drugs, e.g., sorafenib, cabozantinib, or ramucirumab, have been used for the management of HCC. Despite different combinational therapies, there are still no defined biomarkers for an early stage diagnosis of HCC. The current study evaluated the potential of *Bergenia stracheyi*, *Bergenia ciliata*, *Bergenia pacumbis*, and *Bergenia purpurascens*, which belong to the family Saxifragaceae, to treat HCC using an integrated network pharmacology and molecular docking approach. Four active phytochemicals were selected based on oral bioavailability (OB) and drug likeness (DL) parameters. The criteria of phytochemical selection were set to OB > 30% and DL > 0.18. Similarly, the gene targets related to *Bergenia* spp. and the genes related to HCC were retrieved from different databases. The integration of these genes revealed 98 most common overlapping genes, which were mainly interrelated with HCC pathogenesis. Ultimately, the 98 *Bergenia*-HCC associated genes were used for protein–protein interaction (PPI), Kyoto Encyclopedia of Genes and Genomes (KEGG) pathway, and Gene Ontology (GO) enrichment analyses. Finally, the topological analysis revealed the top ten hub genes with maximum degree rank. From the top ten genes, STAT3, MAPK3, and SRC were selected due to their involvement in GO annotation and KEGG pathway. To confirm the network pharmacology results, molecular docking analysis was performed to target STAT3, MAPK3, and SRC receptor proteins. The phytochemical (+)-catechin 3-gallate exhibited a maximum binding score and strong residue interactions with the active amino acids of MAPK3-binding pockets (S-score: −10.2 kcal/mol), SRC (S-score: −8.9 kcal/mol), and STAT3 (S-score: −8.9 kcal/mol) as receptor proteins. (+)-Catechin 3-gallate and β-sitosterol induced a significant reduction in cell viability in HepG2 after 24 h of treatment in a dose-dependent manner. The results of this study explore the potential of (+)-catechin 3-gallate and β-sitosterol, which can be used in the future as potential drug candidates to suppress HCC.

Keywords: hepatitis B virus; hepatitis C virus; (+)-catechin 3-gallate; β-sitosterol; KEGG; protein–protein interactions

Citation: Hussain, S.; Mustafa, G.; Ahmed, S.; Albeshr, M.F. Underlying Mechanisms of *Bergenia* spp. to Treat Hepatocellular Carcinoma Using an Integrated Network Pharmacology and Molecular Docking Approach. *Pharmaceuticals* **2023**, *16*, 1239. https://doi.org/10.3390/ph16091239

Academic Editors: Halil İbrahim Ciftci, Belgin Sever, Hasan Demirci and Einar S Björnsson

Received: 28 June 2023
Revised: 11 August 2023
Accepted: 23 August 2023
Published: 1 September 2023

1. Introduction

Hepatocellular carcinoma (HCC) or liver cancer is the second death-related cancer worldwide with late-stage diagnosis due to its severely fatal tumor [1]. Chronic liver infections such as hepatitis B, hepatitis C, alcoholic abuse, and metabolic disorders later progress into liver inflammation, liver fibrosis, and cirrhosis, which develop symptoms of HCC [2]. HCC is frequently multinodular upon diagnosis and it has a specific proclivity to develop inside the blood vessels and then infiltrate the portal or hepatic veins [3]. The prognosis of HCC is directly associated with tumor stage at the time of diagnosis. The early stage diagnosis of HCC is poorly reported, with a median of 5 years and a 7% survival rate [4]. HCC solely accounts for 75–85% of tumor cases in all liver cancer reports. In a report, the World Health Organization (WHO) predicted 1.3 million deaths by 2040 due to liver cancer [5]. The HCC-linked infection(s) could be recognized and decreased through inhibiting the development of HCC, which in turn increases the life span of the patients through early diagnosis with better combinations [6].

Different pathways including Wnt/ß-catenin pathway, phosphatidylinositol-3-kinase, MET receptor tyrosine kinase pathway, and Hedgehog (Hh) signaling pathway play a leading role in the proliferation of the tumor, which ultimately leads to HCC. Any mutational changes in the genetic makeup and signaling of the metabolic cascade mainly cause the onset of carcinogenesis [7]. Recently, against advanced HCC, sorafenib/lenvatinib and regorafenib/cabozantinib have been administrated as first-line and second-line drugs, respectively. Moreover, the combinational therapy of nivolumab and ipilimumab with pembrolizumab monotherapy has received FDA approval for the treatment of HCC [8]. Despite the combinational therapies and licensed drugs, the survival rate is limited due to the poor diagnosis and severe side effects of such drugs. Many other clinical trials including immune checkpoint inhibitors, chimeric antigen receptor T-cells, and dendritic cell vaccines are in the first stage of testing. Therefore, there is a dire need of drugs with no or fewer side effects for the treatment of HCC.

Plant-based herbal remedies have gained much interest in recent years for the treatment of various cancers. Plants are a natural source of biologically active compounds, which play a leading role as potential drug candidates for the treatment of multiple disorders and infections [9]. *Bergenia* is a genus of flowering plants and belongs to the Saxifragaceae family with about 35 known species. Different Ayurvedic formulations have used *Bergenia* species over the centuries to treat piles, kidney stones, bladder, and pulmonary infections [10]. Almost six species of this genus are present in Pakistan. These are mostly present in the northern areas of Pakistan, particularly in Kashmir or around it. They are present in a large number in temperate Himalayan regions at elevations from 2000 to 2700 m [11].

Network pharmacology is an elaborative domain that predicts the drug mechanism to treat different diseases, which is similar to Chinese medicine's multitargeting functions. Network pharmacology is a multidimensional field in pharmacology, interpreting the network targeting and interrelation of plant phytochemicals to target enormous types of disorders [12]. In this study, the aim to treat HCC using phytochemical constituents of the *Bergenia* species was accomplished via network targeting of multidrug or multi-targeting approach. Using multi-therapeutics with the networking of targeted genes, biologically active phytochemicals have been used as leading drug candidates against key targeted genes with their role in different signaling mechanisms involved in the pathogenesis of HCC.

2. Results

2.1. Active Compounds of Bergenia spp.

A library was constructed which contained 16 phytochemicals from *B. ciliate*, 6 from *B. pacumbis*, 64 from *B. purpurascens*, and 61 from *B. stracheyi*. These phytochemicals were collected from different plant parts (e.g., roots, leaves, rhizome) reported in the literature and IMMPAT database. For network pharmacology analysis, only four compounds (i.e., β-sitosterol, cianidanol, (+)-catechin gallate, and leucocianidol were selected based on their pharmacokinetic criteria of drug likeness (DL > 0.18) and oral bioavailability (OB > 30%). In Table 1, different properties of the four compounds are given.

Table 1. Properties of active phytochemicals.

Sr. No.	Compound	Molecular Formula	Oral Bioavailability (>30%)	Drug Likeness (>0.18)	MW (g/mol)	PubChem ID
1	β-Sitosterol	$C_{29}H_{50}O$	36.91	0.75	414.79	222284
2	Cianidanol	$C_{15}H_{14}O_6$	54.83	0.24	290.29	9064
3	(+)-catechin gallate	$C_{22}H_{18}O_{10}$	53.57	0.75	442.4	5276454
4	Leucocianidol	$C_{15}H_{14}O_7$	30.84	0.27	306.29	440833

MW: Molecular weight.

2.2. Target Prediction for Bergenia spp.

The *Bergenia* spp.-related gene targets were predicted from the SwissTargetPrediction and STITCH database. In total, 313 targets were predicted for the four phytochemicals of *Bergenia* spp. Then, 228 unique drug-related gene targets were predicted after removal of duplicates by aligning the UniprotKB protein IDs.

2.3. Target Prediction for Hepatocellular Carcinoma

A total of 3176 hepatocellular carcinoma-related gene targets were retrieved from GeneCard and DisGeNet databases. After removal of duplicates, a total of 2742 unique gene targets were used for further analysis. The intersection of *Bergenia* spp.-related targets and HCC-related predicted targets was performed for mapping of common overlapping gene targets. Out of these, a total of 98 targets were selected after interaction of drug-related gene targets and HCC-related gene targets (Figure 1).

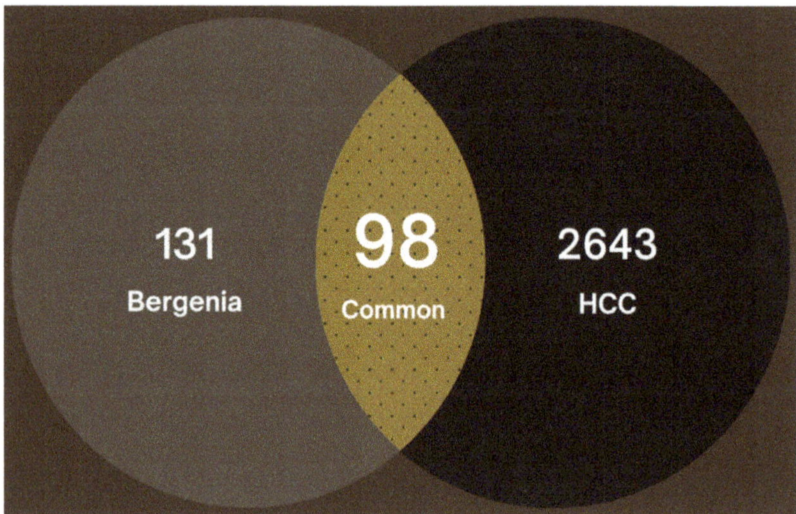

Figure 1. Venn illustration of potential targets.

2.4. Compound-Target Network

The Cytoscape software was used for compound–target network construction for four active plant constituents and 98 potential gene targets. A plug-in Network Analyzer was employed to calculate the topological parameters of the constructed network. The network has 102 nodes and 135 edges representing the active constituents and targeted genes, which are interrelated with lines (Figure 2). The topological analysis represented the network density of 0.026, network centralization of 0.448, and network heterogeneity of

2.694. Furthermore, the active phytochemicals were also categorized by degree method: (+)-catechin gallate (47), β-sitosterol (42), leucocianidol (41), and cianidanol (5), which represented the interactions with multiple targets. In network pharmacology, the network density is a quantitative measure, which is applied to characterize the interconnectedness of nodes (i.e., biological entities such as genes and proteins) within a network. A greater level of interactions between nodes is indicated by a high network density, which results in a more interconnected network. Within a biological network, such as drug–target interaction network or protein–protein interactional network, the network centralization is the degree to which some nodes play influential or important roles compared to other nodes. Similarly, network heterogeneity is considered as the diversity and complexity of interactions within biological networks, specifically, to reveal interactions between drugs, genes, proteins, and other molecules.

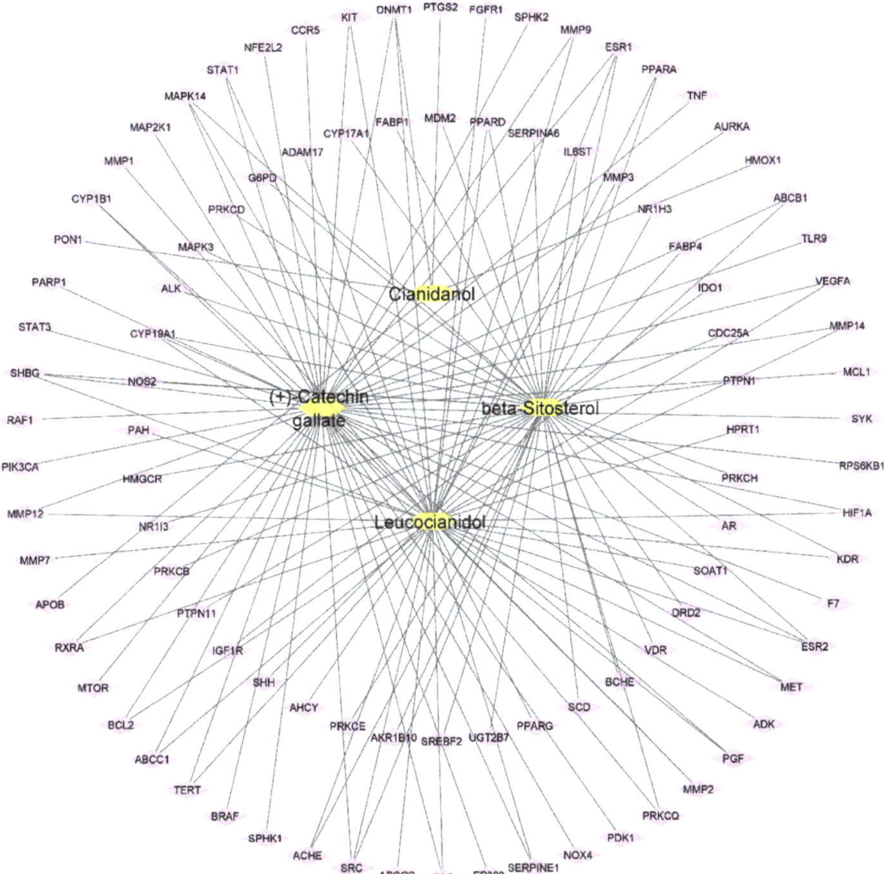

Figure 2. Compound–target network of active plant constituents and predicted targets (yellow: compounds, purple: target genes).

2.5. Protein–Protein Interactions (PPIs)

The 98 potential targets were imported into STRING 11.5 for protein–protein interactions with a high confidence score of 0.700 and by selecting *H. sapiens* as the default organism (Figure 3). In the constructed PPI network, there were 98 nodes, 377 edges with an average node degree of 7.69, and a PPI enrichment p-value of $<1.0 \times 10^{-16}$. The compound–target network of 98 target genes only displayed interactions with (+)-catechin gallate, β-sitosterol, and leucocianidol. Therefore, the phytochemical cianidanol was eliminated from further analysis. In addition, the network density of 0.094, network heterogeneity of 0.907, and network centralization of 0.329 were also calculated by the Network Analyzer tool of the software Cytoscape. The plug-in cytoHubba was also employed to examine the hub genes. The network degree is the number of interactions a node (i.e., compound, gene, protein) makes with other nodes within a biological network. A node with a higher network degree is considered as a hub node, as it shows significant control or influence on the functioning of the network. The degrees of the top targeted genes are represented in Table 2 and Figure 4.

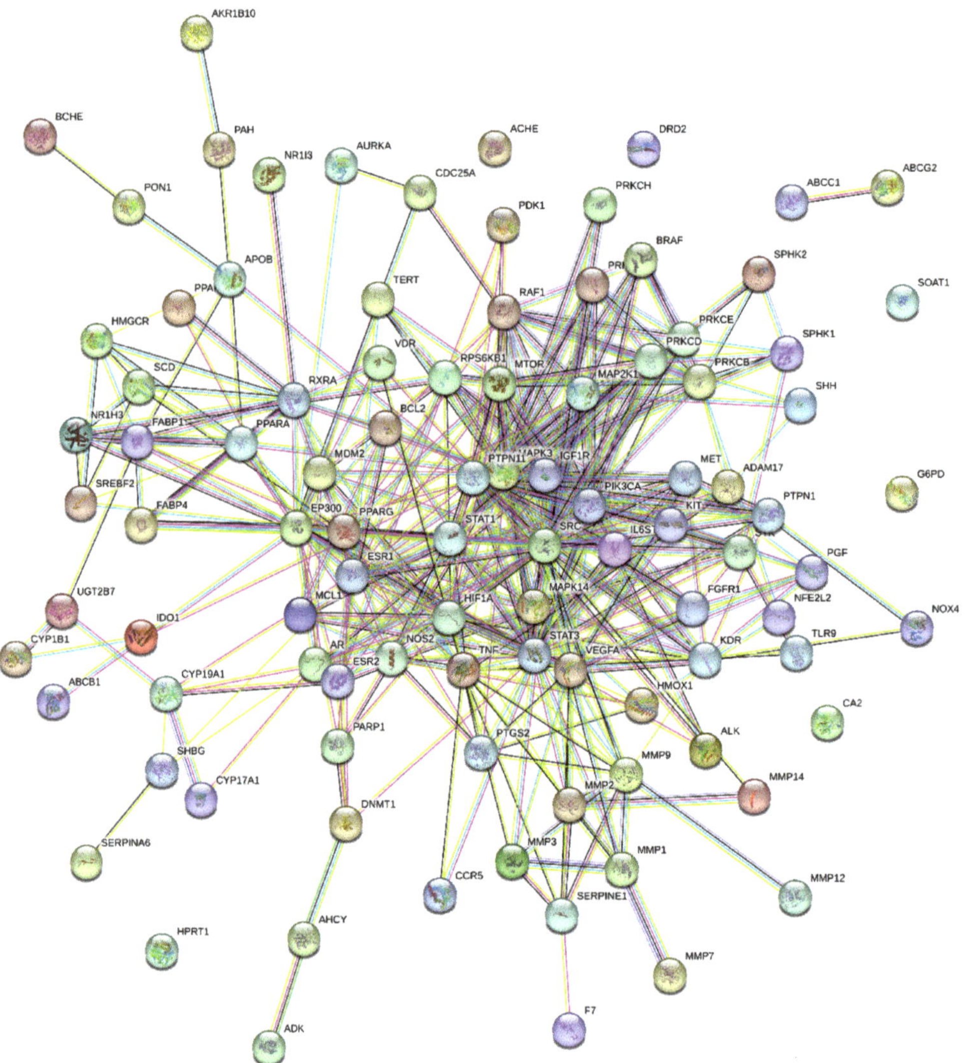

Figure 3. Protein–protein interaction diagram showing the interactions of 98 common target genes.

Table 2. Degrees of hub gene calculated by Cytoscape.

Sr. No.	Hub Genes	Degrees
1	STAT3	37
2	MAPK3	34
3	SRC	33
4	EP300	25
5	VEGFA	22
6	PIK3CA	22
7	TNF	22
8	PTPN11	21
9	ESR1	19
10	HIF1A	19

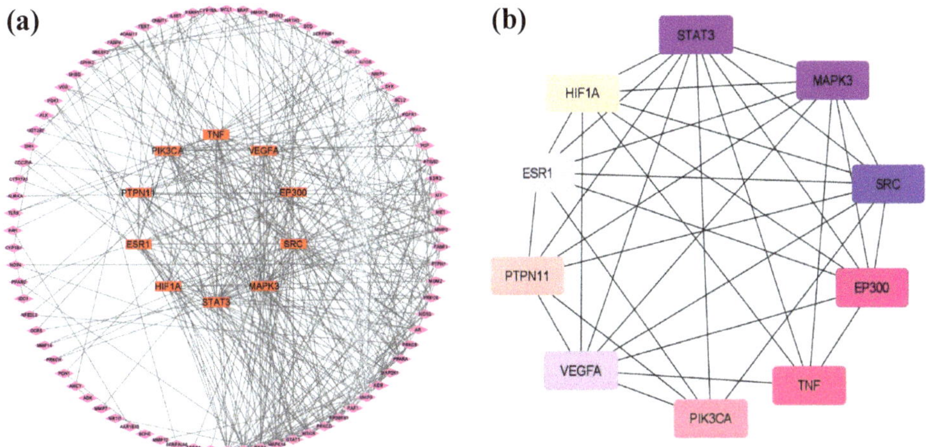

Figure 4. Protein–protein interactions showing: (**a**) interactions of 98 target genes with hub genes in the center (red); (**b**) hub genes with degree evaluation (the darker node is displaying higher rank).

2.6. Analysis of Gene Enrichment

The GO and KEGG enrichment analyses were performed through the DAVID database to predict the functional annotation and pathway enrichment associated with active plant constituents for the treatment of hepatocellular carcinoma. The GO annotation revealed 373 biological processes (BPs), 108 molecular functioning (MF), 40 cellular components (CCs), and 135 KEGG pathways. The top 20 terms in GO and KEGG analyses were identified as mainly involved in cancer pathways (Figure 5). The BPs mainly contain the cellular response toward oxygen-containing compounds, the regulation of programmed cell death, cell proliferation, and responses to stimuli, hormones, and hypoxia. The CC GO annotation was related to mitochondria, ER, receptor complex, chromosome, extracellular matrix, and membrane compartments. The MF was related to phosphotransferase activity, ligand-activated transcription factor activity, nuclear receptor activity, protein kinase activity, and ATP binding. The analysis of the KEGG pathway mainly pointed to the involvement of genes in pathways related to cancer, proteoglycans in cancer, microRNAs in cancer, EGFR tyrosine kinase inhibitor resistance, endocrine resistance, and prostate cancer. These pathways are all co-related directly or indirectly with the onset of hepatocellular carcinoma.

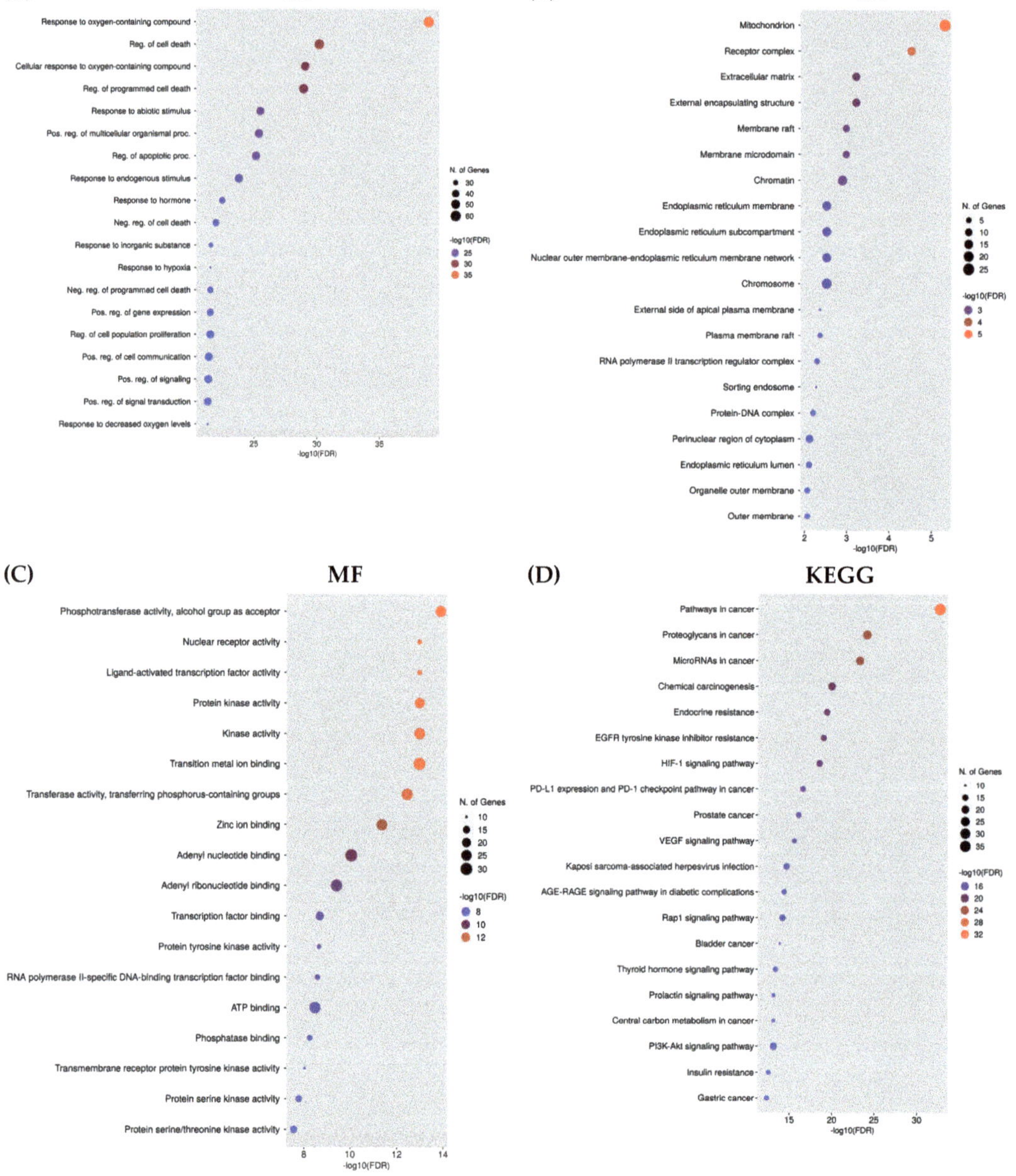

Figure 5. The illustration of functional annotation and enriched pathways in terms of HCC is shown by the bubble plot. (**A**) Gene ontology in terms of biological processes (BP). (**B**) Gene ontology in terms of cellular components (CC). (**C**) Gene ontology in terms of molecular function (MF). (**D**) KEGG pathway analysis.

The ShinyGO tool was used for interpretation and visualization of the top 20 selected pathways in the bar plot. The target–pathway network was constructed with the cystoscope software to fully understand the interrelation of targets with the associated signaling pathways (Figure 6).

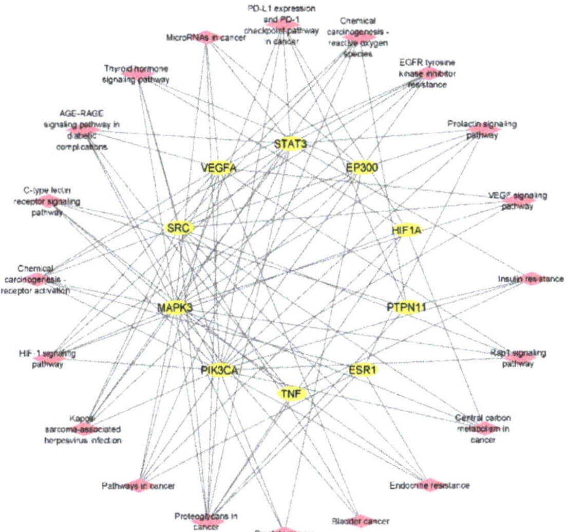

Figure 6. Target–pathway network of hub genes and 20 top enrichment analysis pathways (yellow: hub genes; pink: pathways).

2.7. Construction of Compound–Target–Pathway Network

The Cytoscape software was employed for the integration of the compound–target network and the target–pathway network for the construction of the compound–target–pathway network. The Network Analyzer represents 166 edges and 33 nodes in three active phytochemicals, 10 hub genes, and 20 signaling pathways (Figure 7).

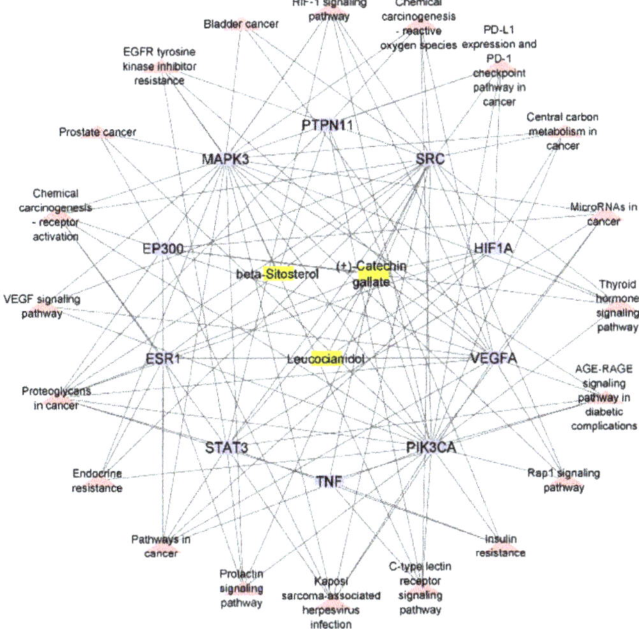

Figure 7. The compound–target–pathway network (yellow: compounds, light purple: hub genes; pink: pathways).

2.8. Molecular Docking Study

The molecular docking approach was used to explore potential drug candidates to target screened genes from a network pharmacology study for the precise targeting of HCC genes for the treatment of liver cancer. The top three genes (i.e., STAT3, MAPK3, SRC) were selected based on their topological analysis, GO, and KEGG enrichment analyses results. These three genes were at the top of the hub genes, sub-gene clustering, and common in the top 20 GO terms and KEGG pathways. The 3D structures of these target proteins STAT3 (with PDB ID 6TLC), MAPK3 (with PDB ID 6GES), and SRC (with PDB ID 2H8H) were retrieved from the Protein Data Bank in PDB format. The removal of solvent molecules and already bound ligand, energy minimization, and 3D protonation of these proteins were performed using the MOE tool. The 3D structures of the selected phytochemicals were retrieved from the PubChem database in .sdf format.

The PyRx software was employed for ligand-based molecular docking of the selected compounds with three target proteins. Among the three phytochemicals, (+)-catechin 3-gallate showed the maximum binding score and the strongest interactions with the active residues of all target proteins. The (+)-catechin 3-gallate, with a docking score of −10.2 kcal/mol, interacted with LysA:71, AspA:128, CysA:183, and AspA:184 residues of the binding pocket of MAPK3 via hydrogen bonding (Figure 8). Similarly, (+)-catechin 3-gallate with a docking score of −8.9 kcal/mol interacted with LysA:295 of the SRC protein and with a docking score of −8 kcal/mol interacted with AlaA:250, GluA:324, GlnA:326, and AspA:334 residues of the STAT3 protein via conventional hydrogen bonds (Figures 9 and 10). The other ligands also showed good energy with substantial binding interactions with the active site residues of binding pockets of target proteins (Table 3). BIOVIA Discovery Studio visualizer was used to visualize the ligand–protein 2D interactions and maps.

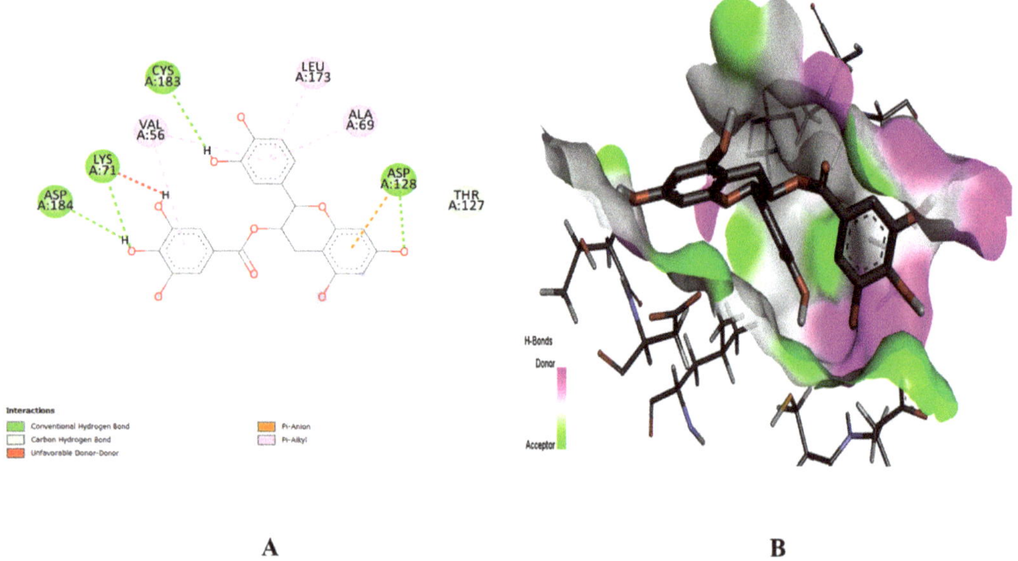

Figure 8. Interaction (**A**) and binding pattern (**B**) of (+)-catechin 3-gallate with active residues of protein MAPK3.

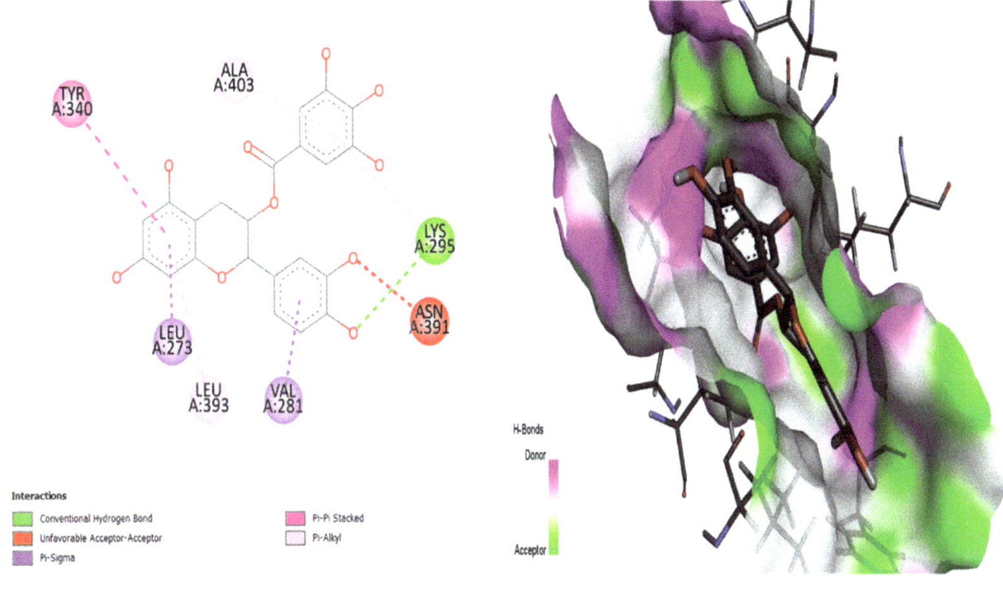

Figure 9. Interaction (**A**) and binding pattern (**B**) of (+)-catechin 3-gallate with active residues of protein SRC.

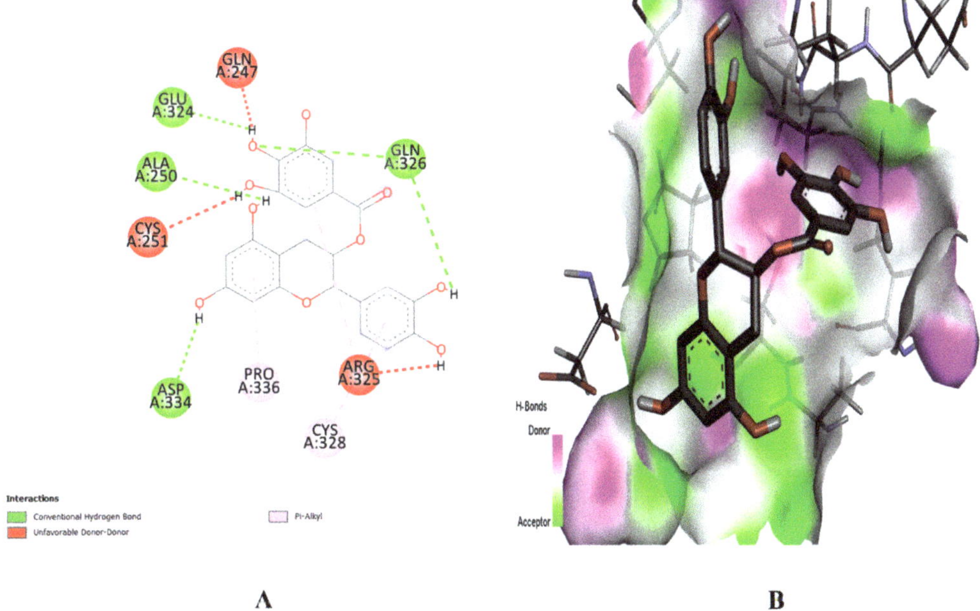

Figure 10. Interaction (**A**) and binding pattern (**B**) of (+)-catechin 3-gallate with active residues of protein STAT3.

Table 3. Binding affinities of phytochemicals with target proteins revealed in the molecular docking study.

Sr. No.	Target Protein	PDB ID	UniProt ID	Phytochemical	Binding Energy (kcal/mol)
1	STAT3	6TLC	P40763	(+)-Catechin 3-gallate	−8.0
				β-sitosterol	−7.4
				Leucocianidol	−7.1
2	MAPK3	6GES	P27361	(+)-Catechin 3-Gallate	−10.2
				β-sitosterol	−9.2
				Leucocianidol	−7.4
3	SRC	2H8H	P12931	(+)-Catechin 3-Gallate	−8.9
				β-sitosterol	−8.4
				Leucocianidol	−7.2

2.9. ADMET Profiling

The ADMET analysis classifies the drug into five parameters (i.e., absorption, distribution, metabolism, excretion, and toxicity). These attributes of a potential drug classify it from the chemical perspective (Table 4). All selected ligands were found to not cross the blood–brain barrier and as being non-Ames toxic. These properties exhibited the potential of these compounds as lead drug candidates for the treatment of HCC.

Table 4. ADMET profiling of lead drug candidates.

ADMET Parameters	Phytochemicals		
	(+)-Catechin 3-Gallate	β-Sitosterol	Leucocianidol
Absorption and distribution			
BBB	No	No	No
Intestinal absorption (human)	62.096%	94.464%	56.712%
PGS	Yes	No	Yes
PGI	No	No	No
Metabolism			
CYP3A4 substrate	No	Yes	No
CYP2D6 substrate	No	No	No
CYP3A4 inhibition	No	No	No
CYP2C9 inhibition	No	No	No
CYP2C19 inhibition	No	No	No
CYP2D6 inhibition	No	No	No
CYP1A2 inhibition	No	No	No
Excretion			
Total Clearance	−0.169 log mL/min/kg	0.628 log mL/min/kg	−0.072 log mL/min/kg
Toxicity			
AMES Toxicity	No	No	No
Hepatotoxicity	No	No	No
Skin Sensitization	No	No	No

Blood–brain barrier (BBB); P-glycoprotein substrate (PGS); P-glycoprotein inhibitor (PGI).

2.10. Cytotoxic Potential of the Best Selected Phytochemicals in HepG2 Cells

To examine the cytotoxicity potential of (+)-catechin 3-gallate, β-sitosterol, and leucocianidol in HepG2 cells, the MTT assay was used. Initially, different concentrations of these compounds, including a standard drug cisplatin (i.e., 1.5625, 3.125, 6.25, 12.50, 25, 50,

100, and 200 µg/mL) were applied to HepG2 cells for 24 h and their cytotoxicity potentials were evaluated through an MTT test. The cytotoxicity potential and percent cell viability of control, (+)-catechin 3-gallate, β-sitosterol, and leucocianidol-treated cells are shown in Figure 11. Treatment with (+)-catechin 3-gallate and β-sitosterol significantly ($p < 0.001$) increased the cytotoxicity of HepG2 cells (Table 5). After treatment with 1.56 µg/mL of (+)-catechin 3-gallate and β-sitosterol, a significant inhibitory effect on the viability of HepG2 cells was observed. After 24 h of treatment in HepG2 cells, the IC_{50} values for (+)-catechin 3-gallate, β-sitosterol, and leucocianidol were estimated to be approximately 5.258, 1.784, and 49.94 µg/mL, respectively, compared to cisplatin (i.e., 2.25 µg/mL) (Figure 11).

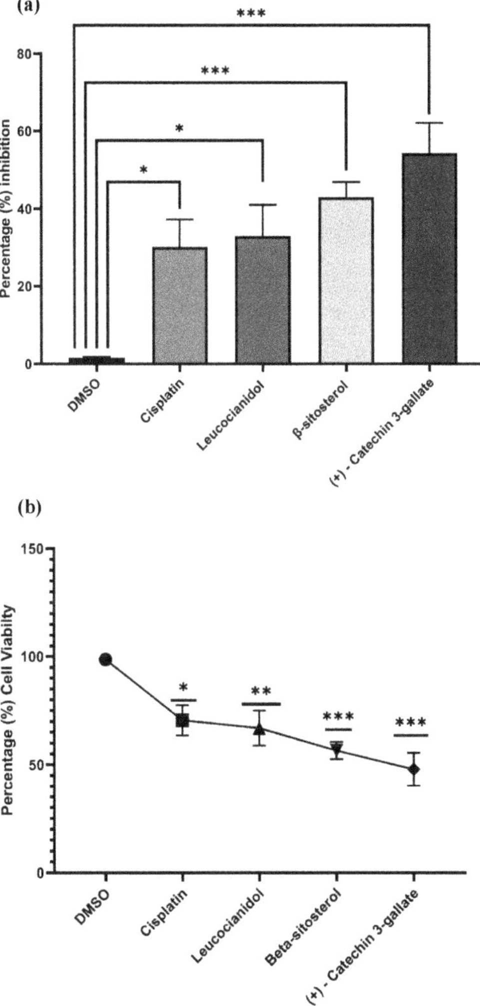

Figure 11. Cytotoxic potential of best selected phytochemicals (i.e., (+)-catechin 3-gallate, β-sitosterol, and leucocianidol). (**a**) Cytotoxicity analysis by MTT assay. The experiment was performed in triplicate and the values are shown as mean ± standard error of mean. (**b**) Percentage of cell viability. If the *p*-value is >0.05, the results were considered statistically significant, represented by * vs. control. ** *p*-value > 0.01 vs. control were considered very significant and *** *p*-value > 0.001 vs. control were considered highly significant. To represent the data, values are presented as mean ± S.E.M.

Table 5. Comparison of percentage inhibition of control groups and treatments at different concentrations.

Concentration (µg/mL)	DMSO	Catechin	β-Sitosterol	(+)-Catechin 3-Gallate
1.5625	0	7 [NS]	19.42 [***]	16.21 [**]
3.125	1.3	12 [NS]	39.3 [****]	34.23 [****]
6.25	1.7	15 [NS]	40.2 [****]	42.65 [****]
12.50	2	29.24 [**]	41.65 [**]	55.92 [***]
25	2	36.95 [***]	49.14 [****]	60.05 [****]
50	2	41.56 [**]	64.86 [****]	69.6 [****]
100	2	43.1 [***]	56.29 [****]	75.63 [****]
200	2	78.4 [****]	46.8 [****]	80.24 [****]
Concentration (µg/mL)	**Cisplatin**	**Catechin**	**β-Sitosterol**	**(+)-Catechin 3-Gallate**
1.5625	5.6	7 [NS]	19.42 [**]	16.21 [*]
3.125	10.5	12 [NS]	39.3 [****]	34.23 [****]
6.25	13.4	15 [NS]	40.2 [***]	42.65 [***]
12.50	27.5	29.24 [NS]	41.65 [NS]	55.92 [**]
25	32.4	36.95 [NS]	49.14 [NS]	60.05 [**]
50	39.5	41.56 [NS]	64.86 [**]	69.6 [**]
100	46.4	43.1 [NS]	56.29 [**]	75.63 [***]
200	65.4	78.4 [NS]	46.8 [NS]	80.24 [****]

NS: Non-significant; *: significant; **: very significant; ***, ****: highly significant.

3. Discussion

The pathogenesis of HCC is complex due to sneaking symptoms which make HCC difficult to diagnose. Hepatocarcinogenesis involves the complex cellular dysfunctioning that predominantly transforms into primary liver carcinoma. The lack of predictable biomarkers and continuous resistance make it limited for treatment and sequential therapies. Conventional anticancer therapies have been associated with severe side effects due to lack of diagnosis and selectivity [13]. The vast diversity and low toxicity make plant-derived compounds a more reliable source of drugs compared to synthetic drugs. Plant-derived compounds are much more effective as anticancer agents counter to multiple hallmarks of cancer [14,15]. In most of the cancer pathways, the triggering of apoptosis is an ideal way to induce tumor death and, in this perspective, plant secondary metabolites are reported as natural triggers of apoptosis signaling in different cancers [16].

In the current study, four plants (i.e., *B. ciliate*, *B. pacumbis*, *B. purpurascens*, and *B. stracheyi*) from the Saxifragaceae family have been used due to their anti-inflammatory history as anticancer therapy. The current study is based on previously used *Bergenia* spp. in different cancer therapies. *B. ciliate*, *B. pacumbis*, *B. purpurascens*, and *B. stracheyi* have been reported with great potential as natural sources of antioxidant, anti-inflammatory, and anticancer compounds. Studies have reported the anticancer effects of *Bergenia* spp. on the inhibition of protein kinase and the induction of apoptosis [17]. Similarly, Faheem et al. [18] reported *Bergenia ligulata* silver nanoparticles for arresting p53-mediated mitochondrial apoptosis in breast cancer. The results of their study reveal the potential of BgAgNps as anticancer agents via the cleavage of caspase-3 and downstream targeting of p53 like Bax In another study, Dulta et al. [19] synthesized zinc oxide NPs from the rhizome extract of *Bergenia ciliate*. The prepared ZnONPs exhibited antibacterial and antioxidant activity against Gram-negative bacterial strains. The ZnONPs with an absorbance band of 340 nm displayed maximum cytotoxic potential in human cervical cancer and human colon cancer cell lines. This indicated the green synthesis of natural NPs to combat with different cancers

In this study, the overlapping and mostly involving gene(s) in each top signaling pathway for the onset of primary liver carcinoma were selected for precise targeting for the selective treatment of HCC. The ten hub genes with their highest degree ranks in topological analysis and PPIs were further selected for pathway and enrichment analysis. The genes STAT3, MAPK3, SRC, EP300, VEGFA, PIK3CA, TNF, PTPN11, ESR1, and HIF1A were on the top of PPIs and mostly involved in the top twenty GO annotations and KEGG pathways. Among these, the genes STAT3, MAPK3, and SRC were evaluated for HCC treatment. Network pharmacology can be used to create a complex integrated network of compound–target–pathways to understand the complex relation of drugs with their respected targets and signaling mechanisms to manage those specific diseases. These networks are based on targets, biologically active compounds, and biological signaling pathways of the gene that addresses the potential of compounds to tackle the involvement of that specific gene to target that pathway. The selection and screening of targets from the pool of genes make it more reliable to point out the involved gene(s) in common cancer pathways [20].

Signal transducer and activator of transcription 3 (STAT3) modulates chronic inflammation in tumor formulation and mediates interactions between tumor cells and stromal cells. STAT3 belongs to the STAT family with seven members which mediate the signal transduction from the plasma membrane toward the nucleus. The overexpression and ubiquitous activation of STAT3 has been associated with metastasis, immune suppression, and tumor progression in liver cancer. The participation of STAT3 in oncogenesis, angiogenesis, anti-apoptosis, and drug resistance has attracted the attention of researchers as a therapeutic target in liver cancer. Different clinical trials have favored STAT3 gene transcription targeting as effective for cancer treatment [21,22].

Mitogen-activated protein kinase 3 (MAPK3) is a member of the MAP kinase family and called extracellular signal-regulated kinases (ERKs). The overexpression or genetic mutation in the MAPK/ERK signaling cascade has been frequently reported in liver cancer. MAPK/ERK acts as a signaling cascade being involved in differentiation, proliferation, and cell cycle signaling in response to outer signals. Any mutation in this signaling cascade leads to tumor initiation, progression, and modulation of the primary liver tumor, thus leading to HCC [23].

SRC kinase is predominantly involved in multiple cellular signaling pathways including mitochondrial oxidative phosphorylation (OXPHOS). Any abhorrent change in the signaling cascade due to SRC kinase mutation ultimately leads to cancer development and metastasis. The change in OXPHOS signaling and expression has been reported in liver cancer biopsies, which showed the involvement of SRC kinase in HCC [24]. Different clinical specimens have indicated a high level of SRC kinase in liver tumor cells compared to non-tumor cells. The SRC expression has been positively related to tumor stage and metastasis has indicated this kinase as a potential target in liver cancer [25].

The results obtained from network pharmacology were further evaluated through experimental work and the cytotoxic effects of (+)-catechin 3-gallate, β-sitosterol, and leucocianidol were explored. The findings show that (+)-catechin 3-gallate and β-sitosterol have cytotoxic effects on HepG2 cell viability in a dose-dependent manner. In a study, Pal et al. [26] assessed the impact of varying concentrations of epigallocatechin gallate (HGCG) on cell viability in normal fibroblasts and hepatocytes, as well as several hepatoma and colon cancer cell lines including HepG2, Huh7, HLF HCC, HCT-116, HCT-115, and HT29. The results demonstrated a significant decrease in cell viability in all hepatoma and colon cancer cell lines ($p < 0.01$), compared to controls, fibroblasts, and hepatocytes in a dose-dependent manner.

The IC_{50} values for (+)-catechin 3-gallate and β-sitosterol were found to be 5.258 and 1.784 μg/mL, respectively, in the current study. In a study, HepG2 cells were treated with EGCG and metformin and their cell viability exhibited a dose-dependent decrease. The IC_{50} values were determined for each treatment. At 24 h of exposure, the IC_{50} values for EGCG and metformin were calculated to be 31.4 μg/mL and 7.57 μg/mL, respectively [27].

Similarly, Ditty et al. [28] conducted a research to examine the potential cytotoxic effects of β-sitosterol on HepG2 cells using the MTT assay. HepG2 cells were exposed to various concentrations of the compound (i.e., 0.2, 0.4, 0.8, and 1 mM/mL) for a duration of 24 h, and their cytotoxicity was evaluated. The results reveal a significant ($p < 0.001$) induction of dose-dependent cytotoxicity in HepG2 cells following β-sitosterol treatment. The highest level of cytotoxicity was observed at a concentration of 1 mM/mL. At 24 h, the IC_{50} value of β-sitosterol in HepG2 cells was determined to be 0.6 mM/mL. Similarly, Raj [29] also conducted a study to investigate the effect of various concentrations (i.e., 2, 4, 6, 8, and 10 ng/mL) of β-sitosterol-assisted silver nanoparticles (BSS-SNPs) on the morphology of HepG2 cells. The HepG2 cells were treated with BSS-SNPs for a duration of 24 h, and the cytotoxicity was assessed. The results demonstrate a significant and dose-dependent cytotoxicity in HepG2 cells following treatment with BSS-SNPs ($p < 0.001$). The IC_{50} value of BSS-SNPs in HepG2 cells was determined to be 7 ng/mL.

In order to investigate the cytotoxic effects of β-amyrin and β-sitosterol-3-O-glucoside, the MTT cell viability assay was employed on two cancer cell lines (HepG2 and Caco-2) in addition to a non-cancer cell line (HEK293). The results reveal a dose-dependent cytotoxicity of the tested compounds on the cancer cell line. Notably, both β-amyrin and β-sitosterol-3-O-glucoside exhibited selective cytotoxicity toward cancer cells, as indicated by their higher IC_{50} values of 156 and 937 µg/mL, respectively, when tested on the control non-cancer cell line. The Caco-2 cell line demonstrated significant cytotoxic activity when exposed to both compounds, with IC_{50} values of 81 µg/mL for β-amyrin and 54 µg/mL for β-sitosterol-3-O-glucoside [30].

Through network pharmacology, three main targets (i.e., MAPK3, STAT3, and SRC) were evaluated in this study as potential targets for (+)-catechin 3-gallate to treat HCC. These proteins are the main parts of different cancer-leading pathways, which make them perfect targets for the treatment of cancer. The molecular docking has confirmed the potential of (+)-catechin 3-gallate as the lead drug candidate for the treatment of HCC. The minimum energy score has displayed the greater binding affinity of (+)-catechin 3-gallate as a ligand for the selected receptor proteins. This study provides a systemic layout that illustrates the key targets and molecular mechanisms as suggestions or recommendations for a detail study of HCC treatment in the future.

4. Materials and Methods

4.1. Active Compounds and Targets Prediction

The biologically active compounds from four *Bergenia* spp. (i.e., *B. ciliate*, *B. pacumbis*, *B. purpurascens*, and *B. stracheyi*) were also retrieved from the literature and the publicly available database of Indian Medicinal Plants, Phytochemistry and Therapeutics (IMP-PAT) [31]. All predicted compounds were virtually screened for their pharmacokinetic parameters of drug likeness (DL) and oral bioavailability (OB) [32]. Only those compounds were selected for further analysis which met the criteria of DL > 0.18 and OB > 30%. Among different pharmacokinetic parameters, the OB is an important one according to the criteria of absorption, distribution, metabolism, and excretion (ADME). For the determination of the DL index of active compounds, a high OB usually serves as a vital indicator. The compounds with OB ≥ 30% are considered for high oral bioavailability [33]. Similarly, the DL index is also an important tool to screen active compounds rapidly, which serves as a qualitative concept that is applied in drug design for the estimation of drugability of a potential compound. The average DL index in the DrugBank is 0.18 and the compound(s) with ≥0.18 DL index are considered to possess high drugability [34].

4.2. Drug Target Profile for Bergenia spp.

The putative gene targets related to selected active phytochemicals were identified and collected by providing SMILES with SwissTargetPrediction tool [35] and STITCH network database [36] by selecting *Homo sapiens* in species option. Protein IDs of each identified protein were aligned with UniProtKB to eliminate duplicates [37].

4.3. HCC-Related Target Screening

Different keywords related to the research studies (i.e., hepatocellular carcinoma, liver cancer) were searched to retrieve HCC-related target genes from GeneCard [38] and DisGeNET databases [39] and aligned with UniProtKB IDs to eliminate duplicates. A Ven-diagram was drawn using Jvenn plug-in [40] to illustrate the common overlapping drug-target related genes.

4.4. Compound–Target Network

The software Cytoscape 3.9.1 [41] was employed to build the compound–target (CT) network of active constituents of *B. ciliate*, *B. pacumbis*, *B. purpurascens*, and *B. stracheyi* with associated target genes. A plug-in "Network Analyzer" was used to access the topological features of the network.

4.5. Protein–Protein Interaction Network

Protein–protein interactions (PPIs) are mandatory to reveal the underlying mechanisms and co-expression of genes [42]. The overlapped genes were imported into the STRING database with a confidence score of 0.7 for PPIs. Multiple protein identifiers were selected with *H. sapiens* as target species to construct the PPI maps. The constructed network was then imported into Cytoscape 3.9.1 software to visualize the topological analysis using Network Analyzer tool. A plug-in "CytoHubba" was used to obtain the hub genes with the highest degree.

4.6. Gene Ontology and KEGG Enrichment Analysis

The Gene Ontology (GO) and Kyoto Encyclopedia of Genes and Genomes (KEGG) gene enrichment analysis of selected genes was performed via the DAVID database [43]. DAVID is a functional annotation database which is used to categorize co-occurrence of sets of genes based on cellular component (CC), biological process (BP), and molecular functioning (MF). The KEGG analysis reveals high-level genome mapping that reveals the biological processes and molecular interactions of genes. The probability value of $p < 0.05$ was set to filter the top twenty enriched pathways for pathway–target network construction through Cytoscape 3.9.1 [41]. Bubble plot illustrations for enrichment analysis of GO and KEGG analyses were created through the online tool ShinyGO 0.77 [44].

4.7. Compound–Target–Pathway Network

Cytoscape 3.9.1 was used to build the compound–target–pathway (C-T-P) network by integration of compound–target and target–pathway networks. The C-T-P network helps to understand the interrelations of each gene with relevant pathways, which are involved in certain biological and cellular signaling cascades. This networking was used to determine the HCC-associated primary key target associations with the active phytochemicals.

4.8. Molecular Docking

The molecular docking study identifies the ligand–target protein interactions to verify the potential of selected ligands as drug candidates [45]. The results of network pharmacology and the potential of selected phytochemicals were further confirmed by the molecular docking approach. The 3D structures of selected receptor proteins were retrieved from the RCSB-PDB database (https://www.rcsb.org/) in .pdb format [46]. Similarly, the chemical structures of selected phytochemicals were retrieved from the PubChem database (https://pubchem.ncbi.nlm.nih.gov/) in .sdf format [47]. The receptor proteins were optimized by removal of ligands, water molecules, and addition of polar hydrogens.

The PyRx software was used for ligand–protein docking to explore the binding patterns of ligands to the active site residues of selected receptor proteins [48]. The docking score was set as selection criterion to choose the best ligands. Finally, the BIOVIA Discovery Studio Visualizer [49] was used to visualize and create 2D/3D figures of interactions and maps of key ligands with target proteins.

4.9. ADMET Profiling

The SwissADME [50] and pkCSM [51] freely available online servers were assessed to evaluate the ADMET profiling of selected compounds. The absorption, distribution, metabolism, excretion, and toxicity (ADMET) parameters play a leading role in drug development for finding potential drug candidates [52].

4.10. Experimental Study

4.10.1. Hep-G2 Cell Culture

The DMEM (Dulbecco's Modified Eagle Medium) with 10% fetal bovine serum (FBS) and 100 μL/mL each of streptomycin and penicillin was used to develop the hepatocellular carcinoma cell line Hep-G2. In a CO_2 incubator, Hep-G2 cells were maintained and allowed to grow at 37 °C with a 5% carbon dioxide source in a moist environment. For treatment purposes, the cells were seeded when sufficient confluence had been reached and 0.25% trypsin-EDTA was added to separate the cells [53].

4.10.2. MTT Cytotoxicity Assay

The MTT assay was used to determine the cytotoxicity-inducing ability of (+)-catechin 3-gallate, β-sitosterol, and leucocianidol. Cisplatin and DMSO were used as a standard drug and control, respectively. Using the MTT assay, the anticancer activities of the best selected phytochemicals were evaluated. For this work, Hep-G2 cells were seeded and planted on 96-well plates. After a 12 h incubation period, different concentrations (1.5625, 3.125, 6.25, 12.50, 25, 50, 100, and 200 μg/mL) of the best selected phytochemicals and cisplatin were delivered to the cancer cells. Following that, cells were treated with 50 μL/mL of MTT solution for 4 h at 37 °C. Then, 0.1% DMSO was also added before aspirating the media Finally, the ELIZA plate reader was used to note the absorbance at 540 nm [54].

$$I\% = \frac{[A540(\text{control}) - A540(\text{treated})]}{A540(\text{control})} \times 100$$

4.10.3. Statistical Analysis

The software Graph Pad Prism 8 was used for the statistical analysis and the significance of the inhibition data was measured using one-way ANOVA. The results with p-value > 0.05 were considered as statistically significant [55].

5. Conclusions

Hepatocellular carcinoma (HCC) is the most lethal cancer type with malignant tumors mostly reported in Asia and Europe. Despite systemic therapies, there is a continuous increase in death cases due to the limited diagnosis at the advanced stages of cancer and lack of diagnosis biomarkers. Moreover, combinational therapies are associated with adverse side effects that increase the mortality rate with the median postdiagnostic survival of 6–12 after an advanced stage. The network pharmacology approach has pointed out the compound-related targets for the management of HCC. The PPI, GO, and KEGG analyses have explored the top genes involved in the pathogenesis of HCC. The viability on HepG2 cells confirmed the cytotoxic effects of (+)-catechin 3-gallate and β-sitosterol in a dose-dependent manner. In the light of the current results, it has been concluded that *Bergenia* spp. could be used as a natural drug source to treat HCC. Furthermore, clinical and in vivo studies would be required to validate the potential of (+)-catechin gallate, specifically, and β-sitosterol and leucocianidol, generally, as the leading drug candidates for the treatment of HCC in the future.

Author Contributions: Conceptualization, G.M.; methodology, S.H. and G.M.; software, S.H. and G.M.; validation, G.M., S.A. and M.F.A.; formal analysis, S.H. and S.A.; investigation, S.H.; resources, G.M. and M.F.A.; data curation, G.M.; writing—original draft, S.H. and S.A.; writing—review and editing, G.M. and M.F.A.; supervision, G.M. All authors have read and agreed to the published version of the manuscript.

Funding: This research was funded by the Researchers Supporting Project Number (RSP2023R436), King Saud University, Riyadh, Saudi Arabia. A part of study was also supported by Higher Education Commission (HEC), Government of Pakistan through National Research Program for Universities (NRPU) with research grant number 20-15244/NRPU/R&D/HEC/2021.

Institutional Review Board Statement: Not applicable.

Informed Consent Statement: Not applicable.

Data Availability Statement: Data is contained within the article.

Acknowledgments: This study was supported by Researchers Supporting Project number (RSP2023R436), King Saud University, Riyadh, Saudi Arabia. Higher Education Commission (HEC), Government of Pakistan is also acknowledged for providing funds for a part of research work.

Conflicts of Interest: The authors declare no conflict of interest.

Sample Availability: Sequences and structures used in this study are available from the corresponding author upon request.

References

1. Singal, A.G.; Lampertico, P.; Nahon, P. Epidemiology and surveillance for hepatocellular carcinoma: New trends. *J. Hepatol.* **2020**, *72*, 250–261.
2. Sakurai, T.; Kudo, M. Molecular link between liver fibrosis and hepatocellular carcinoma. *Liver Cancer* **2013**, *2*, 365. [PubMed]
3. Sangro, B.; Sarobe, P.; Hervás-Stubbs, S.; Melero, I. Advances in immunotherapy for hepatocellular carcinoma. *Nat. Rev. Gastroenterol. Hepatol.* **2021**, *18*, 525–543. [PubMed]
4. Sayiner, M.; Golabi, P.; Younossi, Z.M. Disease burden of hepatocellular carcinoma: A global perspective. *Dig. Dis. Sci.* **2019**, *64*, 910–917.
5. Zhang, H.; Zhang, W.; Jiang, L.; Chen, Y. Recent advances in systemic therapy for hepatocellular carcinoma. *Biomark. Res.* **2022**, *10*, 1–21.
6. Mustafa, G.; Younas, S.; Mahrosh, H.S.; Albeshr, M.F.; Bhat, E.A. Molecular Docking and Simulation-Binding Analysis of Plant Phytochemicals with the Hepatocellular Carcinoma Targets Epidermal Growth Factor Receptor and Caspase-9. *Molecules* **2023**, *28*, 3583.
7. Khalaf, A.M.; Fuentes, D.; Morshid, A.I.; Burke, M.R.; Kaseb, A.O.; Hassan, M.; Hazle, J.D.; Elsayes, K.M. Role of Wnt/β-catenin signaling in hepatocellular carcinoma, pathogenesis, and clinical significance. *J. Hepatocell. Carcinoma* **2018**, *5*, 61–73.
8. Llovet, J.M.; Castet, F.; Heikenwalder, M.; Maini, M.K.; Mazzaferro, V.; Pinato, D.J.; Pikarsky, E.; Zhu, A.X.; Finn, R.S. Immunotherapies for hepatocellular carcinoma. *Nat. Rev. Clin. Oncol.* **2022**, *19*, 151–172.
9. Dutt, R.; Garg, V.; Khatri, N.; Madan, A.K. Phytochemicals in anticancer drug development. *Anti-Cancer Agents Med. Chem.* **2019**, *19*, 172–183.
10. Koul, B.; Kumar, A.; Yadav, D.; Jin, J.-O. Bergenia genus: Traditional uses, phytochemistry and pharmacology. *Molecules* **2020**, *25*, 5555.
11. Ali, I.; Bibi, S.; Hussain, H.; Bano, F.; Ali, S.; Khan, S.W.; Ahmad, V.U.; Al-Harrasi, A. Biological activities of *Suaeda heterophylla* and *Bergenia stracheyi* . *Asian Pac. J. Trop. Dis.* **2014**, *4*, S885–S889.
12. Wang, J.; Shi, J.; Jia, N.; Sun, Q. Network pharmacology analysis reveals neuroprotection of *Gynostemma pentaphyllum* (Thunb.) Makino in Alzheimer'disease. *BMC Complement. Med. Ther.* **2022**, *22*, 57. [CrossRef] [PubMed]
13. Sharif, S.; Atta, A.; Huma, T.; Shah, A.A.; Afzal, G.; Rashid, S.; Shahid, M.; Mustafa, G. Anticancer, antithrombotic, antityrosinase, and anti-α-glucosidase activities of selected wild and commercial mushrooms from Pakistan. *Food Sci. Nutr.* **2018**, *6*, 2170–2176.
14. Mustafa, G.; Ahmed, S.; Ahmed, N.; Jamil, A. Phytochemical and antibacterial activity of some unexplored medicinal plants of Cholistan desert. *Pak. J. Bot.* **2016**, *48*, 2057–2062.
15. Mustafa, G.; Arif, R.; Atta, A.; Sharif, S.; Jamil, A. Bioactive compounds from medicinal plants and their importance in drug discovery in Pakistan. *Matrix Sci. Pharma* **2017**, *1*, 17–26.
16. Ali, M.; Iqbal, R.; Safdar, M.; Murtaza, S.; Mustafa, G.; Sajjad, M.; Bukhari, S.A.; Huma, T. Antioxidant and antibacterial activities of Artemisia absinthium and Citrus paradisi extracts repress viability of aggressive liver cancer cell line. *Mol. Biol. Rep.* **2021**, *48*, 7703–7710. [CrossRef]
17. Spriha, S.E.; Rahman, S. In silico evaluation of selected compounds from *Bergenia ciliata* (haw.) sternb against molecular targets of breast cancer. *Indian J. Pharm. Educ. Res* **2022**, *56*, S105–S114. [CrossRef]

18. Faheem, M.M.; Bhagat, M.; Sharma, P.; Anand, R. Induction of p53 mediated mitochondrial apoptosis and cell cycle arrest in human breast cancer cells by plant mediated synthesis of silver nanoparticles from Bergenia ligulata (Whole plant). *Int. J. Pharm.* **2022**, *619*, 121710. [CrossRef]
19. Dulta, K.; Koşarsoy Ağçeli, G.; Chauhan, P.; Jasrotia, R.; Chauhan, P. A novel approach of synthesis zinc oxide nanoparticles by bergenia ciliata rhizome extract: Antibacterial and anticancer potential. *J. Inorg. Organomet. Polym. Mater.* **2021**, *31*, 180–190.
20. Noor, F.; Tahir ul Qamar, M.; Ashfaq, U.A.; Albutti, A.; Alwashmi, A.S.; Aljasir, M.A. Network pharmacology approach for medicinal plants: Review and assessment. *Pharmaceuticals* **2022**, *15*, 572.
21. Lee, C.; Cheung, S.T. STAT3: An emerging therapeutic target for hepatocellular carcinoma. *Cancers* **2019**, *11*, 1646. [PubMed]
22. Xu, J.; Lin, H.; Wu, G.; Zhu, M.; Li, M. IL-6/STAT3 is a promising therapeutic target for hepatocellular carcinoma. *Front. Oncol.* **2021**, *11*, 760971. [PubMed]
23. Moon, H.; Ro, S.W. MAPK/ERK signaling pathway in hepatocellular carcinoma. *Cancers* **2021**, *13*, 3026. [PubMed]
24. Hunter, C.A.; Koc, H.; Koc, E.C. c-Src kinase impairs the expression of mitochondrial OXPHOS complexes in liver cancer. *Cell. Signal.* **2020**, *72*, 109651.
25. Ren, H.; Fang, J.; Ding, X.; Chen, Q. Role and inhibition of Src signaling in the progression of liver cancer. *Open Life Sci.* **2016**, *11*, 513–518. [CrossRef]
26. Pal, D.; Sur, S.; Roy, R.; Mandal, S.; Kumar Panda, C. Epigallocatechin gallate in combination with eugenol or amarogentin shows synergistic chemotherapeutic potential in cervical cancer cell line. *J. Cell. Physiol.* **2019**, *234*, 825–836.
27. Sabry, D.; Abdelaleem, O.O.; El Amin Ali, A.M.; Mohammed, R.A.; Abdel-Hameed, N.D.; Hassouna, A.; Khalifa, W.A. Anti-proliferative and anti-apoptotic potential effects of epigallocatechin-3-gallate and/or metformin on hepatocellular carcinoma cells: In vitro study. *Mol. Biol. Rep.* **2019**, *46*, 2039–2047.
28. Ditty, M.J.; Ezhilarasan, D. β-sitosterol induces reactive oxygen species-mediated apoptosis in human hepatocellular carcinoma cell line. *Avicenna J. Phytomedicine* **2021**, *11*, 541.
29. Raj, R.K. β-Sitosterol-assisted silver nanoparticles activates Nrf2 and triggers mitochondrial apoptosis via oxidative stress in human hepatocellular cancer cell line. *J. Biomed. Mater. Res. Part A* **2020**, *108*, 1899–1908.
30. Maiyoa, F.; Moodley, R.; Singh, M. Phytochemistry, cytotoxicity and apoptosis studies of β-sitosterol-3-oglucoside and β-amyrin from Prunus africana. *Afr. J. Tradit. Complement. Altern. Med.* **2016**, *13*, 105–112.
31. Vivek-Ananth, R.; Mohanraj, K.; Sahoo, A.K.; Samal, A. IMPPAT 2.0: An enhanced and expanded phytochemical atlas of Indian medicinal plants. *ACS Omega* **2023**, *8*, 8827–8845. [PubMed]
32. Ru, J.; Li, P.; Wang, J.; Zhou, W.; Li, B.; Huang, C.; Li, P.; Guo, Z.; Tao, W.; Yang, Y. TCMSP: A database of systems pharmacology for drug discovery from herbal medicines. *J. Cheminform.* **2014**, *6*, 13.
33. Guo, W.; Huang, J.; Wang, N.; Tan, H.-Y.; Cheung, F.; Chen, F.; Feng, Y. Integrating network pharmacology and pharmacological evaluation for deciphering the action mechanism of herbal formula zuojin pill in suppressing hepatocellular carcinoma. *Front. Pharmacol.* **2019**, *10*, 1185. [PubMed]
34. Tao, W.; Xu, X.; Wang, X.; Li, B.; Wang, Y.; Li, Y.; Yang, L. Network pharmacology-based prediction of the active ingredients and potential targets of Chinese herbal Radix Curcumae formula for application to cardiovascular disease. *J. Ethnopharmacol.* **2013**, *145*, 1–10.
35. Daina, A.; Michielin, O.; Zoete, V. SwissTargetPrediction: Updated data and new features for efficient prediction of protein targets of small molecules. *Nucleic Acids Res.* **2019**, *47*, W357–W364. [CrossRef]
36. Szklarczyk, D.; Santos, A.; Von Mering, C.; Jensen, L.J.; Bork, P.; Kuhn, M. STITCH 5: Augmenting protein–chemical interaction networks with tissue and affinity data. *Nucleic Acids Res.* **2016**, *44*, D380–D384.
37. The UniProt Consortium. UniProt: The universal protein knowledgebase in 2021. *Nucleic Acids Res.* **2021**, *49*, D480–D489.
38. Safran, M.; Rosen, N.; Twik, M.; BarShir, R.; Stein, T.I.; Dahary, D.; Fishilevich, S.; Lancet, D. The genecards suite. In *Practical Guide to Life Science Databases*; Springer: Singapore, 2021; pp. 27–56.
39. Piñero, J.; Ramírez-Anguita, J.M.; Saüch-Pitarch, J.; Ronzano, F.; Centeno, E.; Sanz, F.; Furlong, L.I. The DisGeNET knowledge platform for disease genomics: 2019 update. *Nucleic Acids Res.* **2020**, *48*, D845–D855.
40. Bardou, P.; Mariette, J.; Escudié, F.; Djemiel, C.; Klopp, C. jvenn: An interactive Venn diagram viewer. *BMC Bioinform.* **2014**, *15*, 293. [CrossRef]
41. Shannon, P.; Markiel, A.; Ozier, O.; Baliga, N.S.; Wang, J.T.; Ramage, D.; Amin, N.; Schwikowski, B.; Ideker, T. Cytoscape: A software environment for integrated models of biomolecular interaction networks. *Genome Res.* **2003**, *13*, 2498–2504. [CrossRef]
42. Arif, R.; Zia, M.A.; Mustafa, G. Structural and functional annotation of napin-like protein from momordica charantia to explore its medicinal importance. *Biochem. Genet.* **2021**, *60*, 415–432.
43. Sherman, B.T.; Hao, M.; Qiu, J.; Jiao, X.; Baseler, M.W.; Lane, H.C.; Imamichi, T.; Chang, W. DAVID: A web server for functional enrichment analysis and functional annotation of gene lists (2021 update). *Nucleic Acids Res.* **2022**, *50*, W216–W221. [PubMed]
44. Ge, S.X.; Jung, D.; Yao, R. ShinyGO: A graphical gene-set enrichment tool for animals and plants. *Bioinformatics* **2020**, *36*, 2628–2629. [PubMed]
45. Mustafa, G.; Mahrosh, H.S.; Attique, S.A.; Arif, R.; Farah, M.A.; Al-Anazi, K.M.; Ali, S. Identification of Plant Peptides as Novel Inhibitors of Orthohepevirus A (HEV) Capsid Protein by Virtual Screening. *Molecules* **2023**, *28*, 2675. [PubMed]
46. Bittrich, S.; Rose, Y.; Segura, J.; Lowe, R.; Westbrook, J.D.; Duarte, J.M.; Burley, S.K. RCSB Protein Data Bank: Improved annotation, search and visualization of membrane protein structures archived in the PDB. *Bioinformatics* **2022**, *38*, 1452–1454.

47. Kim, S.; Chen, J.; Cheng, T.; Gindulyte, A.; He, J.; He, S.; Li, Q.; Shoemaker, B.A.; Thiessen, P.A.; Yu, B. PubChem 2019 update: Improved access to chemical data. *Nucleic Acids Res.* **2019**, *47*, D1102–D1109.
48. Dallakyan, S.; Olson, A.J. Small-molecule library screening by docking with PyRx. In *Chemical Biology. Methods in Molecular Biology*; Hempel, J., Williams, C., Hong, C., Eds.; Humana Press: New York, NY, USA, 2015; Volume 1263, pp. 243–250.
49. Sharma, S.; Sharma, A.; Gupta, U. Molecular Docking studies on the Anti-fungal activity of *Allium sativum* (Garlic) against Mucormycosis (black fungus) by BIOVIA discovery studio visualizer 21.1. 0.0. *Res. Sq.* **2021**. [CrossRef]
50. Daina, A.; Michielin, O.; Zoete, V. SwissADME: A free web tool to evaluate pharmacokinetics, drug-likeness and medicinal chemistry friendliness of small molecules. *Sci. Rep.* **2017**, *7*, 42717.
51. Pires, D.E.; Blundell, T.L.; Ascher, D.B. pkCSM: Predicting small-molecule pharmacokinetic and toxicity properties using graph-based signatures. *J. Med. Chem.* **2015**, *58*, 4066–4072.
52. Azeem, M.; Mustafa, G.; Mahrosh, H.S. Virtual screening of phytochemicals by targeting multiple proteins of severe acute respiratory syndrome coronavirus 2: Molecular docking and molecular dynamics simulation studies. *Int. J. Immunopathol. Pharmacol.* **2022**, *36*, 03946320221142793.
53. Rasul, A.; Riaz, A.; Wei, W.; Sarfraz, I.; Hassan, M.; Li, J.; Asif, F.; Adem, Ş.; Bukhari, S.A.; Asrar, M. *Mangifera indica* extracts as novel PKM2 inhibitors for treatment of triple negative breast cancer. *BioMed Res. Int.* **2021**, *2021*, 5514669. [PubMed]
54. Zara, R.; Rasul, A.; Sultana, T.; Jabeen, F.; Selamoglu, Z. Identification of *Macrolepiota procera* extract as a novel G6PD inhibitor for the treatment of lung cancer. *Saudi J. Biol. Sci.* **2022**, *29*, 3372–3379. [PubMed]
55. Abdel-Hamid, N.M.; EL-Gharieb, M.S.; El-Senduny, F.F.; Alnakib, N.A.-A. Effect of Doxorubicin and Cisplatin on Alpha-fetoprotein levels in Hepatocellular Carcinoma Cell lines. *Alfarama J. Basic Appl. Sci.* **2022**, *3*, 35–44.

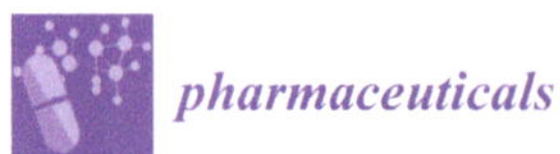

pharmaceuticals

Article

Neuroprotective Properties of Oleanolic Acid—Computational-Driven Molecular Research Combined with In Vitro and In Vivo Experiments

Katarzyna Stępnik [1,2,*], Wirginia Kukula-Koch [2], Wojciech Plazinski [3,4], Magda Rybicka [5] and Kinga Gawel [6]

[1] Department of Physical Chemistry, Institute of Chemical Sciences, Faculty of Chemistry, Maria Curie–Sklodowska University in Lublin, Pl. M. Curie-Skłodowskiej 3, 20-031 Lublin, Poland

[2] Department of Pharmacognosy with Medicinal Plants Garden, Medical University of Lublin, ul. Chodzki 1, 20-093 Lublin, Poland; virginia.kukula@gmail.com

[3] Department of Biopharmacy, Medical University of Lublin, ul. Chodzki 4a, 20-093 Lublin, Poland; wojtek_plazinski@o2.pl

[4] Jerzy Haber Institute of Catalysis and Surface Chemistry, Polish Academy of Sciences, ul. Niezapominajek 8, 30-239 Kraków, Poland

[5] Department of Photobiology and Molecular Diagnostics, Intercollegiate Faculty of Biotechnology, University of Gdansk and Medical University of Gdansk, ul. Abrahama 58, 80-307 Gdańsk, Poland; magda.rybicka@biotech.ug.edu.pl

[6] Department of Experimental and Clinical Pharmacology, Medical University of Lublin, ul. Jaczewskiego Str. 8b, 20-090 Lublin, Poland; kingagawel@umlub.pl

* Correspondence: katarzyna.stepnik@umcs.pl

Citation: Stępnik, K.; Kukula-Koch, W.; Plazinski, W.; Rybicka, M.; Gawel, K. Neuroprotective Properties of Oleanolic Acid—Computational-Driven Molecular Research Combined with In Vitro and In Vivo Experiments. *Pharmaceuticals* **2023**, *16*, 1234. https://doi.org/10.3390/ph16091234

Academic Editors: Halil İbrahim Ciftci, Belgin Sever and Hasan Demirci

Received: 27 July 2023
Revised: 24 August 2023
Accepted: 29 August 2023
Published: 31 August 2023

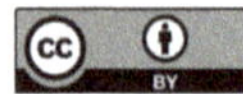

Abstract: Oleanolic acid (OA), as a ubiquitous compound in the plant kingdom, is studied for both its neuroprotective and neurotoxic properties. The mechanism of acetylcholinesterase (AChE) inhibitory potential of OA is investigated using molecular dynamic simulations (MD) and docking as well as biomimetic tests. Moreover, the in vitro SH-SY5Y human neuroblastoma cells and the in vivo zebrafish model were used. The inhibitory potential towards the AChE enzyme is examined using the TLC-bioautography assay (the IC_{50} value is 9.22 μM). The CH-π interactions between the central fragment of the ligand molecule and the aromatic cluster created by the His440, Phe288, Phe290, Phe330, Phe331, Tyr121, Tyr334, Trp84, and Trp279 side chains are observed. The results of the in vitro tests using the SH-SY5Y cells indicate that the viability rate is reduced to 71.5%, 61%, and 43% at the concentrations of 100 μg/mL, 300 μg/mL, and 1000 μg/mL, respectively, after 48 h of incubation, whereas cytotoxicity against the tested cell line with the IC_{50} value is 714.32 ± 32.40 μg/mL. The in vivo tests on the zebrafish prove that there is no difference between the control and experimental groups regarding the mortality rate and morphology ($p > 0.05$).

Keywords: molecular dynamic simulations; molecular docking; neuroprotection; acetylcholinesterase; zebrafish

1. Introduction

The increase in the average life expectancy is associated with the improvement of people's awareness, the availability of medicine, and greater effectiveness of pharmacological treatment results in civilization diseases, including memory disorders, malignant changes, hormonal disturbances, and others. Apart from oncological problems, neurodegenerative diseases constitute a serious therapeutic challenge. Problems associated with neuronal functions are observed with increasing age. These include the deterioration of memory pathways, known as dementia [1,2].

These cognitive impairments are associated with reduced levels of acetylcholine, a neuromodulator secreted by neurons to initiate the action potential necessary for memorizing and retrieving memories. A decrease in the concentration of acetylcholine combined with an increased efficiency of enzymes that break it down prematurely, still in the synaptic cleft before connecting to an appropriate cholinergic receptor, causes the memory process to be disturbed [3].

In addition, with age, beta-amyloid plaques appear on the surface of neurons. They disturb the physiological functioning of neurons, cause inflammation on the surface of neuronal cells, and lead to an accelerated death of nerve cells [4].

Modern medicine has long been trying to find an appropriate therapy to prolong the efficiency of the central nervous system (CNS). Pharmaceuticals available on the market are able to slow down the aging process of neurons, reduce inflammatory conditions in the CNS, and increase the acetylcholine uptake by inhibiting the enzymes that break it down. The latter are the first-line drugs in the treatment of dementia and Alzheimer's disease, which is a consequence of the rapidly progressing neurodegenerative changes in the CNS. Current therapy is able to slow down the course of the disease. However, the available drugs do not reverse their effects. Among the first-line drugs, there are substances of plant origin—the commonly used natural products include galantamine isolated from snowdrop, rivastigmine, a semi-synthetic derivative of physostigmine derived from calabar bean, as well as huperzine A from club moss (*Huperzia serrata*) and berberine from barberry species [5,6]. These plant-derived compounds, together with other synthetic drugs used in the treatment of dementia, have numerous side effects, such as nausea, apathy, low tolerance to the applied dose, short duration of action, and others. Some of them affect the activity of acetylcholinesterase (AChE), which is one of the two enzymes found in the intersynaptic cleft. Inhibition of both enzymes, AChE and the non-specific butyrylcholinesterase, is much more beneficial because it has a greater effect on the memory process [6,7].

In view of the above limitations of the existing therapy, it is necessary to search for new substances, also of plant origin, which could influence memory processes effectively and extend the independent functioning of many patients suffering from dementia.

In the search for new drug candidates, the authors of this paper decided to investigate the pharmacological potential of oleanolic acid (Figure 1)—a plant-derived secondary metabolite from the group of triterpenoid saponins identified in various plant species from the following botanical families: Lamiaceae, Fabaceaae, Myrtaceae, Oleaceae, Rosaceae, Pentaphylaceae, and others [8,9]. It is important to note that OA is one of the most commonly distributed triterpenoids in nature [9], for which several isolation protocols and biosynthetic pathways have been elaborated [10,11].

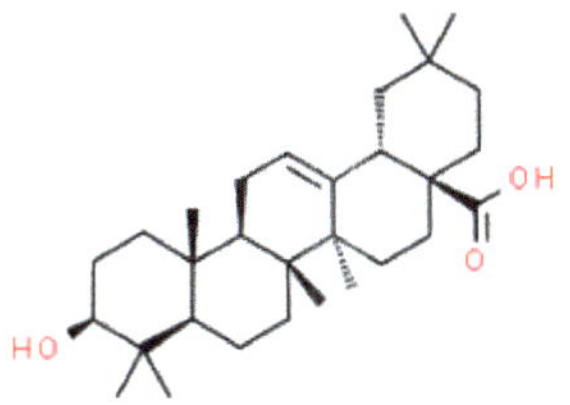

Figure 1. Chemical structure of oleanolic acid.

Oleanolic acid, a pentacyclic triterpenoid, was used in traditional Chinese medicine as an effective drug for the treatment of hepatic disorders. More recent studies have proven its antioxidant, antitumor, weight- and cholesterol-reducing, antidiabetic, and anti-inflammatory properties [9].

Considering the above statement and the good availability of OA, the authors found it important to study its neurological potential. This manuscript aims to determine its inhibitory properties towards acetylcholinesterase enzyme, its neuroprotective properties in the tests carried out on the SH-SY5Y human neuroblastoma cell line, its toxicity that will be tested in the zebrafish model, and finally, its potential mechanism of action that will be modeled by both computational and membrane-like techniques.

2. Results

2.1. The Pharmacokinetic In Silico Studies on BBB Permeation

The BBB pharmacokinetic descriptors were calculated using the ACD/Percepta software. The following were obtained: logBB—the logarithm of blood-to-brain partition coefficient; logPS—the logarithm of permeability–surface area product; logPSFb—the brain/plasma equilibration rate; Fu—the unbound fraction in plasma; Fb—the unbound fraction in the brain (Table 1). In order to extend the interpretation of BBB parameters, there were also calculated some important physicochemical descriptors using the ACD/Percepta software: logPow—the logarithm of n-octanol/water partition coefficient; TPSA—the topological polar surface area; MW—the molecular weight.

Table 1. BBB-pharmacokinetic and physicochemical parameters of OA obtained in silico (ACD/Percepta software).

logBB in silico	logPS	logPS$_{Fb}$	Fu	Fb	logPow	TPSA [Å^2]	MW [g/mol]
−0.45	−4.3	−6.1	0.0055	0.02	11.108	57.53	456.7

2.2. Anisotropic Membrane-like Systems

In order to determine the OA permeability through the BBB, High-Performance Liquid Chromatography (HPLC) was applied using cholesterol-bound (CHOL) as well as Immobilized Artificial Membrane (IAM) and Internal Surface Reverse Phase (ISRP) anisotropic membrane-like stationary phases.

The retention data obtained from these systems allow us to calculate the logarithms of retention factors extrapolated to the pure water (logkw) based on the Soczewiński–Wachtmeister Equation (1) [10]. These values are considered to be an alternative to the logPow (n-octanol/water partition coefficient) lipophilic descriptor [11]. The values obtained from Equation (1) are presented in Table 2.

$$\text{logk} = \text{logkw} - s\varphi \tag{1}$$

where logk is the logarithm of the retention factor; φ is the volume fraction of an organic modifier; s is the slope characteristic of a single solute in the given chromatographic system.

Table 2. The parameters of the Soczewiński–Wachtmeister equation calculated for the chromatographic systems under investigation.

Membrane-like System	logkw	s	R^2
IAM	1.656	1.515	0.991
CHOL	2.361	2.037	0.993
ISRP	0.637	1.853	0.983

2.3. QSAR Analysis for BBB Permeation

Based on our previously established model (2) [12], there was obtained the logBB value. For this purpose, some physicochemical parameters, as well as excess molar refraction from the Linear Free Energy Relationship (LFER) employed by Abraham, were calculated in silico using the ACD/Percepta software (Table 3).

$$\begin{aligned} \text{logBB} = -0.114 - 0.098\,\Delta\text{logP} + 0.278\,\text{logkw} + 0.218\text{E} \\ n = 40, \text{R}^2\text{CV} = 78.25\%, \text{R}^2\text{pred} = 74.02\%, \text{S} = 0.436 \end{aligned} \tag{2}$$

where E is the excess molar refraction and ΔlogP is the hydrogen-binding potential being the difference between the logkw lipophilic descriptor (in this case obtained from the membrane-like systems: logkw$_{ISRP}$, logkw$_{IAM}$, logkw$_{CHOL}$) and the cyclohexane/water (logPcw) partition coefficients values.

Table 3. Parameters for determination of logBB value using the QSAR analysis.

Membrane-like System	Logkw	logPcw	ΔlogP	E
ISRP	0.637		8.358	
IAM	1.656	8.995	7.339	1.46
CHOL	2.361		6.634	

Since the logkw value obtained from the anisotropic membrane-like analysis is widely treated in the chromatographic practice as a lipophilicity descriptor, in this model, it was applied instead of the logPow value used in the previous one. This modification was introduced to the model to examine whether the applied membrane-like analysis proved to be effective in estimating the ability of OA to permeate through the BBB. Figure 2 shows the logBB values obtained based on Equation (2) and the lipophilic logkw values from the anisotropic membrane-like systems.

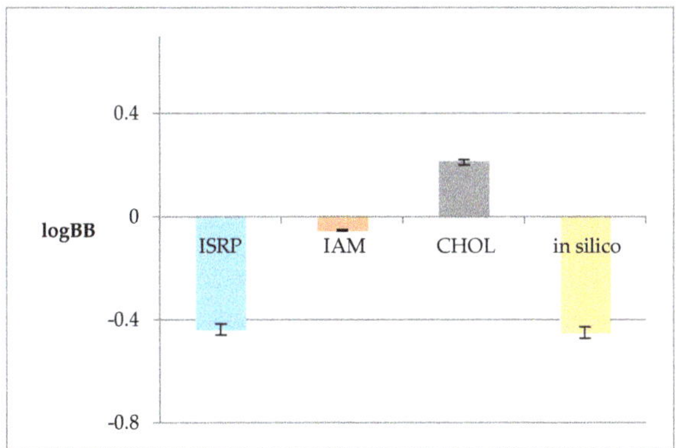

Figure 2. LogBB values calculated based on the QSAR model logkw values from the anisotropic membrane-like systems (ISRP, IAM, CHOL) and that calculated in silico using the ACD/Percepta software.

2.4. Acetylcholinesterase Inhibitory Activity of OA

The TLC-bioautography with the acetylcholinesterase enzyme as a spraying agent was performed to determine the AChE inhibitory properties of OA in the in vitro experiment and to find out whether the computational studies properly predicted the pharmacological properties of the compound. The interactions taking place on a TLC plate resemble those occurring in the brain. Spraying the TLC plate with a compound dispersed on its surface with an enzyme allows for direct contact of the enzyme with the compound of interest. This provides sufficient data to find out whether a compound interacts–inhibits the enzyme by competing with a substrate. The bright inhibition zones being observed on a TLC plate show an effective inhibition of the enzyme by the compound present on the TLC plate. In order to calculate the IC_{50} value, which is a measure of the compound's strength, and demonstrate the concentration of the compound of interest that inhibits the enzyme activity by 50%, five volumes of the OA stock solution (2, 4, 6, and 8 µL) corresponding to 0.002, 0.004, 0.006, and 0.008 mg of OA on the surface of the TLC plate were introduced onto the normal phase TLC plate covered with silica gel (Merck, Darmstadt, Germany). Later, the developed TLC plate was analyzed using an imaging program that transforms the obtained greyish zones, based on their intensity, to numerical value–peak areas. The experiment was repeated three times, and the average value of the obtained peak areas corresponding to different volume injections of OA was taken for the calculation of the IC_{50} value. As a result, there was obtained the following calibration curve equation: $y = 12491x - 12671$ (R^2 0.981). Based on this equation, the IC_{50} of OA was calculated to be 9.22 µM. The respective chromatogram is presented in Figure 3. At the same time, a similar test was performed for the standard of galanthamine. The IC_{50} calculated for this alkaloid was equal to 0.044 µM.

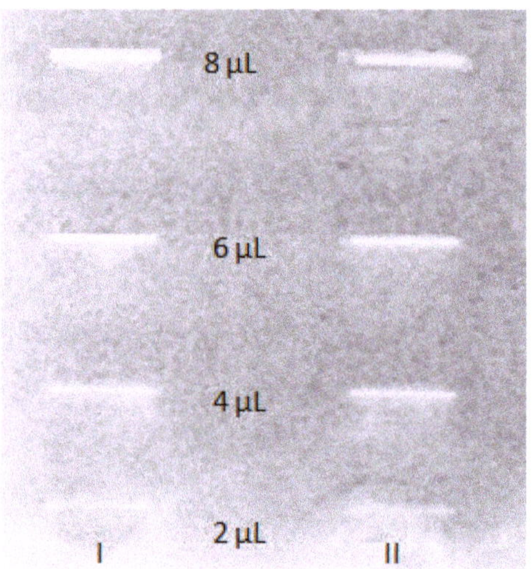

Figure 3. TLC bioautography results for acetylcholinesterase inhibition visualized in daylight. The TLC plate shows different concentrations of OA. I—1st; II—2nd replications.

2.5. Free Energy Calculations and Molecular Docking

Atomistic molecular dynamics simulations were executed to ascertain the affinity between OA and the lipid bilayers of homogeneous composition composed of either POPC or POPG phospholipids. These bilayers, within the scope of the present study, act as simplified representations of the blood–brain barrier. The 1D free energy profiles based on a single coordinate and associated with OA permeation through the bilayer are illustrated in Figure 4.

Both calculated free energy profiles validate OA's strong attraction to the lipid bilayer. This effect is expected due to its positive value of the $logP_{ow}$ parameter (varying from ca. 6.5 to 8.5, depending on the source). In none of the cases, the free energy barrier associated with the immersion into the bilayer was of significant height (<5 kJ/mol). Instead, some barriers of the height of ca. 12–17 kJ/mol appear within the bilayer center. They are associated with the full immersion of whole molecules into the lipid bilayer and disrupting the polar contacts between the hydroxyl and carboxyl groups of OA with the polar head groups of phospholipids. The immersion process is associated with the free energy change of either ca. 43 kJ/mol (POPC) or 23 kJ/mol (POPG), which indicates clearly that OA has a tendency to accumulate in the lipid bilayers and the permeability rate is associated with leaving the bilayer and migrating through it rather than entering it.

When considering interactions with AChE studied using the docking simulations, OA exhibits a high value of binding energy, equal to −61.5 kJ/mol, which indicates a favorable and strong ligand–protein binding.

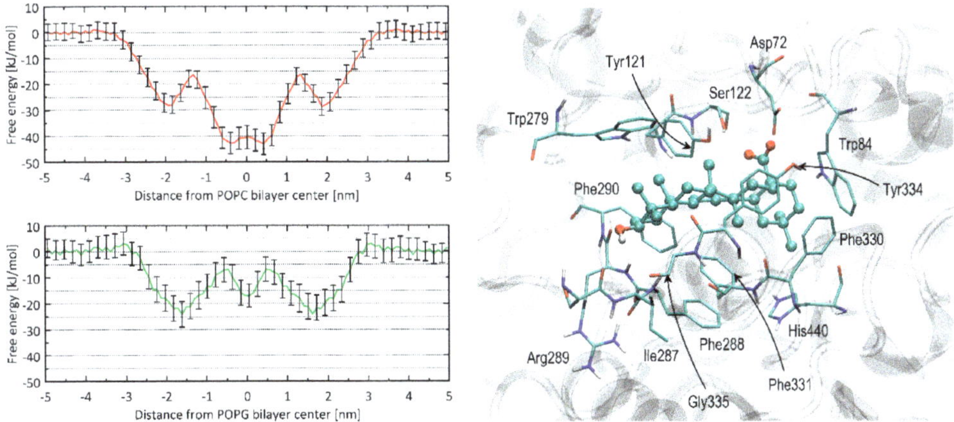

Figure 4. (left) The 1D free energy profiles accompanying the OA molecule movement through the system, including lipid bilayer. The systems contained two types of uniform bilayers: comprising POPC (red lines), or POPG (green lines). The associated error values (shown as vertical bars) were determined using bootstrapping. **(right)** The most favorable binding pose of the OA molecule interacting with AChE. The OA molecule is visualized as ball-and-stick, while amino acid residues in close proximity (within a distance of 0.38 nm) are depicted as thin sticks. Further details about the types of interactions are available in the text. The residue numbering is consistent with the PDB:3EVE record.

The results of the docking study were interpreted in terms of the mechanistic interaction pattern, which is important to understand the origin of the favorable binding energies and the mechanism of inhibition. The summary given below presents the analysis of the ligand–protein contacts that occur when the distance between any pair of corresponding atoms is smaller than the arbitrarily accepted value is 0.38 nm. The latter cutoff value is chosen particularly based on our experience in Vina-based docking and on the nature of the intermolecular interactions expected to occur in the biomolecular systems. Namely, such value allows us to spot all the polar interactions (including hydrogen bonds for which the typical donor-acceptor distance varies 0.25–0.35 nm) but also non-polar contacts characterized by larger interatomic distances (equal to ca. 0.30–0.38 nm in the case of carbon–carbon contact). For the system being presented, no additional amino-acid residues are included in the set of those interacting with the ligand upon increasing the cutoff value up to 0.45 nm.

The essential residues involved in the ligand–protein interactions identified upon accepting such a cutoff value are shown in Figure 4. It should be stressed that the reported results appeared to be reproducible when repeating the docking procedure three times. In particular, exactly the same binding energy values were obtained for the most energetically favorable configurations, and the binding arrangement of the docked ligand differed only by the marginal spatial shifts (<0.02 nm when expressed as RMSD). This is a consequence of the relatively small dimensions of the binding cavity with respect to the size of the ligand molecule; due to the sterically restricted configurational space, the docking algorithm is capable of finding only a single, most favorable pose. The remaining less favorable poses are characterized by significantly higher energy levels (at least 4 kJ/mol in reference to the lowest-energy pose). Thus, they were not considered in the subsequent analysis.

The position of OA in the enzyme cavity allows blocking of the catalytic site. In particular, the ligand molecule is arranged in close proximity to the catalytic His 440 residues. This steric hindrance is further supported by restricting the approach of potential substrates to the catalytic site. This can be attributed to the positioning of the ligand molecule within the vestibule of the binding site. The central fragment of the OA molecule, consisting of aliphatic and cyclic segments, remains in contact with a large aromatic cluster formed by numerous sidechains of the following residues: His440, Phe288, Phe290, Phe330, Phe331, Tyr121, Tyr334, Trp84, and Trp279. These ligand–AChE contacts can be categorized as CH-π interactions. These types of interactions are possible to occur between the aromatic and alkyl moieties; in the present case, the aromatic contribution always comes from the AChE residues (as listed above). The CH-π interactions have been identified as one of the essential driving forces playing a role in ligand–protein binding [13–15], particularly when a ligand molecule of aromatic character interacts with a cluster of aliphatic amino-acid sidechain or the opposite. The two polar moieties of OA, i.e., carboxyl and hydroxyl groups, interact with more polar side chains located closer to the binding cavity entrance. For instance, the carboxyl moiety interacts with Asp72 and Ser122 as well as with the hydroxyl group of Tyr121, whereas the hydroxyl moiety exhibits contact with the backbone fragments of Gly335, Phe290, and Arg289. Some of these contacts occur via hydrogen binding. The close presence of some other residues, e.g., Ile287, seems to be an opportunistic consequence of the previously-listed, more intensive interactions. Thus, the main driving force for binding is the non-polar CH-π interactions, allowing for minimizing the solvent-accessible surface of the aromatic cluster within the binding cavity of AChE; the scarce polar interactions play only a supporting role. Such mechanism of binding is in line with great affinity for the lipid bilayer discussed in the previous subsection as well as with the large, experimental $logP_{ow}$ value.

2.6. Inhibitory Effect of Oleanolic Acid on the SH-SY5Y Cell Viability

Effects of different concentrations of OA on the SH-SY5Y cells were measured using the MTT assays after 48 h of incubation (Figure 5).

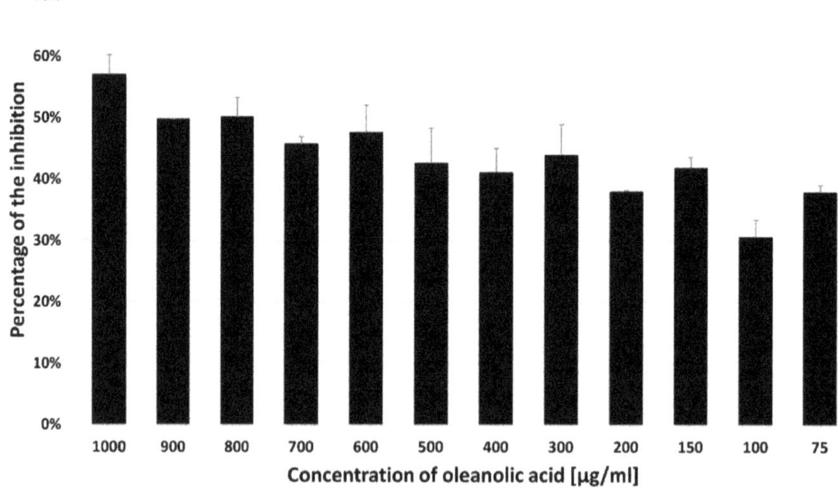

Figure 5. MTT results for the SH-SY5Y cells treated with OA. The OA IC_{50} value was calculated to be 715 µg/mL. The data are presented as the mean ± standard deviation (SD) of 3 independent experiments.

2.7. Effect of Oleanolic Acid on the Cell Cycle Analyzed with the Flow Cytometry

In order to investigate whether OA treatment affected the cell cycle, the SH-SY5Y cells were treated with 715 µg/mL of the compound for 48 h, stained with PI, and subjected to the flow cytometry analysis. The effect on the cell cycle phases in the SH-SY5Y cells treated with OA is shown in Figure 6.

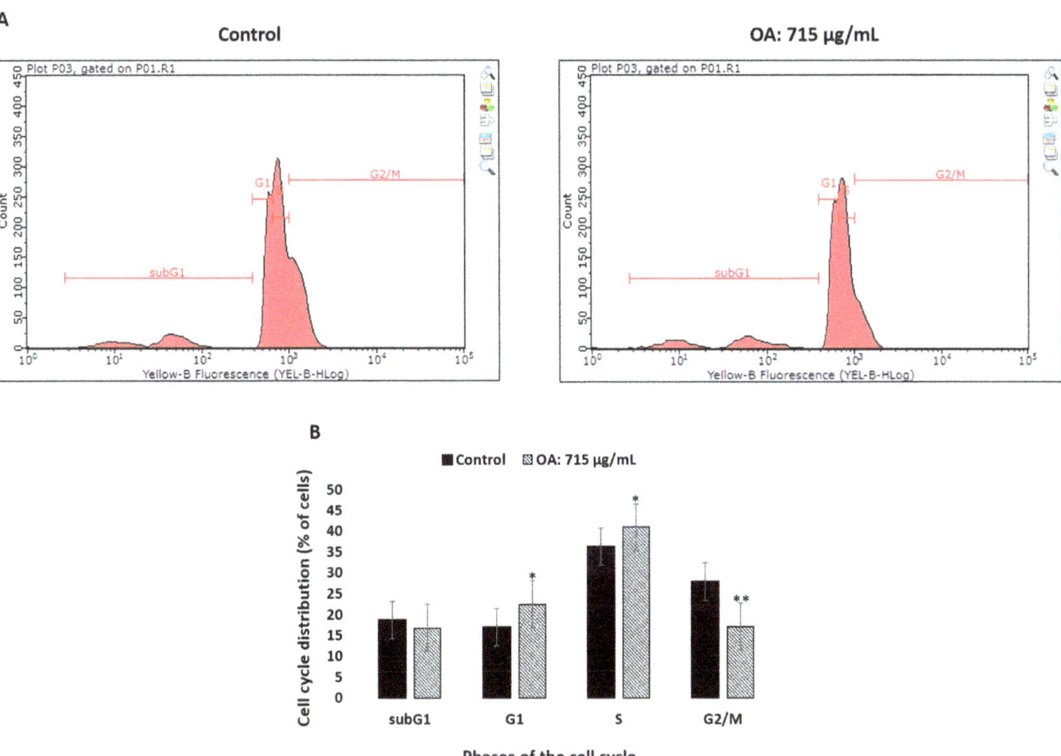

Figure 6. Effect on the phases of cell cycle in the SH-SY5Y cells treated with OA. (**A**)—The cell cycle distribution of PI-labelled cells was analyzed by flow cytometry in the SH-SY5Y control cells and cells treated with OA (715 µg/mL) for 48 h. (**B**)—The histogram shows the percentage of cells that are in different phases of the cell cycle. The results are expressed as the mean ± SD of three independent experiments. The p values below 0.05 (* $p < 0.05$, ** $p < 0.0001$) are considered statistically significant. The treated SH-SY5Y cells were arrested in the G1 phase and the percentage of cells in this phase increased from 16.87 ± 0.68% in the untreated cells to 23.57 ± 1.36% in the cells treated with oleanolic acid. Incubation with OA also caused an increase in the proportion of cells in the S phase (36.18 ± 1.50% vs. 40.85 ± 0.73%, $p = 0.023$) and a significant decrease in the G2/M phase (27.82 ± 0.86% vs. 17.02 ± 1.75%, $p < 0.0001$) of the cell cycle in the treated SH-SY5Y cells in comparison with the control.

2.8. Oleanolic Acid Is Non-Toxic for Developing Zebrafish

The zebrafish embryos were incubated in 715 µg/mL of OA for 95 h, starting at 1 hpf. The representative photo of 4 dpf control and OA-treated larvae is shown in Figure 7. Our study proved that there was no difference between the control and experimental groups as regards the mortality rate in any of the analyzed time points ($p > 0.05$). Furthermore, the larval hatchability was not influenced by OA on 3- and 4-day-old fish ($p > 0.05$). Likewise, taking into account the obtained morphological parameters and the touch-evoked response assay, no difference between the tested groups ($p < 0.05$) was observed. The fish looked similar and reacted to touch, like their control counterparts (Figure 7). Therefore, one may conclude that at the dose of 715 µg/mL, OA is non-toxic in vivo for the developing organism—it does not influence mortality, hatchability, morphology, or muscle performance and its function.

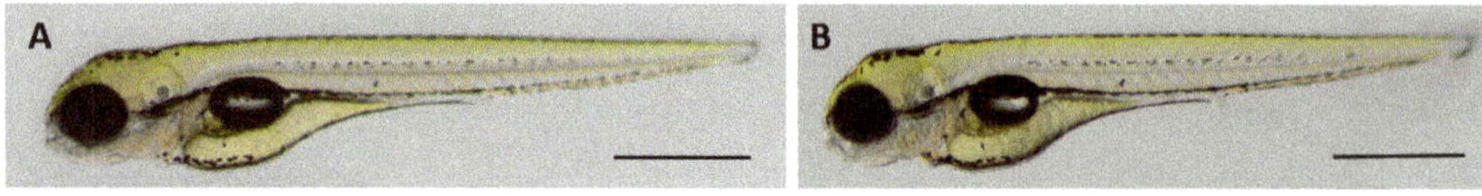

Figure 7. Representative photo of 4 dpf (**A**) control and (**B**) OA-treated larvae. Scale bars 1 mm.

3. Discussion

As mentioned above, neurodegenerative diseases with memory impairment constitute a growing problem mainly in aging societies. The World Health Organization predicts that the number of people suffering from dementia will be 132 million by 2050 [16]. Therefore, new therapeutic agents with possible reversal of memory impairment are constantly being sought. Undoubtedly, the plant kingdom is an interesting source of neuroactive substances, including neuroprotective and pro-cognitive ones.

The traditional Chinese herbs are undeniably a rich source of numerous substances acting on the CNS, e.g., *Ginkgo biloba* L. [17], *Panax ginseng* [18–22], or *Scutellaria baicalensis* [23–26]. Further, other plants grown in different parts of the earth are an invaluable source of neuroactive compounds, e.g., *Berberis integerrima* [27], *Carissa edulis* [28], *Melissa parviflora* [29], *Olea europaea* L. [30–32], *Salvia officinalis* L. [33–36], or *Rosmarinus officinalis* [37]. There are many chemical groups of CNS-active compounds: alkaloids [38,39], flavonoids [40,41], saponins [42,43], tannins [44,45], and terpenoids [46–49]. The mechanism of their action is based on the statement that they could affect both the CNS-nerve cells of the brain and the spinal cord, and thus, they can control, e.g., the mental activities, such as remembering or learning, and the autonomic nervous system, which is involved in the regulation of internal organs, heartbeat, circulation and breathing.

Oleanolic acid with numerous health-promoting properties [50] belongs to a group of pentacyclic triterpenoids whose, among others, cardioprotective [51–54], antioxidant [55], antimicrobial [56,57], anti-inflammatory [58], anticancer [59], pro-cognitive [60], hepatoprotective [61] properties have been proved by many scientific papers.

The in silico studies allowed the determination of the most important BBB-pharmacokinetic parameters, i.e., the distribution of a substance in the blood–brain area (logBB), the rate of passive diffusion/permeability (logPS), the brain/plasma equilibration rate (logPS$_{Fb}$), the fraction unbound in plasma (Fu) and the fraction unbound in the brain (Fb) The blood–brain distribution (BB), frequently expressed as logBB, is defined as the ratio between the concentration in the brain and the concentration in the blood [62,63].

The in silico obtained logBB and Fu values (Table 1) indicate low brain penetration. However, it is proved that OA can affect the CNS, among others, by alleviating brain damage in ischemic stroke and other brain disorders [64] and can also be used as a potential therapeutic agent in the treatment of both the neurodegenerative and neuropsychiatric disorders [65,66]. Taking into account the permeability–surface area product (expressed as logPS) which is closely related to the cerebral blood flow (CBF), it can be stated that OA exhibited even a smaller BBB-permeability potential in comparison with other triterpenoids from the *Terminalia arjuna* bark, i.e., arjunic acid, arjunolic acid, arjunglucoside I, arjunetin, sericic acid, and arjungenin. The CBF ensures the proper delivery of oxygen necessary for the neuronal oxidative metabolism of energy substrates. The PS typically expressed in units of mL blood/(100 g$_{tissue}$·min), or mL blood (100 mL$_{tissue}$·min) [67] or in mL blood/(h·kg) [68] is defined as the blood volume that flows per unit mass and per unit time in the brain tissue.

The smaller the values of the PS or Fb, the longer the time to reach the brain equilibrium is required. Therefore, the time to reach the brain equilibrium can be prolonged when the PS or the Fb decreases [68].

According to the free drug theory, each distribution process of a substance within a living organism depends on the unbound drug concentration [69,70]. As mentioned above,

OA shows the Fu to be only 0.0055. Such a small value of the unbound fraction in plasma could indicate a partial or complete lack of ability to cross the BBB. Nevertheless, it is also hypothesized that drugs that strongly bind to plasma protein can rapidly dissociate and permeate through the BBB into the brain tissues [69].

Taking into account a function of the relative plasma and brain tissue unbound fractions at the distribution equilibrium (Kp, brain), it was observed that OA binds to the plasma proteins more extensively than those in the brain tissues. This lower CNS-distribution potential than those of the other triterpenoids from the *Terminalia arjuna* bark may result from significant impairment in the CNS distribution by, e.g., the efflux transport at the BBB [71]. Analyzing the value of the fraction unbound in plasma in the light of the physicochemical properties of the investigated molecule, it can be stated that Fu depends more on the lipophilic properties of the compounds than on their steric and electronic parameters. This is because the molecule is relatively small (MW less than 500 Da), and the topological polar surface area is less than 100 Å^2. Numerous in silico studies, both earlier and contemporary, proved that there is a relationship between the physicochemical properties of a molecule and its BBB permeability [72–77]. The CNS drugs must cross the endothelium and partition into the aqueous environment of the cerebrospinal fluid and/or brain interstitial fluid [78]. Physicochemical parameters of a molecule, including steric, electronic, and lipophilic ones, are a key factor in this regard [79]. It is assumed that small hydrophilic compounds or those of large molecular weight (macromolecules), even if they are lipophilic, tend to be trapped in the cell membranes, and therefore they cannot cross the BBB passively [78]. The molecules of MW less than 400–500 Da can cross the BBB easily [80]. Besides the lipophilic and steric parameters, the topological polar surface area (TPSA) is of crucial importance for the ability of a substance to cross the BBB [81–83]. It is assumed that the substances that penetrate effectively into the brain tissues have a TPSA value of less than 100 Å^2 or, even smaller, less than 60–70 Å^2 [84].

The starting point for further research was the statement that among the physico-chemical properties of a molecule, lipophilicity is of key importance for the ability to cross biological barriers. Thus, more realistic models for the determination of lipophilicity than the computational ones were applied, i.e., anisotropic membrane-like systems. Taking into account the obtained results (Table 2) of the logkw parameter considered as the lipophilicity descriptor [11], it can be seen that the logkw values are much lower than the logarithm of n-octanol/water partition coefficient determined in silico. This can result from the fact that n-octanol is an isotropic phase contrary to the investigated anisotropic membrane-like systems in which phospholipids are spatially ordered. Further, the electric charge of the phospholipid membrane, which is devoid of n-octanol, makes the membrane-like model more realistic [85].

Based on the Soczewiński–Wachtmeister equation [10], strong linear relationships between the logkw and s values were observed (Table 2) in all the tested membrane-like systems. It is known that higher s values indicate more lipophilic compounds. This is in accordance with the background retention theory where s values correspond to both solute/mobile phase and the solvent/stationary phase net interactions [10]. The obtained logkw values were used to determine the logBB ones based on our QSAR model. As can be seen in Figure 2, the calculated logBB values do not differ significantly. However, the value obtained from the cholesterol-bound column has a negative sign, unlike the other values. This can be due to the retention thermodynamics of OA caused by the lipophilic interactions between the solute and the cholesterol-bound stationary phase ligands, which contribute to the enthalpic changes in the stationary phase [86].

The results of the TLC-bioautography towards the AChE inhibitory potential of OA provided evidence that this property was dependent on the introduced concentration. Taking into account the AChE inhibitory potential of the other compounds of plant origin, it can be observed that OA exhibits a relatively strong inhibitory potential. The comparable IC_{50} values with that obtained for OA (9.22 μM) were determined for the following metabolites: infractopicrin (*Cortinarius infractus* Berk; Cortinariaceae; IC_{50} of 9.72 ± 0.19 μM), hydrohydrastinine (*Corydalis mucronifera* Maxim.; Papaveraceae IC_{50} of 9.13 ± 0.15 μM), jadwarine-A (*Delphinium denudatum*; Ranunculaceae; IC_{50} of 9.2 ± 0.12 μM), or coronaridine (*Ervatamia hainanensis* Tsiang; Apocynaceae; IC_{50} of8.6 μM) [6]. These compounds belong to the alkaloid chemical group. Among triterpenoids of the plant origin, there is 21β-Hydroxyserrat-14-en-3,16-dione from *Lycopodiella cernua* L. Lycopodiaceae) for which a similar IC_{50} value was observed (10.67 ± 0.66 μM) [6]. In comparison to galanthamine (IC_{50} of 3.52 μM [87]) being the first-line drug in the treatment of Alzheimer's disease, it can be stated that OA is a promising compound in this regard.

The results of the AChE inhibition studies inspired the authors to investigate the molecular aspects of BBB permeation and the character of interactions with the AChE enzyme. Due to the fact that only a single compound is considered, we were not able to examine the correlation between the experimentally determined IC_{50} values and the theoretically predicted binding energies, as was performed in our previous study [87]. However, this value is in line with the expectation based on the large dimension of the considered molecule and its more hydrophobic character of OA in comparison to the other previously considered pentacyclic triterpenoid of plant origin, i.e., astragaloside IV [88].

The viability rate of SH-SY5Y cells was reduced to 71.5%, 61%, and 43% at the concentrations of 100 μg/mL, 300 μg/mL, and 1000 μg/mL, respectively, after 48 h of incubation with OA. Cytotoxicity of the compound against the SH-SY5Y cell line with the IC_{50} value was 714.32 ± 32.40 μg/mL. As shown in Figure 6, the treated SH-SY5Y cells were arrested in the G1 phase, and the percentage of cells in this phase increased from $16.87 \pm 0.68\%$ in the untreated cells to $23.57 \pm 1.36\%$ in the cells treated with OA. Incubation with OA also caused an increase in the proportion of cells in the S phase ($36.18 \pm 1.50\%$ vs. $40.85 \pm 0.73\%$, $p = 0.023$) and a significant decrease in the G2/M phase ($27.82 \pm 0.86\%$ vs. $17.02 \pm 1.75\%$, $p < 0.0001$) of the cell cycle in the treated SH-SY5Y cells in comparison with the control.

As regards the in vivo studies, there was no difference between the control and experimental groups as regards the mortality rate in any of the analyzed time points ($p > 0.05$). Furthermore, the larval hatchability was not influenced by OA on 3- and 4-day-old fish ($p > 0.05$). Likewise, taking into account the obtained morphological parameters and the touch-evoked response assay, no difference between the tested groups ($p < 0.05$) was observed. The fish looked similar and reacted to touch, like their control counterparts (Figure 7). Therefore, one may conclude that OA at the dose of 715 μg/mL is non-toxic in vivo for the developing organism—it does not influence mortality, hatchability, morphology, or muscle performance and its function.

4. Materials and Methods

4.1. Chemicals

The OA pharmacopoeial standard was purchased from Sigma Aldrich (Sigma Aldrich, St. Louis, MO, USA; p.a.). All the chromatographic measurements were made using acetonitrile (ACN; Sigma Aldrich, St. Louis, MO, USA; p.a)—water. Distilled water was obtained from the Direct-Q3 UV apparatus (Millipore, Warsaw, Poland). All solvents were >98% pure by the HPLC analysis.

4.2. In Silico Determination of Blood–Brain Barrier (BBB) Pharmacokinetic Descriptors

The BBB-pharmacokinetic descriptors were calculated using the ACD/Percepta software (version 2012, Advanced Chemistry Development, Inc., Toronto, ON, Canada).

4.3. Membrane-like Chromatographic Equipment and Conditions

The HPLC experiments were carried out on a Shimadzu Vp liquid chromatography system (Shimadzu, Kyoto, Japan) equipped with an LC 10AT pump, an SPD 10A UV-Vis detector, an SCL 10A system controller, a CTO-10 AS oven and a Rheodyne injector valve with a 20 μL loop. The solution of the pharmacopoeial OA standard was prepared in methanol (Merck, Darmstadt, Germany; p.a.) at a concentration of 1 mg/mL. The OA was found to be in the neutral form in solution under the experimental conditions. The optimization process was carried out before the chromatographic measurements. The flow rate of the mobile phases was set at 1 mL/min and the temperature at 20 °C. The analyte was detected with UV light at $\lambda = 214$ nm.

Three chromatographic columns, i.e., IAM.PC.DD2 column (IAM; 100×4.6 mm i.d., 10 μm; Regis Technologies, Morton Grove, IL, USA), cholesterol-bound (CHOL; Cosmosil; 75×2 mm i.d., 2.5 μm; Genore, Warsaw, Poland), and Internal Surface Reverse Phase (ISRP) were used as the anisotropic membrane-like stationary phases. The mobile phases were composed of acetonitrile-water as follows: 0.75; 0.80; 0.85; 0.90 *v/v* ACN-water for IAM, 0.70; 0.75; 0.80; 0.85 *v/v* ACN/water for CHOL, and 0.60; 0.65; 0.70; 0.75 *v/v* ACN/water for ISRP system. Each measurement was repeated three times.

The peaks of the citric acid were used as the dead time values. The average value of the obtained retention time was used to calculate the dead time for each system individually. The values of peak asymmetry factor were in the acceptable range.

4.4. Quantitative Structure-Activity Relationship (QSAR) Studies for Estimation of Permeation through the BBB

In order to examine the quantitative relationship between the ability of OA to cross the BBB and its physicochemical properties, the previously set up QSAR model was employed. The selection and multiple division of the dataset were thoroughly described in our previous paper [12]. Briefly, the establishment of a new model was based on the experimentally obtained distribution of the substance in the blood–brain area (logBB) values of 40 chemically diverse compounds [89]. The database was divided randomly into the test set and the training set (10 and 30 compounds, respectively). While setting up the model, the multiple linear regression (MLR) methodology with the backward elimination of variables was applied. This procedure was replicated several times to obtain the best fit between the logBB descriptor and the physicochemical parameters of OA. The predictive potency of the model was investigated based on the leave-ten-out (LTO) cross-validation. Moreover, the applicability domain was applied to evaluate the model's reliability [12]. The following analyses of variance coefficients were performed, including the determination coefficient (R^2), root-mean-square error (RMSE), root-mean-square error of leave-ten-out cross-validation (RMSECV), and predicted residual sum of squares (PRESS).

4.5. TLC-Bioautography Assay toward the Inhibition of Acetylcholinesterase (AChE) Activity

The OA pharmacopoeial standard purchased from Sigma Aldrich (St. Louis, MO, USA) was prepared at the concentration of 1 mg/mL in the double-distilled water: methanol (50:50 *v/v*), and it was applied on the aluminum sheet with the silica gel surface (10 cm $\times$ 10 cm TLC silica gel plate 60 F_{254}, Merck, Darmstadt, Germany) with an autosampler (Camag, Muttenz, Switzerland). The reference solution was applied as 2, 4, 6, 8, and 10 μL volume bands. The measurement was repeated twice, and the average value of the obtained peak areas was taken for IC_{50} value calculation.

According to the previously published protocol [90], the enzymatic assay with some modifications was used, i.e., instead of chromatogram development, the TLC plate was directly sprayed with the substrate (2-naphtyl acetate) dissolved in distilled water with the quantity of 30 mg/20 mL.

The AChE enzyme (from the electric eel type VI-S, Sigma Aldrich, St. Louis, CA, USA) was dissolved in the aqueous solution of trizma buffer (pH 7.8) with bovine serum (500 mg/100 mL, Sigma Aldrich) with the quantity of 3 U/mL. The TLC plate previously dried in cold air was sprayed with the AChE solution and incubated at the temperature of 37 °C for the following 20 min in the humid incubator. After that, the Fast Blue B salt solution was prepared by dissolving the salt in distilled water to obtain a concentration of 0.612 mg/mL. Then, the TLC plate was sprayed with the Fast Blue B solution and visualized active zones as white spots against the violet background. The discolored areas corresponded to the AChE inhibitory activity of the respective zones.

Then, the dried TLC plate was analyzed using the Camag TLC visualizer in visible light. The peak areas of the discolored zones were automatically calculated by the WinCats software (v. 1.4, Camag, Muttenz, Switzerland), and their sizes were used to calculate the IC_{50} values that corresponded to the concentration of the standard providing half maximum inhibition of AChE enzyme.

4.6. Molecular Docking

The molecular docking was performed in accordance with the applied methodology and validated in our previous studies [88]. The OA molecule (deprotonated, as indicated by the corresponding pK_a value) was created using the online SMILES translator [91] and optimized within the UFF force field [92] (5000 steps, steepest descent algorithm) and the Avogadro 1.1.1 software [93]. The optimized ligand molecule was docked into a binding pocket of the protein structure found in the PDB database (PDB:1EVE) according to the flexible docking approach, i.e., the rotatable torsional angles in the ligand molecule were allowed to change their conformation. Docking was performed using the AutoDock Vina 1.1.2 software [94]. The process involved the $22 \times 30 \times 24$ Å^3 cuboid region, which includes the co-crystallized ligand present in the considered PDB entry as well as the nearest amino acid residues being in contact with this ligand. For efficient sampling of possible poses, the exhaustiveness parameter has been increased to 18, whereas the number of generated poses to 20. The exhaustiveness parameter affects the number of iterations in one run, and its increase decreases the probability of not finding the minimum binding energy. As indicated in systematic investigations, elevating the value of this parameter from the default one of 8 leads to results that are more realistic in the context of spatial variation of the docked ligands [95]. Furthermore, the docking procedure followed all standard protocols and algorithms set as default in AutoDock Vina. Alongside the ligand's flexibility, rearrangements in the rotatable torsional angles were permitted for specific amino-acid side chains within the binding cavity. These included Tyr334, Phe288, His440, Gln74, Phe330, Phe75, Trp84, Glu199, Ser200, Tyr70, Tyr121, Trp279, Phe290, Phe331, Leu282, Trp432, Asn85, and Asp285. In order to assess the consistency of outcomes achieved through Vina's inherently non-deterministic algorithm, the docking procedure was repeated three times.

4.7. Free Energy Profiles

Free energy profiles were calculated using the molecular dynamics (MD) approach along the 1D coordinate, which expresses the position of the OA molecule with respect to the homogeneous lipid bilayer. The methodology was analogous to that used in our previous work [88]. The MD simulations were conducted utilizing the GROMOS 53a6 force field [96] and the GROMACS 2016.1 MD package [97]. Each simulation system comprised the deprotonated OA molecule and a lipid bilayer. These components were placed within simulation boxes containing SPC water molecules [98], along with Na^+ and Cl^- ions, to maintain a net charge of zero and an ionic strength of 0.15 M. Two versions of the lipid bilayer were considered: one composed exclusively of 1-palmitoyl-2-oleoyl-sn-glycero-3-phosphocholine (POPC) phospholipids and the other of 1-palmitoyl-2-oleoyl-sn-glycero-3-phosphoglycerol (POPG) phospholipids. The parameters for the phospholipids were sourced from [99], while those for OA were generated using the Automated Topology Builder online server [100]. Simulations were performed under periodic boundary conditions within rectangular computational boxes initially measuring around $8 \times 8 \times 12$ nm. After geometry optimization and equilibration procedures, non-equilibrium pulling simulations were initiated in order to induce the migration of the OA molecule from the bulk solution through the lipid bilayer and back to the bulk solution. The harmonic potential associated with this process had a force constant of 5000 kJ mol^{-1} nm^{-2}, and the pulling rate was set at 0.01 nm ps^{-1}. The Z-axis position of the OA molecule perpendicular to the bilayer served as the pulling coordinate. The reaction coordinate was divided into 40 windows spanning approximately from -5 to 5 nm (with the center of the bilayer corresponding to zero), and 40 independent simulations were initiated. Each simulation employed an umbrella harmonic potential with a force constant of $1000 \text{ kJ mol}^{-1} \text{ nm}^{-2}$, based on the distance between the center of mass of the OA molecule and the box center. Data within each window were collected every 2 ps for a duration of 40 ns. After discarding the initial 5 ns for equilibration, 1D free energy profiles were constructed using the weighted histogram analysis method (WHAM) [101] implemented in GROMACS (as *gmx wham*) [102]. Statistical uncertainties in the energy profiles were determined using Bayesian bootstrapping of complete histograms [102]. Integration of equations of motion was carried out with a timestep of 2 fs. Bond lengths were constrained using the P-LINCS algorithm [103]. Temperature control (310 K) employed the V-rescale thermostat [104], while for pressure control (1 atm, semiisotropic coordinate scaling), the Parrinello–Rahman barostat with a relaxation time of 1 ps [105] was applied. Center of mass motion was removed at each step. Electrostatic interactions were treated using the particle-mesh Ewald (PME) method [106], with a short-range cutoff of 1.2 nm. Van der Waals interactions were gradually switched off at the distance from 1.0 nm to 1.2 nm.

4.8. Cytotoxicity Test in Human Neuroblastoma In Vitro

4.8.1. Cell Culture

The human neuroblastoma SH-SY5Y cells (CRL-2266) obtained from American Type Culture Collection (Manassas, VA, USA) were cultured in the RPMI 1640 medium (Gibco, Invitrogen, Carlsbad, CA, USA) containing 8% FBS (Gibco, Invitrogen, USA), 5% penicillin and streptomycin (Gibco, Invitrogen, USA). At an initial plating density of 0.5 million cells per plate, cells were routinely trypsinized and subcultured.

4.8.2. MTT Assay

The OA cytotoxicity against the SH-SY5Y neuroblastoma cells was determined using the methyl thiazol tetrazolium (MTT) assay. Cells were initially seeded on a 96-well plate with a density of 2×10^4 cells per well and incubated in the CO_2 incubator for 24 h at 37 °C. On the following day, the medium was replaced with a fresh medium supplemented with different concentrations of OA from 100–1000 µg/mL. Each 96-well plate was set up with control (untreated) and blank (medium only) groups. Three biological replicates with four technical replicates each were performed. After 48 h, the culture medium was replaced with fresh medium, and the cells were incubated with 20 µL of MTT working solution (Invitrogen, CA USA) (5 mg/µL) at 37 °C for 3 h. The supernatant was then removed, and purple formazan crystals were solubilized in 100 µL/well of dimethyl sulfoxide (DMSO), followed by incubation (30 min). The absorbance of the formazan solution was measured at 550 nm using a BioTek Epoch 2 Microplate Spectrophotometer (Agilent Technologies, Inc., Santa Clara, CA, USA), and the percentage of cell viability was calculated as follows: [viability (%) = (OD, experimental group − OD, control group)/OD, control group − OD, control group) × 100%]. The cell inhibition ratio (%) = 1 − the cell viability (%)]. The half maximal inhibitory concentration (IC_{50}) was calculated by plotting the graph between the different concentrations of oleanolic acid and the percentage of cell growth inhibition.

4.8.3. Cell Cycle Analysis

Propidium iodide (PI) was used to determine cell cycle progression. SH-SY5Y cells were seeded at 2×10^5 cells/mL in 6-well plates and cultured for 24 h. Subsequently, the culture medium was replaced with the fresh medium (control cells), or cells were exposed to 715 µg/mL OA. Following 48 h incubation, the harvested cells were washed with PBS, centrifuged ($300 \times g$, 6 min, 4 °C), and fixed with ice-cold 70% ethanol at 4 °C overnight. According to the protocol of FxCycle™ PI/Rnase Staining Solution (Thermo Fisher, Scientific, Waltham, MA, USA), three wash steps with PBS were performed. The cells were resuspended to ~1×10^6 cells. Analysis was performed using a Guava easyCyte flowcytometer (Merck, Germany). A total of 10,000 events were obtained per sample.

4.9. Toxicity Analysis in Zebrafish In Vivo

4.9.1. Animals

The embryos of zebrafish (*Danio rerio*) that were used in the study were obtained from the Medical University of Lublin (Poland)–from the Experimental Medicine Centre. The animals were kept in an incubator in a specific zebrafish medium in the following conditions: at the temperature of 28.5 °C $\pm$ 0.5 °C, in the light/dark cycle of 14/10 h, and until the time of 96 h post-fertilization (hpf). The following study was conducted according to the National Institutes of Health Guide for the Care and Use of Laboratory Animals (Directive 2010/63/EU). The aforementioned directive states that there is no ethical approval needed for the yolk-feeding larvae that are up to 120 hpf. Nevertheless, during the experiment, all precautions were taken to limit the number of animals used in the study and to reduce their suffering. For euthanasia, a solution of 15 μM tricaine was used immediately after the completion of the planned experiment.

4.9.2. Zebrafish Embryo Acute Toxicity Test

The OA potential toxicity (715 μg/mL) was examined in the zebrafish embryo acute toxicity test in accordance with the Organization for Economic Cooperation and Development (OECD) recommendation for the testing of chemicals (Test No. 236 [107,108]). Zebrafish embryos were screened for viability, shape, and transparency one hour after fertilization. Only the eggs meeting all criteria, i.e., being viable, completely transparent, and round, were chosen and moved to 12 well plates (Sarstedt, Germany). They were randomly divided into two groups, the control and experimental ones, and kept in each well until the time of experiment elapsed, i.e., up to 96 h. Two batches of embryos (3 wells per batch, n = 5–7 per well) were kept in 3000 μL of the zebrafish medium (control group) or supplemented with 715 μg/mL of OA (experimental group). The mortality rate was scored after 23, 47, 71, and 95 h of incubation. Hatchability was assessed after 71 and 95 h of incubation. The morphological abnormalities were assessed after 95 h of incubation: heartbeat, heart/yolk edema, yolk sac necrosis, hemorrhage [108], jaw development, eye size, and posture. Additionally, for assessing muscle function and performance, the touch-evoked response assay was conducted as described in detail previously [109,110].

4.9.3. Statistical Analysis

The pooled data from the zebrafish experiment were analyzed using the Chi-squared or Fisher's exact test (GraphPad Prism 9.3.1).

5. Conclusions

The results of the studies showed that oleanolic acid may be active towards the AChE enzyme. The in vitro and in vivo tests confirmed its safety in the used doses. Therefore, this can be a novel drug candidate with neuroprotective potential in the treatment of neurodegenerative diseases and an interesting source of further, more profound research in this aspect.

Author Contributions: Conceptualisation, K.S.; methodology, K.S., W.K.-K., W.P., M.R. and K.G.; software, W.P.; validation, K.S., W.K.-K., W.P., M.R. and K.G.; formal analysis, K.S. and W.K.-K.; investigation, K.S., W.K.-K., W.P., M.R. and K.G.; resources, K.S. and W.K.-K.; data curation, K.S.; writing—original draft preparation, K.S.; visualisation, W.P.; supervision, K.S.; project administration, K.S.; funding acquisition, K.S. and W.K.-K. All authors have read and agreed to the published version of the manuscript.

Funding: This research was funded by Union of Lublin Universities in the framework of the program INTERPROJEKT (No. INT/001/2023/II-N).

Institutional Review Board Statement: Not applicable.

Informed Consent Statement: Not applicable.

Data Availability Statement: Data is contained within the article.

Conflicts of Interest: The authors declare no conflict of interest. The funders had no role in the design of the study; in the collection, analyses, or interpretation of data; in the writing of the manuscript; or in the decision to publish the results.

References

1. Tarabasz, D.; Szczeblewski, P.; Laskowski, T.; Płaziński, W.; Baranowska-Wójcik, E.; Szwajgier, D.; Kukula-Koch, W.; Meissner, H.O. The Distribution of Glucosinolates in Different Phenotypes of Lepidium peruvianum and Their Role as Acetyl- and Butyrylcholinesterase Inhibitors—In Silico and In Vitro Studies. *Int. J. Mol. Sci.* **2022**, *23*, 4858. [CrossRef] [PubMed]
2. Kukula-Koch, W.; Koch, W.; Czernicka, L.; Główniak, K.; Asakawa, Y.; Umeyama, A.; Marzec, Z.; Kuzuhara, T. MAO-A Inhibitory Potential of Terpene Constituents from Ginger Rhizomes-A Bioactivity Guided Fractionation. *Molecules* **2018**, *23*, 1301. [CrossRef] [PubMed]
3. Urbain, A.; Simões-Pires, C.A. Thin-Layer Chromatography for the Detection and Analysis of Bioactive Natural Products. In *Encyclopedia of Analytical Chemistry*; Meyers, R.A., Ed.; Wiley: Hoboken, NJ, USA, 2023. [CrossRef]
4. Rajmohan, R.; Reddy, P.H. Amyloid-Beta and Phosphorylated Tau Accumulations Cause Abnormalities at Synapses of Alzheimer's disease Neurons. *J. Alzheimer's Dis. JAD* **2017**, *57*, 975–999. [CrossRef] [PubMed]
5. Abdykerimova, S.; Sakipova, Z.; Nakonieczna, S.; Koch, W.; Biernasiuk, A.; Grabarska, A.; Malm, A.; Kozhanova, K.; Kukula-Koch, W. Superior Antioxidant Capacity of Berberis iliensis-HPLC-Q-TOF-MS Based Phytochemical Studies and Spectrophotometric Determinations. *Antioxidants* **2020**, *9*, 504. [CrossRef] [PubMed]
6. Smyrska-Wieleba, N.; Mroczek, T. Natural Inhibitors of Cholinesterases: Chemistry, Structure–Activity and Methods of Their Analysis. *Int. J. Mol. Sci.* **2023**, *24*, 2722. [CrossRef]
7. Mroczek, T.; Dymek, A.; Widelski, J.; Wojtanowski, K.K. The Bioassay-Guided Fractionation and Identification of Potent Acetylcholinesterase Inhibitors from Narcissus c.v. 'Hawera' Using Optimized Vacuum Liquid Chromatography, High Resolution Mass Spectrometry and Bioautography. *Metabolites* **2020**, *10*, 395. [CrossRef]
8. Ouyang, C.; Ma, X.; Zhao, J.; Li, S.; Liu, C.; Tang, Y.; Zhou, J.; Chen, J.; Li, X.; Li, W. Oleanolic acid inhibits mercury chloride induced-liver ferroptosis by regulating ROS/iron overload. *Ecotoxicol. Environ. Saf.* **2023**, *258*, 114973. [CrossRef]
9. Ayeleso, T.B.; Matumba, M.G.; Mukwevho, E. Oleanolic Acid and Its Derivatives: Biological Activities and Therapeutic Potential in Chronic Diseases. *Molecules* **2017**, *22*, 1915. [CrossRef]
10. Castellano, J.M.; Ramos-Romero, S.; Perona, J.S. Oleanolic Acid: Extraction, Characterization and Biological Activity. *Nutrients* **2022**, *14*, 623. [CrossRef]
11. Lu, C.; Zhang, C.; Zhao, F.; Li, D.; Lu, W. Biosynthesis of ursolic acid and oleanolic acid in *Saccharomyces cerevisiae*. *AIChE J.* **2018**, *64*, 3794–3802. [CrossRef]
12. Soczewiński, E.; Wachtmeister, C.A. The relation between the composition of certain ternary two-phase solvent systems and RM values. *J. Chromatogr.* **1962**, *7*, 311–320. [CrossRef]
13. Janicka, M.; Sztanke, M.; Sztanke, K. Predicting the Blood-Brain Barrier Permeability of New Drug-like Compounds via HPLC with Various Stationary Phases. *Molecules* **2020**, *25*, 487. [CrossRef] [PubMed]
14. Stępnik, K. Biomimetic Chromatographic Studies Combined with the Computational Approach to Investigate the Ability of Triterpenoid Saponins of Plant Origin to Cross the Blood–Brain Barrier. *Int. J. Mol. Sci.* **2021**, *22*, 3573. [CrossRef]
15. Platzer, G.; Mayer, M.; Beier, A.; Brüschweiler, S.; Fuchs, J.E.; Engelhardt, H.; Geist, L.; Bader, G.; Schörghuber, J.; Lichtenecker, R.; et al. PI by NMR: Probing CH–π Interactions in Protein–Ligand Complexes by NMR Spectroscopy. *Angew. Chem. Int. Ed.* **2020**, *59*, 14861. [CrossRef]
16. Ferreira de Freitas, R.; Schapira, M. A systematic analysis of atomic protein–ligand interactions in the PDB. *Med. Chem.Commun.* **2017**, *8*, 1970–1981. [CrossRef] [PubMed]
17. Nishio, M.; Umezawa, Y.; Fantini, J.; Weiss, M.S.; Chakrabarti, P. CH–π hydrogen bonds in biological macromolecules. *Phys.Chem. Chem. Phys.* **2014**, *16*, 12648–12683. [CrossRef]
18. World Health Organization. *Global Action Plan on the Public Health Response to Dementia 2017–2025*; WHO: Geneva, Switzerland, 2017; ISBN 978-92-4-151348-7.
19. Birks, J.; Grimley, E.J. *Ginkgo biloba* for cognitive impairment and dementia. *Cochrane Database Syst. Rev.* **2009**, *21*, CD003120. [CrossRef]
20. Joo, S.S.; Lee, D.I. Potential effects of microglial activation induced by ginsenoside Rg3 in rat primary culture: Enhancement of type a macrophage scavenger receptor expression. *Arch. Pharm. Res.* **2005**, *28*, 1164–1169. [CrossRef]
21. Chen, F.; Eckman, E.A.; Eckman, C.B. Reductions in levels of the Alzheimer's amyloid β peptide after oral administration of ginsenosides. *FASEB J.* **2006**, *20*, 1269–1271. [CrossRef]
22. Li, N.; Liu, B.; Dluzen, D.E.; Jin, Y. Protective effects of ginsenoside Rg2 against glutamate induced neurotoxicity in PC12 cells. *J. Ethnopharmacol.* **2007**, *111*, 458–463. [CrossRef]
23. Joo, S.S.; Yoo, Y.M.; Ahn, B.W.; Nam, S.Y.; Kim, Y.-B.; Hwang, K.W.; Lee, D.I. Prevention of inflammation-mediated neurotoxicity by Rg3 and its role in microglial activation. *Biol. Pharm. Bull.* **2008**, *31*, 1392–1396. [CrossRef] [PubMed]
24. Shieh, P.C.; Tsao, C.W.; Li, J.S.; Wu, H.T.; Wen, Y.J.; Kou, D.H.; Cheng, J.T. Role of pituitary adenylate cyclase-activating polypeptide (PACAP) in the action of ginsenoside Rh2 against betaamyloid-induced inhibition of rat brain astrocytes. *Neurosci. Lett.* **2008**, *434*, 1–5. [CrossRef] [PubMed]

25. Wakabayashi, I.; Yasui, K. Wogonin inhibits inducible prostaglandin E2 production in macrophages. *Eur. J. Pharmacol.* **2000**, *406*, 477–481. [CrossRef]
26. Park, B.K.; Heo, M.Y.; Par, H.; Kim, H.P. Inhibition of TPA-induced cyclooxygenase-2 expression and skin inflammation in mice by wogonin, a plant flavone from *Scutellaria radix*. *Eur. J. Pharmacol.* **2001**, *425*, 153–157. [CrossRef]
27. Nakamura, N.; Hayasaka, S.; Zhang, X.Y.; Nagaki, Y.; Matsumoto, M.; Hayasaka, Y.; Terasawa, K. Effects of baicalein, baicalin, and wogonin on interleukin-6 and interleukin-8 expression, and nuclear factor-kb binding activities induced by interleukin-1beta in human retinal pigment epithelial cell line. *Exp. Eye Res.* **2003**, *77*, 195–202. [CrossRef]
28. Suk, K.; Lee, H.; Kang, S.S.; Cho, G.J.; Choi, W.S. Flavonoid baicalein attenuates activation induced cell death of brain microglia. *J. Pharmacol. Exp. Ther.* **2003**, *305*, 638–645. [CrossRef]
29. Hosseinzadeh, H.; Ramezani, M.; Shafaei, H.; Taghiabadi, E. Anticonvulsant effect of *Berberis integerrima* L. root extracts in mice. *J. Acupunct. Meridian Stud.* **2013**, *6*, 12–17. [CrossRef] [PubMed]
30. Ya'u, J.; Yaro, A.H.; Malami, S.; Musa, M.A.; Abubakar, A.; Yahaya, S.M.; Chindo, B.A.; Anuka, J.A.; Hussaini, I.M. Anticonvulsant activity of aqueous fraction of *Carissa edulis* root bark. *Pharm. Biol.* **2015**, *53*, 1329–1338. [CrossRef]
31. Bhat, J.U.; Nizami, Q.; Asiaf, A.; Parray, S.A.; Ahmad, S.T.; Aslam, M.; Khanam, R.; Mujeeb, M.; Umar, S.; Siddiqi, A. Anticonvulsant activity of methanolic and aqueous extracts of *Melissa parviflora* in experimentally induced Swiss albino mice. *EXCLI J.* **2012**, *11*, 1–6.
32. Tariq, U.; Butt, M.S.; Pasha, I.; Faisal, M.N. Neuroprotective effects of *Olea europaea* L. fruit extract against cigarette smoke-induced depressive-like behaviors in Sprague-Dawley rats. *J. Food Biochem.* **2021**, *45*, e14014. [CrossRef]
33. Angeloni, C.; Malaguti, M.; Barbalace, M.C.; Hrelia, S. Bioactivity of Olive Oil Phenols in Neuroprotection. *Int. J. Mol. Sci.* **2017**, *18*, 2230. [CrossRef] [PubMed]
34. dos Santos-Neto, L.L.; Toledo, M.A.d.V.; Medeiros-Souza, P.; de Souza, G.A. The use of herbal medicine in Alzheimer's disease—A systematic review. *Evid. Based Complement. Altern. Med.* **2006**, *3*, 441–445. [CrossRef]
35. Bozin, B.; Mika-Dukic, N.; Samojlik, I.; Jovin, E. Antimicrobial and antioxidant properties of rosemary and sage (*Rosmarinus officinalis* L. and *Salvia officinalis* L., Lamiaceae) essential oils. *J. Agric. Food. Chem.* **2007**, *55*, 7879–7885. [CrossRef] [PubMed]
36. Imanshahidi, M.; Hosseinzadeh, H. The pharmacological effects of Salvia species on the central nervous system. *Phytother. Res.* **2006**, *20*, 427–437. [CrossRef] [PubMed]
37. Visioli, F.; Grande, S.; Bogani, P.; Galli, C. The role of antioxidant in the Mediterranean diets: Focus on cancer. *Eur. J. Cancer Prev.* **2004**, *13*, 337–343. [CrossRef]
38. Ninfali, P.; Mea, G.; Giorgini, S.; Rocchi, M.; Bacchiocca, M. Antioxidant capacity of vegetables, spices, and dressings relevant to nutrition. *Br. J. Nutr.* **2005**, *93*, 257–266. [CrossRef]
39. Cheung, S.; Tai, J. Anti-proliferative and antioxidant properties of rosemary *Rosmarinus officinalis*. *Oncol. Rep.* **2007**, *17*, 1525–1531. [CrossRef]
40. Lin, S.X.; Curtis, M.A.; Sperry, J. Pyridine alkaloids with activity in the central nervous system. *Bioorg. Med. Chem.* **2020**, *28*, 115820. [CrossRef]
41. Arens, H.; Borbe, H.O.; Ulbrich, B.; Stöckigt, J. Detection of pericine, a new CNS-active indole alkaloid from Picralima nitida cell suspension culture by opiate receptor binding studies. *Planta Med.* **1982**, *46*, 210–214. [CrossRef]
42. Paladini, A.C.; Marder, M.; Viola, H.; Wolfman, C.; Wasowski, C.; Medina, J.H. Flavonoids and the central nervous system: From forgotten factors to potent anxiolytic compounds. *J. Pharm. Pharmacol.* **1999**, *51*, 519–526. [CrossRef]
43. Jäger, A.K.; Saaby, L. Flavonoids and the CNS. *Molecules* **2011**, *16*, 1471–1485. [CrossRef] [PubMed]
44. Sun, A.; Xu, X.; Lin, J.; Cui, X.; Xu, R. Neuroprotection by Saponins. *Phytother. Res.* **2015**, *29*, 187–200. [CrossRef] [PubMed]
45. Yuan, C.S.; Wang, C.Z.; Wicks, S.M.; Qi, L.W. Chemical and pharmacological studies of saponins with a focus on American ginseng. *J. Gins. Res.* **2010**, *34*, 160–167. [CrossRef] [PubMed]
46. Hussain, G.; Huang, J.; Rasul, A.; Anwar, H.; Imran, A.; Maqbool, J.; Razzaq, A.; Aziz, N.; Makhdoom, E.U.H.; Konuk, M.; et al. Putative Roles of Plant-Derived Tannins in Neurodegenerative and Neuropsychiatry Disorders: An Updated Review. *Molecules* **2019**, *24*, 2213. [CrossRef]
47. Takahashi, R.N.; de Lima, T.C.; Morato, G.S. Pharmacological actions of tannic acid; II. Evaluation of CNS activity in animals. *Planta Med.* **1986**, *52*, 272–275. [CrossRef]
48. Awasthi, M.; Upadhyay, A.K.; Singh, S.; Pandey, V.P.; Dwivedi, U.N. Terpenoids as promising therapeutic molecules against Alzheimer's disease: Amyloid beta- and acetylcholinesterase-directed pharmacokinetic and molecular docking analyses. *Mol. Simul.* **2018**, *44*, 1–11. [CrossRef]
49. Min, S.L.; Liew, S.Y.; Chear, N.J.Y.; Goh, B.H.; Tan, W.N.; Khaw, K.Y. Plant Terpenoids as the Promising Source of Cholinesterase Inhibitors for Anti-AD Therapy. *Biology* **2022**, *11*, 307. [CrossRef]
50. Mony, T.J.; Elahi, F.; Choi, J.W.; Park, S.J. Neuropharmacological Effects of Terpenoids on Preclinical Animal Models of Psychiatric Disorders: A Review. *Antioxidants* **2022**, *11*, 1834. [CrossRef]
51. Meckes, M.; Calzada, F.; Tortoriello, J.; González, J.L.; Martínez, M. Terpenoids Isolated from *Psidium guajava* Hexane Extract with Depressant Activity on Central Nervous System. *Phytother. Res.* **1996**, *10*, 600–603. [CrossRef]
52. Mohanty, I.R.; Borde, M.; Kumar, S.; Maheshwari, U. Dipeptidyl peptidase IV Inhibitory activity of Terminalia arjuna attributes to its cardioprotective effects in experimental diabetes: In silico, in vitro and in vivo analyses. *Phytomedicine* **2019**, *57*, 158–165. [CrossRef]

53. Pawar, R.S.; Bhutani, K.K. Effect of oleanane triterpenoids from Terminalia arjuna—A cardioprotective drug on the process of respiratory oxyburst. *Phytomedicine* **2005**, *12*, 391–393. [CrossRef] [PubMed]
54. Kapoor, D.; Vijayvergiya, R.; Dhawan, V. Terminalia arjuna in coronary artery disease: Ethnopharmacology, pre-clinical, clinical & safety evaluation. *J. Ethnopharmacol.* **2014**, *155*, 1029–1045.
55. Sudharsan, P.T.; Mythili, Y.; Selvakumar, E.; Varalakshmi, P. Cardioprotective effect of pentacyclic triterpene, lupeol and its ester on cyclophosphamide-induced oxidative stress. *Hum. Exp. Toxicol.* **2005**, *24*, 313–318. [CrossRef]
56. Pugazhendhi, A.; Shafreen, R.B.; Devi, K.P.; Suganthy, N. Assessment of antioxidant, anticholinesterase and antiamyloidogenic effect of Terminalia chebula, Terminalia arjuna and its bioactive constituent 7-Methyl gallic acid—An in vitro and in silico studies. *J. Mol. Liq.* **2018**, *257*, 69–81. [CrossRef]
57. Gupta, D.; Kumar, M. Evaluation of in vitro antimicrobial potential and GC-MS analysis of *Camellia sinensis* and *Terminalia arjuna*. *Biotechnol. Rep.* **2017**, *13*, 19–25. [CrossRef] [PubMed]
58. Mandal, S.; Patra, A.; Samanta, A.; Roy, S.; Mandal, A.; Das Mahapatra, T.; Pradhan, S.; Das, K.; Nandi, D.K. Analysis of phytochemical profile of Terminalia arjuna bark extract with antioxidative and antimicrobial properties. *Asian Pac. J. Trop. Biomed.* **2013**, *3*, 960–966. [CrossRef]
59. Dube, N.; Nimgulkar, C.; Bharatraj, D.K. Validation of therapeutic anti-inflammatory potential of Arjuna KsheeraPaka—A traditional Ayurvedic formulation of *Terminalia arjuna*. *J. Tradit. Complement. Med.* **2017**, *7*, 414–420. [CrossRef]
60. Ahmad, M.S.; Ahmad, S.; Gautam, B.; Arshad, M.; Afzal, M. *Terminalia arjuna*, a herbal remedy against environmental carcinogenicity: An in vitro and in vivo study. *Egypt. J. Medical Hum. Genet.* **2014**, *15*, 61–67. [CrossRef]
61. Ruszkowski, P.; Bobkiewicz-Kozlowska, T. Natural Triterpenoids and their Derivatives with Pharmacological Activity Against Neurodegenerative Disorders. *Mini-Rev. Org. Chem.* **2014**, *11*, 307–315. [CrossRef]
62. Bhattacharjee, B.; Pal, P.K.; Ghosh, A.K.; Mishra, S.; Chattopadhyay, A.; Bandyopadhyay, D. Aqueous bark extract of *Terminalia arjuna* protects against cadmium-induced hepatic and cardiac injuries in male Wistar rats through antioxidative mechanisms. *Food Chem. Toxicol.* **2019**, *124*, 249–264. [CrossRef]
63. Tanaka, H.; Mizojiri, K. Drug-protein binding and blood-brain barrier permeability. *J. Pharmacol. Exp. Ther.* **1999**, *288*, 912–918. [PubMed]
64. Platts, J.A.; Abraham, M.H.; Zhao, Y.H.; Hersey, A.; Ijaz, L.; Butina, D. Correlation and prediction of a large blood-brain distribution data set--an LFER study. *Eur. J. Med. Chem.* **2001**, *36*, 719–730. [CrossRef] [PubMed]
65. Sapkota, A.; Choi, J.W. Oleanolic Acid Provides Neuroprotection against Ischemic Stroke through the Inhibition of Microglial Activation and NLRP3 Inflammasome Activation. *Biomol. Ther.* **2022**, *30*, 55–63. [CrossRef] [PubMed]
66. Chen, C.; Ai, Q.; Shi, A.; Wang, N.; Wang, L.; Wei, Y. Oleanolic acid and ursolic acid: Therapeutic potential in neurodegenerative diseases, neuropsychiatric diseases and other brain disorders. *Nutr. Neurosci.* **2023**, *26*, 414–428. [CrossRef] [PubMed]
67. Gudoityte, E.; Arandarcikaite, O.; Mazeikiene, I.; Bendokas, V.; Liobikas, J. Ursolic and Oleanolic Acids: Plant Metabolites with Neuroprotective Potential. *Int. J. Mol. Sci.* **2021**, *22*, 4599. [CrossRef]
68. Fantini, S.; Sassaroli, A.; Tga'valekos, K.T.; Kornbluth, J. Cerebral blood flow and autoregulation: Current measurement techniques and prospects for noninvasive optical methods. *Neurophotonics* **2016**, *3*, 031411. [CrossRef]
69. Liu, X.; Smith, B.J.; Chen, C.; Callegari, E.; Becker, S.L.; Chen, X.; Cianfrogna, J.; Doran, A.C.; Doran, S.D.; Gibbs, J.P.; et al. Use of a Physiologically Based Pharmacokinetic Model to Study the Time to Reach Brain Equilibrium: An Experimental Analysis of the Role of Blood-Brain Barrier Permeability, Plasma Protein Binding, and Brain Tissue Binding. *J. Pharmacol. Exp. Ther.* **2005**, *313*, 1254–1262. [CrossRef]
70. Talevi, A.; Bellera, C.L. Free Drug Theory. In *The ADME Encyclopedia*; Springer: Cham, Switzerland, 2022. [CrossRef]
71. Hammarlund-Udenaes, M.; Fridén, M.; Syvänen, S.; Gupta, A. On the rate and extent of drug delivery to the brain. *Pharm. Res.* **2008**, *25*, 1737–1750. [CrossRef]
72. Kalvass, J.C.; Maurer, T.S.; Pollack, G.M. Use of plasma and brain unbound fractions to assess the extent of brain distribution of 34 drugs: Comparison of unbound concentration ratios *to in vivo* p-glycoprotein efflux ratios. *Drug Metab. Dispos.* **2007**, *35*, 660–666. [CrossRef]
73. Banks, W.A.; Kastin, A.J. Peptides and the blood-brain barrier: Lipophilicity as a predictor of permeability. *Brain Res. Bull.* **1985**, *15*, 287–292. [CrossRef]
74. Chikhale, E.G.; Ng, K.-Y.; Burton, P.S.; Borchardt, R.T. Hydrogen bonding potential as a determinant of the in vitro and in situ blood-brain barrier permeability of peptides. *Pharm. Res.* **1994**, *11*, 412–419. [CrossRef] [PubMed]
75. Abbott, N.J. Prediction of blood–brain barrier permeation in drug discovery from in vivo, in vitro and in silico models. *Drug Discov. Today Technol.* **2004**, *1*, 407–416. [CrossRef]
76. Clark, D.E. In silico prediction of blood–brain barrier permeation. *Drug Discov. Today* **2003**, *8*, 927–933. [CrossRef]
77. Stéen, E.J.L.; Vugts, D.J.; Windhorst, A.D. The Application of in silico Methods for Prediction of Blood-Brain Barrier Permeability of Small Molecule PET Tracers. *Front. Nucl. Med.* **2022**, *2*, 853475. [CrossRef]
78. Radan, M.; Djikic, T.; Obradovic, D.; Nikolic, K. Application of in vitro PAMPA technique and in silico computational methods for blood-brain barrier permeability prediction of novel CNS drug candidates. *Eur. J. Pharms. Sci.* **2022**, *168*, 106056. [CrossRef] [PubMed]
79. Yang, R.; Wei, T.; Goldberg, H.; Wang, W.; Cullion, K.; Kohane, D.S. Getting Drugs Across Biological Barriers. *Adv. Mater.* **2017**, *29*, 1606596. [CrossRef]

80. Oldendorf, W.H. Lipid solubility and drug penetration of the blood brain barrier. *Proc. Soc. Exp. Biol. Med.* **1974**, *147*, 813–815. [CrossRef]
81. Aryal, M.; Arvanitis, C.D.; Alexander, P.M.; McDannold, N. Ultrasound-mediated blood-brain barrier disruption for targeted drug delivery in the central nervous system. *Adv. Drug Deliv. Rev.* **2014**, *72*, 94–109. [CrossRef]
82. Feher, M.; Sourial, E.; Schmidt, J.M. A simple model for the prediction of blood-brain partitioning. *Int J. Pharm.* **2000**, *201*, 239–247. [CrossRef]
83. Liu, R.; Sun, H.; So, S.-S. Development of quantitative structure – property relationship models for early ADME evaluation in drug discovery. 2. Blood-brain barrier penetration. *J. Chem. Inf. Comput. Sci.* **2001**, *41*, 1623–1632. [CrossRef]
84. Prasanna, S.; Doerksen, R.J. Topological polar surface area: A useful descriptor in 2D-QSAR. *Curr. Med. Chem.* **2009**, *16*, 21–41. [CrossRef]
85. Van de Waterbeemd, H. In silico models to predict oral absorption. In *Comprehensive Medicinal Chemistry II*; Taylor, J.B., Triggle, D.J., Eds.; Elsevier: Amsterdam, The Netherlands, 2007; pp. 669–697.
86. Barbato, F. The Use of Immobilised Artificial Membrane (IAM) Chromatography for Determination of Lipophilicity. *Curr. Comput. Drug Des.* **2006**, *2*, 341–352. [CrossRef]
87. Ogden, P.B.; Coym, J.W. Retention mechanism of a cholesterol-coated C18 stationary phase: Van't Hoff and Linear Solvation Energy Relationships (LSER) approaches. *J. Chromatogr. A* **2011**, *1218*, 2936–2943. [CrossRef]
88. Stavrakov, G.; Philipova, I.; Lukarski, A.; Atanasova, M.; Zheleva, D.; Zhivkova, Z.D.; Ivanov, S.; Atanasova, T.; Konstantinov, S.; Doytchinova, I. Galantamine-curcumin hybrids as dual-site binding acetylcholinesterase inhibitors. *Molecules* **2020**, *25*, 3341. [CrossRef] [PubMed]
89. Stępnik, K.; Kukula-Koch, W.; Plazinski, W.; Gawel, K.; Gaweł-Bęben, K.; Khurelbat, D.; Boguszewska-Czubara, A. Significance of Astragaloside IV from the Roots of Astragalus mongholicus as an Acetylcholinesterase Inhibitor—From the Computational and Biomimetic Analyses to the In Vitro and In Vivo Studies of Safety. *Int. J. Mol. Sci.* **2023**, *24*, 9152. [CrossRef]
90. Mente, S.; Lombardo, F. A recursive-partitioning model for blood–brain barrier permeation. *J. Comput. Aided Mol. Des.* **2005**, *19*, 465–481. [CrossRef] [PubMed]
91. Kukula-Koch, W.; Mroczek, T. Application of hydrostatic CCC-TLC-HPLC-ESI-TOF-MS for the bioguided fractionation of anticholinesterase alkaloids from *Argemonemexicana* L. roots. *Anal. Bioanal. Chem.* **2015**, *407*, 2581–2589. [CrossRef] [PubMed]
92. Available online: https://cactus.nci.nih.gov/translate (accessed on 10 June 2023).
93. Rappe, A.K.; Casewit, C.J.; Colwell, K.S.; Goddard, W.A.; Skiff, W.M. UFF, a full periodic table force field for molecular mechanics and molecular dynamics simulations. *J. Am. Chem. Soc.* **1992**, *114*, 10024–10035. [CrossRef]
94. Hanwell, M.D.; Curtis, D.E.; Lonie, D.C.; Vandermeersch, T.; Zurek, E.; Hutchison, G.R. Avogadro: An advanced semantic chemical editor, visualization, and analysis platform. *J. Cheminform.* **2012**, *13*, 17. [CrossRef]
95. Agarwal, R.; Smith, J.C. Speed vs Accuracy: Effect on Ligand Pose Accuracy of Varying Box Size and Exhaustiveness in AutoDock Vina. *Mol. Inform.* **2023**, *42*, 2200188. [CrossRef]
96. Trott, O.; Olson, A.J. AutoDock Vina: Improving the speed and accuracy of docking with a new scoring function, efficient optimization, and multithreading. *J. Comput. Chem.* **2010**, *30*, 455–461. [CrossRef]
97. Oostenbrink, C.; Villa, A.; Mark, A.E.; Van Gunsteren, W.F. A biomolecular force field based on the free enthalpy of hydration and solvation: The GROMOS force-field parameter sets 53A5 and 53A6. *J. Comput. Chem.* **2004**, *25*, 1656–1676. [CrossRef] [PubMed]
98. Abraham, M.J.; Murtola, T.; Schulz, R.; Páll, S.; Smith, J.C.; Hess, B.; Lindalhl, E. GROMACS: High performance molecular simulations through multi-level parallelism from laptops to supercomputers. *SoftwareX* **2015**, *1*, 19–25. [CrossRef]
99. Berendsen, H.J.C.; Postma, J.P.M.; van Gunsteren, W.F.; Hermans, J. Interaction models for water in relation to protein hydration. In *Intermolecular Forces*; Pullman, B., Ed.; The Jerusalem Symposia on Quantum Chemistry and Biochemistry; Springer: Dordrecht, The Netherlands, 1981; Volume 14. [CrossRef]
100. Kukol, A. Lipid Models for United-Atom Molecular Dynamics Simulations of Proteins. *J. Chem. Theor. Comput.* **2009**, *5*, 615–626. [CrossRef]
101. Stroet, M.; Caron, B.; Visscher, K.M.; Geerke, D.P.; Malde, A.K.; Mark, A.E. Automated Topology Builder Version 3.0: Prediction of Solvation Free Enthalpies in Water and Hexane. *J. Chem. Theor. Comput.* **2018**, *14*, 5834–5845. [CrossRef] [PubMed]
102. Kumar, S.; Rosenberg, J.M.; Bouzida, D.; Swendsen, R.H.; Kollman, P.A. THE weighted histogram analysis method for free-energy calculations on biomolecules. I. The method. *J. Comput. Chem.* **1992**, *13*, 1011–1021. [CrossRef]
103. Hub, J.S.; de Groot, B.L.; van der Spoel, D. g_wham—A Free Weighted Histogram Analysis Implementation Including Robust Error and Autocorrelation Estimates. *J. Chem. Theor. Comput.* **2010**, *12*, 3713–3720. [CrossRef]
104. Hess, B. P-LINCS: A Parallel Linear Constraint Solver for Molecular Simulation. *J. Chem. Theor. Comput.* **2008**, *4*, 116–122. [CrossRef]
105. Bussi, G.; Donadio, D.; Parrinello, M. Canonical sampling through velocity rescaling. *J. Chem. Phys.* **2007**, *126*, 014101. [CrossRef] [PubMed]
106. Parrinello, M.; Rahman, A. Polymorphic transitions in single crystals: A new molecular dynamics method. *J. Appl. Phys.* **1981**, *52*, 7182–7190. [CrossRef]
107. Essmann, U.; Perera, L.; Berkowitz, M.L.; Darden, T.; Lee, H.; Pedersen, L.G. A smooth particle mesh Ewald method. *J. Chem. Phys.* **1995**, *103*, 8577–8593. [CrossRef]

108. Available online: https://www.oecd-ilibrary.org/environment/test-no-236-fish-embryo-acute-toxicity-fet-test_978926420370 9-en (accessed on 13 June 2023).
109. Nakonieczna, S.; Grabarska, A.; Gawel, K.; Wróblewska-Łuczka, P.; Czerwonka, A.; Stepulak, A.; Kukula-Koch, W. Isoquinoline Alkaloids from *Coptis chinensis* Franch: Focus on Coptisine as a Potential Therapeutic Candidate against Gastric Cancer Cells. *Int. J. Mol. Sci.* **2022**, *23*, 10330. [CrossRef] [PubMed]
110. Gawel, K.; Turski, W.A.; van der Ent, W.; Mathai, B.J.; Kirstein-Smardzewska, K.J.; Simonsen, A.; Esguerra, C.V. Phenotypic Characterization of Larval Zebrafish (*Danio rerio*) with Partial Knockdown of the cacna1a Gene. *Mol. Neurobiol.* **2020**, *57*, 1904–1916. [CrossRef] [PubMed]

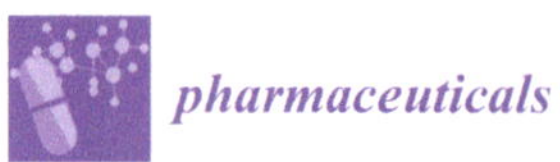*pharmaceuticals*

MDPI

Article

Design, Synthesis, In Silico Studies and In Vitro Evaluation of New Indole- and/or Donepezil-like Hybrids as Multitarget-Directed Agents for Alzheimer's Disease

Violina T. Angelova [1,*], Borislav Georgiev [2], Tania Pencheva [3], Ilza Pajeva [3], Miroslav Rangelov [4], Nadezhda Todorova [2], Dimitrina Zheleva-Dimitrova [5], Elena Kalcheva-Yovkova [6], Iva V. Valkova [1], Nikolay Vassilev [4], Rositsa Mihaylova [7], Denitsa Stefanova [7], Boris Petrov [7], Yulian Voynikov [1] and Virginia Tzankova [7]

[1] Department of Chemistry, Faculty of Pharmacy, Medical University of Sofia, 1000 Sofia, Bulgaria; ivalkova@pharmfac.mu-sofia.bg (I.V.V.); y_voynikov@pharmfac.mu-sofia.bg (Y.V.)
[2] Institute of Biodiversity and Ecosystem Research, Bulgarian Academy of Sciences, 1113 Sofia, Bulgaria; bobogeorgiev5@gmail.com (B.G.); nadeshda@abv.bg (N.T.)
[3] Institute of Biophysics and Biomedical Engineering, Bulgarian Academy of Sciences, 1113 Sofia, Bulgaria; tania.pencheva@biomed.bas.bg (T.P.); pajeva@biomed.bas.bg (I.P.)
[4] Institute of Organic Chemistry with Centre of Phytochemistry, Bulgarian Academy of Sciences, 1113 Sofia, Bulgaria; miroslav.rangelov@orgchm.bas.bg (M.R.); nikolay.vassilev@orgchm.bas.bg (N.V.)
[5] Department of Pharmacognosy, Faculty of Pharmacy, Medical University of Sofia, 1000 Sofia, Bulgaria; dzheleva@pharmfac.mu-sofia.bg
[6] Faculty of Computer Systems and Techologies, Technical University–Sofia, 1000 Sofia, Bulgaria; elena@tu-sofia.bg
[7] Department of Pharmacology, Pharmacotherapy and Toxicology, Faculty of Pharmacy, Medical University of Sofia, 1000 Sofia, Bulgaria; rositsa.a.mihaylova@gmail.com (R.M.); daluani@pharmfac.mu-sofia.bg (D.S.); bobi.stoyanov@abv.bg (B.P.); vtzankova@pharmfac.mu-sofia.bg (V.T.)
* Correspondence: v.stoyanova@pharmfac.mu-sofia.bg

Citation: Angelova, V.T.; Georgiev, B.; Pencheva, T.; Pajeva, I.; Rangelov, M.; Todorova, N.; Zheleva-Dimitrova, D.; Kalcheva-Yovkova, E.; Valkova, I.V.; Vassilev, N.; et al. Design, Synthesis, In Silico Studies and In Vitro Evaluation of New Indole- and/or Donepezil-like Hybrids as Multitarget-Directed Agents for Alzheimer's Disease. *Pharmaceuticals* **2023**, *16*, 1194. https://doi.org/10.3390/ph16091194

Academic Editors: Halil İbrahim Ciftci, Belgin Sever and Hasan Demirci

Received: 25 July 2023
Revised: 13 August 2023
Accepted: 17 August 2023
Published: 22 August 2023

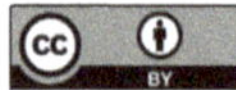

Abstract: Alzheimer's disease (AD) is considered a complex neurodegenerative condition which warrants the development of multitargeted drugs to tackle the key pathogenetic mechanisms of the disease. In this study, two novel series of melatonin- and donepezil-based hybrid molecules with hydrazone (**3a–r**) or sulfonyl hydrazone (**5a–l**) fragments were designed, synthesized, and evaluated as multifunctional ligands against AD-related neurodegenerative mechanisms. Two lead compounds (**3c** and **3d**) exhibited a well-balanced multifunctional profile, demonstrating intriguing acetylcholinesterase (AChE) inhibition, promising antioxidant activity assessed by DPPH, ABTS, and FRAP methods, as well as the inhibition of lipid peroxidation in the linoleic acid system. Compound **3n**, possessing two indole scaffolds, showed the highest activity against butyrylcholinesterase (BChE) and a high selectivity index (SI = 47.34), as well as a pronounced protective effect in H_2O_2-induced oxidative stress in SH-SY5Y cells. Moreover, compounds **3c**, **3d**, and **3n** showed low neurotoxicity against malignant neuroblastoma cell lines of human (SH-SY5Y) and murine (Neuro-2a) origin, as well as normal murine fibroblast cells (CCL-1) that indicate the in vitro biocompatibility of the experimental compounds. Furthermore, compounds **3c**, **3d**, and **3n** were capable of penetrating the blood–brain barrier (BBB) in the experimental PAMPA-BBB study. The molecular docking showed that compound **3c** could act as a ligand to both MT1 and MT2 receptors, as well as to AchE and BchE enzymes. Taken together, those results outline compounds **3c**, **3d**, and **3n** as promising prototypes in the search of innovative compounds for the treatment of AD-associated neurodegeneration with oxidative stress. This study demonstrates that hydrazone derivatives with melatonin and donepezil are appropriate for further development of new AChE/BChE inhibitory agents.

Keywords: AChE/BChE; Alzheimer's disease; neurodegenerative disorders; antioxidants; donepezil; melatonin; neuroprotection; SH-SY5Y; Neuro-2a; BBB; molecular docking; MT1 and MT2

1. Introduction

Alzheimer's disease is a progressive neurodegenerative disorder that primarily affects memory and cognitive functions [1,2]. The etiology of AD has not been fully elucidated; however, several pathological mechanisms have been recognized in the development of the disease: the deposition of amyloid β (Aβ) plaques, hyperphosphorylation of microtubule-associated protein tau (MAPT), oxidative stress, inflammation, impaired homeostasis of bio metals, reduction in acetylcholine (ACh) levels, neuronal loss, and dysfunction of the cholinergic system [3]. A key hallmark in AD pathogenesis, which can exacerbate its progression, is oxidative stress, especially in cortical and hippocampal tissues of the brain [4,5]. As a result, elevated lipid levels in the brain render it susceptible to the detrimental effects of oxidative stress; the appropriate application of antioxidants can slow down the progression of AD, consequently minimizing neuronal degeneration [6].

Current approaches in AD pharmacotherapy based on the cholinergic hypothesis aim to increase the level of ACh. This can be achieved by influencing the activity of the cholinesterase enzymes (ChE). There are two isoenzymes which play a key role in hydrolyzing the mediator: ACh–acetylcholinesterase (AChE) and butyrylcholinesterase (BChE). AChE activity is prominent in a healthy brain; however, in the case of AD, it remains unchanged or is slightly lowered, whereas BChE function may increase [7]. The vast majority of modern pharmaceuticals for the treatment of AD rely on AChE inhibition, however, newer approaches are oriented towards dual targeting of both enzymes, partly to more effectively restore the AchE balance, but also on the account that both enzymes take part in Aβ aggregation [4,8]. In addition, AchE can form an AchE-Aβ complex, which is more neurotoxic than Aβ alone [9]. Donepezil, rivastigmine, and galanthamine are the first-line treatment options used to enhance brain ACh levels in AD patients. The mechanisms by which AChE inhibitors block the catalytic action of the enzyme fall into three major categories: competitive inhibition, pseudo-irreversible inhibitions, and irreversible inhibition [10]. Donepezil is a selective, noncompetitive, and rapidly reversible inhibitor [11]; galanthamine acts as a reversible and competitive acetylcholinesterase inhibitor that also up-regulates the expression of nicotinic receptors [12]; rivastigmine is pseudo-irreversible and also inhibits BChE [7,13]. Tacrine, the first reversible dual AChE and BChE inhibitor used in AD therapy, has been withdrawn from the market due to its hepatotoxicity [14].

In light of this, researchers continue to make efforts in the design and development of small molecules with good activity towards AChE because of their favorable "drug-like" properties, i.e., low molecular mass and good pharmacokinetic profiles, but also continue the quest for multi-target-directed ligands (MTDLs) with low hepatotoxicity and a good safety profile [15,16].

MTDLs are organic scaffolds designed to target multiple biological pathways simultaneously with the goal of synergistic enhancement of the therapeutic efficacy [15]. Due to the complex pathogenesis of AD, MTDLs currently represent the most promising solution in AD therapy, and their design has generated considerable research interest [17,18].

Over the years, molecules containing both melatonin scaffold and a donepezil fragment have been demonstrated to possess strong inhibitory activity against acetylcholinesterase [19–22]. Melatonin holds promise as a potential therapeutic agent for developing new multitarget hybrids against neurodegeneration, including AD, because it can modulate the balance of Aβ production/clearance and mitigate Aβ neurotoxicity [23–25]. It is well known that melatonin modulates ADAM10, BACE1, PIN1, and GSK3 levels and reduces Aβ production; promotes Aβ clearance systems, such as glymphatic/lymphatic drainage, and blood–brain barrier (BBB) transportation and autophagy; acts on the PrPc/mGluR5/Fyn/Pyk2 and Ca^{2+}/mitochondria pathways to ameliorate Aβ oligomer-induced neurotoxicity; and improves cognitive function and sleep quality in AD patients [23]. The neuromodulator melatonin synchronizes circadian rhythms and related physiological functions through the actions of two G-protein-coupled receptors: MT1 and MT2 [26]. In this context, the indole scaffold is also one of the preferable pharmacophores and is considered an essential mediator between the gut-brain axis due to its neuroprotective, anti-inflammatory, β-amyloid anti-aggregation and antioxidant activities [27]. Additionally, the molecules carrying melatonin scaffold and hydrazone or sulfonyl hydrazone moieties have been shown to exhibit significant antioxidant properties [28] as well as AChE inhibitory activity [29–32].

Therefore, the new derivatives designed in this work aimed to act as potential AChE and BChE inhibitors with significant additional pharmacological properties. With the aim to improve the antioxidant activity of the designed hybrid molecules, we synthesized a series of 30 target compounds by variation in indole and/or donepezil fragments, supported by the preliminary molecular docking results. Thus, we prepared three families of hydrazine–hydrazone-based compounds as well as sulfonyl hydrazone analogues. The effectiveness of the new compounds was predicted by using in silico approaches.

This study employed molecular docking, ADME/Tox computer prediction, and biological assays to determine the potential of the new hybrids for AChE/BChE inhibition and in vitro neuroprotection against oxidative stress on human dopaminergic neuroblastoma SH-SY5Y cells. The antioxidant activity of the hybrid molecules was assessed using various methods, including free radical scavenging (DPPH), cation radical scavenging activity (ABTS), investigation of lipid peroxidation activity using a β-carotene-linoleic acid assay and the FRAP method. Additionally, the effect of the compounds on specific brain cells, such as human and mouse normal and malignant cell lines (CCL-1, SH-SY5Y, NEURO-2A), was also studied because the biocompatibility of the newly synthesized compounds is an integral part of their characterization. Furthermore, the most perspective compounds identified as promising AChE and/or BChE inhibitors were tested by in vitro PAMPA assay to evaluate their ability to access the brain.

2. Results and Discussion

2.1. Chemistry and Design Strategy of the Multifunctional Donepezil–Melatonin Hybrids

In this study, we developed novel melatonin–donepezil hybrids by combining two fragments that possess complementary properties. The melatonin and/or indole scaffold, in addition to its above-mentioned neurogenic profile, could demonstrate antioxidant and neuroprotective features and could also interact with the AChE-PAS via pie–pie interactions (π–π or aromatic–aromatic are stacking interactions between aromatic ring systems of the ligand and of the residue side chain of the receptor). The protonable *N*-benzyl piperidine which is present in the well-known AChE inhibitor donepezil can interact with AChE-CAS through cation–pie interaction (electrostatic interactions between a cationic atom or a positively charged functional group and the p-electron cloud of the aromatic ring). The last feature of the designed compounds is the linker between the groups interacting with the PAS and CAS sites: the hydrazone and sulfonyl hydrazone fragments. It is known that the crystallographic structure of AChE includes a peripheral cationic site (PAS) at the entrance and a catalytic active site (CAS) at the bottom of the receptor cavity. Hence, inhibitors that bind to either site could inhibit the AChE.

The 30 target compounds from two series hydrazide–hydrazones **3a–r** and sulfonyl hydrazones **5a–l** were synthesized from appropriate aldehydes **1a–n** and hydrazides **2a–f** and/or sulfonyl hydrazides **4a–c** by a one-step synthesis [33], shown in Scheme 1. Thus, the designed aroylhydrazone **3a–r** or sulfonyl hydrazone **5a–l** framework (Figure 1) was made in two parts: substituted indole or *N*-benzyl piperidine/*N*-benzyl pirrolidine, or substituted phenyl as a mainstay and substituted indole heterocycle at the fifth position as well as phenyl-substituted aromatic rings, connected to hydrazide or sulfonyl hydrazide moiety to intensify the desired pharmacophoric behavior with drug-like properties as well as antioxidant activities, cholinesterase inhibition, and neuroprotective effects.

The precise structure elucidation of all the synthesized scaffolds was carried out utilizing HREI-MS and NMR (^{1}H- and ^{13}C-NMR) spectroscopic tools. The spectral analyses were in accordance with the designed structures. (See the Supporting Information, ^{1}H NMR, ^{13}C NMR and HRMS spectra, Figures S12–S80). The ^{1}H-NMR spectra of hydrazide–hydrazones (**3e–r**) showed single signals corresponding to resonances of azomethine protons (CH=N) at 7.27–7.67 ppm with the exception of compounds with donepezyl fragment **3a–d** which showed a doublet corresponding to the resonances of azomethine protons (CH=N) at 7.85–8.49 ppm. For the sulfonyl hydrazones (**5a–l**), the azomethine protons (CH=N) were in the range from 7.19 to 8.10 ppm. The NH protons were observed at 10.75–11.54 ppm, respectively. ^{13}C-NMR spectra of **5a–g** exhibited resonances of azomethine (HC=N) carbons at 149.22 to 155.26 and hydrazide/hydrazone (C=O) carbons for the compounds **3a–r** at 165.28–175.01, respectively. 2D homonuclear correlation (COSY), DEPT-135 and 2D inverse detected heteronuclear (C–H) correlation (HMQC and HMBC) NMR experiments were used for the precise structure elucidation of all new compounds.

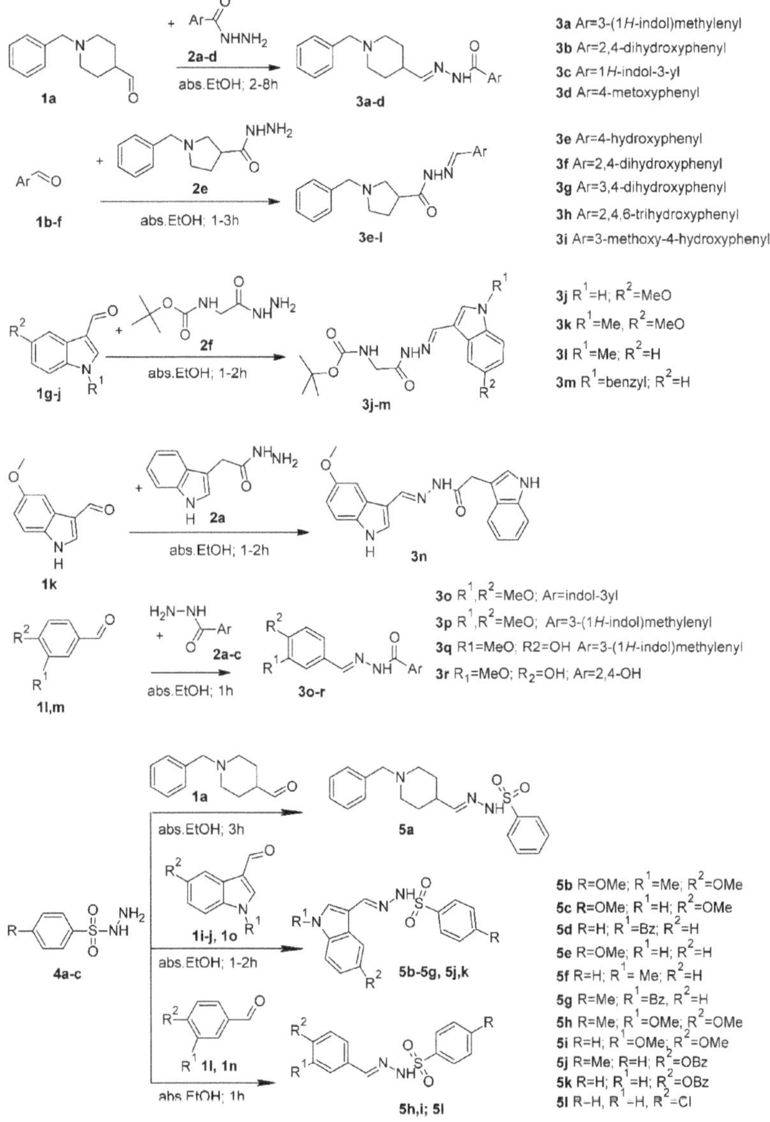

Scheme 1. Preparation of hydrazide–hydrazones **3a–r** and sulfonylhydrazone series **5a–l** in one pot method.

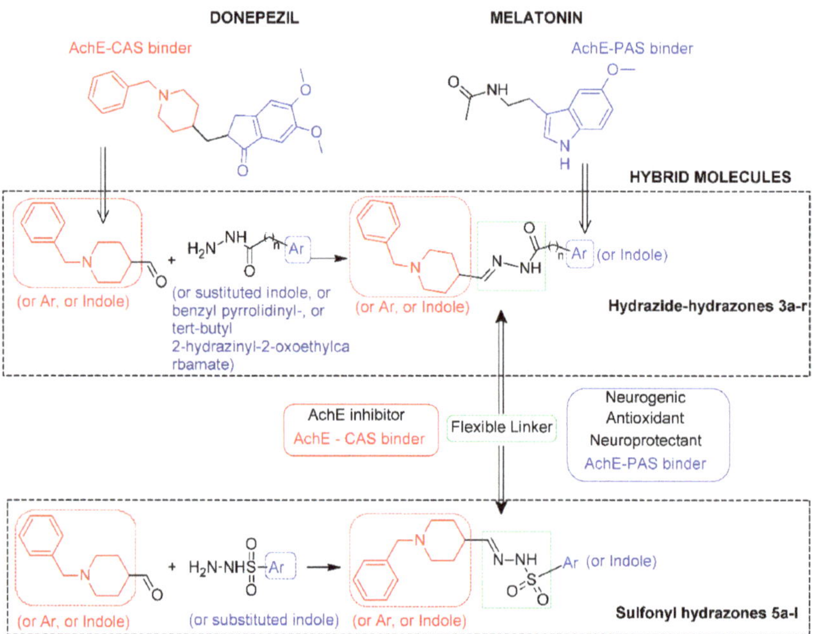

Figure 1. Design strategy and synthesis of the new multifunctional donepezil–melatonin hybrids with hydrazide–hydrazone (**3a–r**) and sulfonyl hydrazone (**5a–l**) linker.

The stereochemistry of hydrazide–hydrazones **3a–r** was unambiguously confirmed with the help of cross-peak intensities observed in the 2D NOESY (nuclear Overhauser effect spectroscopy) spectrum. Although the four isomers were considered (Figure S1 in the Supporting Information) [34,35] for the aroylhydrazones with indole scaffold, *E/Z* isomerization was generally not observed and the *Z* geometric isomers were absent. Only the ^{1}H NMR spectrum of compound **3c** and **3o** taken in DMSO-d$_6$ at 20 °C shows a 1:1 mixture of conformers. According to the confirmed nuclear Overhauser effect (NOE) between the methylidene proton and the NH proton, the most stable were the *E* isomers around the C=N double bond and the synperiplanar conformer around the amide O=C–N–N bond. Therefore, we concluded that a single *E* geometrical isomer was observed and the duplication pattern in the novel hydrazone derivatives to be due to the presence of syn/anti amide conformers in DMSO-d$_6$. Additionally, for the purposes of structure elucidation, the NMR spectra of compound **3c** were measured at 363 K (compound of **3o** at 353 K) to achieve a fast exchange. After cooling down to 293 K, the ^{1}H NMR spectra of **3a** and **3o** remained unchanged.

2.2. In Vitro AChE and BChE Inhibition Assays

The AChE and BChE inhibitory activity results of the synthesized compounds from two series, hydrazones **3a–r** and sulfonyl hydrazones **5a–l,** are provided in Tables 1 and 2. To assess the selectivity of all the final synthesized compounds, the improved Ellman spectrophotometric method was employed, with certain modifications [36,37]. Donepezil and galanthamine were used as reference compounds. The results are presented by the IC$_{50}$ as the mean of three measurements $\pm$ standard deviation. The enzyme inhibition percentage at 1 mM of the compounds is also given (Tables 1 and 2).

Table 1. AChE and BChE inhibitory activity of hydrazide hydrazone derivatives **3a–r**.

Compd.	Formula	Activity [a] [%]	AChE IC$_{50}$ [μM]	Activity [b] [%]	BChE IC$_{50}$ [μM]	SI [c] AChE	SI [d] BChE
3a	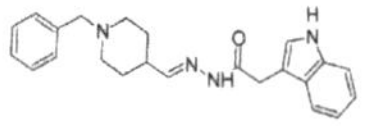	78.93	76.51 ± 3.04	80.43	56.50 ± 0.20	-	1.35
3b	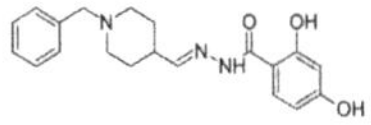	89.27	19.84 ± 0.95	75.94	262.40 ± 8.75	13.22	-
3c	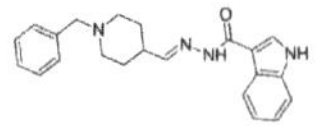	72.02	10.76 ± 1.66	76.95	26.32 ± 3.11	2.45	-
3d	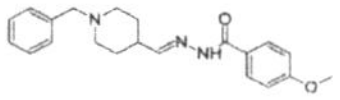	81.16	9.77 ± 0.76	72.88	197.27 ± 18.65	20.19	
3e	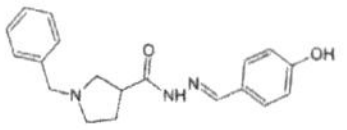	3.84	>1000	12.44	>1000	-	-
3f	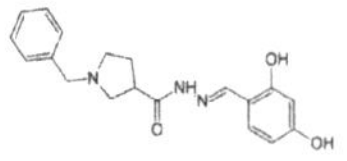	64.07	549.73 ± 37.08	57.16	708.73 ± 41.32	1.28	-
3g	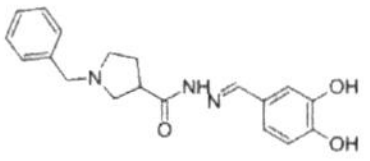	2.74	>1000	28.19	>1000	-	-
3h	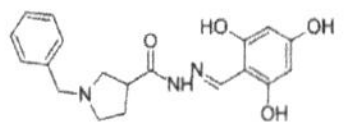	73.31	351.37 ± 17.93	76.49	178.60 ± 11.54	-	1.96
3i	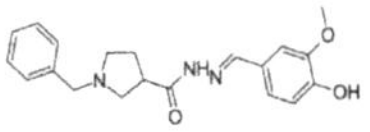	20.64	>1000	17.57 ± 2.45	>1000	-	-
3j	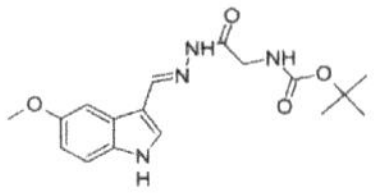	na	>1000	17.39	>1000	-	-
3k	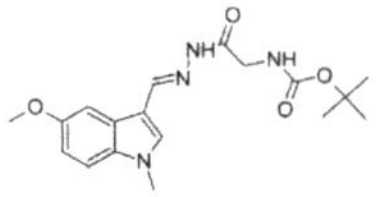	3.26	>1000	30.28	>1000	-	-
3l	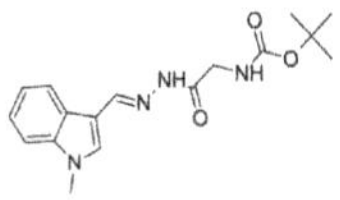	na	>1000	39.09	>1000	-	-
3m	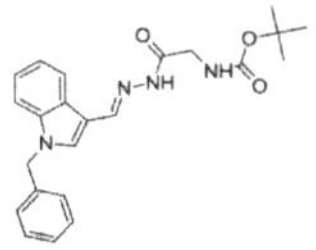	2.01	>1000	59.40	326.90 ± 34.35	-	3.05
3n	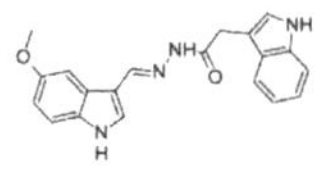	29.24	>1000	73.65	21.12 ± 1.48	-	47.34
3o	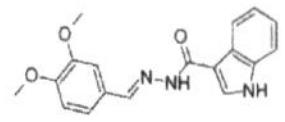	na	>1000	na	>1000	-	-

Table 1. *Cont.*

Compd.	Formula	Activity [a] [%]	AChE IC$_{50}$ [μM]	Activity [b] [%]	BChE IC$_{50}$ [μM]	SI [c] AChE	SI [d] BChE
3p	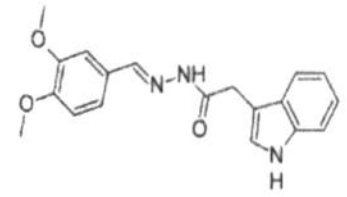	na	>1000	23.96	>1000	-	-
3q	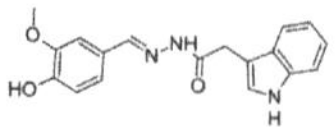	12.85	>1000	13.90	>1000	-	-
3r	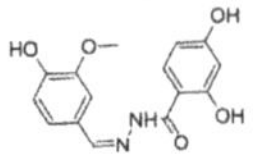	na	>1000	16.89	>1000	-	-
Donepezil	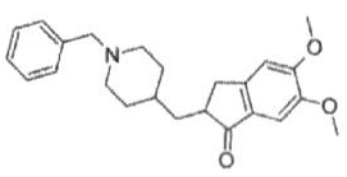	65.64	0.20 ± 0.04	69.14	1.83 ± 0.35	9.15	-
Galanthamine	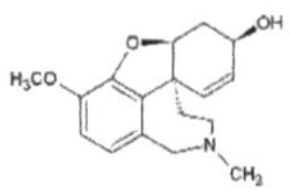	85.22	1.48 ± 0.11	85.83	29.55 ± 0.96	16.5	-
Melatonin	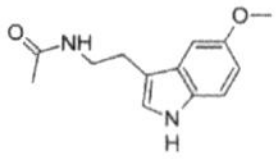	1.24	>1000	4.21 ± 0.88	>1000	-	-

[a] Inhibition percentage of AChE/BChE by 1 mM solution of the tested compounds. [b] Inhibitor concentration (means ± SD of three experiments) for 50% inactivation of AChE/BChE. [c] Selectivity for AChE is defined as IC$_{50}$(BChE)/IC$_{50}$(AChE). [d] Selectivity for BChE is defined as IC$_{50}$(AChE)/IC$_{50}$(BChE).

Table 2. AChE and BChE inhibitory activity of sulfonyl hydrazone derivatives **5a–l**.

Compd.	Formula	Activity [a] [%]	AChE IC$_{50}$ [μM]	Activity [b] [%]	BChE IC$_{50}$ [μM]	SI [c] AChE	SI [d] BChE
5a	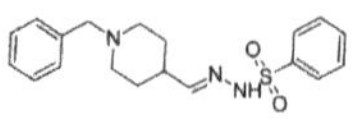	76.99	162.83 ± 10.73	79.44	259.20 ± 4.90	1.81	-
5b	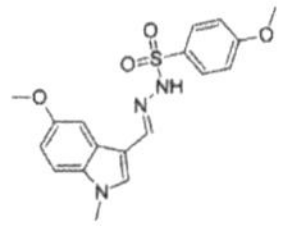	na	>1000	na	>1000	-	-
5c	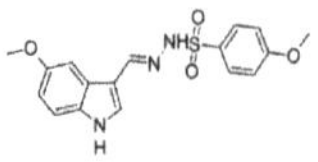	na	>1000	18.21	>1000	-	-
5d	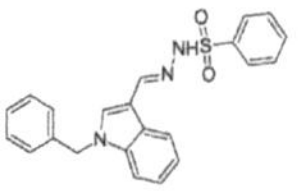	41.72	>1000	na	>1000	-	-
5e	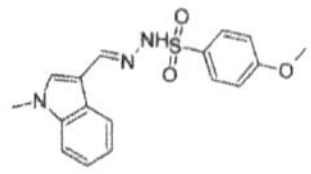	na	>1000	na	>1000	-	-
5f	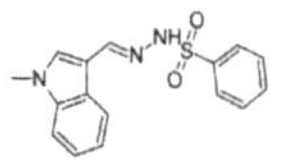	na	>1000	na	>1000	-	-

Table 2. *Cont.*

Compd.	Formula	Activity [a] [%]	AChE IC$_{50}$ [μM]	Activity [b] [%]	BChE IC$_{50}$ [μM]	SI [c] AChE	SI [d] BChE
5g	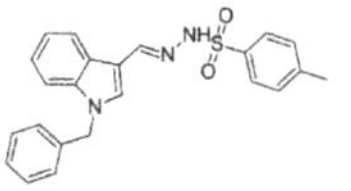	2.18	>1000	40.65	>1000	-	-
5h	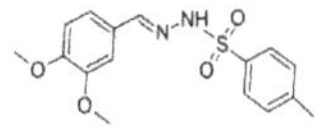	10.53	>1000	26.65 ± 5.11	>1000	-	-
5i	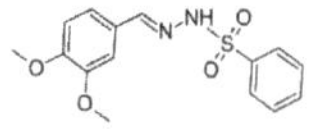	2.63	>1000	7.67 ± 0.99	>1000	-	-
5j	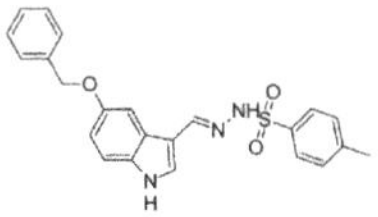	13.17	>1000	56.92	865.40 ± 159.28	-	1.15
5k	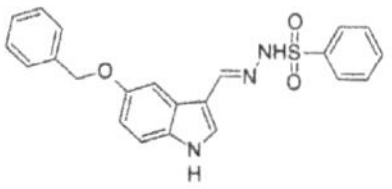	35.41	>1000	4.97	>1000	-	-
5l	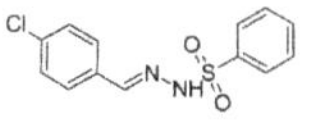	na	>1000	na	>1000	-	-
Donepezil	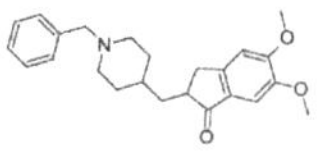	65.64	0.20 ± 0.04	69.14	1.83 ± 0.35	9.15	-
Galanthamine	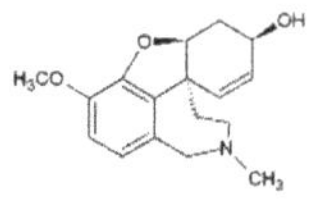	85.22	1.48 ± 0.11	85.83	29.55 ± 0.96	16.5	-
Melatonin	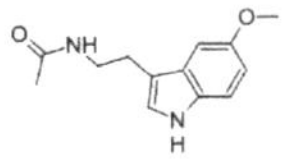	1.24	>1000	4.21 ± 0.88	>1000	-	-

[a] Inhibition percentage of AChE/BChE by 1 mM solution of the tested compounds. [b] Inhibitor concentration (means ± SD of three experiments) for 50% inactivation of AChE/BChE. [c] Selectivity for AChE is defined as IC$_{50}$(BChE)/IC$_{50}$(AChE). [d] Selectivity for BChE is defined as IC$_{50}$(AChE)/IC$_{50}$(BChE).

None of the 30 tested compounds proved to be a more potent AChE inhibitor than the positive controls galanthamine and donepezil. The piperidinyl-containing derivatives (**3a–d** and **5a**) belonging to the first family showed relatively high IC$_{50}$ values (76.51 ± 3.04, 19.84 ± 0.95, 10.76 ± 1.66, 9.77 ± 0.76 and 162.83 ± 10.73 μM, respectively). The derivative **3d** with a p-MeO benzene ring had the lowest IC$_{50}$ (9.77 ± 0.76) in the family. The presence of the methoxy group on the appropriate position in the benzene ring (**3d**) lead to more of an increase in inhibitory activity than the *o*-, *p*-disubstituted benzene ring (**3b**) and indole containing hybrids **3a** and **3c**, increasing the selectivity index for the compound **3d** (SI = 20.19). Also, replacing the indole moiety in **3c** with a 2,4-dihydroxy benzene ring in compound **3b** caused a decrease in the AChE inhibitory activity. It is impressive that the introduction of a methylene group in the connecting hydrazone fragment in compound **3a**, compared to the indole-donepezil hybrid **3c** with the same moieties, lead to a loss of inhibitory activity towards AchE and an increase in activity towards the butyrylcholinesterase enzyme; the selective index is in favor of BChE (SI BChE = 1.35). The SAR, including molecular modelling studies, disclosed that the benzyl moiety provided interaction with CAS residues, while the indole moiety was oriented within PAS. On the other hand, compound **5a** with sulfonyl hydrazone linkage showed the best IC_{50} (162.83 ± 10.73 μM) from this family, indicating that the sulfonyl hydrazone fragment probably decreased the inhibitory activity.

Pyrrolidine-containing derivatives **3e–i** from the second family displayed highly variable results. Among them, the derivatives **3f** and **3h** exhibited moderate inhibitory activity with IC_{50} values of 549.73 ± 37.08 and 351.37 ± 17.93 μM, respectively. However, derivatives **3e**, **3g**, and **3i** showed significantly lower inhibitory activity and were practically inactive. It appeared that reducing the size of the piperidine ring to pyrrolidine, as well as the turn of the hydrazide hydrazone bond, resulted in a drastic decrease in inhibitory activity for both acetyl and butyrylcholinesterase. Comparing the compounds containing *p*-hydroxy groups and *m*-, *p*-dihydroxy groups in benzene rings (**3f** and **3h**) with *o*-, *p*-dihydroxy and *o-p*- trihydroxy benzene rings (**3e** and **3i**), it seemed that a combination of two hydroxyl groups at the ortho- and para-position assisted AChE inhibition. The presence of three hydroxyl groups in the *o*- and *para*- position of the benzene ring led to increased BChE inhibitory activity (SI BChE = 1.96).

Other *tert*-butyl-2-hydrazinyl-2-oxoethylcarbamate derivatives from the third family with different substitutions in the indole ring (**3j–m**) did not show significant inhibitory activity towards both AchE and BchE in the measured concentration, compared with the results obtained from H. Zhang et al., 2022 [38].

Finally, derivatives from the fourth family (**3n–r**) with different substitutions in the indole ring and hydrazide hydrazone linkage as well as their analogues with sulfonyl hydrazone linkage (**5b–l**) did not show satisfactory AChE inhibitory activity either, probably due to a lack of protonated nitrogen-containing moiety to ensure binding with CAS residues. Two sets of compounds inhibited BChE more than AChE: those containing a tosyl group (**5j**, **5g**, **5h**) and those with a *tert*-butyl-2-hydrazinyl-2-oxoethylcarbamate group (**3j–m**). All compounds containing a vanillin moiety (**3i**, **3q**, and **3r**) showed very weak to no inhibition to both AChE and BChE. Surprisingly, the compound **3n** with two indole scaffolds showed the highest activity against BChE (IC_{50} = 21.12 ± 1.48 μM) and a high selectivity index (SI = 47.34) (Table 1). The difference in BChE inhibition between **3n** and another melatonin-containing derivatives might be due to the presence of a melatonin fragment and other indole rings in the molecule.

As can be seen, compounds **3c**, **3f**, and **5a** did not show a remarkable selectivity for the AChE enzyme more than BChE and, thus, they can be considered non-selective cholinesterase inhibitors. From the above-mentioned results, it can be concluded that those compounds are non-selective AChE/BChE inhibitors with moderate activity against AChE

2.3. Cytotoxicity of the Compounds

A series of MTT experiments were conducted against normal murine fibroblast cells (CCL-1) and malignant neuroblastoma cell lines of human (SH-SY5Y) and murine (Neuro-2a) origin to accommodate the in vitro biocompatibility of the experimental compounds. The results obtained from the cell viability assays are presented in Table 3.

The estimated half-inhibitory concentrations indicate a favorable cytotoxic profile of most compounds in both series with IC_{50} values ranging near or exceeding 100 μM in all three cellular test systems. However, the highest biocompatibility was observed in the hydrazide hydrazone series, where benzylpiperadine- (**3a–d**), pyrrolidine- (**3e**, **3g**, **3h**), *tert*-butyl- (**3j**, **3k**, **3l**) and vanillin- (**3r**) carrying representatives of all families were virtually devoid of cytotoxic activity (prevailing IC_{50} values were >300 and >800 μM, as seen from Table 3, many times exceeding the correspondent ones for the referent drug donepezil). In the alternative sulfonyl hydrazone series, the weakest effect on cell viability was again observed for the benzylpiperadine-substituted analogue **5a**, followed by **5d**, **5f**, **5k**, and **5l**.

The cytotoxicity profiles of the newly designed 30 hybrid compounds are in a good correlation with their antioxidant capacity, evaluated in several in vitro settings and presented in the section below. In a complimentary manner, the leading compounds with prominent free radical scavenging and cholinesterase inhibitory activity (**3a–d, 3h–l, 5a**) did not affect cell viability of neither normal nor malignant cell cultures.

Table 3. In vitro cytotoxicity IC_{50} [$\mu M \pm SD$] of the experimental hydrazide–hydrazones **3a–r**, sulfonyl hydrazones **5a–l**, and the reference drugs donepezil and galanthamine against the tested cell lines.

Compd	Neuro-2a IC_{50} μM	SH-SY5Y IC_{50} μM	CCL-1 IC_{50} μM
3a	>300	129 ± 7.5	138.5 ± 9.8
3b	>300	138.4	153.5 ± 7.3
3c	>300	97.3	167.8 ± 10.4
3d	>300	122.3 ± 9.2	220
3e	>300	170.2 ± 10.6	>300
3f	12.5 ± 2.4	35.8 ± 5.5	150 ± 11.2
3g	110.5 ± 9.1	>300	>300
3h	>300	>300	>300
3i	>300	178.1 ± 15.7	>800
3j	>300	150.4 ± 12.3	>300
3k	>300	130.8 ± 11.8	>300
3l	>300	106.7 ± 8.9	>300
3m	108.7 ± 9.1	7.2 ± 1.8	65.4 ± 5.1
3n	83.7 ± 8.3	107.8 ± 9.4	48.2 ± 6.4
3o	125.8 ± 10.7	70.0 ± 7.2	>300
3p	115.5 ± 12.8	87.4 ± 7.7	>300
3q	254.5 ± 13.7	140.8 ± 8.8	170.2 ± 14.0
3r	>300	155.6 ± 11.1	>300
5a	>300	142.0 ± 13.1	156.9 ± 8.5
5b	30.5 ± 3.2	70.4 ± 4.9	38.1 ± 3.5
5c	7.5 ± 2.4	48.3 ± 5.2	25.7 ± 2.9
5d	117.4 ± 11.5	99.5 ± 7.8	140.3 ± 8.4
5e	19.9 ± 1.7	83.3 ± 4.9	180 ± 9.6
5f	134.9 ± 10.9	131.8 ± 10.3	167.4 ± 11.8
5g	134.9 ± 10.9	92.1 ± 9.3	50.7 ± 3.6
5h	135.5 ± 12.6	42.0 ± 5.2	159.6
5i	109.2 ± 5.1	40.3 ± 6.1	147.3
5j	65.4 ± 0.1	33.1 ± 0.1	41.2 ± 4.2
5k	77.7 ± 6.9	134.7 ± 14.0	321.4 ± 16.2
5l	117.4 ± 11.5	99.5 ± 7.8	131.4 ± 11.4
Donepezil	248.1 ± 15.4	79.3 ± 6.2	52.0 ± 5.3
Galanthamine	>300	>300	>300

2.4. Determination of Antioxidant Activity

The antioxidant activity of the most perspective synthesized compounds was studied using three different spectrophotometric methods. The results are presented in Tables 4 and 5.

2.5. DPPH Radical Scavenging Activity

The DPPH (2,2-diphenyl-1-picryl-hydrazyl-hydrate) free radical scavenging activity method is based on the neutralization of the DPPH radical by an antioxidant. Four compounds **5k, 5j, 5g**, and **3r** revealed the highest DPPH activity, with means from 45.17 ± 4.65% to 47.36 ± 2.75% (Table 4). Significant antioxidant activity was shown by the hydrazone compound **3r** (45.17 ± 4.65), characterized by the presence of three hydroxyl groups in the benzene ring and a vanillin moiety. The hydrazone-containing compound with a vanillin fragment and pyrrolidine scaffold, **3i** (6.56 ± 0.78), demonstrated noteworthy activity. The presence of multiple hydroxyl substituents attached to both aromatic rings created rich conjugated systems, making the hydrazones strong antioxidant agents. This ability allows them to effectively scavenge free radicals in their solutions by readily undergoing hydrogen radical abstraction (H), transforming into free radicals themselves. The present results are in agreement with the results obtained by other researchers [39,40] which showed that conjugated systems resulting from aromatic Schiff bases containing multi-hydroxyl groups have much higher antioxidant activities. Other hydrazone-containing compounds with moderate antioxidant activity better than BHT (butylated hydroxytoluene) were **3m**, **3c**, and **3d**. The displacement of the hydrazone with sulfonyl hydrazone linkage produced a consistent increase in the activity, as seen for compounds **5g**, **5j**, and **5k** with 1-benzyl-1*H*-indol-3-yl or 5-(benzyloxy)-3-methyl-1*H*-indole fragments.

Table 4. DPPH, ABTS-radical scavenging, and FRAP of the most perspective synthesized compounds.

Compd.	DPPH Activity	ABTS Activity		FRAP
	[%]	[%]	IC_{50} [mM]	μMTE
3a	5.74 ± 0.39	27.44 ± 2.57	27.44 ± 2.57	15.42 ± 0.74
3b	13.30 ± 0.83	93.22 ± 0.30	2.57 ± 0.10	16.63 ± 0.98
3c	30.05 ± 0.55	36.69 ± 0.70	>5	38.97 ± 3.58
3d	40.80 ± 3.10	≥100	1.05 ± 0.04	15.87 ± 1.41
3i	6.56 ± 0.78	≥100	2.37 ± 0.05	14.67 ± 1.14
3m	32.06 ± 4.70	36.20 ± 1.40	>5	19.06 ± 1.96
3n	40.62 ± 0.83	≥100	0.77 ± 0.06	14.30 ± 0.56
3q	20.40 ± 0.83	≥100	2.38 ± 0.07	15.60 ± 0.90
3r	45.17 ± 4.65	91.41 ± 0.47	2.50 ± 0.23	14.30 ± 0.56
5a	6.56 ± 0.78	43.80 ± 0.23	>5	17.48 ± 0.90
5g	45.72 ± 1.38	≥100	2.08 ± 0.10	15.87 ± 1.13
5h	16.94 ± 1.09	≥100	1.85 ± 0.03	20.37 ± 0.90
5i	16.21 ± 3.01	65.29 ± 2.34	3.74 ± 0.05	14.67 ± 0.81
5j	47.36 ± 2.75	≥100	2.18 ± 0.16	18.59 ± 2.28
5k	47.18 ± 1.14	≥100	2.57 ± 0.13	22.52 ± 1.29
Donepezil	na	na	>5	20.09 ± 0.16
Melatonin	na	≥100	0.50 ± 0.02	13.73 ± 0.84
BHT	7.78 ± 0.77	29.53 ± 1.65	>5	15.79 ± 0.58

Table 5. Lipid peroxidation activity of the tested synthesized compounds.

Compd.	Absorbance				
	Day 1	Day 2	Day 3	Day 4	Day 5
3a	0.87 ± 0.03	0.87 ± 0.08	0.72 ± 0.07	0.72 ± 0.05	0.71 ± 0.08
3b	0.92 ± 0.06	0.93 ± 0.09	0.95 ± 0.05	0.96 ± 0.01	1.00 ± 0.02
3c	0.89 ± 0.07	0.87 ± 0.02	0.85 ± 0.05	0.85 ± 0.07	0.74 ± 0.05
3d	0.85 ± 0.02	0.86 ± 0.02	0.88 ± 0.05	0.85 ± 0.07	0.84 ± 0.09
3i	0.80 ± 0.09	0.83 ± 0.04	0.08 ± 0.07	0.82 ± 0.03	0.84 ± 0.07
3m	0.89 ± 0.09	0.89 ± 0.01	0.92 ± 0.05	0.95 ± 0.01	0.96 ± 0.08
3n	0.85 ± 0.05	0.87 ± 0.07	0.89 ± 0.04	0.90 ± 0.01	0.92 ± 0.06
3q	0.76 ± 0.03	0.77 ± 0.08	0.79 ± 0.03	0.84 ± 0.05	0.91 ± 0.09
3r	0.80 ± 0.04	0.81 ± 0.01	0.82 ± 0.02	0.87 ± 0.09	0.86 ± 0.09
5a	0.83 ± 0.02	0.88 ± 0.08	0.89 ± 0.04	1.00 ± 0.04	1.10 ± 0.05
5g	0.82 ± 0.04	0.87 ± 0.09	0.88 ± 0.09	0.87 ± 0.05	0.88 ± 0.03
5h	0.70 ± 0.09	0.82 ± 0.06	0.83 ± 0.05	0.83 ± 0.06	0.80 ± 0.05
5i	0.81 ± 0.08	0.83 ± 0.01	0.83 ± 0.09	0.81 ± 0.02	0.83 ± 0.03
5j	0.83 ± 0.01	0.83 ± 0.08	0.84 ± 0.02	0.83 ± 0.05	0.82 ± 0.02
5k	0.80 ± 0.04	0.80 ± 0.09	0.83 ± 0.05	0.84 ± 0.08	0.87 ± 0.09
Donepezil	0.79 ± 0.08	0.82 ± 0.08	0.84 ± 0.04	1.19 ± 0.24	2.00 ± 0.18
Melatonin	0.75 ± 0.07	0.80 ± 0.09	0.89 ± 0.05	0.89 ± 0.02	0.94 ± 0.01
BHT	0.74 ± 0.07	0.77 ± 0.03	0.78 ± 0.06	0.80 ± 0.06	0.81 ± 0.09
Control	0.83 ± 0.08	0.84 ± 0.07	0.85 ± 0.03	0.92 ± 0.02	1.02 ± 0.2

2.6. ABTS Radical Scavenging Assay

These compounds were also tested for their antioxidant activities by using the ABTS [2,2′-azinobis (3-ethylbenzothiazoline-6-sulfonic acid)] cation radical decolorization method

(Table 4). The BHT [41] was used for comparison. The ABTS cation radical is produced by oxidation of the ABTS molecule with strong oxidizing agents, such as potassium persulfate in water. The produced greenish solution of this radical absorbs light at a wavelength of 734 nm. The advantage of this radical is the solubility in inorganic and organic solvents. Therefore, by using this assay, both hydrophilic and hydrophobic compounds can be tested. Another advantage of the ABTS assay is that the bulky compounds can approach this molecule to transfer electrons easier, compared to the DPPH molecule. It is well known that as a result of the polar effect of the substituents, the N-H bond in the structure of hydrazones and sulfonyl hydrazones is weakened, which increases the tendency of reacting with the ABTS molecule and more polar hydrazones were more amenable to react with ABTS, compared to less polar ones. In the ABTS assay, among the tested compounds, sulfonyl hydrazones exhibited higher cation radical scavenging activity. As shown in Table 4, most of the compounds demonstrated superior antioxidant activities than BHT and similar to melatonin, where hydrazine derivatives **3i**, **3d**, and **5h** showed the lowest values of IC_{50}, followed by sulfonyl hydrazones **5j**, **5g**, **5k**, and hydrazones **3q**, **3n**, **3r**.

2.7. Ferric Reducing Antioxidant Power (FRAP)

The Ferric Reducing Antioxidant Power (FRAP) test measures the reduction in the complex of ferric ions (Fe^{3+})-ligand to the intensely blue ferrous complex (Fe^{2+}) by means of antioxidants in acidic environments. Unlike other methods, the FRAP test is carried out in acidic pH conditions (pH = 3.6) to maintain solubility of iron complexes. Thus, the FRAP assay utilizes an SET (single electron transfer) mechanism to determine the capacity of an antioxidant in the reduction of an oxidant. With respect to the FRAP method, compound **3c** has the strongest activity, followed by **5a**, **5h**, donepezil, **3m** and **5j**.

The FRAP values of the tested compounds, as displayed in Table 1, showed a different trend than the DPPH radical scavenging results. Some of the compounds had lower activity in the DPPH assay but exhibited high activities in the FRAP assay. Compound **3c**, which was mildly active in the DPPH assay, showed the highest ferric reducing activity while compounds **5j** and **5g**, which were highly active in the DPPH assay, showed an unusually low FRAP value. The probable reason for these differences is that the reducing capacity of a sample in FRAP test is not directly related to its radical scavenging capability. Also, not all antioxidants reduce ferric ions at a fast rate.

In this study, according to the antioxidant activity assay results of the synthesized compounds, most of the hydrazones and sulfonyl hydrazones with indole and vanillin aromatic rings exhibited good antioxidant activity with the potential of forming free radicals by weakening the N-H bond in the hydrazone group.

2.8. Determination of Antioxidant Activity in Linoleic Acid System by the FTC Method

In the present study, the inhibition of lipid peroxidation of the synthesized compounds (10 mM) was determined using the FTC method in the linoleic acid system (Table 5). During lipid peroxidation, peroxides were formed and oxidized Fe^{2+} to Fe^{3+}. The Fe^{3+} ions formed a complex with SCN^-, with an absorption maximum of 500 nm. Thus, a high absorbance was an indication of high peroxide formation during the emulsion incubation. The presence of compounds with antioxidant properties in the mixture decreased the linoleic acid oxidation and reduced absorption, respectively. The highest significant diminution was demonstrated by **3a** followed by **3c**, **5h**, and **5j**. Moreover, most of the studied compounds demonstrated activity close to that of BHT, but inhibited lipid peroxidation stronger than the donepezil, melatonin, and control (Table 5).

The presented data of direct and indirect antioxidant activities as measured by the DPPH, ABTS, FRAP, and FTC methods (Tables 4 and 5) demonstrate that aromatic hydrazones and sulfonyl hydrazones are promising antioxidant agents. The compound **3c**, which was a promising acetylcholinesterase inhibitor from all new derivatives, showed the best antioxidant activity in the three tested methods FRAP, ABTS, and FTC. As a future perspective, hydrazone **3c** will be evaluated in vivo in models of Alzheimer's disease and melatonin deficiency as well as Aβ (1–42) aggregation.

Consequently, the prioritized structures (**3a–d**, **3n** and **5a**) were further subjected to an in vitro evaluation of their neuroprotective properties against H_2O_2-induced oxidative stress damage.

2.9. Neuroprotection against Oxidative Stress

The SH-SY5Y cell line is a commonly utilized human neuronal cell model that holds significant value in elucidating the mechanisms underlying neurotoxicity within neurodegenerative disorders [42,43]. It serves as an essential tool for investigating and comprehending the intricate processes involved in neurotoxicity associated with such diseases. To assess the potential neuroprotective properties of new compounds, an experimental setup was conducted where SH-SY5Y cells were subjected to pre-treatment with varying concentrations (0.1, 1, 5, 10, 25, 50 μM) for a duration of 90 min. Subsequently, the cells were exposed to 1 mM H_2O_2, resulting in a notable reduction in cell viability, confirming its toxicity (Figure 2). The mechanism of toxicity of H_2O_2 (hydrogen peroxide) in vitro involves oxidative stress and damage to cellular components. H_2O_2 can readily cross cell membranes and generate reactive oxygen species (ROS) through its spontaneous decomposition. ROS, including hydroxyl radicals and peroxyl radicals, can cause damage to DNA, proteins, and lipids, leading to cellular dysfunction and injury [44].

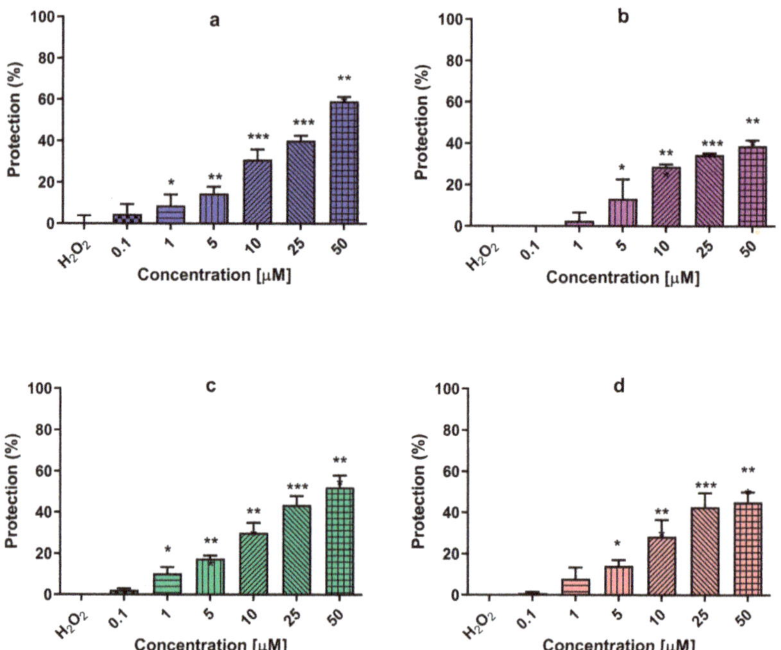

Figure 2. Protective effects of (**a**) compound **3n**, (**b**) donepezil, (**c**) reference melatonin, and (**d**) rasagiline at different concentrations (0.1, 1, 5, 10, 25, and 50 μM) in a model of H_2O_2-induced oxidative stress in human neuroblastoma SH-SY5Y cells. Data are presented as means from three independent experiments ± SD. * $p < 0.05$, ** $p < 0.01$, *** $p < 0.001$, vs. H_2O_2-treated cells (one-way analysis of variance with Dunnet's post hoc test).

Therefore, we performed an investigation to assess the potential protective effects of the newly synthesized compounds using an in vitro model of hydrogen peroxide-induced oxidative stress.

The application of melatonin, a reference compound, in a pre-treatment regimen for a duration of 90 min exhibited remarkable benefits in enhancing the resilience of SH-SY5Y cells against H_2O_2-induced damage. This was evidenced by a substantial increase in cell viability compared to the H_2O_2 group, with percentages of 10%, 18%, 30%, 44%, and 52%, for melatonin concentrations of 1, 5, 10, 25, and 50 µM, respectively. A statistical analysis revealed significant differences ($p < 0.05$; $p < 0.001$) when compared to the H_2O_2 group. Likewise, the compound rasagiline exhibited a protective influence at concentrations of 5, 10, 25, and 50 µM, resulting in viability percentages of 14%, 28%, 43%, and 45%, respectively. The pre-incubation with compound **3n** effectively preserved the integrity of SH-SY5Y cells, indicating a potential neuroprotective effect. Notably, compound **3n** displayed a more pronounced protective effect when compared to the reference compound donepezil. Furthermore, at the highest concentration employed, it demonstrates the most significant neuroprotective activity among the three reference compounds, providing 60% protection ($p < 0.001$).

In summary, although none of the 30 tested compounds proved to be a more potent AChE inhibitor than donepezil than the compounds designed from Wang et al. [45] based on the fusion of donepezil and melatonin, our lead molecule **3c** manifests itself as a potential multifunctional agent with antioxidant activity better than donepezil–melatonin in the DPPH and FRAP methods, inhibited lipid peroxidation stronger than donepezil–melatonin and the control, showed better biocompatibility than donepezyl, and also displayed very low cytotoxic activity against normal murine fibroblast cells (CCL-1) and malignant neuroblastoma cell lines of human (SH-SY5Y) and murine (Neuro-2a). Additionally, the pharmacokinetic properties and the blood–brain barrier (BBB) permeability of compound 3c were favorable and suitable for further study in vivo. Additionally, the compound 3n with two indole scaffolds showed the highest activity against BChE (IC_{50} = 21.12 ± 1.48 µM), a high selectivity index (SI = 47.34), and effectively preserved the integrity of SH-SY5Y cells in the in vitro model of hydrogen peroxide-induced oxidative stress, indicating a more pronounced protective effect than the reference compound donepezil.

2.10. Molecular Docking of Human AChE and of Human BChE

The thirty hydrazide hydrazone and sulfonyl hydrazone derivatives were subjected to molecular docking in AChE and BChE crystallographic structures. Studies were conducted using the X-ray crystallographic structures of human AChE (PDB ID 4EY7) and human BChE (PDB ID 6QAA). Figure 3 presents the 2D protein–ligand interaction (PLIs) diagrams of the co-crystalized ligands in AChE (Figure 3a) and BChE (Figure 3b), respectively.

The PLI diagrams of the reference compounds clearly demonstrate that water molecules mediate some of the PLIs in the active sites of the enzymes. Thus, the applied docking protocol involves water (solvent) molecules. In addition, the PLIs outline several amino acid residues that participate in specific interactions with the ligands. These residues were taken into account when analyzing the PLIs of the studied hydrazide hydrazones and sulfonyl hydrazones derivatives.

Molecular docking studies of the investigated compounds in AChE and BChE were performed by applying a "triangle matcher" option as a placement method and London dG scoring function. Different docking protocols were explored to follow the effect of docking parameters on the docking results. The following docking protocols (DP) were applied depending on the type of the post-placement refinement and the final scoring methodologies: DP 1: rigid receptor/no final scoring; DP 2: rigid receptor/London dG final scoring; DP 3: rigid receptor/GBVI/WSA final scoring; DP 4: induced fit/no final scoring; DP 5: induced fit/London dG final scoring; DP 6: induced fit/GBVI/WSA final scoring. For both targets, very similar results were obtained between DP 1 and DP 4, DP 2 and DP 5, and between DP 3 and DP 6, respectively (Figure 4). The analysis of the obtained results shows that the rankings obtained with DP 1 and DP 4 (Figure 4), lower charts) are in best agreement with the experimentally reported activities (Tables 1 and 2). For clarity,

Figure 4a shows the obtained results from rigid receptor docking (DP 1, DP 2 and DP 3) in AChE and from induced fit docking (DP 4, DP 5 and DP 6), in BChE (Figure 4b).

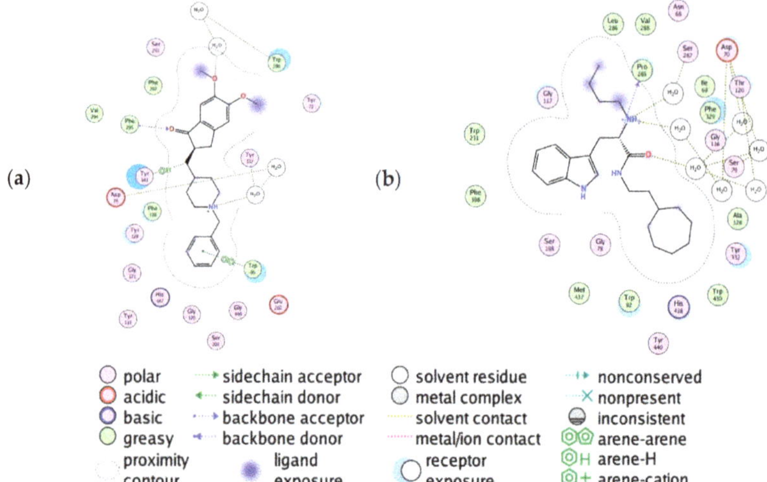

Figure 3. 2D protein-ligand interaction diagrams of the co-crystalized ligands: (**a**) E20 (donepezil) in AChE, and (**b**) HUN in BChE.

The docking protocols have been validated by inspecting the binding energies and the RMSD values of the redocked reference ligand (donepezil). The reported docking scores of donepezil (Figure 4) correspond to the poses with the lowest RMSD (between 0.367 and 1.053 Å for docking protocols DP1 to DP6) illustrating the ability of the applied protocols to reproduce the experimental pose of the reference ligand in very similar orientations and conformations. The parallel runs resulted in the same docking scores and poses. In addition, the ranking of compounds according to their activities and docking scores show good correspondence (Figure 4), thus confirming the ability of the applied docking protocols to approximate the binding energies of the studied compounds.

As seen from Figure 4, hydrazide hydrazone derivatives (3* compounds) show more favorable binding energies in comparison with sulfonyl hydrazone derivatives (5* compounds). The lower charts in Figure 4 show separately the results obtained by DP 1, where the most active compounds (see Tables 1 and 2) are presented in magenta. In the case of AChE, the most active compounds occupy the positions with highest binding energies following donepezil. In the case of BChE, this tendency is less pronounced; however, all active compounds are classified in the top half.

In addition to the analysis based on the docking scores (binding energies) (Figure 4), a visual inspection of the poses of the most active compounds, along with those of donepezil, were also performed to ensure that the poses with the lowest docking scores correspond to the most reasonable binding modes of the compounds (the best overlap to the reference compound, similar orientations of the interacting functional groups and atoms of the ligand). Figure 5 illustrates the best poses of donepezil and of the active compounds **3a**, **3b**, **3c**, and **3d** in the binding site of AChE. As seen, the most active compounds overlay well with donepezil and especially in the CAS region of the pocket.

Figure 6 represents the PLIs diagrams of the best poses after docking (except for compound **3a**, where the third scored pose of binding energy −53.91 kcal/mol towards −57.88 kcal/mol of the best scored pose, as shown in Figure 4) of the most active compounds in AChE performed with DP 1 chosen as the most reliable one after a thorough analysis of the obtained results.

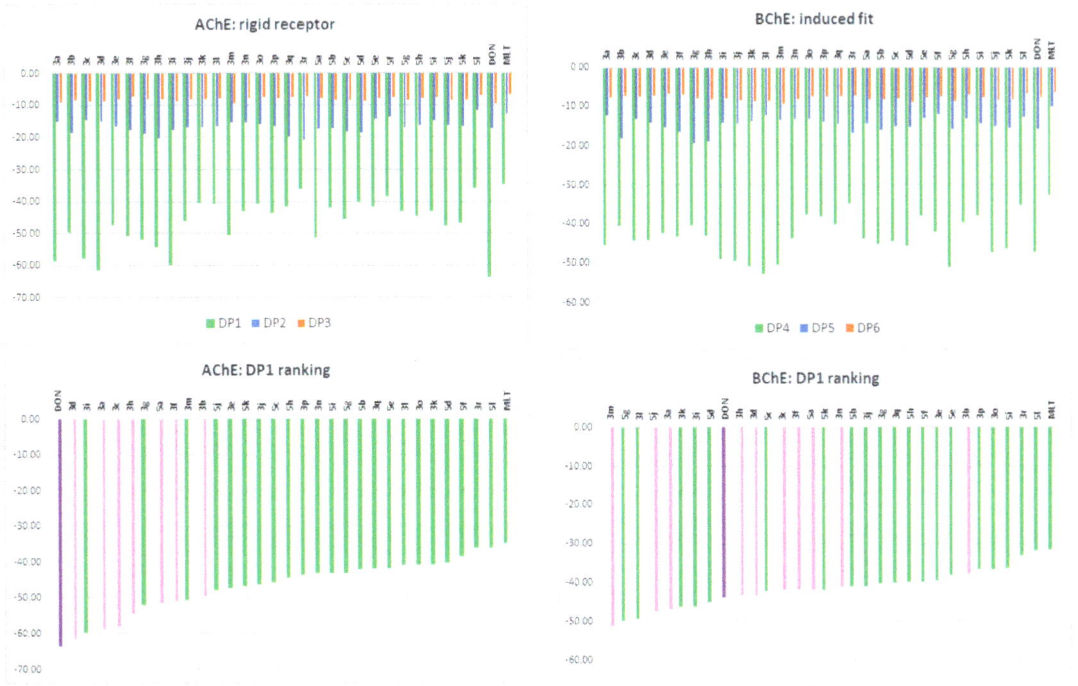

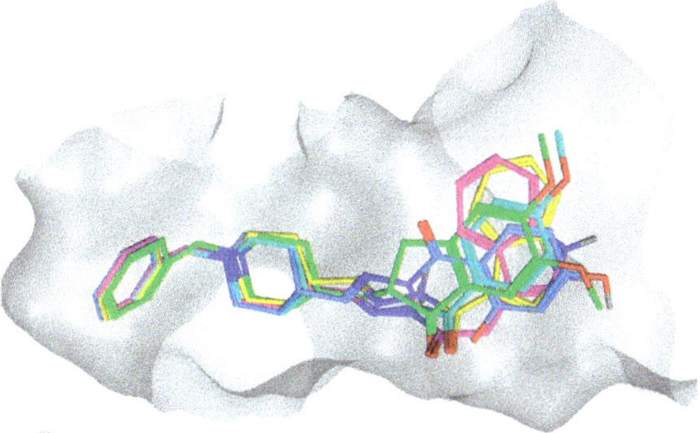

Figure 4. Docking results of all 30 synthesized compounds along with donepezil and melatonin, respectively, for: (**a**) AChE, and (**b**) BChE. The docking scores (Y-axis) approximate the binding energies of the compounds (lower docking scores correspond to better binding energies, in kcal/mol). The order of compounds (X-axis) in the upper charts is in accordance with Tables 1 and 2 and donepezil (DON) and melatonin (MLT) are shown last; in the lower charts, the compounds are ranked according to their docking scores. Colors used for docking scores: green—DP 1 and DP 4; blue—DP 2 and DP 5; red—DP 3 and DP 6; magenta—active compounds (Tables 1 and 2); violet—donepezil.

Figure 5. The best poses of donepezil (C-atoms in green) and the active compounds **3a** (C-atoms in magenta), **3b** (C-atoms in blue), **3c** (C-atoms in yellow), **3d** (C-atoms in cyan) in the active site of AChE (PDB ID 4EY7); O-atoms are colored in red and N-atoms in dark blue.

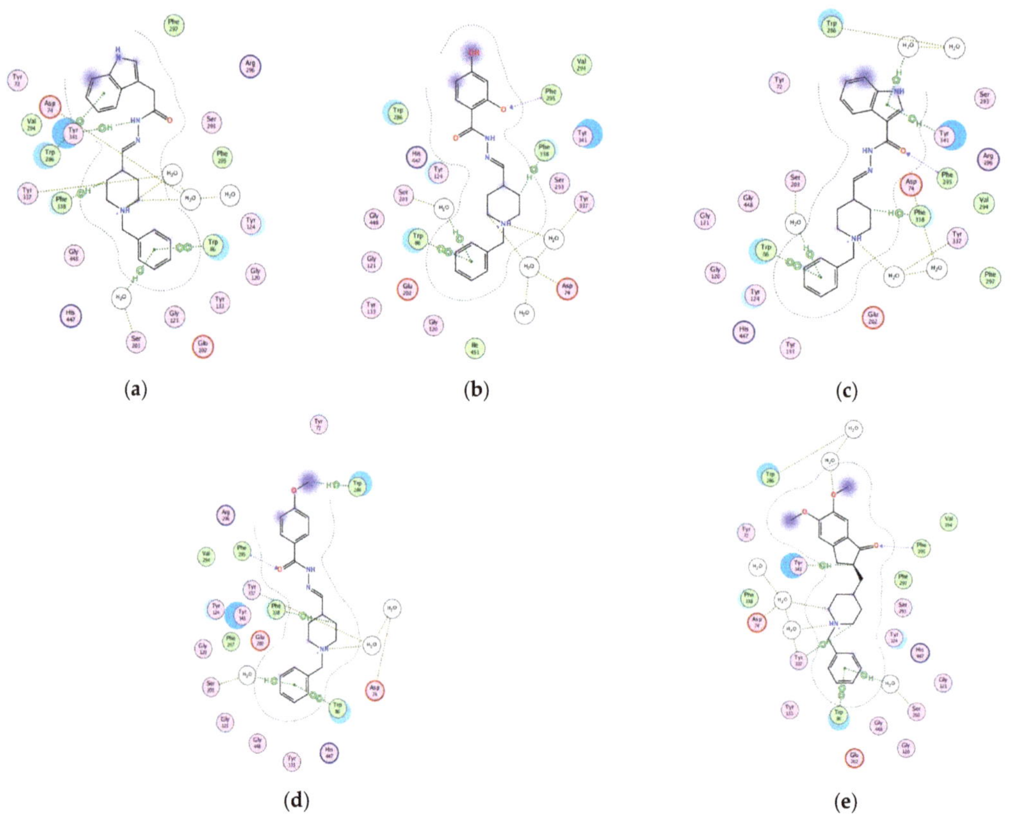

Figure 6. PLI of (**a**) **3a**, (**b**) **3b**, (**c**) **3c**, (**d**) **3d**, and (**e**) donepezil in the ligand-binding domain of AChE (PDB ID 4EY7). For the type of interactions, see the legend in Figure 3.

As seen from Figure 3a, the co-crystalized AChE donepezil demonstrated six PLIs: one H-bond with Phe295, two H-bonds mediated by water with Asp74 and Tyr337, one arene-arene interaction with Trp86, one arene-H interaction with Tyr341 and one arene-H interaction mediated by water with Trp286. The donepezil, after docking (Figure 6e), repeated all the PLIs of the co-crystalized ligand, showing one newly appeared PLI—an arene-H interaction with Ser203. As seen from Figure 6a–d, the most active compounds **3a**, **3b**, **3c**, and **3d** repeated the aforementioned PLIs of donepezil after docking with Asp74, Trp86, Ser203, and Tyr337. Almost all of the shown compounds repeated the arene-H interaction with Trp86, except compound **3b**, where this interaction appeared directly with Trp286 without mediating water. Almost all of the shown compounds performed the H-bond with Phe295, except compound **3a**. Two out of four shown compounds (**3a** and **3d**) repeated the arene-H interaction with Tyr341. All four compounds demonstrated a newly appeared interaction of type arene-H with Phe338. The results obtained by the molecular docking studies are in agreement with the results shown by Alov et al., [46] demonstrating the interactions with Trp86, Trp286, and Phe295 as of high importance for AChE. The interaction with Trp286 is one of the most frequent intermolecular interactions between AChE and donepezil, therefore its engagement in the interaction of our ligands and AChE mimics the natural ligand interaction.

The binding modes of the compounds of series 5 were also analyzed on the example of the best ranked and most active sulfonyl hydrazone derivative **5a** (Supporting information, Figure S2a,b). In contrast to hydrazide hydrazone derivatives, the preferable ionized form of the compound at physiological pH (73% of all possible forms) was with a polarized =N-N- group, potentially due to the neighboring -SO$_2$ group (Supporting information, Figure S2a). In addition, except the best one, the remaining binding poses showed an opposite orientation in the receptor pocket with the benzyl-piperadine part directed to the PAS region of the cavity. Figure S2b in the Supporting information illustrates these results on the example of the first two highest ranked poses of compound 5a. Although the best ranked pose has an orientation similar to that of donepezil, the other poses (with similar docking scores) had opposite orientations in the binding site. Thus, the lower activity values and docking scores of the compounds of series 5 can be related to the above discussed structural peculiarities; however, additional studies should prove these suggestions.

Figure 7 represents the PLIs of compounds **3a**, **3c**, **3d**, and **3n** after docking performed with DP 1, respectively, in AChE and BChE. The compounds **3a**, **3c**, and **3n** were chosen as the most active ones in BChE, while the compound **3d** was chosen instead of the next most active compound **3h**, due to its highest activity in AChE. The best poses of compounds **3c** and **3n** are shown, while Figure 5a depicts the second scored pose of compound **3a** with a binding energy −45.11 towards −46.88 of the best scored pose; Figure 6c depicts the fifth scored pose of compound 3d with a binding energy −40.34 towards −43.22 of the best scored pose.

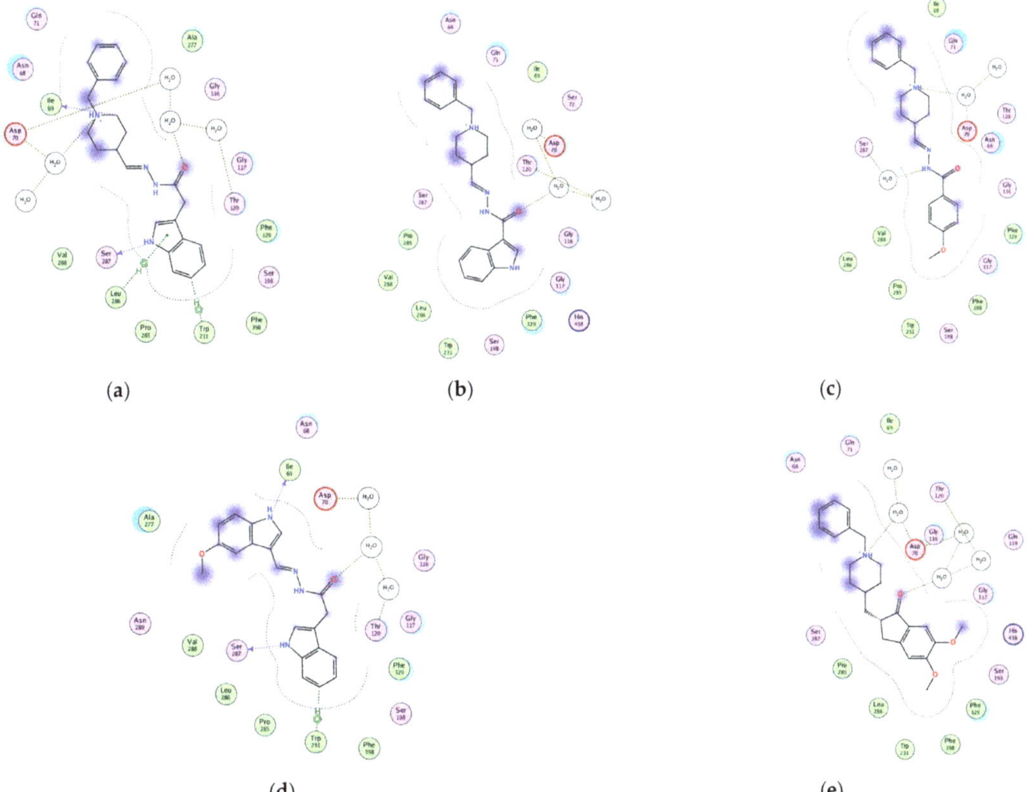

Figure 7. PLI of (**a**) **3a**, (**b**) **3c**, (**c**) **3d**, (**d**) **3n**, and (**e**) donepezil, in the ligand-binding domain of BChE (PDB ID 6QAA). For the type of interactions, see the legend in Figure 3.

As seen from Figure 7e, the best scored pose of donepezil after docking in BChE demonstrated water-mediated H-bonds with Asp70 and Thr120. In Figure 7a–d, all compounds **3a**, **3c**, **3d**, and **3n** repeated the H-bond with Asp70, while the compounds **3a** and **3c** repeated the PLI with Thr120 as well. In addition, compounds **3a**, **3d**, and **3n** demonstrated a H-bond mediated by water (except **3a**) with Ser287. Compounds **3a** and **3n** demonstrated a H-bond with Ile69, as well as an arene-H interaction with Trp231.

The above analysis illustrates that the most active compounds in the series have similar binding modes to that of donepezil and perform specific interactions with residues involved in donepezil binding. Thus, based on the binding energies and protein–ligand interactions, the donepezil-based derivatives appear to be promising lead structures as inhibitors of the studied cholinesterases.

2.11. Docking of Ligand Set in MT1 and MT2 Receptors

The neuromodulator melatonin synchronizes circadian rhythms and related physiological functions through the actions of two G-protein-coupled receptors: MT1 and MT2. Because MLT exerts neuroprotective and anti-apoptotic effects by the activation of MT1 receptors—probably through the induction of the expression of several antioxidant enzymes and the modulation of mitochondrial function by MT1 receptors localized on mitochondria in mouse models of neurodegenerative disorders—we docked the most promising AchE and BchE inhibitors from the molecular docking results discussed above to an MT1and MT2 crystal structure, prioritizing structural fit and chemical novelty.

2.12. MT1 Receptor Docking Results

The pocket in the MT1 receptor is mostly isolated from the outside media and its widest dimension is in the plane, perpendicular to spirals forming channels. There also exists a narrow protuberance in the inside of the cell. A visualization of the pocket of the MT1 receptor (Figure S1), as well as detailed data of the docking results, are presented in the supplementary materials (Tables S1, S2 and S5; Figures S4, S5 and S10).

To present interactions between receptors and our ligands at their best poses, we prepared interaction maps at which polar amino acids are depicted with pink, while lipophilic ones are in green (Figure 8), acidic amino acids are circled with red, while the basic ones are circled with blue. Side chain interactions are depicted with green arrows, and the interaction with the backbone is in blue, where the arrowhead points to the hydrogen bond acceptor. Exposure to the solvent is depicted with a blue halo around the ligand atoms and by blue circles around the amino acids of the receptor. The proximity contour of the pocket is depicted by a gray dotted line.

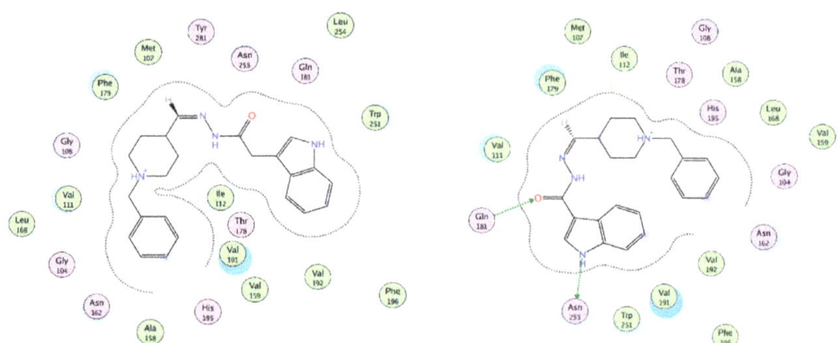

Figure 8. Interaction maps of best performing ligands with MT1: **3a** (**left**) and **3c** (**right**).

The best interaction with MT1 is by **3a** (Table S5 in Supplementary Materials). The best interaction energy in this case is due to its best fit in the active site cavity without big sterical hindrances and its major term is hydrophobic energy. Unfortunately, there are no formed hydrogen bonds or relatively high electrostatic interactions. It is worth mentioning that in the very close vicinity to the ligand are some key amino acids, of which the unique configuration is characteristic of the active form of the receptor. The interaction of Asn162

(N162 4.60), according to Ballesteros–Weinstein nomenclature [47], with neighboring amino acids and, thus, the formation of a H-bond, leads to modulation and a reduction in the entrance of the ligand. His195 (H195 5.46) is well known to be crucial for the formation of the "longitudinal channel" for ligands in MT1 and its mutation is deleterious [48]. Tyr281 (Y281 7.39) with two adjacent residues also participating in forming smaller pockets in MT1, allowing more accommodation in the MT1 of different ligands than MT2, thus helping in subtype specificity between them.

The next of the best interacting ligands is **3c**, which has a low hydrophobic energy gain due to the less hydrophobic solvent-accessible surface based on the lack of one CH_2 group. It forms two hydrogen bonds with the amide group of Gln181 (Q181 ECL2) and with Asn255 (N255 6.52) that will lead to increased selectivity of that ligand to the pocket of MT1. Ramelteon, a well known agonist used for insomnia treatment, forms hydrogen bonds with Gln181 [49]; mutational studies confirm its importance for the binding of natural ligand melatonin and receptor activation. Gln181, together with closely situated Phe179 (F179 ECL2), is positioned in the ECL2 (extra cellular loop) with part of the receptor forming a "lid" structure, participating in ligand recognition and positioning it right for further activation. It is recognized in mutation analysis that the replacement of Gln181 severely diminished the function of the MT1 receptor to its natural ligand, therefore highlighting its importance. What is also impressive is the formed hydrogen bond with Asn255, the amino acid, known to form the only significant polar interaction of melatonin in the MT1 receptor [50].

An analysis of the best 50 poses of our ligands inside the MT1 cavity shows that most of the ligands interact by surface contact with Phe179 followed by arene contact with Phe196 (F196 5.47), side chain hydrogen bond forming with Asn255 (as donor), hydrogen bond forming with the backbone of Gly104 (G104 3.29) (as donor), and interacting with the side chain of Gln181 as a hydrogen bond acceptor.

Phe179 and Gln181 as part of ECL2 and their role in receptor activation, as well as Asn255 interaction, are discussed above. Stauch et al. [51] stated that the ligands interact with MT1 "mainly by strong aromatic stacking with Phe179 and auxiliary hydrogen bonds with Asn162 and Gln181". Phe196 (F196 5.47) is one of the three most frequent intermolecular interactions between the MT1 receptor and melatonin, therefore its engagement in the interaction with our ligands and MT1 mimics the natural ligand interaction [50].

2.13. MT2 Receptor Docking Results

The widest dimension of the active site pocket of MT2 is in the plane, perpendicular to the spirals forming the channel. A narrow protuberance is formed inside of the cell that is bigger compared to the one in MT1and highly hydrophilic. A visualization of the pocket of the MT2 receptor (Figure S5) as well as detailed data of the docking results (see Supporting information, Tables S3, S4 and S6; Figures S4, S7 and S8) are presented in the supplementary materials. Interaction maps of the best ligands by their interaction energy are presented in Figure 9.

An analysis of the best 50 poses of our ligands inside the MT2 cavity (supplementary materials Figures S6 and S7) shows that most of the ligands interact by surface contact with Phe192 (F192 ECL2) followed by interactions with Gln194 (Q194 ECL2), of which the side chain acts as an acceptor of the hydrogen bond. In most cases, Phe209 (F209 5.47) interacts by its arene ring and Ala117 (A117 3.29) acts as a donor of the hydrogen bond with its backbone atoms. Tyr294 (Y294 7.39) interacts as an acceptor of the hydrogen bond with its phenolic group.

Tyr 294 (Y294 7.39) is one of the amino acid residues that, together with Tyr 298 (Y298 7.43) and Leu295 (L295 7.40), is the reason for the formation of larger pockets in the MT2 receptor, allowing the accommodation of bigger ligands. Therefore, Tyr 294 is one of the amino acids participating in the formation of molecular structure and is selective for MT2 agonists [48].

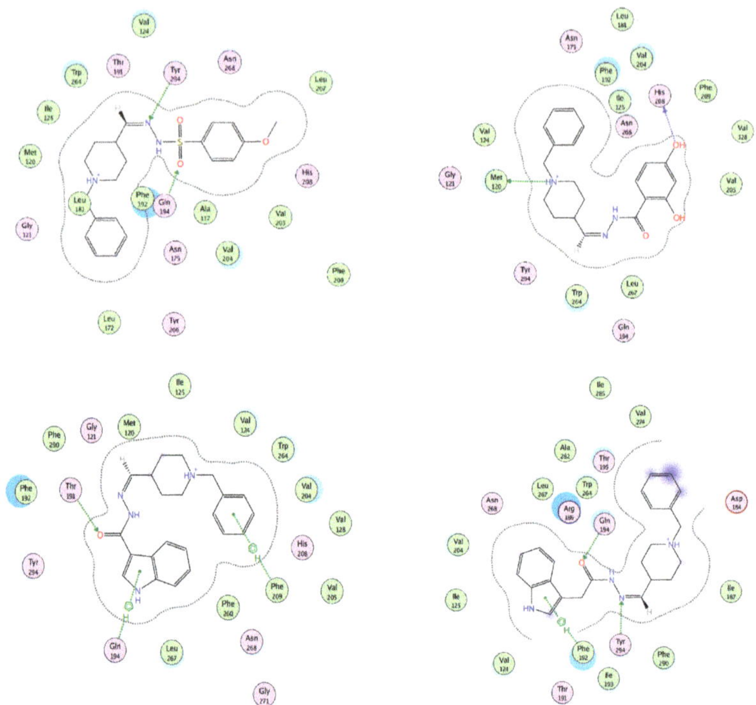

Figure 9. Interaction maps of our best ligands and MT2 receptor interior **3d** (**upper left**), **3b** (**upper right**), **3c** (**lower left**), **3a** (**lower right**).

A number of direct and water-mediated hydrogen bonds with the polar side chains of Gln194 ECL2, Asn162 (N162 4.60), and Asn268 (N268 6.52) are reported for simulations of ligand binding specific to the MT2 receptor [52], and Asn268 (N268 6.52) and Leu295 (L295 7.40) are reported in expression studies as essential for natural ligand binding to MT2 [52]. Phe209, on the other hand, is participating in the formation of the MT2 receptor specifically to the hydrophobic subpocket [53].

Ala117 is found to be one of the bulkier amino acids that is different in MT2 in comparison to MT1 and, thus, interaction with them could aid in the larger and more specific accommodation of MT2ligands [54]. Phe 192 from ECL2 is known to form an "aromatic sandwich" in interactions with specific ligands for MT2, thus is involved in the agonist specificity of the MT2 receptor [55]. As can be seen in Figure S11 (See Supporting information), with the exception of **5a** and **3i**, the ligands with a clear preference towards one of the receptors prefer the MT2 receptor. Only two of the ligands, **3a** and **3c**, do not discriminate between MT1 and MT2 receptors, but bind strongly to both of them. These ligands are the best binders for the MT1 receptor and are in the first four of the best binders for MT2 receptors.

Since MLT inhibits Aβ generation and prevents their aggregation and formation into amyloid fibrils through its neuroprotective and antioxidant properties in the brain via the activation of MT1 and MT2 receptors, we hope that newly synthesized compounds, especially **3c**, similarly to MLT would mediate antifibrillogenic effects and prevent cells from β Amyloid (Aβ)-mediated toxicity, the pathogenic process underlying AD.

2.14. In Silico ADME/Tox Study

The synthesized compounds were subjected to in silico ADME screening using the SwissADME online tool. Specific molecular and physicochemical properties were analyzed in comparison to available drugs used to treat AD (Table 6 for the hydrazide hydrazones and Table 7 for the sulfonyl hydrazones). These included molecular weight (MW), number of heavy atoms, number of aromatic heavy atoms, number of rotatable bonds, hydrogen bond donors (HBD), hydrogen bond acceptors (HBA), topological polar surface area (TPSA), molar refractivity (MR), octanol/water ratio (WLOGP), solubility, BBB permeability, PgP substrate, and gastro-intestinal absorption (GIA).

Table 6. In silico ADME properties of the new hydrazide hydrazones.

Compd.	MW	Heavy Atoms	Arom. Heavy Atoms	RB	HBA	HBD	TPSA	MR	WLOGP	ESOL Class	BBB Perm.	Pgp Subs	GIA
3a	374.48	28	15	7	3	2	60.49	117.59	3.19	Moderately soluble	Yes	Yes	High
3b	353.41	26	12	6	5	3	85.16	105.2	2.19	Soluble	No	Yes	High
3c	360.45	27	15	6	3	2	60.49	113.01	3.26	Moderately soluble	Yes	Yes	High
3d	351.44	26	12	7	4	1	53.93	107.64	2.79	Soluble	Yes	No	High
3e	323.39	24	12	6	4	2	64.93	98.14	1.83	Soluble	Yes	Yes	High
3f	339.39	25	12	6	5	3	85.16	100.17	1.54	Soluble	No	Yes	High
3g	339.39	25	12	6	5	3	85.16	100.17	1.46	Soluble	No	Yes	High
3h	355.39	26	12	6	6	4	105.39	102.19	1.24	Soluble	No	Yes	High
3i	353.41	26	12	7	5	2	74.16	104.64	1.84	Soluble	Yes	Yes	High
3j	346.38	25	9	9	5	3	104.81	94.61	2.15	Soluble	No	Yes	High
3k	360.41	26	9	9	5	2	99.51	93.95	2.16	Soluble	No	Yes	High
3l	330.38	24	9	8	4	2	84.72	93.02	2.15	Soluble	No	No	High
3m	406.48	30	15	10	4	2	84.72	117.5	3.66	Moderately soluble	No	No	High
3n	346.38	26	18	6	3	3	82.27	102.4	3.35	Soluble	No	Yes	High
3o	323.35	24	15	6	4	2	75.71	92.45	2.95	Soluble	Yes	No	High
3p	337.37	25	15	7	4	2	75.71	97.04	2.88	Soluble	Yes	No	High
3q	323.35	24	15	6	4	3	86.71	92.57	2.57	Soluble	No	No	High
3r	302.28	22	12	5	6	4	111.38	80.17	1.58	Soluble	No	No	High
donepezil	379.49	28	12	6	4	0	38.77	115.31	3.83	Moderately soluble	Yes	Yes	High
melatonin	232.28	17	9	5	2	2	54.12	67.18	1.86	Soluble	Yes	No	High

The obtained results showed average molecular weight (MW) levels below 450 for all newly synthesized compounds, which is essential for drugs that need to cross into and affect the central nervous system (CNS). The TPSA values were in the range of 60 Å^2 to 112 Å^2, which also fell within the limit below 140 Å^2 for active absorption of the molecules, good permeability, and oral bioavailability. In all derivatives, the rotatable bonds were between 5 and 7, except for compound **3m** where there were 10 [56]. Most CNS affecting compounds have 5 or fewer rotatable bonds, and more than 10 have been shown in rats to reduce the oral bioavailability [56].

The formation of hydrogen bonds is primarily associated with the bonding of oxygen and nitrogen in molecules. Thus, the probability of the molecule entering the CNS increases when the sum of nitrogen and oxygen atoms is less than five. The analysis showed that the number of proton acceptors was less than six and the number of proton donors was less than three for both hydrazide hydrazones and sulfonyl hydrazones.

The n-octanol/water ratio (logPo/w) is a key physicochemical parameter related to the lipophilicity of compounds. The biological activity of drugs is almost entirely due to their logP, and the rate at which they are metabolized is linearly related to logP. LogP values between two and four were recommended for drugs used to treat neurological diseases where higher log p values indicate a higher rate of brain penetration of compounds, as well as the opposite [57]. From the obtained data shown in Table 6, we found that compound

3m (3.66) had the highest WLOGP value among the hydrazide hydrazones followed by **3n** (3.35), both values being under that of donepezil (3.83). Most of the sulfonyl hydrazones (Table 7) showed acceptable values less than 4, except for a few molecules with higher values: **5g** (5.39), **5j** (5.30), and **5d** (5.08).

Table 7. In silico ADME properties of the new sulfonyl hydrazones.

Compd.	MW	Heavy Atoms	Arom.Heavy Atoms	RB	HBA	HBD	TPSA	MR	WLOGP	ESOL Class	BBB Perm.	Pgp Subs	GIA
5a	357.47	25	12	6	4	1	70.15	104.05	3.41	Soluble	Yes	No	High
5b	373.43	26	15	6	5	1	90.3	100.25	3.59	Soluble	No	No	High
5c	359.4	25	15	6	5	2	101.16	95.35	3.53	Soluble	No	No	High
5d	389.47	28	21	6	3	1	71.84	111.75	5.08	Moderately soluble	No	No	High
5e	343.4	24	15	5	4	1	81.07	93.76	3.58	Soluble	No	No	High
5f	313.37	22	15	4	3	1	71.84	87.27	3.57	Soluble	Yes	No	High
5g	403.5	29	21	6	3	1	71.84	116.72	5.39	Moderately soluble	No	No	High
5h	334.39	23	12	6	5	1	85.37	88.46	3.41	Soluble	No	No	High
5i	320.36	22	12	6	5	1	85.37	83.49	3.1	Soluble	No	No	High
5j	419.5	30	21	7	4	2	91.93	118.31	5.3	Moderately soluble	No	No	High
5k	405.47	29	21	7	4	2	91.93	113.35	4.99	Moderately soluble	No	No	High
5l	294.76	19	12	4	3	1	66.91	75.52	3.73	Soluble	Yes	No	High
donepezil	379.49	28	12	6	4	0	38.77	115.31	3.83	Moderately soluble	Yes	Yes	High
melatonin	232.28	17	9	5	2	2	54.12	67.18	1.86	Soluble	Yes	No	High

Molar refractivity (MR) is another important descriptor frequently used in QSAR studies in drug design. To increase the drug similarity, logP values were recommended to be in the range of −0.4 to +5.6 and for molar refractivity from 40 to 130. The values of the relevant descriptors for all compounds fell within these indicated ranges (Tables 6 and 7).

The results of the studies on the solubility of the proposed newly synthesized compounds were also presented in Tables 6 and 7 Most of the hydrazide hydrazones were classified as soluble, except **3a**, **3c**, and **3m** (Table 6) that were marked as moderately soluble. In the group of the sulfonyl hydrazones (Table 7), eight compounds were predicted to be soluble (**5a**, **5b**, **5c**, **5e**, **5f**, **5h**, **5i**, and **5l**) and the rest as moderately soluble, according to the classic ESOL model.

2.15. Drug-Likeness Properties

Lipinski's rule is important for the development of new drugs because initial screening with this rule allows optimization of the chemical structure of promising molecules in the preliminary analysis. Lipinski's rule is a heuristic approach to predict drug similarity and determines that molecules with MM > 500, logP > 5, proton donors >5, and proton acceptors >10 have both poor absorption and permeability. From Tables 6 and 7, it can be seen that the molecular weights of the new compounds were within the range 294.7–419.5 Da. The logP values of most of the hydrazones were smaller than 5 (in the range of 2.49–4.67), except for compounds **5d** (5.03), **5g** (5.39), and **5j** (5.30). The number of groups that accepted hydrogen atoms (n-ON) was less than 10, and the groups that donated hydrogen atoms (n-OHNH) were less than 5, which were within Lipinski's rules.

2.16. In Silico Prediction of BBB Permeability

Drugs that target the CNS must first cross the blood–brain barrier (BBB). The inability of therapeutic molecules to penetrate the BBB is a key obstacle for CNS drug candidates and needs to be addressed quickly in the drug development process; predicting the BBB permeability of new CNS drugs is therefore crucial [54]. A SwissADME webserver was used to predict the BBB permeability [56]. The study confirmed that all compounds can penetrate the BBB, and this facilitates their action inside the CNS for treating AD. From the prediction results obtained (Tables 6 and 7), it can be seen that only some of the proposed compounds meet the requirements for possible transfer to the brain: **3a, 3c, 3d, 3e, 3i, 3o, 3p, 5a, 5f,** and **5l**. Most of the hydrazide hydrazone structures were predicted to have the ability to act as a substrate for P-gp except compounds **3d, 3l, 3m,** and **3o–3r**. Unlike hydrazide hydrazones, none of the sulfonyl hydrazones showed properties of a P-gp substrate. The predicted GI data of the 30 compounds and the two control drugs are also presented in Tables 6 and 7. All of them showed a high degree of GI absorption.

2.17. Predicted Toxicity

The results from the toxicity prediction experiments performed over the proposed hydrazide and sulfonyl hydrazones are presented in Table 8. The predicted values of the median lethal dose (LD_{50}), the toxicity class, the logP value, and the main toxicological pathways and endpoints were calculated and presented along with the corresponding mean value of the probability (Prob). The predictive results indicated that almost all compounds are defined as Inactive with regard to hepatotoxicity, mutagenicity, immunotoxicity, and cytotoxicity. Weak activity (in blue) with a relatively low level of probability was established for compounds **3o** and **3r**, similar to the control drug donepezil. In terms of carcinogenicity, most compounds were determined to be weakly active (in blue) with low probability levels between 0.50 and 0.63. Only one of the tested compounds, **3r,** showed high activity (in red) in the immunotoxicity study with a probability level of 0.94, as well as donepezil itself (0.95).

2.18. BBB Permeability by In Vitro PAMPA Test

Compounds **3a, 3b, 3c, 3m, 3n,** and **5a** were considered as promising CNS-acting agents based on their AChE and/or BChE inhibition potencies, selectivity, and favorable cytotoxicity profiles. At the same time, they needed to fulfill the requirement for good BBB permeation in order to achieve sufficient brain exposure. Although transport across the BBB is quite a complex phenomenon, passive diffusion is still the primary route for exogenous substances to access that target [58]. So, the selected compounds were subjected to an in vitro PAMPA-BBB assay, relying on the capacity of the method in distinguishing the candidates with good BBB passive permeabilities [59]. The results (Table 9) showed that five amongst the six tested compounds had a high BBB permeability of logPe < 5, and only 3b was moderately permeable with logPe = 5.873.

Our experimental PAMPA-BBB study was accompanied by in silico calculations of the physicochemical properties responsible for an optimal BBB passage [37]. For the purposes of the present discussion, the following parameters were calculated by ACD/logD software v. 9.08, ACD Inc., Benton, AR, Canada: molecular weight (Mw), the most basic $pKa_{,MB}$ value, logP, pH dependent octanol/water distribution coefficient calculated at pH 7.4 ($logD_{7.4}$), polar surface area (PSA), number of free rotatable bonds (FRB), counts of hydrogen bond donors (HBD), and hydrogen bond acceptors (HBA) (Table 7).

All compounds except **3m** fulfill Lipinski's rule of five, which is an indication of good gastro-intestinal permeability. Because of the anatomical and functional specificities of the BBB, more stringent criteria are applied to compounds aimed at action in the brain. The molecular weights of tested compounds are around the upper limit of 400 g/mol, proposed as a threshold for good BBB permeability [60]. With logP values between 3.16 and 5.05, $logD_{7.4}$ in the range 2.56–5.05, 5–8 free rotatable bonds (FRB), 1–3 H-bond donors (HBD) and 5–7 H-bond acceptors (HBA), most of the compounds meet the requirements for the given properties and agreed well with the PAMPA-BBB experimental results [61,62].

Compounds **3a** and **3c** are moderate bases, **3m** is a week acid with pKa 10.85, **3b, 3n,** and **5a** are amphoteric. Compounds **3a, 3b, 3c,** and **5a** are partially ionized at physiological pH 7.4 which is reflected by the difference between logP and $logD_{7.4}$ values, while **3m** and

3n exist mainly in a neutral state. Only **3c** and **5a** satisfy the polarity restriction criterion (PSA < 79 Å^{2}) [61]. Compounds **3a**, **3c**, and **5a** were also suggested as capable of escaping the P-gp mediated-efflux in the brain. The sum of nitrogen and oxygen atoms in their molecules is five (counted from the structure) and only slightly exceeds the proposed cut-off of four, but they completely obey the other two requirements of the rule of four, namely pKa$_{,MB}$ < 8 and and MW < 400 [63]. The moderate BBB permeability of **3b** is undoubtedly attributed to its higher polarity and more extensive ionization, about 80% at pH 7.4.

Table 8. Results from the toxicity prediction study.

Comp.	LD$_{50}$ (mg/kg) (Pred)	Toxicity Class (Pred)	Octanol/Water Partition coeff. (logP)	Organ Toxicity (Hepatotoxicity)		Carcinogenicity		Immunotoxicity		Mutagenicity		Cytotoxicity	
				Pred	Prob	Pred	Prob	Pred	Prob	Pred	Prob	Pred	Prob
3a	225	3	4.05	I	0.64	A	0.65	I	0.99	I	0.59	I	0.56
3b	1000	4	3.05	I	0.63	A	0.57	I	0.86	I	0.57	I	0.67
3c	370	4	4.12	I	0.6	A	0.63	I	0.99	I	0.54	I	0.56
3d	2000	4	3.65	I	0.69	A	0.63	I	0.88	I	0.57	I	0.63
3e	1962	4	2.69	I	0.62	A	0.62	I	0.98	I	0.55	I	0.66
3f	1962	4	2.64	I	0.57	A	0.54	I	0.74	I	0.58	I	0.65
3g	1962	4	2.4	I	0.59	A	0.56	I	0.71	I	0.59	I	0.6
3h	1962	4	2.1	I	0.57	A	0.52	I	0.97	I	0.59	I	0.66
3i	1250	4	2.7	I	0.59	A	0.57	A	0.79	I	0.59	I	0.6
3j	1120	4	2.93	I	0.5	I	0.52	A	0.5	I	0.58	I	0.61
3k	1120	4	2.94	I	0.53	I	0.54	A	0.64	I	0.57	I	0.55
3l	498	4	2.93	I	0.53	I	0.53	I	0.96	I	0.59	I	0.58
3m	498	4	4.45	I	0.52	I	0.54	I	0.98	I	0.58	I	0.55
3n	900	4	3.74	A	0.58	A	0.61	A	0.81	I	0.6	I	0.69
3o	4540	5	3.34	A	0.64	A	0.65	A	0.57	A	0.51	I	0.67
3p	6000	6	3.27	A	0.57	A	0.67	A	0.5	I	0.54	I	0.64
3q	6000	6	2.97	A	0.59	A	0.6	A	0.6	I	0.56	I	0.62
3r	4920	5	1.97	A	0.6	A	0.63	A	0.94	A	0.5	I	0.74
5a	1398	4	4.27	I	0.71	A	0.53	I	0.99	I	0.61	I	0.62
5b	500	4	3.98	A	0.5	A	0.5	I	0.8	I	0.51	I	0.74
5c	500	4	3.97	I	0.5	A	0.52	I	0.84	I	0.54	I	0.82
5d	500	4	5.47	I	0.6	A	0.5	I	0.99	I	0.56	I	0.61
5e	500	4	3.97	I	0.5	I	0.51	I	0.96	I	0.5	I	0.72
5f	500	4	3.96	I	0.53	A	0.51	I	0.99	I	0.55	I	0.63
5g	500	4	5.78	I	0.62	A	0.51	I	0.99	I	0.55	I	0.63
5h	500	4	3.8	I	0.51	A	0.54	I	0.99	I	0.54	I	0.86
5i	500	4	3.49	I	0.51	A	0.54	I	0.99	I	0.55	I	0.88
5j	500	4	5.84	I	0.51	I	0.52	I	0.99	I	0.54	I	0.8
5k	500	4	5.53	I	0.5	I	0.53	I	0.99	I	0.55	I	0.78
5l	500	4	4.12	I	0.63	I	0.6	I	0.99	I	0.66	I	0.7
donepezil	505	4	4.3	I	0.98	A	0.5	A	0.95	I	0.53	A	0.63
melatonin	963	4	2.25	I	0.84	I	0.68	I	0.51	I	0.9	I	0.73

From the viewpoint of the lead discovery process, compounds **3c** and **5a** were considered as the most prospective for further optimization since they most closely cover the rule of three recommendations [64].

Table 9. Experimentally measured BBB permeability and in silico calculated physicochemical properties of compounds selected for PAMPA analysis: logP; logD$_{7.4}$—distribution coefficient at pH 7.4; pK$_{a,MB}$—the most basic pKa value; PSA—polar surface area; FRB—free rotatable bonds; HBD—hydrogen bond donors; HBA—hydrogen bond acceptors; Ro4—violation of Rule of 4, Ro5—violation of Lipinski's rule of 5.

Compd.	PAMPA BBB −logPe	logP	logD$_{7.4}$	pK$_{a,MB}$	PSA, Å^2	FRB	HBD	HBA	Ro5
3a	4.420	3.33	2.74	7.86	82.27	6	3	5	0
3b	5.873	3.3	2.56	8.00	85.16	7	3	6	0
3c	4.466	3.31	2.72	7.85	60.49	5	2	5	0
3m	4.377	5.05	5.05	-	84.72	8	2	7	1
3n	4.084	3.52	3.52	0.83	82.27	5	3	6	0
5a	4.749	3.16	2.58	7.83	70.15	5	1	5	0

3. Materials and Methods

3.1. Chemistry

All solvents, chemicals, and reagents were obtained commercially and used without purification. Thin layer chromatography (TLC) was used to monitor the reactions. All melting points were determined in open glass capillaries and are uncorrected. ^{1}H spectra were recorded using DMSO-d$_6$ as a solvent on a Brucker Advance III 600 MHz spectrometer with tetramethylsilane as an internal standard. Chemical shifts (δ) are given in parts per million (ppm). High resolution mass spectrometry (HRMS) analysis was performed with the use of Agilent Accurate-Mass Q-TOF LC/MS G6520B system with dual electrospray (DESI) source (Agilent Technologies, Santa Clara, CA, USA). Microplate reader EZ Read 800, Biochrom and Shimatzu 1203 UV-VIS spectrophotometer (Japan) were used for antioxidant activity. All determinations were performed in triplicate (n = 3).

3.2. General Procedure for the Synthesis of Compounds **3a–r**

The solution of 20 mmol of the corresponding carbonyl compounds (**1a–n**) in 10 mL of absolute ethanol was mixed with a hot solution of 20 mmol (60 °C) aroylhydrazide (**2a–f**) in 10 mL of absolute ethanol and stirred for 1–8 h. The obtained crystalline precipitates were filtered, washed with ethanol-ether, recrystallized from ethanol.

N′-[(E)-(1-benzylpiperidin-4-yl)methylidene]-2-(1H-indol-3-yl)acetohydrazide, **3a** Yield: 68%; m.p. 167–168 °C. ^{1}H NMR (400 MHz, DMSO-d$_6$): 1:0.83 mixture of conformers; signals for major *synperiplanar* conformer around the amide bond: δ = 1.42–1.53 (m, 2H, CH2), 1.67–1.78 (m, 2H, CH2), 1.94–2.04 (m, 2H, CH2), 2.17–2.24 (m, 1H, H-4′), 2.77–2.82 (m, 2H, CH2), 3.46 (s, 2H, CH2), 3.90 (s, 2H, CH2), 6.98 (ddd, J = 1.00, 7.0, 8.0 Hz, 1H, H-5), 7.05 (ddd, J = 1.0, 7.0, 5.0 Hz, 1H, H-6), 7.17 (d, J = 2.3 Hz, 1H, H-2), 7.22–7.33 (m, 10H, H-2″, H-3″, H-4″, H-5″, and H-6″), 7.35 (d, J = 7.0 Hz, 1H, H-7), 7.44 (d, J = 5.3 Hz, 1H, CH), 7.53 (d, J = 8.2 Hz, 1H, H-4), 10.84 (s, 1H, NH), 10.85 (bs, 1H, NH); resolved signals for minor *antiperiplanar* conformer around the amide bond: 3.45 (s, 2H, CH2), 3.53 (s, 2H, CH2), 6.96 (ddd, J = 1.0, 7.0, 8.0 Hz, 1H, H-5), 7.07 (ddd, J = 1.0, 7.0, 5.0 Hz, 1H, H-6), 7.20 (d, J = 2.3 Hz, 1H, H-2), 10.89 (bs, 1H, NH), 11.06 (s, 1H, NH); ^{13}C NMR (100 MHz, DMSO-d6): signals for major *synperiplanar* conformer around the amide bond: δ = 28.85 (CH2), 29.06 (CH2), 38.10 (C-4′), 52.45 (CH2), 62.39 (CH2), 108.22 (C-3), 111.24 (C-7), 118.19 (C-5), 118.65 (C-4), 120.84 (C-6), 120.95 (C-5), 123.83 (C-2), 126.80 (C-4″), 127.14 (C-4a), 127.39 (C-4a), 128.11 (C-3″ and C-5″), 128.73 (C-2″ and C-6″), 135.95 (C-7a), 138.51 (C-1″), 149.21 (CH), 166.66 (C=0); resolved signals for minor *antiperiplanar* conformer around the amide bond: 152.96 (CH), 172.20 (C=O). HRMS (ESI) m/z: calcd: [M+H]$^+$ 375.217938. Found: [M+H]$^+$ 375.2178.

N′-[(E)-(1-benzylpiperidin-4-yl)methylidene]-2,4-dihydroxybenzohydrazide, **3b** Yield: 59%; m.p. 201–203 °C. ^{1}H NMR (400 MHz, DMSO-d$_6$): δ = 1.46 (dd, J = 3.1, 11.7, 1H) and 1.52 (dd, J = 3.1, 11.7 Hz, 1H, CH$_2$), 1.74 (dd, J = 2.7, 13.5 Hz, 2H, CH$_2$), 2.00–2.05 (m, 2H, CH$_2$), 2.22–2.34 (m, 1H, H-4′), 2.82 (d, J = 11.4 Hz, 2H, CH$_2$), 3.48 (s, 2H, CH$_2$), 6.27 (d, J = 2.3 Hz, 1H, H-3), 6.32 (dd, J = 2.3, 8.7 Hz, 1H, H-5), 7.23–7.35 (m, 5H, Ar), 7.67 (d,

J = 5.0 Hz, 1H, CH), 7.72 (d, J = 8.7 Hz, 1H, H-6), 10.17 (bs, 1H, OH), 11.32 (bs, 1H, NH), 12.44 (bs, 1H, OH). ^{13}C NMR (100 MHz, DMSO-d$_6$): δ = 29.00 (C-3$'$ and C-5$'$), 38.53 (C-4$'$), 52.42 (C-2$'$ and C-6$'$), 62.36 (CH$_2$), 102.81 (C-3), 105.87 (C-1), 107.19 (C-5), 126.86 (C-4$''$), 128.13 (C-3$''$ and C-5$''$), 128.78 (C-2$''$ and C-6$''$), 129.35 (C-6), 138.41 (C-1$''$), 155.26 (CH), 162.49 and 162.53 (C-2 and C-4), 165.44 (C=O). HRMS (ESI) *m/z*: calcd: [M+H]+ 354.181218. Found: [M+H]+ 354.1811.

N$'$-[(E)-(1-benzylpiperidin-4-yl)methylidene]-1H-indole-3-carbohydrazide, **3c** Yield: 72%; m.p. 249–250 °C. ^{1}H NMR (400 MHz, DMSO-d$_6$, 363K): δ = 1.51 (dd, J = 3.7, 11.3 Hz, 1H, CH$_2$), 1.57 (dd, J = 3.7, 11.1 Hz, 1H, CH$_2$), 1.79 (dd, J = 3.4, 12.9 Hz, 2H, CH$_2$), 2.09 (dt, J = 2.6, 11.3 Hz, 2H, CH$_2$), 2.23–2.32 (m, 1H, H-4$'$), 2.82 (td, J = 3.5, 11.7 Hz, 1H, CH$_2$), 3.49 (s, 2H, CH$_2$), 7.12 (dt, J = 1.2, 10.9 Hz, 1H, H-5), 7.16 (dt, J = 1.4, 7.5 Hz, 1H, H-6), 7.21–7.26 (m, 1H, H-4$''$), 7.29–7.32 (m, 4H, C-3$''$, C-5$''$, C-2$''$, and C-6$''$), 7.44 (d, J = 7.9 Hz, 1H, H-7), 7.55 (d, J = 4.8 Hz, 1H, CH), 8.12 (bs, 1H, H-2), 8.17 (d, J = 7.3 Hz, 1H, H-4), 10.53 (bs, 1H, NH), 11.36 (bs, 1H, NH). ^{13}C NMR (100 MHz, DMSO-d$_6$, 363K): δ = 29.01 (C-3$'$ and C-5$'$), 37.97 (C-4$'$), 52.19 (C-2$'$ and C-6$'$), 62.11 (CH$_2$), 108.42 (C-3), 111.44 (C-7), 120.21 (C-5), 120.95 (C-4), 121.73 (C-6), 126.43 (C-4$''$), 126.63 (C-4a), 127.74 (C-3$''$ and C-3$''$), 128.44 (C-2$''$ and C-6$''$), 129.27 (C-2), 135.69 (C-7a), 138.34 (C-1$''$), 150.89 (CH), 162.35 (C=O). HRMS (ESI) *m/z*: calcd: [M+H]+ 361.202288. Found: [M+H]+ 361.2021.

N$'$-[(E)-(1-benzylpiperidin-4-yl)methylidene]-4-methoxybenzohydrazide, **3d** Yield: 82%; m.p. 138–140 °C. ^{1}H NMR (600 MHz, DMSO-d$_6$): δ = 1.49 (q, J = 10.9 Hz, 2H) and 1.74 (d, J = 11.6 Hz, 2H, H-2$'$, and H6$'$), 2.01 (t, J = 11.0 Hz, 2H) and 2.82 (d, J = 11.2 Hz, 2H, H-3$'$, and H-5$'$), 2.25 (d, J = 4.7 Hz, 1H, H-1$'$), 3.47 (s, 2H, CH$_2$), 3.82 (s, 3H, OCH$_3$), 7.02 (d, J = 8.6 Hz, 2H, H-3, and H-5), 7.25 (tt, J = 2.0, 6.7 Hz, 1H, H-4$''$), 7.30–7.34 (m, 4H, H-2$''$, H-3$''$, H-5$''$, and H-6$''$), 7.67 (d, J = 5.1 Hz, 1H, CH), 7.84 (d, J = 8.8 Hz, 2H, H-2, and H-6), 11.28 (s, 1H, NH). ^{13}C NMR (151 MHz, DMSO-d$_6$): δ = 29.14 (C-2$'$ and C-6$'$), 38.57 (C-1$'$), 52.48 (C-3$'$ and C-5$'$), 55.37 (OCH$_3$), 62.42 (CH$_2$), 113.60 (C-3 and C-5), 125.58 (C-1), 126.82 (C-4$''$), 128.12 (C-3$''$ and C-5$''$), 128.76 (C-2$''$ and C-6$''$), 129.34 (C-2 and C-6), 138.51 (C-1$''$), 154.21 (CH), 161.80 (C-4), 162.23 (C=O). HRMS (ESI) *m/z*: calcd: [M+H]+ 352.201953. Found: [M+H]+ 352.20115.

1-benzyl-N$'$-[(E)-(4-hydroxyphenyl)methylidene]pyrrolidine-3-carbohydrazide, **3e** Yield: 84%; m.p. 240–241 °C. ^{1}H NMR (600 MHz, DMSO-d$_6$): 1:0.77 mixture of conformers; signals for major *synperiplanar* conformer around the amide bond: δ = 1.94–2.03 (m, 2H, H-4$'$), 2.40–2.42 (m, 2H, H-5$'$), 2.62–2.69 (m, 1H, 1/2H-2$'$), 2.88–2.91 (m, 1H, 1/2H-2$'$), 3.55–3.62 (m, 2H, CH$_2$), 3.61–3.66 (m, 1H, H-3$'$), 6.79 (d, J = 8.6 Hz, 2H, H-3, and H-5), 7.22–7.26 (m, 1H, H-4$''$), 7.30–7.33 (m, 4H, H-2$''$, H-3$''$, H-5$''$, and H-6$''$), 7.44 (d, J = 8.7 Hz, 2H, H-2, and H-6), 7.85 (s, 1H, CH), 9.84 (bs, 1H, OH), 11.05 (s, 1H, NH); resolved signals for minor *antiperiplanar* conformer around the amide bond: 8.04 (s, 1H, CH), 9.87 (bs, 1H, OH), 11.10 (s, 1H, NH). ^{13}C NMR (151 MHz, DMSO-d$_6$): signals for major *synperiplanar* conformer around the amide bond: δ = 26.95 (C-4$'$), 41.47 (C-3$'$), 53.58 (C-5$'$), 56.43 (C-2$'$), 59.30 (CH$_2$), 115.65 (C-3 and C-5), 125.37 (C-1), 126.75 (C-4$''$), 128.11 (C-2$''$ and C-6$''$), 128.28 (C-2 and C-6), 128.65 (C-3$''$ and C-5$''$), 139.16 (C-1$''$), 142.74 (CH), 158.99 (C-4), 175.01 (C=O); resolved signals for minor *antiperiplanar* conformer around the amide bond: 146.34 (CH), 159.22 (C-4), 169.78 (C=O). HRMS (ESI) *m/z*: calcd: [M+H]+ 324.170653. Found: [M+H]+ 324,1705.

1-benzyl-N$'$-[(E)-(2,4-dihydroxyphenyl)methylidene]pyrrolidine-3-carbohydrazide, **3f** Yield: 81%; m.p. 224–225 °C. ^{1}H NMR (600 MHz, DMSO-d$_6$): δ = 1:0.39 mixture of conformers; signals for major *synperiplanar* conformer around the amide bond: δ = 1.92–2.04 (m, 2H, H-4$'$), 2.41–2.48 (m, 2H, H-5$'$), 2.66–2.69 (m, 1H, 1/2H-2$'$), 2.82–2.94 (m, 1H, 1/2H-2$'$), 3.52–3.57 (m, 1H, H-3$'$), 3.57–3.61 (m, 2H, CH$_2$), 6.29 (d, J = 2.3 Hz, 1H, H-3), 6.33 (dd, J = 8.4, 2.3 Hz, 1H, H-5), 7.25 (d, J = 8.5 Hz, 1H, H-6), 7.29–7.33 (m, 5H, Ar), 8.21 (s, 1H, CH), 9.91 (bs, 1H, OH), 11.32 (s, 1H, OH), 11.36 (s, 1H, NH); resolved signals for minor *antiperiplanar* conformer around the amide bond: 8.11 (s, 1H, CH), 9.79 (bs, 1H, OH), 10.11 (bs, 1H, OH), 11.04 (s, 1H, NH). ^{13}C NMR (151 MHz, DMSO-d$_6$): signals for major *synperiplanar* conformer around the amide bond: δ = 27.47 (C-4$'$), 41.23 (C-3$'$), 53.52 (C-5$'$),

56.83 (C-2′), 59.17 (CH$_2$), 102.58 (C-3), 107.57 (C-5), 110.41 (C-1), 126.81 (C-4″), 128.14 (C-2″ and C-6″), 128.51 (C-3″ and C-5″), 131.16 (C-6), 139.17 (C-1″), 147.58 (CH), 159.27 (C-2), 160.52 (C-4), 169.58 (C=O); resolved signals for minor *antiperiplanar* conformer around the amide bond: 141.95 (CH), 157.97 (C-2), 160.22 (C-4), 174.44 (C=O). HRMS (ESI) *m*/*z*: calcd: [M+H]+ 340.165568. Found: [M+H]+ 340.1655.

1-benzyl-N′-[(E)-(3,4-dihydroxyphenyl)methylidene]pyrrolidine-3-carbohydrazide, **3g** Yield: 72%; m.p. 199–201 °C. ^{1}H NMR (600 MHz, DMSO-d$_6$): 1:0.65 mixture of conformers; signals for major *synperiplanar* conformer around the amide bond: δ = 2.57 (m, J = 8.3 Hz, 2H, H-4′), 2.63 (d, J = 8.45 Hz, 2H, H-5′), 3.32–3.37 (m, 1H, H-2′), 3.57 (t, J = 9.5 Hz, 1H, H-2′), 3.91 (dq, J = 6.2, 8.6 Hz, 1H, H-3′), 4.35 (d, J = 15.0 Hz, 1H) and 4.46 (d, J = 15.0 Hz, 1H, CH$_2$), 6.75 (dd, J = 0.6, 7.7 Hz, 1H, H-5), 6.89 (dd, J = 1.2, 8.3 Hz, 1H, H-6), 7.09 (s, 1H, H-2), 7.23–7.25 (m, 2H, H-2″ and H-6″), 7.27–7.30 (m, 1H, H-4″), 7.34–7.37 (m, 2H, H-3″ and H-5″), 7.80 (s, 1H, CH), 9.15 (bs, 1H, OH), 9.39 (bs, 1H, OH), 11.23 (s, 1H, NH); resolved signals for minor *antiperiplanar* conformer around the amide bond: 7.96 (s, 1H, CH), 9.24 (bs, 1H, OH), 9.37 (bs, 1H, OH), 11.26 (s, 1H, NH). ^{13}C NMR (151 MHz, DMSO-d$_6$): signals for major *synperiplanar* conformer around the amide bond: δ = 33.54 (C-3′), 35.41 (C-4′), 45.79 (CH$_2$), 48.98 (C-5′), 49.37 (C-2′), 113.21 (C-2), 116.05 (C-5), 120.37 (C-6), 126.02 (C-1), 127.73 (C-4″), 128.05 (C-2″ and C-6″), 129.06 (C-3″ and C-5″), 137.24 (C-1″), 144.49 (CH), 146.11 (C-3), 148.17 (C-4), 172.83 (C=O); resolved signals for minor *antiperiplanar* conformer around the amide bond: 147.81 (CH), 146.15 (C-3), 148.43 (C-4), 173.81 (C=O). HRMS (ESI) *m*/*z*: calcd: [M+H]+ 340.165568. Found: [M+H]+ 340.1646.

1-benzyl-N′-[(E)-(2,4,6-trihydroxyphenyl)methylidene]pyrrolidine-3-carbohydrazide, **3h** Yield: 65%; m.p. 215–217 °C. ^{1}H NMR (600 MHz, DMSO-d$_6$): 1:0.19 mixture of conformers; signals for major *synperiplanar* conformer around the amide bond: δ = 1.91–2.03 (m, 2H, H-4′), 2.41–2.47 (m, 2H, H-5′), 2.66–2.69 (m, 1H, H-2′), 2.81–2.85 (m, 1H, H-2′), 2.85–2.91 (m, 1H, H-3′), 3.57 (d, J = 12.8 Hz, 1H) and 3.60 (d, J = 13.0 Hz, 1H, CH$_2$), 5.81 (s, 2H, H-3 and H-5), 7.23–7.27 (m, 1H, H-4″), 7.30–7.33 (m, 4H, H-2″, H-3″, H-5″ and H-6″), 8.49 (s, 1H, CH), 9.77 (bs, 1H, OH), 10.95 (bs, 2H, OH), 11.33 (s, 1H, NH); resolved signals for minor *antiperiplanar* conformer around the amide bond: 8.37 (s, 1H, CH), 9.80 (bs, 1H, OH), 10.51 (bs, 2H, OH), 11.12 (s, 1H, NH). ^{13}C NMR (151 MHz, DMSO-d$_6$): signals for major *synperiplanar* conformer around the amide bond: δ = 27.47 (C-3′), 41.19 (CH$_2$), 53.50 (C-4′), 56.81 (C-5′), 59.16 (C-2′), 94.29 (C-3 and C-5), 98.80 (C-1), 126.81 (C-4″), 128.14 (C-2″ and C-6″), 128.51 (C-3″ and C-5″), 139.12 (C-1″), 145.15 (CH), 159.48 (C-2 and C-6), 161.34 (C-4), 169.21 (C=O). HRMS (ESI) *m*/*z*: calcd: [M+H]+ 356.160483. Found: [M+H]+ 356.1604.

tert-butyl(2-{(2E)-2-[(1-benzyl-1H-indol-3-yl)methylidene]hydrazinyl}-2-oxoethyl) carbamate, **3i** ^{1}H NMR, ^{13}C NMR and HRMS spectra of compound **3i** were published elsewhere [33].

tert-butyl(2-{(2E)-2-[(5-methoxy-1-methyl-1H-indol-3-yl)methylidene]hydrazinyl}-2-oxoethyl)carbamate, **3j** Yield: 48%; m.p. 203–206 °C. ^{1}H NMR (600 MHz, DMSO-d$_6$): 1:0.28 mixture of conformers; signals for major *synperiplanar* conformer around the amide bond: δ = 1.41 (s, 9H, CH$_3$), 3.79 (s, 3H, OCH$_3$), 4.16 (d, J = 6.0 Hz, 2H, CH$_2$), 6.76 (t, J = 5.9 Hz, 1H, H-4), 6.85 (dd, J = 2.6, 8.8 Hz, 1H, H-6), 7.34 (d, J = 8.8 Hz, 1H, H-7), 7.62 (d, J = 2.4 Hz, 1H, H-4), 7.72 (d, J = 2.9 Hz, 1H, C-2), 8.14 (s, 1H, CH), 11.00 (s, 1H, NH), 11.40 (bs, 1H, NH); resolved signals for minor *antiperiplanar* conformer around the amide bond: 8.35 (s, 1H, CH), 11.09 (s, 1H, NH), 11.40 (bs, 1H, NH). ^{13}C NMR (151 MHz, DMSO-d$_6$): signals for major *synperiplanar* conformer around the amide bond: δ = 28.22 (CH$_3$), 41.39 (CH$_2$), 55.05 (OCH$_3$), 77.88 (OC), 103.48 (C-4), 111.10 (C-3), 112.16 (C-7), 112.53 (C-6), 124.63 (C-3a), 130.50 (C-2), 131.93 (C-7a), 140.68 (CH), 154.37 (C-5), 155.89 (OC=O), 169.74 (C=O). HRMS (ESI) *m*/*z*: calcd: [M+H]+ 347.171382. Found: [M+H]+ 347.1712.

tert-butyl(2-{(2E)-2-[(5-methoxy-1H-indol-3-yl)methylidene]hydrazinyl}-2-oxoethyl) carbamate, **3k** Yield: 83%; m.p. 197–199 °C. ^{1}H NMR (600 MHz, DMSO-d$_6$): 1:0.33 mixture of conformers; signals for major *synperiplanar* conformer around the amide bond: δ = 1.41 (s, 9H, CH$_3$), 3.78 (s, 3H, NCH$_3$), 3.80 (s, 3H, OCH$_3$), 4.16 (d, J = 5.9 Hz, 2H, CH$_2$), 6.76 (t, J = 5.9 Hz, 1H, NH), 6.92 (dd, J = 2.6, 8.8 Hz, 1H, H-6), 7.41 (d, J = 8.8 Hz, 1H, H-7),

7.62 (d, J = 2.5 Hz, 1H, H-4), 7.71 (s, 1H, C-2), 8.11 (s, 1H, CH), 11.07 (s, 1H, NH); resolved signals for minor *antiperiplanar* conformer around the amide bond: 8.32 (s, 1H, CH), 11.00 (1H, s), ^{13}C NMR (151 MHz, DMSO-d_6): signals for major *synperiplanar* conformer around the amide bond: δ = 28.01 (CH$_3$), 32.91 (NCH$_3$), 41.38 (CH$_2$), 55.11 (OCH$_3$), 77.88 (OC), 103.66 (C-4), 109.95 (C-3), 111.05 (C-7), 112.10 (C-6), 125.01 (C-3a), 132.65 (C-7a), 134.03 (C-2), 140.20 (CH), 154.65 (C-5), 155.89 (OC=O), 169.72 (C=O). HRMS (ESI) *m/z*: calcd: [M+H]+ 361.187032. Found: [M+H]+ 361.1869.

tert-butyl(2-{(2E)-2-[(1-methyl-1H-indol-3-yl)methylidene]hydrazinyl}-2-oxoethyl) carbamate, **3l** Yield: 54%; m.p. 178–179 °C. ^{1}H NMR (600 MHz, DMSO-d_6): 1:0.40 mixture of conformers; signals for major *synperiplanar* conformer around the amide bond: δ = 1.41 (s, 9H, CH$_3$), 3.82 (s, 3H, NCH$_3$), 4.12 (d, J = 6.1 Hz, 2H, CH$_2$), 6.83 (t, J = 6.1 Hz, 1H, NH), 7.22 (ddd, J = 0.7, 7.1, 7.8 Hz, 1H, H-5), 7.28 (ddd, J = 1.2, 7.0, 8.2 Hz, 1H, H-6), 7.51 (d, J = 7.5 Hz, 1H, H-7), 7.77 (s, 1H, C-2), 8.08 (d, J = 7.8 Hz, 1H, H-4), 8.13 (s, 1H, CH), 11.06 (s, 1H, NH); resolved signals for minor *antiperiplanar* conformer around the amide bond: 8.34 (s, 1H, CH), 11.02 (s, 1H, NH). ^{13}C NMR (151 MHz, DMSO-d_6): signals for major *synperiplanar* conformer around the amide bond: δ = 28.24 (CH$_3$), 32.76 (NCH$_3$), 41.42 (CH$_2$), 77.87 (OC), 110.27 (C-7), 110.38 (C-3), 120.83 (C-5), 121.55 (C-4), 122.66 (C-6), 124.43 (C-3a), 133.90 (C-2), 137.56 (C-7a), 140.22 (CH), 155.96 (OC=O), 169.78 (C=O). HRMS (ESI) *m/z*: calcd: [M+H]+ 331.176467. Found: [M+H]+ 331.1764.

tert-butyl(2-{(2E)-2-[(1-benzyl-1H-indol-3-yl)methylidene]hydrazinyl}-2-oxoethyl) carbamate, **3m** Yield: 90%; m.p. 207–208 °C. ^{1}H NMR (600 MHz, DMSO): 1:0.40 mixture of conformers; signals for major *antiperiplanar* conformer around the amide bond: δ 11.10 (s, 1H, NH), 8.15 (s, 1H, CH), 8.08 (d, J = 8.3 Hz, 1H, H-4), 7.95 (s, 1H, H-2), 7.50 (d, J = 7.4 Hz, 1H, H-7), 7.30 (d, J = 7.5 Hz, 2H, o-Ph), 7.26–7.22 (m, 1H, H-6), 7.21–7.18 (m, 1H, H-5), 7.24 (t, J = 8.7 Hz, 2H, m-Ph), 7.20 (t, J = 8.0 Hz, 1H, p-Ph), 6.85 (t, J = 6.1 Hz, 1H, NH), 5.44 (s, 2H, CH$_2$), 4.10 (d, J = 6.1 Hz, 2H, CH$_2$), 1.40 (s, 9H, CH$_3$); resolved signals for minor *antiperiplanar* conformer around the amide bond: 7.05 (t, J = 6.0 Hz, 1H, NH), 8.21 (d, J = 7.9 Hz, 1H, H-4), 8.34 (s, 1H, CH), 3.62 (d, J = 6.1 Hz, 2H, CH$_2$). ^{13}C NMR (151 MHz, DMSO): signals for major *antiperiplanar* conformer around the amide bond: δ 170.03 (C=O), 156.16 (O-C=O), 140.39 (CH), 137.68 (i-Ph), 137.02 (C-7a), 133.54 (C-2), 128.79 (C-o), 127.72 (p-Ph), 127.27 (m-Ph), 124.85 (C-3a), 123.03 (C-5), 121.87 (C-4), 121.18 (C-6), 111.15 (C-3), 110.93 (C-7), 78.12 (C), 49.45 (CH$_2$), 42.56 (CH$_2$), 28.38 (CH$_3$); resolved signals for minor *synperiplanar* conformer around the amide bond: 143.22 (CH), 122.29 (C-2), 78.27 (C), 41.57 (CH$_2$), 28.35 (CH$_3$). HRMS (ESI) *m/z*: calcd: [M+H]+ 407.207767. Found: [M+H]+ 407.2078.

2-(1H-indol-3-yl)-N'-[(E)-(5-methoxy-1H-indol-3-yl)methylidene]acetohydrazide, **3n** ^{1}H NMR, ^{13}C NMR and HRMS spectra of compound **3n** were published elsewhere [65].

N'-[(E)-(3,4-dimethoxyphenyl)methylidene]-1H-indole-3-carbohydrazide, **3o** Yield: 78%; m.p. 267–270 °C. ^{1}H NMR (400 MHz, DMSO-d_6, 353K): δ = 3.83 (s, 3H, OCH$_3$), 3.84 (s, 3H, OCH$_3$), 7.03 (d, J = 8.3 Hz, 1H, H-5'), 7.14 (ddd, J = 1.3, 7.0, 7.7 Hz, 1H, H-5), 7.18 (dt, J = 1.6, 6.6 Hz, 1H, H-6), 7.20 (dd, J = 1.6, 7.2 Hz, 1H, H-6'), 7.35 (d, J = 1.9 Hz, 1H, H-2'), 7.48 (d, J = 8.0 Hz, 1H, H-7), 8.21 (d, J = 7.6 Hz, 1H, H-4), 8.26 (s, 1H, CH), 10.98 (bs, 1H, NH), 11.52 (bs, 1H, NH). ^{13}C NMR (151 MHz, DMSO-d_6, 353K): δ = 55.48 (CH$_3$), 55.56 (CH$_3$), 108.45 (C-3), 109.14 (C-2'), 111.45 (C-5'), 112.05 (C-7), 120.22 (C-4), 120.74 (C-5), 120.89 (C-6'), 121.73 (C-6), 126.53 (C-1'), 127.66 (C-3a), 129.17 (C-2), 135.69 (C-7a), 144.03 (CH), 149.15 (C-3'), 150.35 (C-4'), 162.13 (C=O). HRMS (ESI) *m/z*: calcd: [M+H]+ 324.134268. Found: [M+H]+ 324.13358.

N'-[(E)-(3,4-dimethoxyphenyl)methylidene]-2-(1H-indol-3-yl)acetohydrazide, **3p** Yield: 92%; m.p. 177–180 °C. ^{1}H NMR (600 MHz, DMSO-d_6): 1:0.80 mixture of conformers; signals for major *antiperiplanar* conformer around the amide bond: δ = 3.80 (s, 3H, OCH$_3$), 3.81 (s, 3H, OCH$_3$), 4.05 (s, 2H, CH$_2$), 6.95 (t, J = 7.5 Hz, 1H, H-5), 7.01 (d, 8.5 Hz, 2H, H-5'), 7.06 (t, J = 7.0 Hz, 1H, H-6), 7.17 (dt, J = 1.8, 8.7 Hz, 2H, H-6'), 7.28 (d, J = 1.7 Hz, 1H, H-2'), 7.35 (d, J = 2.42 Hz, 1H, H-2), 7.36 (d, J = 9.27 Hz, 1H, H-7), 7.60 (dd, J = 3.46, 7.85 Hz, 1H, H-4), 7.91 (s, 1H, CH), 10.87 (bs, 1H, NH), 11.18 (s, 1H, NH); resolved signals for minor *antiperiplanar* conformer around the amide bond: 8.15 (s, 1H, CH), 10.91 (bs, 1H, NH), 11.40

(s, 1H, NH) ^{13}C NMR (151 MHz, DMSO-d$_6$): signals for major *antiperiplanar* conformer around the amide bond: δ = 29.24 (CH$_2$), 55.40 (OCH$_3$), 108.22 (C-2′), 108.25 (C-3), 111.30 (C-5′), 111.56 (C-7), 118.28 (C-4), 118.66 (C-5), 120.97 (C-6′), 121.59 (C-6), 123.86 (C-2), 127.13 (C-1′), 127.39 (C-3a), 135.98 (C-7a), 142.46 (CH), 148.99 (C-3′), 150.56 (C-4′), 172.52 (C=O). HRMS (ESI) *m/z*: calcd: [M+H]+ 338.149918. Found: [M+H]+ 338.14902.

N′-[(E)-(4-hydroxy-3-methoxyphenyl)methylidene]-2-(1H-indol-3-yl)acetohydrazide, **3q** Yield: 72%; m.p. 246–247 °C. ^{1}H-NMR (400 MHz, DMSO-d$_6$): 0.54: 0.46 mixture of two conformers; signals for major conformer: δ = 3.81 (s, 3H, CH$_3$), 4.04 (s, 2H, CH$_2$), 6.82 (d, J = 8.1 Hz, 1H, H-5′), 6.96–7.00 (m, 1H, H-5), 7.02–7.09 (m, 2H, H-6, and H-6′), 7.22 (d, J = 2.3 Hz, 1H, H-2), 7.29 (d, J = 1.8 Hz, 1H, H-2′), 7.33 (d, J = 6.8 Hz, 1H, H-7), 7.59 (d, J = 7.9 Hz, 1H, H-4), 7.87 (s, 1H, CH), 9.46 (s, 1H, OH), 10.86 (s, 1H, NH), 11.10 (s, 1H, NH); Signals for minor conformer: δ(ppm): 3.61 (s, 2H, CH$_2$), 3.79 (s, 3H, CH$_3$), 6.81 (d, J = 8.1 Hz, 1H, H-5′), 6.93–6.97 (m, 1H, H-5), 7.02–7.09 (m, 2H, H-6, and H-6′),7.24 (d, J = 1.9 Hz, 2H, H-2, and H-2′), 7.35 (d, J = 7.0 Hz, 1H, H-7), 7.59 (d, J = 7.9 Hz, 1H, H-4), 8.11 (s, 1H, CH), 9.48 (s, 1H, OH), 10.90 (s, 1H, NH), 11.33 (s, 1H, NH). ^{13}C-NMR (151 MHz, DMSO-d$_6$): 0.54:0.46 mixture of two conformers; signals for major conformer: δ = 29.20 (CH$_2$), 55.51 (CH$_3$), 108.33 (C-3), 109.10 (C-2′), 111.30 (C-7), 115.37 (C-5′), 118.27 (C-5), 118.68 (C-4), 120.88 (C-6′), 121.11 (C-6), 123.86 (C-2), 125.82 (C-1′), 127.42 (C-4a), 135.98 (C-7a), 142.81 (CH), 147.97 (C-3′), 148.51 (C-4′), 172.43 (C=O); signals for minor conformer: δ(ppm): 31.69 (CH$_2$), 55.51 (CH$_3$), 108.31 (C-3), 108.93 (C-2′), 111.35 (C-7), 115.52 (C5′), 118.36 (C-5), 118.68 (C-4), 121.00 (C-6′), 121.87 (C-6), 123.86 (C-2), 125.73 (C-1′), 127.14 (C-4a), 136.10 (C-7a), 146.65 (CH), 147.97 (C-3′), 148.78 (C-4′), 166.79 (C=O). HRMS (ESI) *m/z*: calcd: [M+H]+ 324.134268. Found: [M+H]+ 324.1341.

2,4-dihydroxy-N′-[(E)-(4-hydroxy-3-methoxyphenyl)methylidene]benzohydrazide, **3r** Yield: 76%; m.p. 242–243 °C. ^{1}H NMR (400 MHz, DMSO-d$_6$): 3.36 (s, 3H, CH$_3$), 6.31 (d, J = 2.4 Hz, 1H, H-3), 6.37 (dd, J = 2.4, 8.7 Hz, 1H, H-5), 6.85 (d, J = 8.1 Hz, 1H, H-6′), 7.10 (dd, J = 1.8, 8.1 Hz, 1H, H-5′), 7.32 (d, J = 1.8 Hz, 1H, H-2′), 7.80 (d, J = 8.7 Hz, 1H, H-6), 8.33 (s, 1H, CH), 9.56 (s, 1H, OH), 10.19 (s, 1H, OH), 11.54 (s, 1H, NH), 12.45 (s, 1H, OH). ^{13}C NMR (100 MHz, DMSO-d$_6$): 55.55 (CH$_3$), 102.86 (C-3), 106.20 (C-1), 107.33 (C-5), 108.99 (C-2′), 115.45 (C-6′), 122.27 (C-5′), 125.59 (C-1′), 129.49 (C-6), 148.05 (C-4′), 148.61 (CH), 149.09 (C-3′), 162.31 (C-4), 162.57 (C-2), 165.28 (C=O). HRMS (ESI) *m/z*: calcd: [M+H]+ 303.097548. Found: [M+H]+ 303.0974.

3.3. General Procedure for the Synthesis of Compounds **5a–5l**

The solution of 20 mmol of the corresponding carbonyl compounds (**1a, 1i, 1j, 1k, 1l, 1o**) in 10 mL of absolute ethanol was mixed with a hot solution of 20 mmol (60 °C) benzene-sulfonohydrazide (**4a**) or 4-methylbenzenesulfonohydrazide (**4b**) and 4-methoxylbenzenesulfonohydrazide (**4c**) in 10 mL of absolute ethanol and stirred for 1–3 h. The obtained crystalline precipitates were filtered, washed with ethanol-ether, recrystallized from ethanol.

N′-[(E)-(1-benzylpiperidin-4-yl)methylidene]benzenesulfonohydrazide, **5a** Yield: 59%; m.p. 110–111 °C. ^{1}H NMR (400 MHz, DMSO-d$_6$): δ = 1.26–1.36 (m, 2H, CH$_2$), 1.54–1.58 (m, 2H, CH$_2$), 1.91–1.97 (m, 2H, CH$_2$), 2.05–2.14 (m, 1H CH), 2.65–2.68 (m, 2H, CH$_2$), 3.40 (s, 2H, CH$_2$), 7.19 (d, J = 4.8 Hz, 1H, CH), 7.21–7.27 (m, 3H, H-2″, H-4″ and H-6″), 7.29–7.33 (m, 2H, H-3″, and H-5″), 7.59–7.63 (m, 2H, H-3′, and H-5′), 7.65–7.69 (m, 1H, H-4′), 7.78–7.81 (m, 2H, H-2′, and H-6′), 10.93 (1H, s). ^{13}C NMR (DMSO) (100 MHz, DMSO-d$_6$): δ = 27.62 (CH$_2$), 36.94 (CH), 51.11 (CH$_2$), 61.25 (CH$_2$), 125.85 (C-4″), 126.12 (C-2′ and C-6′), 127.11 (C-3″ and C-5″), 127.75 (C-2″ and C-6″), 128.07 (C-3′ and C-5′), 131.86 (C-4′), 137.28 (C-1″), 137.94 (C-1′), 153.47 (CH). HRMS (ESI) *m/z*: calcd: [M+H]+ 358.158373. Found: [M+H]+ 358.1581.

4-methoxy-N′-[(E)-(5-methoxy-1-methyl-1H-indol-3-yl)methylidene]benzenesulfon ohydrazide, **5b** Yield: 78%; m.p. 145–146 °C. ^{1}H NMR (600 MHz, DMSO-d$_6$): δ = 3.74 (s, 3H, NCH$_3$), 3.77 (s, 3H, OCH$_3$), 3.80 (s, 3H, OCH$_3$), 6.86 (dd, J = 2.6, 8.8 Hz, 1H, H-6), 7.11 (d, J = 9.0 Hz, 2H, H-3′, and H-5′), 7.36 (d, J = 8.8 Hz, 1H, H-7), 7.47 (d, J = 2.5 Hz, 1H, H-4), 7.64 (s, 1H, H-2), 7.85 (d, J = 8.8 Hz, 2H, H-2′, and H-6′), 8.05 (s, 1H, CH), 10.75 (s,

1H, NH). ^{13}C NMR (151 MHz, DMSO-d$_6$): δ = 32.90 (NCH$_3$), 55.22 (OCH$_3$), 55.64 (OCH$_3$), 103.31 (C-4), 109.71 (C-3), 111.01 (C-7), 112.54 (C-6), 114.20 (C-3′ and C-5′), 124.90 (C-3a), 129.49 (C-1′), 130.83 (C-2′ and C-6′), 132.52 (C-7a), 134.20 (C-2), 145.01 (CH), 154.66 (C-4), 162.45 (C-4′). HRMS (ESI) *m/z*: calcd: [M+H]+ 374.11597. Found: [M+H]+ 374.1169.

4-methoxy-N′-[(E)-(5-methoxy-1H-indol-3-yl)methylidene]benzenesulfonohydrazide, **5c** Yield: 53%; m.p. 159–163 °C. ^{1}H NMR (400 MHz, DMSO-d$_6$): δ = 3.76 (s, 3H, OCH$_3$), 3.80 (s, 3H, OCH$_3$), 6.80 (dd, J = 2.6, 8.8 Hz, 1H, H-6), 7.11 (d, J = 9.0 Hz, 2H, H-3′, and H-5′), 7.29 (d, J = 8.8 Hz, 1), 7.46 (d, J = 2.6 Hz, 1H, H-4), 7.66 (d, J = 2.8 Hz, 1H, H-2), 7.85 (d, J = 9.0 Hz, 2H, H-2′ and H-6′), 8.08 (s, 1H, CH), 10.76 (s, 1H, NH), 11.37 (d, J = 2.2 Hz, 1H, NH).^{13}C NMR (100 MHz, DMSO-d$_6$): δ = 55.15 (OCH$_3$), 55.63 (OCH$_3$), 103.12 (C-4), 110.85 (C-3), 112.48 (C-7), 112.59 (C-6), 114.19 (C-3′ and C-5′), 124.49 (C-3a), 129.48 (C-1′), 130.73 (C-2′ and C-6′), 130.84 (C-7a), 131.78 (C-2), 145.46 (CH), 154.35 (C-4), 162.43 (C-4′). HRMS (ESI) *m/z*: calcd: [M+H]+ 360.10125. Found: [M+H]+ 360.10037.

N′-[(E)-(1-benzyl-1H-indol-3-yl)methylidene]benzenesulfonohydrazide, **5d** Yield: 89%; m.p. 146–149 °C. ^{1}H NMR (600 MHz, DMSO-d$_6$): δ = 5.41 (s, 3H, CH$_2$), 7.15 (t, J = 7.4 Hz, 1H, H-5), 7.18 (ddd, J = 1.2, 7.1, 8.2 Hz, 1H, H-6), 7.21 (d, J = 7.0 Hz, 2H, H-2′, and H-6′), 7.24 (t, J = 7.3 Hz, 1H, H-4′), 7.30 (t, J = 7.3 Hz, 2H, H-3′, and H-5′), 7.48 (d, J = 8.1 Hz, 1H, H-7), 7.59–7.65 (m, 3H, H-3″, H-4″, and H-5″), 7.90 (s, 1H, H-2), 7.93 (dd, J = 1.0, 7.6 Hz, 2H, H-2″, and H-6″), 7.97 (d, J = 7.8 Hz, 1H, H-4), 8.10 (s, 1H, CH), 11.01 (s, 1H, NH).^{13}C NMR (151 MHz, DMSO-d$_6$): δ = 49.27 (CH$_2$), 110.65 (C-3), 110.67 (1C, s), 120.89 (C-5), 121.78 (C-4), 122.79 (C-6), 124.61 (C-3a), 127.09 (C-2′ and C-6″), 127.28 (C-2″ and C-6″), 127.51 (C-4′), 128.59 (C-3′ and C-5′), 129.05 (C-3″ and V-5″), 132.82 (C-4″), 133.50 (C-2), 136.75 (C-7a), 137.44 (C-1′), 139.13 (C-1″), 144.60 (CH). HRMS (ESI) *m/z*: calcd: [M+H]+ 390.127073. Found: [M+H]+ 390.12604.

4-methoxy-N′-[(E)-(1-methyl-1H-indol-3-yl)methylidene]benzenesulfonohydrazide, **5e** Yield: 66%; m.p. 170–175 °C. ^{1}H NMR (600 MHz, DMSO-d$_6$): δ = 3.78 (s, 3H, NCH$_3$), 3.79 (s, 3H, OCH$_3$), 7.11 (d, J = 9.0 Hz, 2H, H-3′ and H-5′), 7.17 (t, J = 7.5 Hz, 1H, H-5), 7.24 (ddd, J = 1.1, 7.1, 8.1 Hz, 1H, H-6), 7.46 (d, J = 8.2 Hz, 1H, H-7), 7.69 (s, 1H, H-2), 7.84 (d, J = 9.0 Hz, 2H, H2′, and H-6′), 7.97 (d, J = 7.9 Hz, 1H, H-4), 8.05 (s, 1H, CH), 10.76 (s, 1H, NH). ^{13}C NMR (151 MHz, DMSO-d$_6$): δ = 32.73 (NCH$_3$), 55.61 (OCH$_3$), 110.11 (C-3), 110.17 (C-7), 114.18 (C-3′ and H-5′), 120.74 (C-5), 121.66 (C-4), 122.62 (C-6), 124.40 (C-3a), 129.48 (C-2′ and C-6′), 130.81 (C-2′ and C-6′), 133.89 (C-1′), 137.42 (C-7a), 144.44 (CH), 162.44 (C-4′).HRMS (ESI) *m/z*: calcd: [M+H]+ 344.106338. Found: [M+H]+ 344.1055.

N′-[(E)-(5-methoxy-1-methyl-1H-indol-3-yl)methylidene]benzenesulfonohydrazide, **5f** ^{1}H NMR, ^{13}C NMR and HRMS spectra of compound **5f** were published elsewhere [66].

N′-[(E)-(1-benzyl-1H-indol-3-yl)methylidene]-4-methylbenzenesulfonohydrazide, **5g** Yield: 79%; m.p. 145–146 °C.^{1}H NMR (400 MHz, DMSO-d$_6$): δ = 2.34 (s, 3H, CH$_3$), 5.41 (s, 2H, CH$_2$), 7.13–7.32 (m, 7H, H-5, H6, H-2″, H-3″, H-4″, H-5″, and H-6″), 7.39 (d, J = 7.9 Hz, 2H, H-3′, and H-5′), 7.48 (dd, J = 1.3, 7.1 Hz, 1H, H-7), 7.81 (d, J = 8.2 Hz, 2H, H-2′, and H-6′), 7.89 (s, 1H, H-2), 7.99 (d, J = 7.3 Hz, 1H, H-4), 8.08 (s, 1H, CH), 10.92 (s, 1H, NH).^{13}C NMR (100 MHz, DMSO-d$_6$): δ = 20.95 (CH$_3$), 49.26 (CH$_2$), 110.66 (C-7), 110.72 (C-3), 120.88 (C-5), 121.83 (C-4), 122.78 (C-6), 124.63 (C-4a), 127.08 (C-2″ and C-6″), 127.33 (C-2′ and C-6′), 127.51 (C-4″), 128.59 (C-3″ and C-5″), 129.47 (C-3′ and C-5′), 133.41 (C-2), 136.26 (C-1′), 136.74 (C-7a), 137.46 (C-1″), 143.16 (C-4′), 144.32 (C-H). HRMS (ESI) *m/z*: calcd: [M+H]+ 404.142723. Found: [M+H]+ 404.1425.

N′-[(E)-(3,4-dimethoxyphenyl)methylidene]-4-methylbenzenesulfonohydrazide, **5h** ^{1}H NMR, ^{13}C NMR and HRMS spectra of compound **5h** were published elsewhere [66].

N′-[(E)-(3,4-dimethoxyphenyl)methylidene]benzenesulfonohydrazide, **5i** ^{1}H NMR, ^{13}C NMR and HRMS spectra of compound **5i** were published elsewhere [66].

N′-{(E)-[5-(benzyloxy)-1H-indol-3-yl]methylidene}-4-methylbenzenesulfonohydrazide, **5j** Yield: 67%; m.p. 222–223 °C. ^{1}H NMR (400 MHz, DMSO-d$_6$): δ = 2.28 (s, 3H, CH$_3$), 5.03 (s, 2H, CH$_2$), 6.88 (dd, J = 2.5, 8.8 Hz, 1H, H-6), 7.30 (d, J = 8.8 Hz, 1H, H-7), 7.34 (d, J = 8.1 Hz, 2H, H-3′, and H-5′), 7.36 (t, J = 7.2 Hz, 1H, H-4″), 7.43 (t, J = 7.4 Hz, 2H, H-3″, and H-5″), 7.53 (d, J = 7.2 Hz, 2H, H-2″, and H-6″), 7.57 (d, J = 2.4 Hz, 1H, H-4), 7.68 (d,

J = 2.8 Hz, 1H, H-2), 7.81 (d, J = 8.2 Hz, 2H, H-2', and H-6'), 8.09 (s, 1H, CH), 10.84 (s, 1H, NH), 11.40 (d, J = 2.0 Hz, 1H, NH). ^{13}C NMR (100 MHz, DMSO-d$_6$): δ = 20.90 (CH$_3$), 69.68 (CH$_2$), 104.82 (C-4), 110.81 (C-3), 112.50 (C-6), 113.02 (C-7), 124.48 (C-4a), 127.37 (C-2' and C-6'), 127.84 (C-4''), 127.93 (C-2'' and C-6''), 128.46 (H-3'' and H-5''), 129.41 (C-3' and C-5'), 130.96 (C-2), 131.98 (C-7a), 136.33 (C-1'), 137.35 (C-1''), 143.08 (C-4'), 145.68 (CH), 153.38 (C-5). HRMS (ESI) *m/z*: calcd: [M+H]+ 404.142723. Found: [M+H]+ 420.1373.

N'-((E)-[5-(benzyloxy)-1H-indol-3-yl]methylidenebenzenesulfonohydrazide, **5k**^{1}H NMR, ^{13}C NMR and HRMS spectra of compound **5k** were published elsewhere [67].

N'-[(E)-(4-chlorophenyl)methylidene]benzenesulfonohydrazide, 5l^{1}H NMR, ^{13}C NMR and HRMS spectra of compound **5l** were published elsewhere [66].

3.4. Biological Evaluation

Assessment of AChE and BChE Inhibitory Activity

AChE and BChE inhibitory activity was measured using the microplate assay described by Ellman et al. [68] with the modifications added by López et al. [36]. The compounds were tested at concentrations between 10^{-3} and 10^{-8} M. First, all compounds were dissolved in 1% DMSO in a concentration of 1 mg/mL. Then, they were serially diluted using phosphate buffer (PBS) (8 mM K$_2$HPO$_4$, 2.3 mM NaH$_2$PO$_4$, 0.15 M NaCl, pH 7.5) to provide the concentration range needed. Acetylcholinesterase from *Electrophorus electricus* and butyrylcholinesterase from equine serum (Sigma-Aldrich, Hamburg, Germany) were used with a substrate solution of 5,5'-dithiobis(2-nitrobenzoic acid) (DTNB) with acetylthiocholine iodide (ATCI) or butyrylthiocholine iodide (BuTCI), respectively (0.04 M Na$_2$HPO$_4$, 0.2 mM DTNB, 0.24 mM ATCI or BuTCI, pH 7.5).

Then, 50 microliters of AchE or BchE (0.25 U/mL) dissolved in phosphate buffer and 50 µL of the tested compound solution were added to the wells. Incubation of the plates was performed at room temperature for 30 min. Then, 100 µL of substrate solution were added to start the enzymatic reaction. The absorbances were read in a microplate reader (BIOBASE, ELISA-EL10A, China) at 405 nm after 3 min for AChE and 10 min for BChE. Enzyme activity was calculated as an inhibition percentage compared to an assay including buffer instead of an inhibitor. Galanthamine and donepezil were used as positive controls. All data were analyzed with the software package Prism 3 (Graph Pad Inc., San Diego, CA, USA). The IC$_{50}$ values were measured in triplicate and the results are presented as means ± SD. For the less active compounds instead of IC$_{50}$, an inhibition percentage of 1 mM is presented (1 mM is the maximal tested concentration).

3.5. Cytotoxicity of the Compounds

3.5.1. Cell Lines and Culture Conditions

To evaluate the biocompatibility of the experimental compounds, their in vitro cytotoxicity was assessed against malignant neuroblastoma cells of human (SH-SY5Y) and murine (NEURO-2A) origin, as well as normal fibroblast murine cells (CCL-1). All cell lines were purchased from the German Collection of Microorganisms and Cell Cultures (DSMZ GmbH, Braunschweig, Germany). Cell cultures were cultivated in a growth medium RPMI 1640 supplemented with 10% fetal bovine serum (FBS), 5% L-glutamine, and incubated under standard conditions of 37 °C and 5% humidified CO2 atmosphere.

3.5.2. MTT Assay

The effects of the newly synthesized hydrazide hydrazone and sufonyl hydrazone derivatives on cell viability were measured using a standard MTT colorimetric assay. The method is based on the biotransformation of the yellow tetrazole salt MTT (3-(4,5-dimethyliazol-2-yl)-2,5-diphenyltetrazole bromide) to violet formazan under the action of mitochondrial succinate dehydrogenases of vital cells. Exponential phased cells were harvested and seeded (100 µL/well) in 96-well plates at the appropriate density (1.5×10^5). On the following day, cell cultures were treated with different concentrations of the experimental compounds and after 72 h exposure time, filter sterilized MTT substrate solution

(5 mg/mL in PBS) was added to each well of the culture plate. A further 4 h incubation allowed for the formation of purple insoluble formazan precipitates. The latter were dissolved in isopropyl alcohol solution containing 5% formic acid prior to absorbance measurement at 580 nm on a Labexim LMR1 automated ELISA reader. Collected absorbance values were blanked against MTT and isopropanol solution and normalized to the mean value of untreated control (100% cell viability).

3.6. Determination of Antioxidant Activity

3.6.1. DPPH Radical Scavenging Activity

Free radical scavenging activity was measured using DPPH method [69,70] with slight modification. Here, 300 µL of 5 mM solutions of tested compounds in MeOH were added to 2 mL methanolic solution of DPPH (2 mg/mL). The absorbance was measured at 517 nm after 30 min. Results were evaluated as percentage scavenging of radical:

$$\text{DPPH radical scavenging activity (\%)} = ((\text{Abs}_{\text{contr.}} - \text{Abssample})/\text{Abs}_{\text{scontr.}}) \times 100,$$

where $\text{Abs}_{\text{scontr.}}$ is the absorbance of DPPH radical with 300 µL MeOH, Abssample is the absorbance of DPPH radical solution mixed with sample. BHT was used as positive control

3.6.2. ABTS Radical Scavenging Assay

For ABTS assay, the procedure followed the method of Arnao et al. [71] with some modifications. The stock solutions included 7 mM ABTS solution and 2.4 mM potassium persulfate solution. The working solution was then prepared by mixing the two stock solutions in equal quantities and allowing them to react for 14 h at room temperature in the dark. The solution was then diluted by mixing 2 mL ABTS solution with 50 mL methanol to obtain an absorbance of 0.605 ± 0.01 units at 734 nm using a spectrophotometer. A fresh ABTS solution was prepared for each assay. Different concentrations (5, 2.5, 1, 1.25, 0.5 mM) (10 µL) of compounds were allowed to react with 2 mL of the ABTS solution and the absorbance was taken at 734 nm after 5 min. The ABTS scavenging capacity of the compound was calculated as follows:

$$\text{ABTS radical scavenging activity (\%)} = ((\text{Abs}_{\text{contr.}} - \text{Abs}_{\text{sample}})/\text{Abs}_{\text{contr.}}) \times 100,$$

where $\text{Abs}_{\text{contr.}}$ is the absorbance of DPPH radical with 300 µL MeOH, Abssample is the absorbance of DPPH radical solution mixed with the sample. The IC_{50} value (concentration of sample where absorbance of ABTS decreases 50% with respect to absorbance of blank) of the sample was determined. BHT was used as positive control.

3.6.3. Ferric Reducing/Antioxidant Power (FRAP)

The FRAP assay was done according to the method described by Benzie and Strain [72] with some modifications. The stock solutions included 300 mM acetate buffer pH 3.6, 10 mM TPTZ solution in 40 mM HCl, and 20 mM $FeCl_3.6H_2O$ solution. The fresh working solution was prepared by mixing 25 mL acetate buffer, 2.5 mL TPTZ solution, and 2.5 mL $FeCl_3.6H_2O$ solution and then warmed at 37 °C before use. Then, 150 µL of compounds in MeOH (5 mM) were allowed to react with 2 mL of the FRAP solution for 30 min in the dark. Readings of the colored product (ferrous tripyridyltriazine complex) were then taken at 593 nm. Results are expressed in mM Trolox equivalent (TE/mM). BHT was used as positive control.

3.6.4. Determination of Antioxidant Activity in Linoleic Acid System by the FTC Method

The antioxidant activity of studied compounds against lipid peroxidation was measured through ammonium thiocyanate assay as described by Takao et al. [66] with some modifications. The reaction solution, containing 200 µL of the compound (10 mM) in MeOH, 200 µL of linoleic acid emulsions (25 mg/mL in 99% ethanol), and 400 µL of 50 mM phosphate buffer (pH 7.6) was incubated in the dark at room temperature. A 10 µL aliquot of the reaction solution was then added to 200 µL of 70% (*v/v*) ethanol and 10 µL of 30% (*w/v*) ammonium thiocyanate. Precisely 3 min after the addition of 10 µL of 20 mM ferrous chloride in 3.5% (*v/v*) hydrochloric acid to the reaction mixture, the absorbance of the resulting red color was measured at 500 nm. Aliquots were assayed every 24 h until the day after the absorbance of the control solution (without compound) reached maximum value. BHT (10 mM) was used as positive control.

3.7. Model of H_2O_2-Induced Oxidative Stress in SH-SY5Y Cell Line

The human neuroblastoma cell line SH-SY5Y (94030304) was acquired from the European Collection of Cell Cultures (ECACC, Salisbury, UK). SH-SY5Y cells were cultured in RPMI medium supplemented with 10% heat-inactivated fetal bovine serum (FBS), 2 mM L-glutamine, and penicillin/streptomycin. The cells were maintained in a humidified atmosphere at 37 °C with 5% CO2. The culture medium was refreshed every 2–3 days to ensure optimal conditions for cell growth and viability.

3.7.1. Model

The SH-SY5Y cells were seeded at a density of 3.5×104 cells per well (100 µL of RPMI) in 96-well plates. After 24 h, the cell medium was aspirated and the cells were treated with different concentrations of the test compounds (0.1, 1, 5, 10, 25, 50 µM) for 90 min. Thereafter, SH-SY5Y cells were washed with phosphate-buffered saline (PBS) and exposed to hydrogen peroxide (1 mM) for 10 min. The solution of H_2O_2 in PBS was aspirated and changed with cell medium. After 24 h, cell viability was evaluated by the MTT assay. Cells not treated with hydrogen peroxide (negative controls) were considered a measure for 100% protection, and cells treated with hydrogen peroxide (positive controls) for 0% protection. Melatonin and rasagiline (Sigma-Aldrich Chemie GmbH) were used as references due to the abundance of data on their antioxidant and neuroprotective activity [73,74]. Considering the structural similarity of the newly synthesized compound to donepezil, it was included as a reference compound in the study.

3.7.2. Statistical Analysis

Statistical analysis was conducted using GraphPad Prism 6 Software. A one-way ANOVA followed by Dunnett's multiple comparisons post-test was utilized to compare the data between the control and treatment groups. A significance level of 0.05 was selected for all comparisons.

3.8. In Silico Studies

3.8.1. Molecular Docking of Human AChE and of Human BChE

Molecular docking studies were performed using Docking tool of Molecular Operating Environment of Chemical Computing Group (MOE, version 2022.02).

Selection of PDB structures: The following crystallographic structures of human acetylcholinesterase (AChE) and human butyrylcholinesterase (BChE) have been chosen for molecular docking studies:

(1)　AChE, complexed with 1-Benzyl-4-[(5,6-dimethoxy-1-indanon-2-yl)methyl]piperidine (E20) and co-factor 2-acetamido-2-deoxy-beta-D-glucopyranose (NAG), retrieved from Protein Data Bank (http://www.rcsb.org/) with PDB ID 4EY7;

(2)　BChE, complexed with butyl-[(2~(S))-1-(2-cycloheptylethylamino)-3-(1~(H)-indol-3-yl)-1-oxidanylidene-propan-2-yl]azanium (HUN) and NAD again (PDB ID 6QAA).

The choice of aforementioned crystallographic structures followed previous investigations of Alov et al. [46], who, aiming at multi-target hit compounds for neurodegenerative disease drug development, performed molecular docking in AChE (PDB ID 4EY7). Aktar et al. [75] have investigated the enzyme inhibition activities of new sulfonyl hydrazones performing molecular docking simulations in BChE (PDB ID 6QAA).

Structures preparation: The 3D structures of the investigated compounds were built and optimized with AMBER10:EHT in MOE. The R enantiomers (a chiral carbon atom in the pyrrolidine ring) of compounds **3e–3i** were used in docking. These forms correspond to the extended conformations of the compounds, thus fitting better to the deep and narrow binding cavity of the cholinesterases. The PDB complexes were prepared using the "Quick preparation" procedure in MOE. In addition to adding hydrogens and assigning protonation states of titratable protein groups by the Generalized Born electrostatics model at physiologically relevant conditions (temperature of 300 K; pH = 7; ion concentration of 0.1 mol/L), tethers were added to the receptor heavy atoms and distant atoms were fixed. Following this, the system refinement was performed applying Amber10: EHT force field and the default RMS gradient of 0.1 kcal/mol/$Å^2$.

Prediction of the protonation state of the investigated structures. The "Protomer" panel in MOE was used to explore the possible ionization states of the molecules that can be populated at physiological pH. The resulting ionization states were sorted in order of decreasing population and the ionization state with the highest % of population at the physiological pH was used for docking.

Docking simulations: Molecular docking studies were performed in the "Docking" module in MOE. The following settings were applied in the docking protocol: (I) in the set of atoms defining the receptor, the receptor and solvent atoms were included. (II) "Triangle Matcher" placement to generate poses by aligning ligand triplets of atoms on triplets of alpha spheres in the most systematic way; the London dG scoring function was used to rank the poses (30 placement poses). (III) Subsequent refinement using "Rigid receptor" or "Induced fit" (flexible side chains) tools based on London dG and GBVI/WSA scoring functions (5 poses as the final output following the refinement step). London dG is the default scoring function in MOE that estimates the free energy of binding of the ligand from a given pose combining enthalpy and entropy terms. The GBVI/WSA dG is the default force field-based scoring function that is used after rescoring for the final refinement of the docking poses. The protein–ligand interactions in the active site of the complexes were visualized using the "Ligand Interactions" MOE tool.

3.8.2. In Silico Docking Studies of MT1 and MT2 Receptors

We prepared a model of human melatonin receptors MT1 and MT2 which we employed as docking templates in order to propose the possible molecular mechanism of action of our ligands. XRD structures of human MT1 and MT2 receptors were selected for our modeling on the base of resolution and completeness of crystallized deposited data in Protein Data Bank.

If more than one copy of the receptor structure in the PDB existed, we used all of them in further analysis.

In all selected PDB structures, the minor structural improprieties were corrected, followed by removal of all nonprotein species. For the purpose of attaining the right protonation state at 7.0 pH, which was the physiological one, we used Labute's protonate 3D algorithm (Labute 2008) at 300K and 0.154 M/l salt concentration as it is implemented in MOE software package.

The codes of selected PDB for MT1 were 6ME2, 6ME3, 6ME4, 6ME5, 7DB6, 7VGY, 7VGZ.

Although only 2 amino acids in the active site differ between these structures ALA104 in 6ME2, 6ME3, 6ME4, 6ME5 is GLY104 in 7DB6, 7VGY, 7VGZ and PHE251 in 6ME2, 6ME3, 6ME4, 6ME5 is TRP251 in 7DB6, 7VGY, 7VGZ, we prepared our model for docking by homology modeling the sequence of NCBI NP005949.1 melatonin receptor type 1A [Homo Sapiens] on consensus model formed by all of the PDB structures. The above-mentioned differences are due to the point mutations for increased thermostability of the protein introduced by Stauch et al. [51].

Active site for docking was defined by natural position of ligands inside crystallized structures.

The PDB codes of selected structures for MT2 were 6ME6, 6ME7, 6ME8, 6ME9, 6PS8, 7VH0. In this set, only PHE264 from the residues forming active site is replaced with TRP264 in 7VH0, based on the point mutations introduced by Stauch et al. [51].

In the case of MT2 receptor, we prepared our model for further docking by homology modeling the sequence of NCBI NP.005950.1 melatonin receptor 1B [Homo Sapiens] on consensus model formed by all of the selected PDB structures.

Fortunately, all of the selected XRD structures were crystallized with their natural-like ligands in the cavity, therefore presenting the active state of MT1 and MT2 receptors.

All newly synthesized ligands were protonated according to their protonation state at 7 pH. Due to the low amount of rotatable bonds, the systematic approach was used in formation of ligand library. Every generated structure was further energy minimized using AMBER12EHT [MOE] force field in gas phase. All unique conformational structures within 10 kcal/mol from the lowest structure of every ligand were used for further docking.

All conformations of all ligands were docked in active site of the MT1 and MT2 receptors using AlphaPMI algorithm [MOE] for initial placement of every structure. These poses were scored by London dG [MOE] function, which estimates the free energy of binding of the ligand from a given pose and consists of terms that estimate average gain/loss of rotational and translational entropy, measures the geometric imperfections of hydrogen bonds and the desolvation energy of atoms.

The best 100 poses for every ligand for every pocket were further optimized with Induced Fit methodology using AMBER12EHT force field and Generalized Born solvation model with optimization cutoff of 5A from the ligand. The GBVI/WSA dG [MOE] was used as a rescoring function and the best 30 poses were collected for the next coming analysis.

In all cases, the original ligands from the PDB files were also used in our docking study as they were subjected to the same ligand preparation methodology as our ligands. Placement of the original ligands in the receptor cavities from the placement algorithm in a position similar to that in the intact PDB was used as a criterion for the adequacy of our docking methodology.

RMSD of alpha carbons of the active site residues between aligned chains of selected PDB structures for MT1 and MT2 structures are presented in supplementary materials as Tables S3 and S5. Differences in sequences of selected structures according to BLOSSUM62 are presented also in supporting materials as Tables S4 and S6.

The difference between *Z* and *E* isomers in some of the ligands discussed in the text was calculated using B3LYP/6–311++G** hybrid functional and basis set as they are implemented in GAUSSIAN 09 software suite.

As a verification of our docking study, we included in our ligand set the original ligands from the used pdb files. These ligands were treated in the same way as our structures and were used to expand the ligand set for docking. Analysis of their interaction energies shows that all the structures studied have better interaction energies than the original ligands and the docking procedure used positions the original ligands in the receptor cavities in the same way as they are in the original PDB files.

3.8.3. ADME/Tox

In silico ADME studies were performed by using the online tool SwissADME/Tox of the Swiss Institute of Bioinformatics (https://www.sib.swiss, accessed on 20 April 2022).

3.8.4. In Silico Prediction of BBB Permeability

The webserver was used to predict BBB permeability of compounds, SwissADME (https://www.sib.swiss, accessed on 20 April 2022).

3.8.5. BBB Permeability by In Vitro PAMPA Test

The blood–brain barrier permeabilities were measured by PAMPA Permeability Analyzer (pIONInc, Billerica, MA, USA). The tested compounds and reference standards were prepared as 10 mM stock solutions in DMSO and further diluted in Prisma HT buffer pH 7.4. The experiment followed the BBB Protocol: 200 µL sample's aliquots in the donor compartment, Brain Sink Buffer aliquots (200 µL) in the acceptor wells, BBB-1 lipid for coating the permeation membranes, "sandwich" assembly with the acceptor plate on top of the donor one, and incubation at temperature 25 °C for 4 h under humidity control without stirring. For permeability assessment, UV spectra of the blank, reference, donor, and acceptor plates were collected at wavelength 250–500 nm. Effective permeability Pe (10^{-6} cm/s) of the compounds was calculated and presented as $-\log Pe$. Samples were analyzed in triplicate and average values were reported. Highly permeable compounds were indicated by values of $-\log$Pe < 5, the medium permeable by $-\log$Pe between 5 and 6, and if $-\log$Pe > 6, the compound was considered as low permeable [76]. Theophylline, corticosterone, and propranolol HCl were used as reference standards to control the quality and consistency of the BBB permeability experiment [77].

4. Conclusions

Alzheimer's disease (AD) is a significant concern for chemistry researchers seeking new multi-target compounds to address this complex neurodegenerative condition. Focusing on melatonin/donepezil hybrids as potential candidates for AD treatment, we synthesized 30 new derivatives. Among them, compounds **3c** and **3d** displayed the most promising AChE inhibitory activity (10.76 ± 1.66 µM and 9.77 ± 0.76 µM, respectively), while compound **3n**, containing melatonin, exhibited notable BChE inhibitory activity (21.12 ± 1.48 µM).

The in vitro antioxidant activities for the most promising molecules were investigated by the DPPH, FRAP, ABTS, and FTC methods. All tested compounds hold potential as therapeutic neuroprotective agents for neurodegenerative disorders. The sulfonylhydrazones **5k**, **5j**, **5g**, and hydrazone 3r revealed the highest DPPH activity and hydrazones **3i**, **3d**, **3c**, and **5h** showed the lowest values of IC_{50} in the ABTS test. With respect to the FRAP method, compound 3c has the strongest activity, followed by **5a**, **5h**, donepezil, **3m**, and **5j**. In the FTC method, the highest significant diminution was demonstrated by **3a** followed by **3c**, **5h**, and **5j**, compared with BHT. Thus, compound **3c**, a promising acetylcholinesterase inhibitor among the new derivatives, demonstrated very good antioxidant activity across the three tested methods (FRAP, ABTS, and FTC). Additionally, in vitro studies revealed that the melatonin derivative **3n** efficiently prevents oxidative stress-induced injury in SH-SY5Y cells, exhibiting the best BChE inhibitory activity. As a future perspective, we plan to evaluate hydrazones **3c**, **3d**, **3a**, **3n**, and **5a** in vivo using models of Alzheimer's disease and melatonin deficiency, as well as Aβ (1–42) aggregation.

Importantly, the new series of melatonin derivatives containing the donepezil fragment showed low cytotoxicity and a good in vitro safety profile. Compounds **3a–d** (IC_{50} 129, 138.4, 97.3, 122.3 µM, respectively), **3k** (130.8 µM), and **5a** (142.0 µM) exhibited the best bioavailability, with IC_{50} values twice as high as the reference donepezil (79.3 ± 6.2 µM) in the human neuroblastoma cell line SH-SY5Y and three times higher in normal mouse fibroblasts. Notably, the most active compounds **3a–d** and **5a** displayed negligible cytotoxic activity in the mouse neuroblastoma cell culture Neuro-2a (IC_{50} > 300 µM); making them promising structures for further study in AD. An in silico pharmacokinetics analysis predicted that all tested hybrids could be well absorbed, metabolized, and excreted, with most of them capable of crossing the BBB. Additionally, the most promising compounds were measured by PAMPA for blood–brain barrier permeabilities.

Finally, docking studies suggest potential future applications of the MTDL **3c** in complex diseases such as major depression and AD, which involve targeting AChE and/or BChE enzymes and melatonin MT1 and MT2 receptors.

Supplementary Materials: The following supporting information can be downloaded at: https://www.mdpi.com/article/10.3390/ph16091194/s1, Figure S1: Key NOESY correlations of hydrazide-hydrazones **3c** and **3o**; Figure S2: Docking results of compound 5a: (a) left–PLIs of the highest ranked pose; right–PLI of the second highest ranked pose; (b) the best pose of donepezil (green), the highest ranked pose (light pink) and the second highest ranked pose (dark pink) in the active site of AChE (PDB ID 4EY7); Table S1: RMSD of CA of the active site residues between aligned chains of selected PDB structures for MT1 modeling; Table S2: Similarity of PDB sequences of selected PDB structures for modeling MT1 receptor according to BLUSSUM62; Table S3: RMSD of CA of the active site residues between aligned chains of selected PDB structures for MT2 modeling, Table S4: Similarity of PDB sequences of selected PDB structures for modeling MT2 receptor according to BLUSSUM62; Figure S3: Side, up and down view, respectively, of the pocket that forms the active site in our model of the MT1 receptor (lipophilic parts of the pocket are in green, while hydrophilic are represented in pink); Table S5: The best results from induced fit docking of ligands on MT1 receptor according to GBVI/WSA scoring function (kcal/mol); Figure S4: The best interaction energies of our ligands with the MT1 (blue) and MT2 (red) receptors according to GBVI/WSA scoring function (kcal/mol); Figure S5: PLIF Barcode map of interaction between the best 50 ligands poses and amino acids of the active site cavity of the MT1 receptor; Figure S6: Population histogram of the interactions of the first 50 ligand poses with residues inside active site of the receptor according to PLIF analysis (Phe179); Figure S7: Side, up and down view, respectively, of the pocket that forms the active site in our model of the MT2 receptor (lipophilic parts of the pocket are in green, while hydrophilic are represented in pink); Table S6: The best results from induced fit docking of ligands on MT2 receptor according to GBVI/WSA scoring function (kcal/mol); Figure S8: Barcode map of interaction between best 50 ligands poses and amino acids of the active site cavity of the MT2 receptor; Figure S9: Population histogram of the interactions of the first 50 ligand poses with residues inside the active site of the receptor according to PLIF analysis; Figure S10: Interaction maps of the best poses of the third (5a left) and forth (3i right) of the best ligands for MT1 receptor; Figure S11: Difference between MT2 and MT1 receptor binding energies of our ligands (kcal/mol). Ligands with negative values prefer to bind to MT1, while ligands with positive values prefer to bind to MT2; From Figure S12 to Figure S80—^{1}H NMR, ^{13}C NMR and HRMS spectra.

Author Contributions: Conceptualization, V.T.A.; methodology, V.T.A.; software, T.P., I.P., N.T., M.R. and E.K.-Y.; validation, N.T., I.P., T.P. and M.R.; investigation, V.T.A., B.G., T.P., I.P., D.Z.-D., I.V.V., N.V., R.M., D.S., B.P. and Y.V.; writing original draft preparation, V.T.A.; writing review and editing, V.T.A., R.M., Y.V., B.G. and V.T.; visualization, V.T.A., T.P., N.V., N.T. and M.R.; supervision, V.T.A. and V.T.; project administration, V.T.A.; funding acquisition, V.T.A. All authors have read and agreed to the published version of the manuscript.

Funding: This research was funded by the Bulgarian national plan for recovery and resilience through the Bulgarian National Science Fund, grant number KP-06-N63/11; 14.12.2022.

Institutional Review Board Statement: Not applicable.

Informed Consent Statement: Not applicable.

Data Availability Statement: Data is contained within the article and Supplementary Material.

Acknowledgments: Research equipment of Distributed Research Infrastructure INFRAMAT, part of the Bulgarian National Roadmap for Research Infrastructures, supported by the Bulgarian Ministry of Education and Science, was used in this investigation. The authors express their thankfulness to Teodora Atanasova, Paraskev Nedyalkov, and Kaloyan Krastev for their valuable assistance.

Conflicts of Interest: The authors declare no conflict of interest. The funders had no role in the design of the study; in the collection, analyses, or interpretation of data; in the writing of the manuscript, or in the decision to publish the results.

Sample Availability: Samples of the compounds are available from the authors.

References

1. World Health Organization. Multiregional workshop on the implementation of the global action plan on public health response to dementia. *East. Mediterr. Health J.* **2023**, *29*, 302–303. [CrossRef] [PubMed]
2. Walsh, S.; Wallace, L.; Kuhn, I.; Mytton, O.; Lafortune, L.; Wills, W.; Mukadam, N.; Brayne, C. Are Population-Level Approaches to Dementia Risk Reduction Under-Researched? A Rapid Review of the Dementia Prevention Literature. *J. Prev. Alzheimer's Dis.* **2023**, 1–8. [CrossRef]
3. Sheppard, O.; Coleman, M. *Alzheimer's Disease: Etiology, Neuropathology and Pathogenesis*; Exon Publications: Brisbane, QLD, Australia, 2020; pp. 1–21.
4. Nasb, M.; Tao, W.; Chen, N. Alzheimer's Disease Puzzle: Delving into Pathogenesis Hypotheses. *Aging Dis.* **2023**, *15*, 2.
5. Tönnies, E.; Trushina, E. Oxidative stress, synaptic dysfunction, and Alzheimer's disease. *J. Alzheimer's Dis.* **2017**, *57*, 1105–1121. [CrossRef] [PubMed]
6. Buccellato, F.R.; D'Anca, M.; Fenoglio, C.; Scarpini, E.; Galimberti, D. Role of oxidative damage in Alzheimer's disease and neurodegeneration: From pathogenic mechanisms to biomarker discovery. *Antioxidants* **2021**, *10*, 1353. [CrossRef]

7. Fernández-Bolaños, J.G.; López, Ó. Butyrylcholinesterase inhibitors as potential anti-Alzheimer's agents: An updated patent review (2018–present). *Expert Opin. Ther. Pat.* **2022**, *32*, 913–932. [CrossRef]

8. Meghana, G.; Gowda, D.; Chidambaram, S.B.; Osmani, R.A. Amyloid–β pathology in Alzheimer's Disease: A Nano delivery Approach. *Vib. Spectrosc.* **2023**, *126*, 103510. [CrossRef]

9. Carvajal, F.J.; Inestrosa, N.C. Interactions of AChE with Aβ aggregates in Alzheimer's brain: Therapeutic relevance of IDN 5706. *Front. Mol. Neurosci.* **2011**, *4*, 19. [CrossRef]

10. Moss, D.E. Improving anti-neurodegenerative benefits of acetylcholinesterase inhibitors in Alzheimer's disease: Are irreversible inhibitors the future? *Int. J. Mol. Sci.* **2020**, *21*, 3438. [CrossRef]

11. Zeb, M.W.; Riaz, A.; Szigeti, K. Donepezil: A review of pharmacological characteristics and role in the management of Alzheimer disease. *Clin. Med. Insights. Geriatr.* **2017**, *10*, 1–14.

12. Lee, C.-H.; Hung, S.-Y. Physiologic Functions and Therapeutic Applications of α7 Nicotinic Acetylcholine Receptor in Brain Disorders. *Pharmaceutics* **2022**, *15*, 31. [CrossRef] [PubMed]

13. Jann, M.W. Rivastigmine, a new-generation cholinesterase inhibitor for the treatment of Alzheimer's disease. *Pharmacother. J. Hum. Pharmacol. Drug Ther.* **2000**, *20*, 1–12. [CrossRef] [PubMed]

14. Marucci, G.; Buccioni, M.; Dal Ben, D.; Lambertucci, C.; Volpini, R.; Amenta, F. Efficacy of acetylcholinesterase inhibitors in Alzheimer's disease. *Neuropharmacology* **2021**, *190*, 108352. [CrossRef] [PubMed]

15. de Freitas Silva, M.; Dias, K.S.; Gontijo, V.S.; Ortiz, C.J.C.; Viegas, C., Jr. Multi-target directed drugs as a modern approach for drug design towards Alzheimer's disease: An update. *Curr. Med. Chem.* **2018**, *25*, 3491–3525. [CrossRef] [PubMed]

16. Papagiouvannis, G.; Theodosis-Nobelos, P.; Kourounakis, P.N.; Rekka, E.A. Multi-target directed compounds with antioxidant and/or anti-inflammatory properties as potent agents for alzheimer's disease. *Med. Chem.* **2021**, *17*, 1086–1103. [CrossRef]

17. Grosjean, S.; Pachón-Angona, I.; Dawra, M.; Refouvelet, B.; Ismaili, L. Multicomponent reactions as a privileged tool for multitarget-directed ligand strategies in Alzheimer's disease therapy. *Future Med. Chem.* **2022**, *14*, 1583–1606. [CrossRef]

18. Ramalakshmi, N.; RS, R.; CN, N. Multitarget directed ligand approaches for Alzheimer's disease: A Comprehensive Review. *Mini Rev. Med. Chem.* **2021**, *21*, 2361–2388. [CrossRef]

19. Eissa, K.I.; Kamel, M.M.; Mohamed, L.W.; Kassab, A.E. Development of new Alzheimer's disease drug candidates using donepezil as a key model. *Arch. Der Pharm.* **2023**, *356*, 2200398. [CrossRef]

20. Gulcan, H.O.; Kosar, M. The hybrid compounds as multi-target ligands for the treatment of Alzheimer's disease: Considerations on donepezil. *Curr. Top. Med. Chem.* **2022**, *22*, 395–407. [CrossRef]

21. Luo, Z.; Sheng, J.; Sun, Y.; Lu, C.; Yan, J.; Liu, A.; Luo, H.-b.; Huang, L.; Li, X. Synthesis and evaluation of multi-target-directed ligands against Alzheimer's disease based on the fusion of donepezil and ebselen. *J. Med. Chem.* **2013**, *56*, 9089–9099. [CrossRef]

22. Pravin, N.; Jozwiak, K. Effects of linkers and substitutions on multitarget directed ligands for Alzheimer's diseases: Emerging paradigms and strategies. *Int. J. Mol. Sci.* **2022**, *23*, 6085. [CrossRef]

23. Li, Y.; Zhang, J.; Wan, J.; Liu, A.; Sun, J. Melatonin regulates Aβ production/clearance balance and Aβ neurotoxicity: A potential therapeutic molecule for Alzheimer's disease. *Biomed. Pharmacother.* **2020**, *132*, 110887. [CrossRef] [PubMed]

24. Ramos, E.; Egea, J.; de Los Ríos, C.; Marco-Contelles, J.; Romero, A. Melatonin as a versatile molecule to design novel multitarget hybrids against neurodegeneration. *Future Med. Chem.* **2017**, *9*, 765–780. [CrossRef] [PubMed]

25. Verma, A.K.; Singh, S.; Rizvi, S.I. Therapeutic potential of melatonin and its derivatives in aging and neurodegenerative diseases. *Biogerontology* **2023**, *24*, 183–206. [CrossRef]

26. Brunner, P.; Sozer Topcular, N.; Jockers, R.; Ravid, R.; Angeloni, D.; Fraschini, F.; Eckert, A.; Muller Spahn, F.; Savaskan, E. Pineal and cortical melatonin receptors MT1 and MT2 are decreased in Alzheimer's disease. *Eur. J. Histochem.* **2006**, *50*, 311–316. [PubMed]

27. Halder, A.K.; Mitra, S.; Cordeiro, M.N.D. Designing multi-target drugs for the treatment of major depressive disorder. *Expert Opin. Drug Discov.* **2023**, *18*, 643–658. [CrossRef]

28. Anastassova, N.; Stefanova, D.; Hristova-Avakumova, N.; Georgieva, I.; Kondeva-Burdina, M.; Rangelov, M.; Todorova, N.; Tzoneva, R.; Yancheva, D. New Indole-3-Propionic Acid and 5-Methoxy-Indole Carboxylic Acid Derived Hydrazone Hybrids as Multifunctional Neuroprotectors. *Antioxidants* **2023**, *12*, 977. [CrossRef]

29. Aslanhan, Ö.; Kalay, E.; Tokalı, F.S.; Can, Z.; Şahin, E. Design, synthesis, antioxidant and anticholinesterase activities of novel isonicotinic hydrazide-hydrazone derivatives. *J. Mol. Struct.* **2023**, *1279*, 135037. [CrossRef]

30. Bozbey, İ.; Özdemir, Z.; Uslu, H.; Özçelik, A.B.; Şenol, F.S.; Orhan, İ.E.; Uysal, M. A series of new hydrazone derivatives: Synthesis, molecular docking and anticholinesterase activity studies. *Mini Rev. Med. Chem.* **2020**, *20*, 1042–1060. [CrossRef]

31. Demurtas, M.; Baldisserotto, A.; Lampronti, I.; Moi, D.; Balboni, G.; Pacifico, S.; Vertuani, S.; Manfredini, S.; Onnis, V. Indole derivatives as multifunctional drugs: Synthesis and evaluation of antioxidant, photoprotective and antiproliferative activity of indole hydrazones. *Bioorg. Chem.* **2019**, *85*, 568–576. [CrossRef]

32. Tchekalarova, J.; Ivanova, N.; Nenchovska, Z.; Tzoneva, R.; Stoyanova, T.; Uzunova, V.; Surcheva, S.; Tzonev, A.; Angelova, V.T.; Andreeva-Gateva, P. Evaluation of neurobiological and antioxidant effects of novel melatonin analogs in mice. *Saudi Pharm. J.* **2020**, *28*, 1566–1579. [CrossRef] [PubMed]

33. Angelova, V.T.; Pencheva, T.; Vassilev, N.; Simeonova, R.; Momekov, G.; Valcheva, V. New indole and indazole derivatives as potential antimycobacterial agents. *Med. Chem. Res.* **2019**, *28*, 485–497. [CrossRef]

34. Martins, F.; Santos, S.; Ventura, C.; Elvas-Leitão, R.; Santos, L.; Vitorino, S.; Reis, M.; Miranda, V.; Correia, H.F.; Aires-de-Sousa, J. Design, synthesis and biological evaluation of novel isoniazid derivatives with potent antitubercular activity. *Eur. J. Med. Chem.* **2014**, *81*, 119–138. [CrossRef]

35. Oliveira, P.F.; Guidetti, B.; Chamayou, A.; André-Barrès, C.; Madacki, J.; Korduláková, J.; Mori, G.; Orena, B.S.; Chiarelli, L.R.; Pasca, M.R. Mechanochemical synthesis and biological evaluation of novel isoniazid derivatives with potent antitubercular activity. *Molecules* **2017**, *22*, 1457. [CrossRef] [PubMed]

36. López, S.; Bastida, J.; Viladomat, F.; Codina, C. Acetylcholinesterase inhibitory activity of some Amaryllidaceae alkaloids and Narcissus extracts. *Life Sci.* **2002**, *71*, 2521–2529. [CrossRef] [PubMed]

37. Rankovic, Z. CNS drug design: Balancing physicochemical properties for optimal brain exposure. *J. Med. Chem.* **2015**, *58*, 2584–2608. [CrossRef]

38. Zhang, H.; Wang, Y.; Liu, D.; Li, J.; Feng, Y.; Lu, Y.; Yin, G.; Li, Z.; Shi, T.; Wang, Z. Carbamate-based N-Substituted tryptamine derivatives as novel pleiotropic molecules for Alzheimer's disease. *Bioorg. Chem.* **2022**, *125*, 105844. [CrossRef]

39. Al-Mamary, M.; Al-Habori, M.; Al-Zubairi, A.S. The in vitro antioxidant activity of different types of palm dates (*Phoenix dactylifera*) syrups. *Arab. J. Chem.* **2014**, *7*, 964–971. [CrossRef]

40. Alam, M.K.; Rana, Z.H.; Islam, S.N.; Akhtaruzzaman, M. Total phenolic content and antioxidant activity of methanolic extract of selected wild leafy vegetables grown in Bangladesh: A cheapest source of antioxidants. *Potravinarstvo* **2019**, *13*, 287–293. [CrossRef]

41. Dai, S.; Yu, C.; Liang, M.; Cheng, H.; Li, W.; Lai, F.; Ma, L.; Liu, X. Oxidation characteristics and thermal stability of Butylated hydroxytoluene. *Arab. J. Chem.* **2023**, *16*, 104932. [CrossRef]

42. Hoffmann, L.F.; Martins, A.; Majolo, F.; Contini, V.; Laufer, S.; Goettert, M.I. Neural regeneration research model to be explored: SH-SY5Y human neuroblastoma cells. *Neural Regen. Res.* **2023**, *18*, 1265. [PubMed]

43. Lopez-Suarez, L.; Al Awabdh, S.; Coumoul, X.; Chauvet, C. The SH-SY5Y human neuroblastoma cell line, a relevant in vitro cell model for investigating neurotoxicology in human: Focus on organic pollutants. *Neurotoxicology* **2022**, *92*, 131–155. [CrossRef] [PubMed]

44. Valko, M.; Leibfritz, D.; Moncol, J.; Cronin, M.T.; Mazur, M.; Telser, J. Free radicals and antioxidants in normal physiological functions and human disease. *Int. J. Biochem. Cell Biol.* **2007**, *39*, 44–84. [CrossRef] [PubMed]

45. Wang, J.; Wang, Z.-M.; Li, X.-M.; Li, F.; Wu, J.-J.; Kong, L.-Y.; Wang, X.-B. Synthesis and evaluation of multi-target-directed ligands for the treatment of Alzheimer's disease based on the fusion of donepezil and melatonin. *Bioorg. Med. Chem.* **2016**, *24*, 4324–4338. [CrossRef] [PubMed]

46. Alov, P.; Stoimenov, H.; Lessigiarska, I.; Pencheva, T.; Tzvetkov, N.T.; Pajeva, I.; Tsakovska, I. In Silico Identification of Multi-Target Ligands as Promising Hit Compounds for Neurodegenerative Diseases Drug Development. *Int. J. Mol. Sci.* **2022**, *23*, 13650. [CrossRef]

47. Ballesteros, J.A.; Weinstein, H. [19] Integrated methods for the construction of three-dimensional models and computational probing of structure-function relations in G protein-coupled receptors. In *Methods in Neurosciences*; Elsevier: Amsterdam, The Netherlands, 1995; Volume 25, pp. 366–428.

48. Wang, Q.; Lu, Q.; Guo, Q.; Teng, M.; Gong, Q.; Li, X.; Du, Y.; Liu, Z.; Tao, Y. Structural basis of the ligand binding and signaling mechanism of melatonin receptors. *Nat. Commun.* **2022**, *13*, 454. [CrossRef] [PubMed]

49. Okamoto, H.H.; Miyauchi, H.; Inoue, A.; Raimondi, F.; Tsujimoto, H.; Kusakizako, T.; Shihoya, W.; Yamashita, K.; Suno, R.; Nomura, N. Cryo-EM structure of the human MT1–Gi signaling complex. *Nat. Struct. Mol. Biol.* **2021**, *28*, 694–701. [CrossRef]

50. Clement, N.; Renault, N.; Guillaume, J.L.; Cecon, E.; Journé, A.S.; Laurent, X.; Tadagaki, K.; Cogé, F.; Gohier, A.; Delagrange, P. Importance of the second extracellular loop for melatonin MT1 receptor function and absence of melatonin binding in GPR50. *Br. J. Pharmacol.* **2018**, *175*, 3281–3297. [CrossRef]

51. Stauch, B.; Johansson, L.C.; McCorvy, J.D.; Patel, N.; Han, G.W.; Huang, X.-P.; Gati, C.; Batyuk, A.; Slocum, S.T.; Ishchenko, A. Structural basis of ligand recognition at the human MT1 melatonin receptor. *Nature* **2019**, *569*, 284–288. [CrossRef]

52. Herrera-Arozamena, C.; Estrada-Valencia, M.; Perez, C.; Lagartera, L.; Morales-Garcia, J.A.; Perez-Castillo, A.; Franco-Gonzalez, J.F.; Michalska, P.; Duarte, P.; Leon, R. Tuning melatonin receptor subtype selectivity in oxadiazolone-based analogues: Discovery of QR2 ligands and NRF2 activators with neurogenic properties. *Eur. J. Med. Chem.* **2020**, *190*, 112090. [CrossRef]

53. Boutin, J.A.; Witt-Enderby, P.A.; Sotriffer, C.; Zlotos, D.P. Melatonin receptor ligands: A pharmaco-chemical perspective. *J. Pineal Res.* **2020**, *69*, e12672. [CrossRef] [PubMed]

54. Pala, D.; Lodola, A.; Bedini, A.; Spadoni, G.; Rivara, S. Homology models of melatonin receptors: Challenges and recent advances. *Int. J. Mol. Sci.* **2013**, *14*, 8093–8121. [CrossRef] [PubMed]

55. Farce, A.; Chugunov, A.O.; Logé, C.; Sabaouni, A.; Yous, S.; Dilly, S.; Renault, N.; Vergoten, G.; Efremov, R.G.; Lesieur, D. Homology modeling of MT1 and MT2 receptors. *Eur. J. Med. Chem.* **2008**, *43*, 1926–1944. [CrossRef] [PubMed]

56. Pajouhesh, H.; Lenz, G.R. Medicinal chemical properties of successful central nervous system drugs. *NeuroRx* **2005**, *2*, 541–553. [CrossRef] [PubMed]

57. Vucicevic, J.; Nikolic, K.; Dobričić, V.; Agbaba, D. Prediction of blood–brain barrier permeation of α-adrenergic and imidazoline receptor ligands using PAMPA technique and quantitative-structure permeability relationship analysis. *Eur. J. Pharm. Sci.* **2015**, *68*, 94–105. [CrossRef] [PubMed]

58. Di, L.; Artursson, P.; Avdeef, A.; Ecker, G.F.; Faller, B.; Fischer, H.; Houston, J.B.; Kansy, M.; Kerns, E.H.; Krämer, S.D. Evidence-based approach to assess passive diffusion and carrier-mediated drug transport. *Drug Discov. Today* **2012**, *17*, 905–912. [CrossRef]

59. Reis, M.; Sinko, B.; HR Serra, C. Parallel artificial membrane permeability assay (PAMPA)-Is it better than Caco-2 for human passive permeability prediction? *Mini Rev. Med. Chem.* **2010**, *10*, 1071–1076. [CrossRef]

60. van de Waterbeemd, H.; Camenisch, G.; Folkers, G.; Chretien, J.R.; Raevsky, O.A. Estimation of blood-brain barrier crossing of drugs using molecular size and shape, and H-bonding descriptors. *J. Drug Target.* **1998**, *6*, 151–165. [CrossRef] [PubMed]

61. Daina, A.; Zoete, V. A boiled-egg to predict gastrointestinal absorption and brain penetration of small molecules. *ChemMedChem* **2016**, *11*, 1117–1121. [CrossRef]

62. Ghose, A.K.; Herbertz, T.; Hudkins, R.L.; Dorsey, B.D.; Mallamo, J.P. Knowledge-based, central nervous system (CNS) lead selection and lead optimization for CNS drug discovery. *ACS Chem. Neurosci.* **2012**, *3*, 50–68. [CrossRef]

63. Didziapetris, R.; Japertas, P.; Avdeef, A.; Petrauskas, A. Classification analysis of P-glycoprotein substrate specificity. *J. Drug Target.* **2003**, *11*, 391–406. [CrossRef] [PubMed]

64. Congreve, M.; Carr, R.; Murray, C.; Jhoti, H. A'rule of three'for fragment-based lead discovery? *Drug Discov. Today* **2003**, *8*, 876–877. [CrossRef] [PubMed]

65. Karabeliov, V.R.; Kondeva-Burdina, M.S.; Vassilev, N.G.; Elena, K.; Angelova, V.T. Neuroprotective evaluation of novel substituted 1, 3, 4-oxadiazole and aroylhydrazone derivatives. *Bioorg. Med. Chem. Lett.* **2022**, *59*, 128516. [CrossRef] [PubMed]

66. Angelova, V.T.; Tatarova, T.; Mihaylova, R.; Vassilev, N.; Petrov, B.; Zhivkova, Z.; Doytchinova, I. Novel Arylsulfonylhydrazones as Breast Anticancer Agents Discovered by Quantitative Structure-Activity Relationships. *Molecules* **2023**, *28*, 2058. [CrossRef] [PubMed]

67. Angelova, V.T.; Pencheva, T.; Vassilev, N.; K-Yovkova, E.; Mihaylova, R.; Petrov, B.; Valcheva, V. Development of new antimycobacterial sulfonyl hydrazones and 4-methyl-1, 2, 3-thiadiazole-based hydrazone derivatives. *Antibiotics* **2022**, *11*, 562 [CrossRef]

68. Ellman, G.; Coutney Jr, K.V. Anders and RM Featherstone. *Biochem. Pharmacol.* **1961**, *7*, 85–95.

69. Blois, M.S. Antioxidant determinations by the use of a stable free radical. *Nature* **1958**, *181*, 1199–1200. [CrossRef]

70. Grochowski, D.M.; Uysal, S.; Aktumsek, A.; Granica, S.; Zengin, G.; Ceylan, R.; Locatelli, M.; Tomczyk, M. In vitro enzyme inhibitory properties, antioxidant activities, and phytochemical profile of Potentilla thuringiaca. *Phytochem. Lett.* **2017**, *20*, 365–372 [CrossRef]

71. Arnao, M.B.; Cano, A.; Acosta, M. The hydrophilic and lipophilic contribution to total antioxidant activity. *Food Chem.* **2001**, *73*, 239–244. [CrossRef]

72. Benzie, I.F.; Strain, J.J. The ferric reducing ability of plasma (FRAP) as a measure of "antioxidant power": The FRAP assay. *Anal. Biochem.* **1996**, *239*, 70–76. [CrossRef]

73. Jaworek, A.K.; Szepietowski, J.C.; Hałubiec, P.; Wojas-Pelc, A.; Jaworek, J. Melatonin as an antioxidant and immunomodulator in atopic dermatitis—A new look on an old story: A Review. *Antioxidants* **2021**, *10*, 1179. [CrossRef] [PubMed]

74. Un, H.; Ugan, R.A.; Kose, D.; Yayla, M.; Tastan, T.B.; Bayir, Y.; Halici, Z. A new approach to sepsis treatment by rasagiline: A molecular, biochemical and histopathological study. *Mol. Biol. Rep.* **2022**, *49*, 3875–3883. [CrossRef]

75. Aktar, B.S.K.; Sıcak, Y.; Tatar, G.; Oruç-Emre, E.E. Synthesis, Antioxidant and Some Enzyme Inhibition Activities of New Sulfonyl Hydrazones and their Molecular Docking Simulations. *Pharm. Chem. J.* **2022**, *56*, 559–569. [CrossRef]

76. Doytchinova, I.; Atanasova, M.; Valkova, I.; Stavrakov, G.; Philipova, I.; Zhivkova, Z.; Zheleva-Dimitrova, D.; Konstantinov, S.; Dimitrov, I. Novel hits for acetylcholinesterase inhibition derived by docking-based screening on ZINC database. *J. Enzym. Inhib. Med. Chem.* **2018**, *33*, 768–776. [CrossRef] [PubMed]

77. Di, L.; Kerns, E.H.; Fan, K.; McConnell, O.J.; Carter, G.T. High throughput artificial membrane permeability assay for blood–brain barrier. *Eur. J. Med. Chem.* **2003**, *38*, 223–232. [CrossRef]

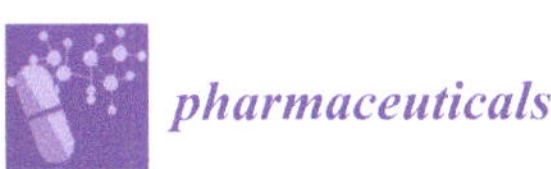

Article

Discovery of Potential Noncovalent Inhibitors of Dehydroquinate Dehydratase from Methicillin-Resistant *Staphylococcus aureus* through Computational-Driven Drug Design

César Millán-Pacheco [1,†], Lluvia Rios-Soto [2,†], Noé Corral-Rodríguez [2], Erick Sierra-Campos [3], Mónica Valdez-Solana [3], Alfredo Téllez-Valencia [2,*] and Claudia Avitia-Domínguez [2,*]

[1] Facultad de Farmacia, Universidad Autónoma del Estado de Morelos, Cuernavaca, Morelos 62209, Mexico; cmp@uaem.mx

[2] Facultad de Medicina y Nutrición, Universidad Juárez del Estado de Durango, Av. Universidad y Fanny Anitua S/N, Durango 34000, Mexico; lluviarios.soto@gmail.com (L.R.-S.); noe.corral.96@outlook.com (N.C.-R.)

[3] Facultad de Ciencias Químicas, Universidad Juárez del Estado de Durango Campus Gómez Palacio, Avenida Artículo 123 S/N, Fracc. Filadelfia, Gómez Palacio 35010, Mexico; ericksier@gmail.com (E.S.-C.); valdezandyval@gmail.com (M.V.-S.)

* Correspondence: atellez@ujed.mx (A.T.-V.); claudia.avitia@ujed.mx (C.A.-D.)

† These authors contributed equally to this work.

Citation: Millán-Pacheco, C.; Rios-Soto, L.; Corral-Rodríguez, N.; Sierra-Campos, E.; Valdez-Solana, M.; Téllez-Valencia, A.; Avitia-Domínguez, C. Discovery of Potential Noncovalent Inhibitors of Dehydroquinate Dehydratase from Methicillin-Resistant *Staphylococcus aureus* through Computational-Driven Drug Design. *Pharmaceuticals* **2023**, *16*, 1148. https://doi.org/10.3390/ph16081148

Academic Editors: Halil İbrahim Ciftci, Belgin Sever and Hasan Demirci

Received: 30 June 2023
Revised: 10 August 2023
Accepted: 10 August 2023
Published: 12 August 2023

Abstract: Bacteria resistance to antibiotics is a concerning global health problem; in this context, methicillin-resistant *Staphylococcus aureus* (MRSA) is considered as a high priority by the World Health Organization. Furthermore, patients with a positive result for COVID-19 received early antibiotic treatment, a fact that potentially encourages the increase in antibiotic resistance. Therefore, there is an urgency to develop new drugs with molecular mechanisms different from those of the actual treatments. In this context, enzymes from the shikimate pathway, a route absent in humans, such as dehydroquinate dehydratase (DHQD), are considered good targets. In this work, a computer-aided drug design strategy, which involved exhaustive virtual screening and molecular dynamics simulations with MM-PBSA analysis, as well as an in silico ADMETox characterization, was performed to find potential noncovalent inhibitors of DHQD from MRSA (SaDHQD). After filtering the 997 million compounds from the ZINC database, 6700 compounds were submitted to an exhaustive virtual screening protocol. From these data, four molecules were selected and characterized (**ZINC000005753647 (1)**, **ZINC000001720488 (2)**, **ZINC000082049768 (3)**, and **ZINC000644149506 (4)**). The results indicate that the four potential inhibitors interacted with residues important for substrate binding and catalysis, with an estimated binding free energy like that of the enzyme's substrate. Their ADMETox-predicted properties suggest that all of them support the structural characteristics to be considered good candidates. Therefore, the four compounds reported here are excellent option to be considered for future in vitro studies to design new SaDHQD noncovalent inhibitors and contribute to the search for new drugs against MRSA.

Keywords: MRSA; shikimate pathway; dehydroquinate dehydratase; virtual screening; molecular dynamics; computer-aided drug design

1. Introduction

Bacterial resistance to antibiotics is a concerning global health problem [1] that is constantly evolving, where the emergence of antibiotic resistance is an outcome of a repertoire of factors in various environmental and clinical settings that have important repercussions on the health of the population [2–4]. Furthermore, increased exposure to healthcare and invasive procedures implies expanded antibiotic use, which further increases the risk for resistant pathogens to emerge [5]. Moreover, another situation is currently taking place; reports are emerging that pose a concerning situation; the intensity with which the COVID-19 pandemic is affecting healthcare and community environments is threatening [6–8]. High volumes of patients are becoming infected over short periods of time, resulting in a spike in antimicrobial consumption. According to a review of the data on COVID-19 cases, approximately 70% of patients with a positive result of COVID-19 received early antibiotic treatment when only approximately 8% needed it [9,10], a fact that could potentially encourage the increase of antibiotic resistance.

Even though effective antibiotics are a cornerstone of modern medicine, few bacteria can be as threatening as *Staphylococcus aureus*, a pathogen considered a high priority by the World Health Organization [11,12] and implicated in skin and soft tissue infections. One of the principal challenges is the methicillin-resistant *S. aureus* (MRSA) strains, because this pathogen is resistant to most of the actual treatments, which in turn results in high rates of mortality [13]. Therefore, new treatments are required to be able to manage this increasing threat. Under this light, a fundamental metabolic pathway for bacteria's survival is the Shikimate Pathway (SK), a biosynthetic route that links carbohydrate metabolism through glycolysis and the pentose phosphate pathway, which has been considered an excellent target for antibacterial drug design, furthermore, this pathway is absent in humans [14]. This pathway consists of seven enzymatic steps that conclude with the formation of chorismate, a precursor of aromatic compounds, folates, and ubiquinone, as the final product [15,16].

One of these enzymes is 3-dehydroquinate dehydratase, which exists in two isoforms denoted as Type I and Type II. Structurally, Type I enzymes are homodimers, whilst Type II are dodecamers [17,18]. Type I 3-dehydroquinate dehydratase (DHQD) is encoded by the gene aroD and is found in fungi, plants, and bacteria, including the pathogenic *Salmonella* (*typhi* and *enterica*), *Escherichia coli*, *Clostridium difficile*, and *Staphylococcus aureus* [19–21]. DHQD catalyzes the reversible conversion of 3-dehydroquinate to 3-dehydroshikimate by a syn-elimination of water, another difference with Type II, which performs it through an Anti-elimination of water [22,23].

In addition to the biosynthetic role of DHQD, deletions in the aroD gene in *S. typhi*, *S. flexneri*, and *S. auerus* have suggested that this enzyme may act as a virulence factor [24]. In the same context, in *S. aureus*, a Small Colony Variant (SCV) phenotype was isolated. This strain supports an Ochre mutation in the aroD gene, being auxotrophic for all aromatic amino acids and less virulent than the wild type [25]. Furthermore, aroD gene mutants have been proposed as vaccines for *Francisella tularensis*, the causative agent of Tularemia [26]. Therefore, this enzyme has been considered a promising target not only for antibiotic drug design but also for the design of new antivirulence drugs [24].

In this work, a computer-aided drug design strategy, including exhaustive virtual screening, molecular dynamics, MM/PBSA analysis, and in silico ADMETox predictions, was followed to find potential noncovalent inhibitors of DHQD from methicillin-resistant *Staphylococcus aureus* (SaDHQD). The molecules reported here potentially bind to the active site of the enzyme and support the structural characteristics to be considered promising drug candidates to fight against antibacterial resistance.

2. Results and Discussion

2.1. Database Filtering and Virtual Screening

Nowadays, only a few covalent (irreversible) inhibitors of SaDHQD have been reported [27]. Noncovalent (reversible) inhibitors of DHQD have been reported only from other bacteria such as *C. difficile* and *E. faecalis* [28,29]. With the aim of obtaining the first potential noncovalent inhibitors from SaDHQD, a computer-aided drug design protocol was implemented (Figure 1). By the time the ZINC database was consulted, 997 million compounds were included in the TRANCHES 3D section. The first filtering criteria was to select structures with physicochemical characteristics similar to those of the substrate of the enzyme (3-dehydroquinate, MW = 198 Da and Log p = −1.7), therefore, compounds with a MW in the range of 200–250 Da, and a Log p value of −1 were included. Additionally, the highest reactivity clean criteria (without reactive groups) were applied, keeping only 123,000 molecules. Thereafter, Lipinski's rule of five compliance, toxicity risk assessment,

Topological Surface Area (TPSA), and rotatable bond filters were applied, leaving a final set of 6700 compounds. Nowadays, a lot of works using different virtual screening protocols to filter large chemical libraries have been published, but the challenge is always to select the best candidates for further experimental studies [30]. In this context, approximations such as consensus docking or rescoring functions have been used [31]. Here, with the aim to select molecules that potentially recognize the catalytic site of SaDHQD and to ensure that each result was consistent, three independent virtual screening assays over the same database (6700 compounds) were conducted using Autodock Vina (Table S1). It is important to mention that stereoisomers from compounds with chiral centers in their structure were included. The goal of this was to use molecular docking to find the compounds with the best binding pose according to their docking score for further computational characterization, not to perform binding free energy determinations [32]. The data show that four compounds met the requirement: **ZINC000005753647 (1)**, **ZINC000001720488 (2)**, **ZINC000082049768 (3)**, and **ZINC000644149506 (4)** (Table 1).

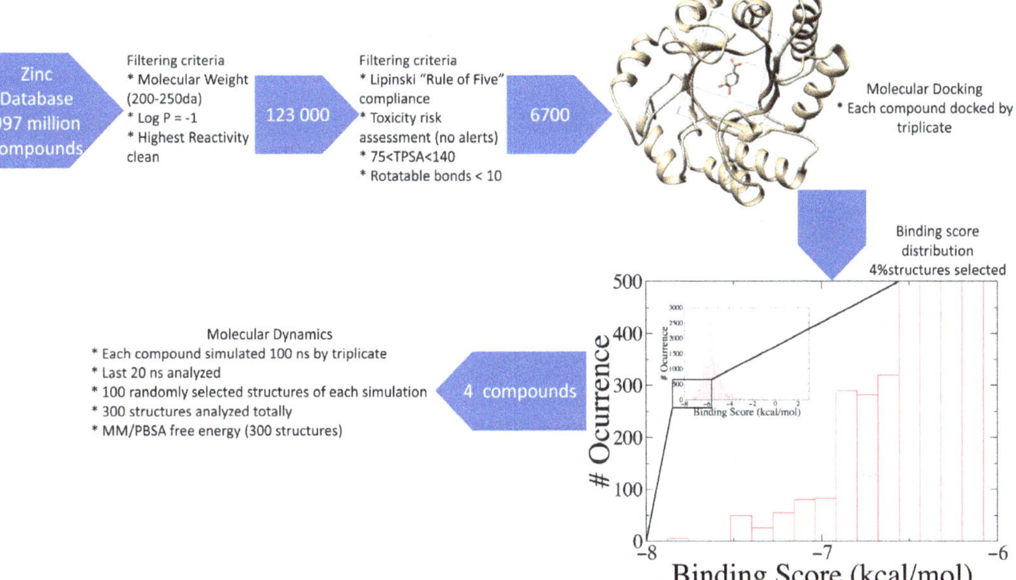

Figure 1. Workflow to obtain potential SaDHQD noncovalent inhibitors.

Table 1. Autodock Vina docking score for the best ligands.

Ligand	Docking Score (kcal/mol)	Structure
3-dehydroquinate	-6.1 ± 0.0	

Table 1. *Cont.*

Ligand	Docking Score (kcal/mol)	Structure
Compound **1**	−7.5 ± 0.0	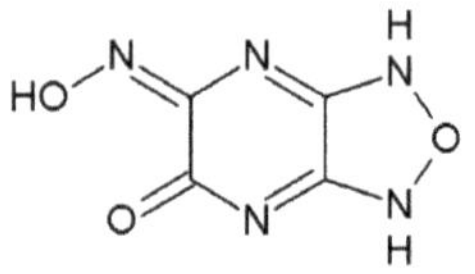
Compound **2**	−7.5 ± 0.0	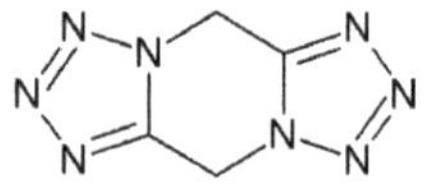
Compound **3**	−7.5 ± 0.0	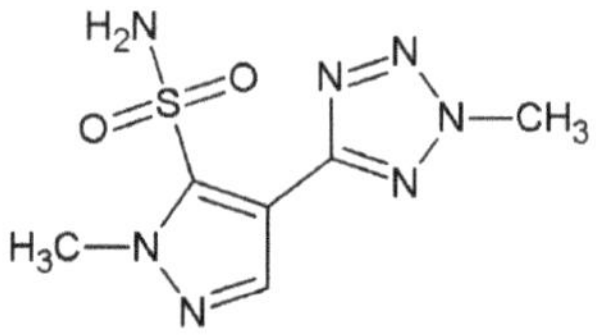
Compound **4**	−7.8 ± 0.0	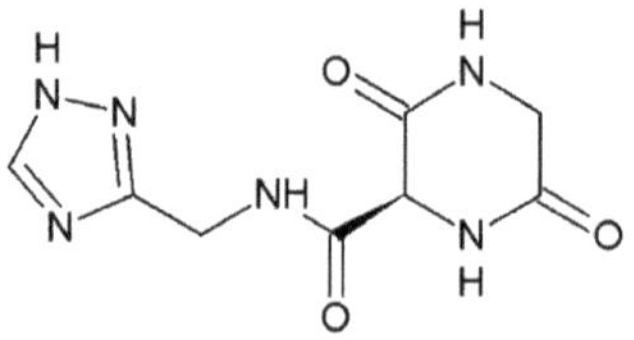

2.2. Molecular Dynamics Simulations

At this moment, we have a set of possible compounds that might bind to SaDHQD. However, those ligands were selected using molecular docking that does not include sidechain and/or protein conformational changes that may influence the ligand's binding to the enzyme [33]. To gain more information about the enzyme-ligand interaction, three independent 100 ns molecular dynamics simulations were conducted on each system, including the crystallographic ligand (3-dehydroquinate) (Figure 2). With the aim of performing the analysis on the period when the simulations were stable over time, the last 20 ns were used for the analysis of each trajectory. Results show that the α-carbon Root Mean Square Deviation (RMSD) for most of the systems simulated was stable along the last 20 ns, but there were a couple of systems where RMSD fluctuations indicate that they may not be stable or higher than the other replicas. However, fluctuations observed for those systems were lower than 3.5 Å when compared to all systems; in fact, all systems had a RMSD variation against the initial of no more than 3.5 Å (see, for example, the green line on the 3-dehydroquinate complex and compare it with the red line from compound 4 on Figure 2); therefore, those trajectories were included and analyzed.

The same situation was observed when the position of the ligands along the simulations was analyzed. In this case, 3-dehydroquinate shows the highest variations, followed by compounds **3** and **4**. However, the variations were so small that it can be said that all the ligands kept their binding sites. In fact, when ligand movement is observed in the binding site, complexes corresponding to substrate and compounds **3** and **4** show more variations (Figure 3).

On the other hand, no important changes were observed in Root Mean Square Fluctuations (RMSF) plots, which are used to explore the flexibility of each residue during simulations [34]. Therefore, the binding of the potential inhibitors did not provoke substantial alterations in the lateral chains of amino acids (Figure 4).

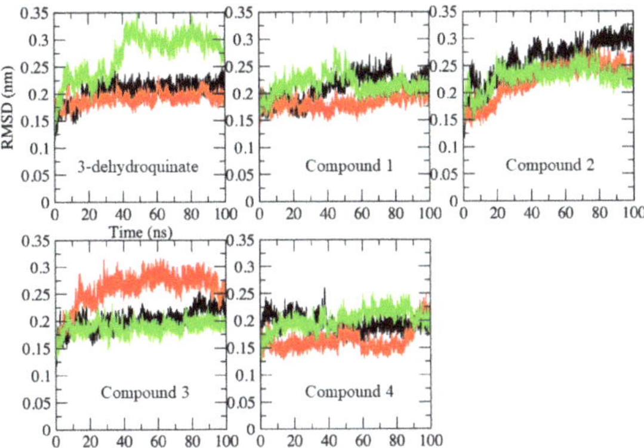

Figure 2. Alpha carbon-RMSD along the 100 ns of simulated time in each complex. Replicates are shown in different colors (black, replicate 1; red, replicate 2; and green, replicate 3). Axis labels are shown only on the first graph to avoid confusion.

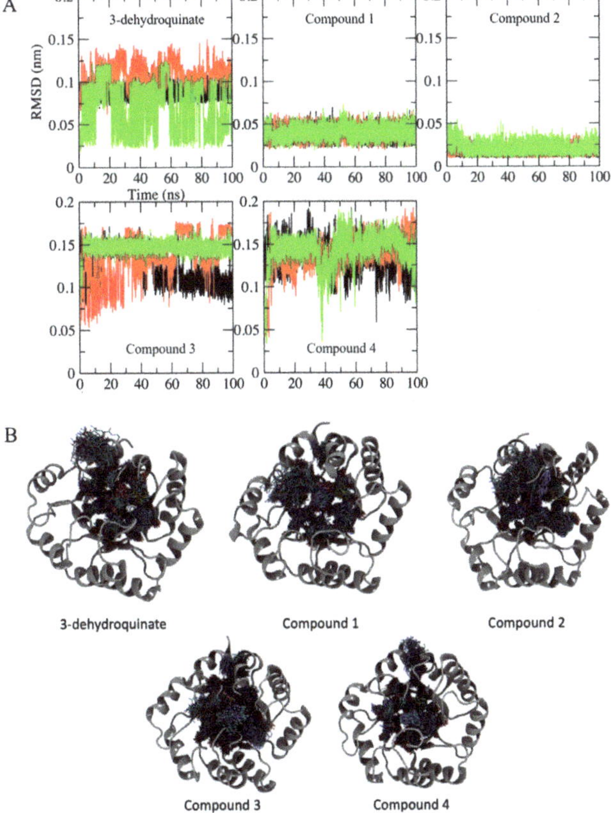

Figure 3. Ligand-RMSD. (**A**) RMSD along the 100 ns of simulated time in each complex. Replicates and axes labels are shown as described in Figure 2. (**B**) Ligand movement (brighter atoms at the center of each image) on the binding site (darker atoms on each image) in SaDHQD during the last 20 ns. The image also shows the movement of the lateral chains from the amino acids in the binding site.

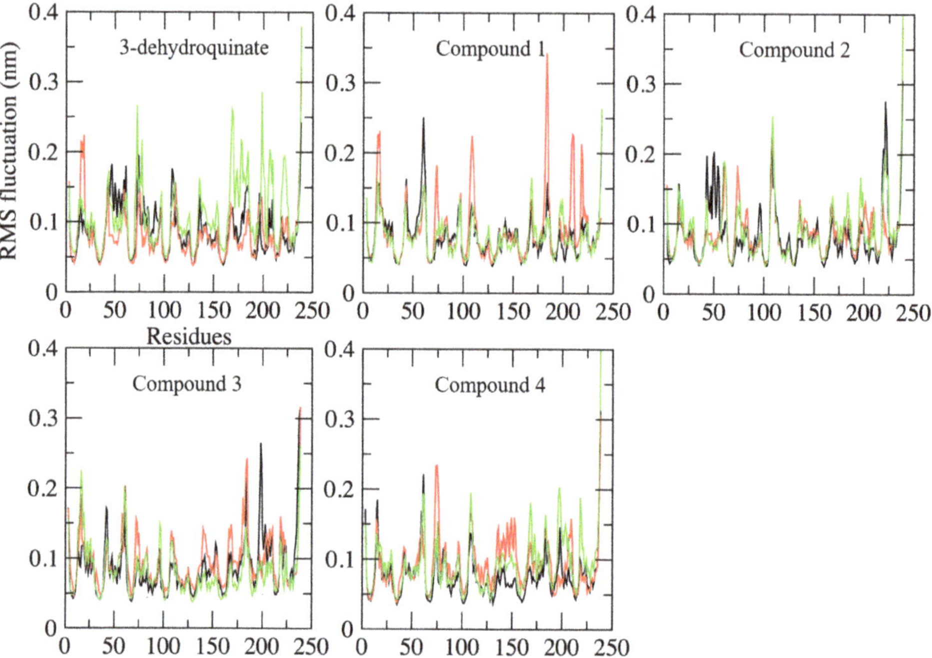

Figure 4. Root mean square fluctuation along the 100 ns of simulated time in each complex. Replicates and axes labels are shown as described in Figure 2.

This is in consonance with data obtained from Radius of Gyration (RoG) plots. RoG is a quantity that can be related to the natural protein "breathing". A high value of RoG might be an indication of a possible denaturation of the protein; the opposite might be related to a compaction of the protein. Initial RoG was 1.72 ± 0.003 nm. RoG values over time show fluctuations with increments above 1.8 nm. These fluctuations might indicate that the protein had an opening that can be related to the natural movement of the amino or carboxyl terminal. However, RoG distributions show that (even in the worst case: 3-dehydroquinate simulation in green), these values are located around 1.76 and 1.77 nm. These values show an increment of 0.4 Å when compared to the initial value. Therefore, no effect was observed in the compactness of the protein structure, i.e., the binding of the compounds did not generate a crucial conformational change (Figure 5).

In respect to hydrogen bond formation, as was expected, none of the compounds made as many hydrogen bonds as the substrate (Figure 6). This is the logic: when the structure of the potential inhibitors is analyzed, the number of hydrogen bond donors or acceptors is limited, contrary to what is observed in the substrate. Therefore, the binding of these compounds was governed (as shown later) by Van der Waals interactions, which are the most common type of interactions and influence the stability of the complex [35].

According to a representative structure of the most populated cluster obtained from clustering the last 20 ns of each replicate, compound **1** made a hydrogen bond with Glu35, whilst compound **2** did not make any interaction. Compound **3** made hydrogen bonds with Pro223 and Gln225, and compound **4** formed the same type of interaction with Glu35, Arg37, Arg70, His133, Lys160, and Gln225. Some of these interactions were shared by the substrate, such as Glu35, Lys160, and Gln225, additionally, a hydrogen bond with Arg37 and Arg202 was established by the substrate (Figure 7). Therefore, it can be said that compounds **1**, **3**, and **4** were able to make some of the same interactions as the substrate.

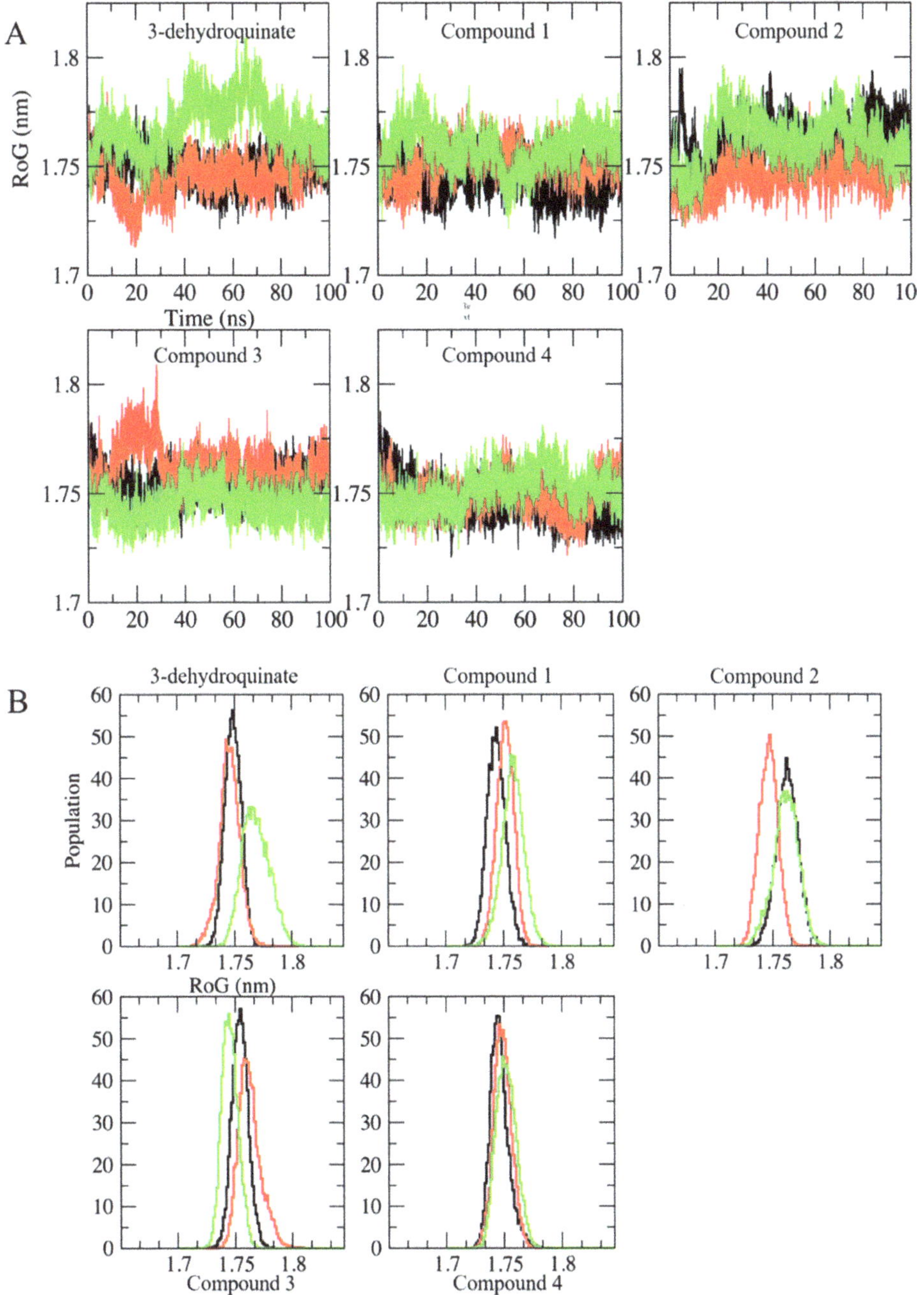

Figure 5. Radius of gyration along the 100 ns of simulated time in each complex. Replicates and axes labels are shown as described in Figure 2. (**A**) RoG of the systems herein simulated along 100 ns. (**B**) Normalized distribution of the RoG for all the systems.

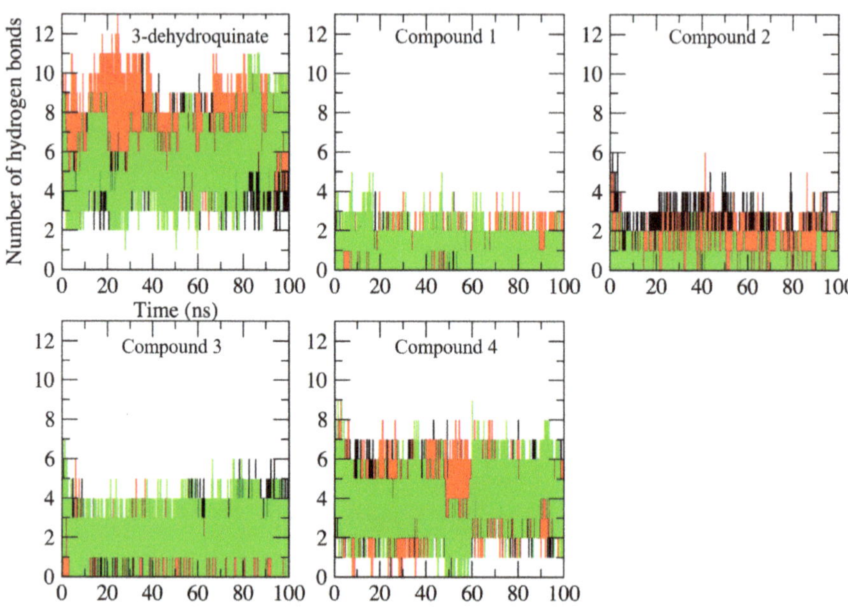

Figure 6. Number of hydrogen bonds formed along the 100 ns of simulated time in each complex. Replicates and axes labels are shown as described in Figure 2.

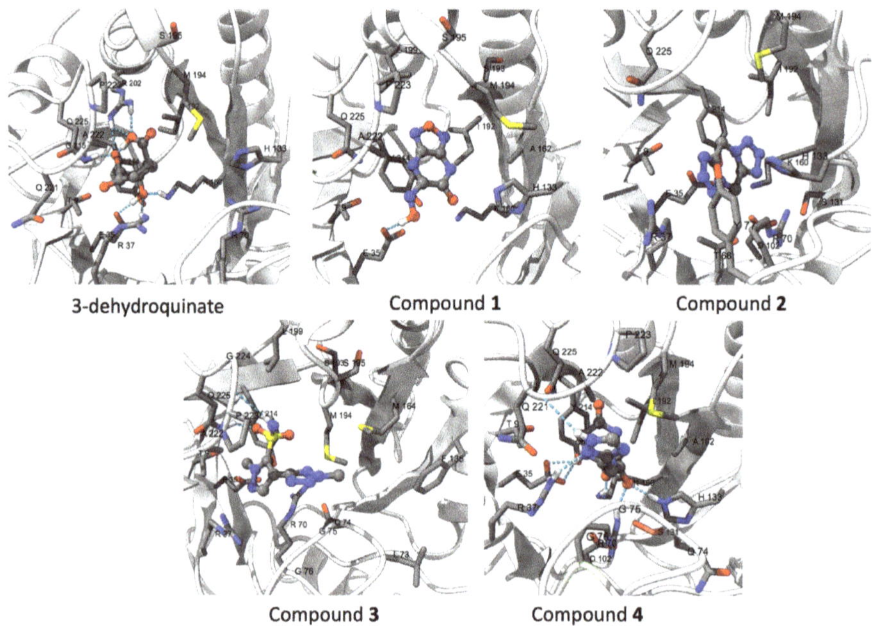

Figure 7. 3D interaction map of each complex; the image shows a representative structure. Residues in the binding site were Thr9, Glu35, Arg37, Thr68, Arg70, Asp102, Ser131, His133, Lys160, Ala162, Ile192, Met194, Arg202, Tyr214, Gln221, Ala22, and Gln225 (thin lines). Ligands are on thicker lines at the center of each image. Hydrogen bonds are depicted as blue dashed lines.

2.3. Binding Free and Interaction Energies

To study the stability of each complex, binding free energy was calculated using the MM/PBSA approximation. MM/PBSA is a computational way to estimate relative binding affinities at a reduced computational cost that could be used to obtain a qualitative ranking of the compounds tested [36–40]. Even when there are more robust ways to calculate these affinities, such as free energy perturbation [41] or thermodynamic integration [42,43], those methodologies are very time- and resource-consuming. Herein, we used the MM/PBSA method, performing three independent replicas (100 ns) for each complex obtained from the molecular docking screening (also realized in triplicate). Clustering analysis was used to choose 100 random structures from each system, concatenate them, and treat them as a single system (300 structures) using GMXPBSA 2.1 scripts. The energy calculations suggest that the complex with 3-dehydroquinate was stabilized by polar contributions (solvation energy terms), whilst in the case of the four potential inhibitors, their complexes were stabilized through apolar contributions (nonsolvation energy terms) (Table 2). These agree with ligand structure; substrate (3-dehydroquinate) has three alcohols and a carboxyl group that allow it to be an acceptor or donor of hydrogen bonds. On the other hand, compound **1** has only one hydroxyl and one carbonyl group, while compound **2** has no hydrogen donor atoms and, as can be seen in Figure 3, has basically hydrophobic interactions with SaDHQD. Compound **3** possesses a hydrogen bond donor and acceptor atom; however, its binding was dominated by apolar contributions. Finally, compound **4** has three carbonyl groups and a 1, 2, 4-triazole ring that might be acting as hydrogen bond acceptors, but like in the other inhibitors, the hydrophobic interactions were the principal component (Figure 3 and Table 2).

Table 2. Binding free energy from potential SaDHQD inhibitors.

Ligand	Total (kcal/mol)	Polar Contribution	Apolar Contribution
3-dehydroquinate	0.00 ± 0.00	0.00 ± 0.00	0.00 ± 0.00
Compound 1	86.88 ± 8.96	219.17 ± 7.68	−132.29 ± 4.61
Compound 2	68.67 ± 9.39	218.77 ± 8.51	−150.10 ± 4.04
Compound 3	29.08 ± 9.33	237.14 ± 8.41	−208.06 ± 4.09
Compound 4	4.80 ± 8.90	172.73 ± 7.85	−168.03 ± 4.15

Note: Compound binding energies were referenced with respect to substrate binding energies. Positive energy values in compounds mean that the substrate has a higher value (more negative) than the respective compound. On the other hand, a negative energy value means that compounds have a higher value than the substrate.

To gain more information about the interactions made between the compounds and the protein through dynamic simulations, interaction energy was estimated for each residue at the binding site. The same 300 frames used for the binding free energy were used to calculate the interaction energy between the corresponding amino acid and compound (Figure 8, Table S2). Additionally, interactions with more than 50% appearance along the simulation time were considered for the analysis (Table 3). As can be observed, the interactions with Arg70, Lys160, Met194, and Ala222 were the only ones shared among potential inhibitors and the substrate crystallographic complex even with the 3-dehydroquinate complex simulated, having additionally high percentages of appearance [19]. The above highlights the importance of these residues as hot spots to interact with the enzyme. Furthermore, from an energetic point of view, compound **4** shows the highest interaction energies at residue level and the highest total interaction energy among the four potential inhibitors. It is important to mention that the total interaction energy includes not only the residues shown in Table 3, but also considers interactions with residues that have less than 50% appearance.

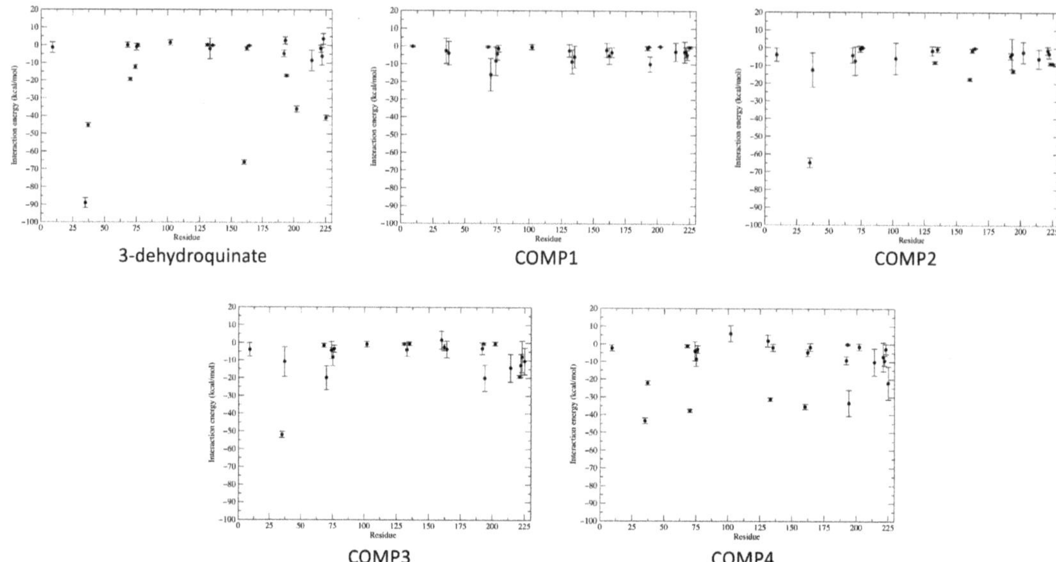

Figure 8. Interaction energy (kcal/mol) between the substrate and each potential inhibitor with residues at 5 Å in the binding site. The residue number and interaction energy values are shown in x and y-axes, respectively. Each point indicates the mean ± SD.

Table 3. Protein/ligand interaction energy over structures used for MM/PBSA analysis.

	3-dehydroquinate	Compound 1	Compound 2	Compound 3	Compound 4
THR9 *	−1.35 ± 2.96 (88.67)		−3.97 ± 3.75 (65.33)	−3.93 ± 3.77 (89.33)	−2.28 ± 1.71 (73.67)
GLU35 *	−89.04 ± 48.34 (88.67)		64.91 ± 47.03 (67.00)	−52.03 ± 29.74 (88.33)	−43.42 ± 27.92 (85.67)
ARG37 *	−45.26 ± 21.24 (88.67)		−12.50 ± 9.63 (67.00)	−10.91 ± 8.45 (89.33)	−22.15 ± 21.41 (72.67)
THR68 *	0.08 ± 1.48 (52.67)		−4.34 ± 4.27 (63.00)		
ARG70 *	−19.21 ± 16.73 (71.67)	−16.05 ± 9.22 (89.33)	−7.47 ± 8.01 (74.33)	−19.87 ± 6.70 (89.33)	−37.71 ± 15.75 (86.00)
GLN74		−8.36 ± 8.11 (86.67)		−4.28 ± 4.86 (59.00)	−3.99 ± 5.35 (59.33)
GLY75		−4.38 ± 3.40 (83.67)		−8.05 ± 5.10 (89.33)	−8.45 ± 4.22 (85.67)
GLY76				−3.42 ± 2.00 (86.33)	−2.98 ± 2.13 (67.33)
ASP102 *			−6.03 ± 8.87 (57.00)		5.97 ± 4.50 (57.67)
SER131 *					1.93 ± 3.36 (78.33)
HIS133 *		−8.65 ± 6.69 (97.33)		−3.83 ± 3.84 (61.67)	−31.24 ± 16.88 (86.00)
PHE135		−5.86 ± 6.24 (70.00)			−1.90 ± 2.03 (62.33)
LYS160 *	−65.90 ± 21.63 (88.67)	−2.07 ± 3.98 (58.67)	−17.53 ± 14.40 (68.67)	1.60 ± 5.04 (62.67)	−35.25 ± 25.62 (86.00)
ALA162 *	−1.81 ± 1.02 (67.00)	−5.34 ± 4.63 (80.00)		−2.42 ± 1.81 (58.33)	−4.63 ± 1.99 (86.00)
MET164		−3.36 ± 2.73 (63.00)			
ILE192 *	−4.65 ± 1.96 (88.00)		−4.46 ± 1.73 (83.00)		−9.06 ± 2.36 (86.00)
SER193	2.73 ± 2.05 (59.33)				
MET194 *	−16.97 ± 10.48 (87.33)	−9.89 ± 4.22 (98.67)	−12.99 ± 13.97 (91.33)	−19.99 ± 7.40 (89.33)	−33.32 ± 7.31 (86.00)
ARG202 *	−35.99 ± 29.86 (76.00)				
TYR214 *	−8.48 ± 5.76 (88.33)		−6.06 ± 5.32 (91.67)	−14.17 ± 7.95 (89.33)	−10.07 ± 7.73 (86.00)
GLN221 *				−19.07 ± 13.41 (73.67)	−7.14 ± 8.21 (55.33)
ALA222 *	−6.12 ± 4.98 (60.67)	−3.28 ± 2.88 (61.33)	−3.12 ± 2.48 (56.67)	−12.81 ± 6.59 (86.67)	−9.28 ± 2.89 (86.00)
PRO223	3.71 ± 3.00 (55.67)	−4.76 ± 2.70 (83.33)			−2.74 ± 2.81 (83.33)
GLN225 *	−40.92 ± 27.09 (72.67)		−8.89 ± 11.19 (72.67)	−10.35 ± 7.63 (89.33)	−22.02 ± 9.30 (86.00)
Total interaction energy	−345.01 ± 12.26	−90.67 ± 22.37	−181.24 ± 21.01	−202.39 ± 23.87	−284.03 ± 19.98

Note: Protein/ligand interaction energy was calculated from any atom of the ligand to any residue of the protein within a 5 Å radius. Only interactions with more than 50% appearance are shown (number in parenthesis). Residues identified in the crystallographic complex are highlighted (*).

2.4. ADMETox Properties

Finally, an important point in the first steps of the drug design process is to predict the drug-like characteristics of the potential inhibitors. In this context, the ADMETox properties of each compound were analyzed through an in silico approach (Table S3). This analysis was performed considering additional properties to those taken for initial filtering; these included Pharmacokinetics, Druglikeness, and Medicinal Chemistry characteristics. In respect to Pharmacokinetics, compounds **1** and **4** show low GI absorption, whilst in Druglikeness, the best evaluated were compounds **3** and **4** with only one violation of Ghose rules. On the other hand, predictions classified in Medicinal Chemistry are interesting because they involve aspects such as Pan-assay interference compounds (PAINS) and Brenk alerts that analyze the presence of undesirable substructures; synthetic accessibility, a characteristic that becomes important if the molecules reach the lead optimization step; Blood Brain Barrier penetration (BBB); and CYP450 inhibition, among others. From the fifteen characteristics evaluated, none of the compounds received a positive score in all of them; however, the four potential inhibitors approved the majority, highlighting PAINS alerts, synthetic accessibility, BBB, and Pgp inhibition (Table 4). Therefore, considering all the predictions performed, in general, the four compounds meet the commitments to be considered good candidates.

Table 4. The most relevant ADMETox predicted properties from the SaDHQD potential inhibitors.

Parameter	Compound 1	Compound 2	Compound 3	Compound 4
		Pharmacokinetics		
GI absortion	Low	High	High	Low
Log K_p (Skin permeation)	−7.36 cm/s	−8.33 cm/s	−8.27 cm/s	−8.90 cm/s
		Druglikeness		
Ghose	No; 2 violations: WLOGP < −0.4, #atoms < 20	No; 3 violations: WLOGP < −0.4, MR < 40, #atoms < 20	No; 1 violation: WLOGP < −0.4	No; 1 violation: WLOGP < −0.4
Veber	Yes	Yes	Yes	Yes
Egan	Yes	Yes	Yes	Yes
Muegge	No; 2 violations: MW < 200, #C < 5	No; 2 violations: MW < 200, #C < 5	Yes	Yes
Bioavailability score	0.55	0.55	0.55	0.55
		Medicinal chemistry		
PAINS	0 alert	0 alert	0 alert	0 alert
Brenk	3 alerts: imine_1, oxime_1, oxygen-nitrogen_single_bond	0 alert	0 alert	1 alert: beta_keto_anhydride
Leadlikeness	No; 1 violation: MW < 250	No; 1 violation: MW < 250	No; 1 violation: MW < 250	No; 1 violation: MW < 250
Synthetic accesibility	3.60	2.42	2.78	2.61
BBB	0.31	0.08	0.05	0.05
In vitro Caco2 cell permeability	3.94	0.73	1.28	6.54
In vitro CYP 2C19 inhibition	Inhibitor	Inhibitor	Non	Inhibitor
In vitro CYP 2C9 inhibition	Non	Non	Non	Non
In vitro CYP 2D6 inhibition	Non	Non	Non	Non
In vitro CYP 2D6 substrate	Non	Non	Non	Non
In vitro CYP 3A4 inhibition	Non	Non	Non	Inhibitor
In vitro CYP 3A4 substrate	Weakly	Non	Substrate	Non
HIA	40.23	70.25	70.86	27.24
MDCK	1.42	0.72	0.60	0.59
Pgp inhibition	Non	Non	Non	Non
Plasma Protein Binding	2.68	14.37	60.17	5.91

Note: All values were calculated with the SwissADME web tool and PreADMET server. Skin Permeability: in vitro skin permeability-transdermal delivery (logKp, cm/h), Ghose, Veber, Egan, and Muegge (Filters that determine the druglikeness of a compound: no violations are considered ideal). Bioavailability score: it predicts the probability of a compound having at least 10% oral bioavailability in rats, Number of Brenk alerts and PAINS alerts (number of alerts for undesirable substructures/substructures; a result with no alerts is ideal). Leadlikeness: molecules are evaluated according to three parameters: ≤250 MW ≤350, XLOGP ≤3.5, and number of rotatable bonds ≤7; there should be no violations; Synthetic accessibility: refers to the ease of chemical synthesis from 1 (very easy) to 10 (very difficult). BBB: in vivo blood-brain barrier penetration (C.brain/C.blood); Caco2: in vitro Caco−2 cell permeability (nm/s); values > 500 nm s^{-1} indicate a good permeability, and values < 25 nm s^{-1} indicate a low permeability; CYP 2C19 inhibition: in vitro Cytochrome P450 2C19 inhibition; CYP 2C9 inhibition: in vitro Cytochrome P450 2C9 inhibition; CYP 2D6 inhibition: in vitro Cytochrome P450 2D6 inhibition; CYP 2D6 substrate: in vitro Cytochrome P450 2D6 substrate; CYP 3A4 inhibition: in vitro Cytochrome P450 3A4 inhibition; CYP 3A4 substrate: in vitro Cytochrome P450 3A4 substrate; HIA: Human intestinal absorption (HIA, %); a high intestinal abortion percentage is desirable, as indicated by values closest to 100%; MDCK: in vitro MDCK (Mandin Darby Canine Kidney) cell permeability (nm/s), values > 500 nm s^{-1} indicate a good permeability, and values < 25 nm s^{-1} indicate a low permeability; Pgp inhibition: in vitro P-glycoprotein inhibition; Plasma Protein Binding: in vitro plasma protein binding (%); a value of >90% is desirable.

3. Materials and Methods

3.1. Compound Selection and Filtering

Compound selection was performed from the TRANCHES 3D collection in the ZINC15 database (https://zinc15.docking.org/ accessed on 30 September 2020) [44], which consisted of over 997 million compounds by the time the database was consulted. From this library, compounds with a molecular weight up to 250 Da and a Log p value of -1 considering 3-dehydroquinate properties (MW = 198 Da and Log p = -1.7), as well as structures without reactive groups (highest reactivity clean), were selected; this process resulted in a database of 123,000 compounds. Thereafter, additional filtering criteria including physicochemical characteristics in accordance with the Lipinski rule of five, compounds with predicted toxicological parameters (mutagenicity, reproductive, tumorigenic, and irritant effects) were eliminated, structural aspects (such as the number of rotatable bonds <5, number of aromatic rings <4, a polar surface area >75 and <140), and an adequate "druglike" value (-2 to 5) that indicates the potential that a certain compound had in order to become a drug, were applied using Data Warrior V.5.2.1 software (http://www.openmolecules.org/datawarrior/) [45]. Finally, 6700 compounds were selected for the virtual screening process.

3.2. Exhaustive Virtual Screening

To perform the virtual screening, the SaDHQD crystal structure (PDBID: 1SFJ, chain A) was used as a receptor [19]. The structure was prepared by removing the crystallographic ligand 3-dehydroquinate, and energy was minimized with 100 steps using the steepest descent method and 10 steps using conjugate gradient as implemented in Chimera UCSF [46]. Compounds were processed with Openbabel 3.1.1 [47] to convert the SDF library to individual pdb files, and then each pdb file was converted to a pdbqt file using prepare_ligand4.py as distributed on MGLTools 1.5.7 [48]. Molecular docking was performed using Autodock Vina [49]. The crystallographic ligand was used as the center of the grid box (104.40, -17.89, -107.70) with a size of $15 \times 15 \times 15$ Å^3. To validate docking results, a crystallographic ligand was redocked, obtaining an RMSD value of 2.35 ± 0.00 Å. To consider a correct molecular docking study, the RMSD between the crystallographic and the redocked ligand must be lower than 2 Å. Our study had a higher RMSD value, but it is important to point out that we are not doing covalent docking, which is the case for 3-dehydroquinate. Nonetheless, the number and type of interactions found on the crystal and the redocked ligand remain at 82%. Only three interactions were missing on the redocked 3-dehydroquinate (Thr68, Asp102, and Ser131). Three independent docking experiments were made on each ligand (6700×3), and all outputs were clustered by binding score. Ligands with a binding score lower than the average minus two standard deviations (4% of the normal distribution) were selected for molecular dynamics simulations (Figure 1).

3.3. Exhaustive Molecular Dynamics Simulations

Complexes generated on Autodock Vina for each compound and the crystallographic ligand 3-dehydroquinate were used to perform molecular dynamics simulations using GROMACS 2019 [50,51]. To this end, ligand parameters were obtained from the Automated Topology Builder and Repository (ATB) [52]. Each system was immersed in an orthorhombic cell with SPC water molecules and 0.15 M NaCl to neutralize. Every system was energy minimized with 1000 steepest descent steps, followed by 50,000 steps of molecular dynamics on the NVT and NPT ensembles to equilibrate the system. Finally, 100 ns molecular dynamics simulations were performed using a 2 fs timestep, periodic boundary conditions (PBC), Particle Mesh Ewald (PME) for electrostatics, velocity rescale temperature coupling, and Parrinello–Rahman (NPT ensemble) for pressure coupling. Molecular dynamics simulations were carried out in triplicate for a total of 15 systems (1.5 µs total simulation time). The last 20 ns of every system (2000 frames) were used for clustering structures using α-carbons with the gromacs gmx cluster utility. Clustering was made using a cutoff of 1.25 Å with the GROMOS method [53], which allowed that at least 50% of the structures were clustered on the first cluster.

3.4. Binding Free Energy

Additionally, binding free interaction energies of 300 random structures (100 structures of each replica) of the most populated cluster (for every replica) were calculated using the Molecular Mechanics/Poisson-Boltzmann Accessible Area (MM-PBSA) approximation [36,37,54]. MM-PBSA binding-free energies were calculated using GMXPBSA 2.1 scripts [55]. Binding free energy was obtained from the equation:

$$\Delta G_{binding} = G_{complex} - \left(G_{protein\ in\ complex} + G_{ligand\ in\ complex} \right)$$

Each free energy value was calculated as follows:

$$< G > = E_{MM} + G_{SOLV} - T < S_{MM} >$$

Entropy was not calculated; therefore, binding free energies reported are the enthalpic contribution to the total binding free energy.

3.5. ADMETox Properties

ADMETox properties prediction (Absorption, Distribution, Metabolism, Excretion, and Toxicity) of the selected compounds was carried out using the SwissADME [56] and PREADMET online servers [57] (Bioinformatics and Molecular Design Research Center; 2004). Different parameters, including gastrointestinal absorption, permeability of the blood-brain barrier, potential substrate or inhibitor of G-glycoprotein, inhibitor of the cytochrome family, and artificial synthesis accessibility, were estimated.

4. Conclusions

In the present work, a computer-aided drug design strategy was applied to report potential noncovalent SaDHQD inhibitors. After an exhaustive virtual screening protocol, four compounds were selected and characterized (**ZINC000005753647 (1)**, **ZINC000001720488 (2)**, **ZINC000082049768 (3)**, and **ZINC000644149506 (4)**). Clustering molecular dynamics show that these molecules were able, potentially, to interact with residues important for substrate binding and catalysis when compared to the crystallographic ligand. The interaction energy calculation for each residue in the binding site helped to detect hotspots for potential enzyme inhibition. Finally, the ADMETox properties prediction suggests that these compounds can be considered good candidates. Therefore, the four compounds reported here are excellent options to be considered for future in vitro studies to design new SaDHQD noncovalent inhibitors and contribute to the search for new drugs against MRSA.

Supplementary Materials: The following supporting information can be downloaded at: https://www.mdpi.com/article/10.3390/ph16081148/s1, Table S1: Molecular docking scores from the three independent runs: Excell_datasheet; Table S2: Interaction energy (kcal/mol) between ligands and those residues at 5 Å. Table S3: ADMETox predicted properties from the SaDHQD potential inhibitors.

Author Contributions: Conceptualization, A.T.-V. and C.A.-D.; methodology, C.M.-P., L.R.-S., N.C.-R., A.T.-V. and C.A.-D.; formal analysis, C.M.-P., L.R.-S., N.C.-R., M.V.-S. and E.S.-C.; writing—original draft preparation, C.M.-P. and L.R.-S.; writing—review and editing, A.T.-V. and C.A.-D. All authors have read and agreed to the published version of the manuscript.

Funding: This research received no external funding.

Institutional Review Board Statement: Not applicable.

Informed Consent Statement: Not applicable.

Data Availability Statement: Not applicable.

Acknowledgments: The authors acknowledge the Laboratorio de Quimioinformática y Diseño de Fármacos, CIDC, UAEM, for providing partial computational time to complete this work.

Conflicts of Interest: The authors declare no conflict of interest.

References

1. O'Neill, J. Tackling Drug-Resistant Infections Globally: Final Report and Recommendations, Government of the United Kingdom. Available online: https://apo.org.au/node/63983 (accessed on 23 December 2021).
2. Pärnänen, K.M.M.; Narciso-da-Rocha, C.; Kneis, D.; Berendonk, T.U.; Cacace, D.; Do, T.T.; Elpers, C.; Fatta-Kassinos, D.; Henriques, I.; Jaeger, T.; et al. Antibiotic resistance in European wastewater treatment plants mirrors the pattern of clinical antibiotic resistance prevalence. *Sci. Adv.* **2019**, *5*, eaau9124. [CrossRef] [PubMed]
3. Prestinaci, F.; Pezzotti, P.; Pantosti, A. Antimicrobial resistance: A global multifaceted phenomenon. *Pathog. Glob. Health* **2015**, *109*, 309–318. [CrossRef] [PubMed]
4. Frost, I.; Van Boeckel, T.P.; Pires, J.; Craig, J.; Laxminarayan, R. Global geographic trends in antimicrobial resistance: The role of international travel. *J. Travel. Med.* **2019**, *26*, taz036. [CrossRef]
5. Abushaheen, M.A.; Muzaheed; Fatani, A.J.; Alosaimi, M.; Mansy, W.; George, M.; Acharya, S.; Rathod, S.; Divakar, D.D.; Jhugroo, C.; et al. Antimicrobial resistance, mechanisms and its clinical significance. *Dis. Mon.* **2020**, *66*, 100971. [CrossRef]
6. Adebisi, Y.A.; Alaran, A.J.; Okereke, M.; Oke, G.I.; Amos, O.A.; Olaoye, O.C.; Oladunjoye, I.; Olanrewaju, A.Y.; Ukor, N.A.; Lucero-Prisno, D.E., 3rd. COVID-19 and Antimicrobial Resistance: A Review. *Infect. Dis.* **2021**, *14*, 11786337211033870. [CrossRef]
7. Ghosh, S.; Bornman, C.; Zafer, M.M. Antimicrobial Resistance Threats in the emerging COVID-19 pandemic: Where do we stand? *J. Infect. Public Health* **2021**, *14*, 555–560. [CrossRef] [PubMed]
8. Founou, R.C.; Blocker, A.J.; Noubom, M.; Tsayem, C.; Choukem, S.P.; Van Dongen, M.; Founou, L.L. The COVID-19 pandemic: A threat to antimicrobial resistance containment. *Future Sci. OA* **2021**, *7*, FSO736. [CrossRef] [PubMed]
9. Rawson, T.M.; Moore, L.S.P.; Zhu, N.; Ranganathan, N.; Skolimowska, K.; Gilchrist, M.; Satta, G.; Cooke, G.; Holmes, A. Bacterial and Fungal Coinfection in Individuals with Coronavirus: A Rapid Review to Support COVID-19 Antimicrobial Prescribing. *Clin. Infect. Dis.* **2020**, *71*, 2459–2468. [CrossRef] [PubMed]
10. Clancy, C.J.; Nguyen, M.H. Coronavirus Disease 2019, Superinfections, and Antimicrobial Development: What Can We Expect? *Clin. Infect. Dis.* **2020**, *71*, 2736–2743. [CrossRef] [PubMed]
11. WHO. Media Centre. News Release. WHO Publishes List of Bacteria for which New Anti-Biotics are Urgently Needed. Available online: http://www.who.int/mediacentre/news/releases/2017/bacteria-antibiotics-needed/en/ (accessed on 25 June 2022).
12. Tacconelli, E.; Carrara, E.; Savoldi, A.; Harbarth, S.; Mendelson, M.; Monnet, D.L.; Pulcini, S.; Kahlmeter, G.; Kluytmans, J.; Carmeli, Y.; et al. Discovery, research, and development of new antibiotics: The WHO priority list of antibiotic-resistant bacteria and tuberculosis. *Lancet Infect. Dis.* **2018**, *18*, 318–327. [CrossRef] [PubMed]
13. Nandhini, P.; Kumar, P.; Mickymaray, S.; Alothaim, A.S.; Somasundaram, J.; Rajan, M. Recent Developments in Methicillin-Resistant *Staphylococcus aureus* (MRSA) Treatment: A Review. *Antibiotics* **2022**, *11*, 606. [CrossRef] [PubMed]
14. Bentley, R. The shikimate pathway a metabolic tree with many branches. *Crit. Rev. Biochem. Mol. Biol.* **1990**, *25*, 307–384. [CrossRef] [PubMed]
15. Nunes, J.A.; Duque, M.A.; De Freitas, T.F.; Galina, L.; Timmers, L.F.S.M.; Bizarro, C.V.; Machado, P.; Basso, L.A.; Ducati, R.G. *Mycobacterium tuberculosis* Shikimate Pathway Enzymes as Targets for the Rational Design of Anti-Tuberculosis Drugs. *Molecules* **2020**, *25*, 1259. [CrossRef] [PubMed]
16. Ducati, R.G.; Basso, L.A.; Santos, D.S. Mycobacterial shikimate pathway enzymes as targets for drug design. *Curr. Drug Targets* **2007**, *8*, 423–435. [CrossRef] [PubMed]
17. Roszak, A.W.; Robinson, D.A.; Krell, T.; Hunter, I.S.; Fredrickson, M.; Abell, C.; Coggins, J.R.; Lapthorn, A.J. The structure and mechanism of the type II dehydroquinase from *Streptomyces coelicolor*. *Structure* **2002**, *10*, 493–503. [CrossRef] [PubMed]
18. Liu, C.; Liu, Y.M.; Sun, Q.L.; Jiang, C.Y.; Liu, S.J. Unraveling the kinetic diversity of microbial 3-dehydroquinate dehydratases of shikimate pathway. *AMB Express* **2015**, *5*, 7. [CrossRef] [PubMed]
19. Nichols, C.E.; Lockyer, M.; Hawkins, A.R.; Stammers, D.K. Crystal structures of *Staphylococcus aureus* type I dehydroquinase from enzyme turnover experiments. *Proteins* **2004**, *56*, 625–628. [CrossRef] [PubMed]
20. Light, S.H.; Minasov, G.; Shuvalova, L.; Duban, M.E.; Caffrey, M.; Anderson, W.F.; Lavie, A. Insights into the mechanism of type I dehydroquinate dehydratases from structures of reaction intermediates. *J. Biol. Chem.* **2015**, *290*, 19008. [CrossRef] [PubMed]
21. Lee, W.H.; Perles, L.A.; Nagem, R.A.; Shrive, A.K.; Hawkins, A.; Sawyer, L.; Polikarpov, I. Comparison of different crystal forms of 3-dehydroquinase from *Salmonella typhi* and its implication for the enzyme activity. *Acta Crystallogr. D Biol. Crystallogr.* **2002**, *58*, 798–804. [CrossRef] [PubMed]
22. Hanson, K.R.; Rose, I.A. The absolute stereochemical course of citric acid biosynthesis. *Proc. Natl. Acad. Sci. USA* **1963**, *50*, 981–988. [CrossRef] [PubMed]
23. Shneier, A.; Kleanthous, C.; Deka, R.; Coggins, J.R.; Abell, C. Observation of an imine intermediate on dehydroquinase by electrospray mass spectrometry. *J. Am. Chem. Soc.* **1991**, *113*, 9416–9418. [CrossRef]

24. González-Bello, C.; Tizón, L.; Lence, E.; Otero, J.M.; van Raaij, M.J.; Martinez-Guitian, M.; Beceiro, A.; Thompson, P.; Hawkins, A.R. Chemical Modification of a Dehydratase Enzyme Involved in Bacterial Virulence by an Ammonium Derivative: Evidence of its Active Site Covalent Adduct. *J. Am. Chem. Soc.* **2015**, *137*, 9333–9343. [CrossRef] [PubMed]
25. Zhang, P.; Wright, J.A.; Osman, A.A.; Nair, S.P. An aroD Ochre Mutation Results in a *Staphylococcus aureus* Small Colony Variant That Can Undergo Phenotypic Switching via Two Alternative Mechanisms. *Front. Microbiol.* **2017**, *8*, 1001. [CrossRef] [PubMed]
26. Cunningham, A.L.; Mann, B.J.; Qin, A.; Santiago, A.E.; Grassel, C.; Lipsky, M.; Vogel, S.N.; Barry, E.M. Characterization of Schu S4 aro mutants as live attenuated tularemia vaccine candidates. *Virulence* **2020**, *11*, 283–294. [CrossRef]
27. González-Bello, C.; Harris, J.M.; Manthey, M.K.; Coggins, J.R.; Abell, C. Irreversible inhibition of type I dehydroquinase by substrates for type II dehydroquinase. *Bioorg. Med. Chem. Lett.* **2000**, *10*, 407–409. [CrossRef]
28. Ratia, K.; Light, S.H.; Antanasijevic, A.; Anderson, W.F.; Caffrey, M.; Lavie, A. Discovery of selective inhibitors of the *Clostridium difficile* dehydroquinate dehydratase. *PLoS ONE* **2014**, *9*, e89356. [CrossRef] [PubMed]
29. Cheung, V.W.; Xue, B.; Hernandez-Valladares, M.; Go, M.K.; Tung, A.; Aguda, A.H.; Robinson, R.C.; Yew, W.S. Identification of polyketide inhibitors targeting 3-dehydroquinate dehydratase in the shikimate pathway of *Enterococcus faecalis*. *PLoS ONE* **2014**, *9*, e103598. [CrossRef] [PubMed]
30. Scior, T.; Bender, A.; GTresadern, G.; Medina-Franco, J.L.; Martínez-Mayorga, K.; Langer, T.; Cuanalo-Contreras, K.; Agrafiotis, D.K. Recognizing pitfalls in virtual screening: A critical review. *J. Chem. Inf. Model.* **2012**, *52*, 867–881. [CrossRef] [PubMed]
31. Cerón-Carrasco, J.P. When Virtual Screening Yields Inactive Drugs: Dealing with False Theoretical Friends. *Chem. Med. Chem.* **2022**, *17*, e202200278. [CrossRef] [PubMed]
32. Breznik, M.; Ge, Y.; Bluck, J.P.; Briem, H.; Hahn, D.F.; Christ, C.D.; Mortier, J.; Mobley, D.L.; Meier, K. Prioritizing Small Sets of Molecules for Synthesis through in-silico Tools: A Comparison of Common Ranking Methods. *ChemMedChem* **2023**, *18*, e202200425. [CrossRef] [PubMed]
33. Warren, G.L.; Webster Andrews, C.; Capelli, A.-N.; Clarke, B.; LaLonde, J.; Lambert, M.H.; Lindvall, M.; Nevins, N.; Semus, S.F.; Senger, S.; et al. A critical assessment of docking programs and scoring functions. *J. Med. Chem.* **2006**, *49*, 5912–5931. [CrossRef] [PubMed]
34. Benson, N.C.; Daggett, V. A comparison of multiscale methods for the analysis of molecular dynamics simulations. *J. Phys. Chem. B* **2012**, *116*, 8722–8731. [CrossRef] [PubMed]
35. De Freitas, R.F.; Schapira, M. A systematic analysis of atomic protein–ligand interactions in the PDB. *MedChemComm* **2017**, *8*, 1970–1981. [CrossRef] [PubMed]
36. Hou, T.; Wang, J.; Li, Y.; Wang, W. Assessing the performance of the MM/PBSA and MM/GBSA methods. 1. The accuracy of binding free energy calculations based on molecular dynamics simulations. *J. Chem. Inf. Model* **2011**, *51*, 69–82. [CrossRef] [PubMed]
37. Wang, C.; Greene, D.; Xiao, L.; Qi, R.; Luo, R. Recent Developments and Applications of the MMPBSA Method. *Front. Mol. Biosci.* **2018**, *4*, 87. [CrossRef]
38. Wang, S.; Sun, X.; Cui, W.; Yuan, S. MM/PB(GB)SA benchmarks on soluble proteins and membrane proteins. *Front. Pharmacol.* **2022**, *13*, 1018351. [CrossRef] [PubMed]
39. Tuccinardi, T. What is the current value of MM/PBSA and MM/GBSA methods in drug discovery? *Expert Opin. Drug Discov.* **2021**, *16*, 1233–1237. [CrossRef] [PubMed]
40. El Khoury, L.; Santos-Martins, D.; Sasmal, S.; Eberhardt, J.; Bianco, G.; Ambrosio, F.A.; Solis-Vasquez, L.; Koch, A.; Forli, S.; Mobley, D.L. Comparison of affinity ranking using AutoDock-GPU and MM-GBSA scores for BACE-1 inhibitors in the D3R Grand Challenge 4. *J. Comput. Aided Mol. Des.* **2019**, *33*, 1011–1020. [CrossRef] [PubMed]
41. Jorgensen, W.L. Free Energy Calculations: A Breakthrough for Modeling Organic Chemistry in Solution. *Acc. Chem. Res.* **1989**, *22*, 184–189. [CrossRef]
42. Kirkwood, J.G. Statistical Mechanics of Fluid Mixtures. *J. Chem. Phys.* **1935**, *3*, 300–313. [CrossRef]
43. Genheden, S.; Nilsson, I.; Ryde, U. Binding affinities of factor Xa inhibitors estimated by thermodynamic integration and MM/GBSA. *J. Chem. Inf. Model* **2011**, *51*, 947–958. [CrossRef] [PubMed]
44. Sterling, T.; Irwin, J.J. ZINC 15 Ligand Discovery for Everyone. *J. Chem. Inf. Model* **2015**, *55*, 2324–2337. [CrossRef] [PubMed]
45. Sander, T.; Freyss, J.; von Korff, M.; Rufener, C. DataWarrior: An open-source program for chemistry aware data visualization and analysis. *J. Chem. Inf. Model* **2015**, *55*, 460–473. [CrossRef] [PubMed]
46. Pettersen, E.F.; Goddard, T.D.; Huang, C.C.; Couch, G.S.; Greenblatt, D.M.; Meng, E.C.; Ferrin, T.E. UCSF Chimera--a visualization system for exploratory research and analysis. *J. Comput. Chem.* **2004**, *25*, 1605–1612. [CrossRef] [PubMed]
47. O'Boyle, N.M.; Banck, M.; James, C.A.; Morley, C.; Vandermeersch, T.; Hutchison, G.R. Open Babel: An open chemical toolbox. *J. Cheminform.* **2011**, *3*, 33. [CrossRef] [PubMed]
48. Morris, G.M.; Huey, R.; Lindstrom, W.; Sanner, M.F.; Belew, R.K.; Goodsell, D.S.; Olson, A.J. AutoDock4 and AutoDockTools4: Automated docking with selective receptor flexibility. *J. Comput. Chem.* **2009**, *30*, 2785–2791. [CrossRef] [PubMed]
49. Trott, O.; Olson, A.J. AutoDock Vina: Improving the speed and accuracy of docking with a new scoring function, efficient optimization, and multithreading. *J. Comput. Chem.* **2010**, *31*, 455–461. [CrossRef] [PubMed]
50. Hess, B.; Kutzner, C.; van der Spoel, D.; Lindahl, E. GROMACS 4: Algorithms for Highly Efficient, Load-Balanced, and Scalable Molecular Simulation. *J. Chem. Theory Comput.* **2008**, *4*, 435–447. [CrossRef] [PubMed]

51. Abraham, M.J.; Murtola, T.; Schulz, R.; Páll, S.; Smith, J.C.; Hess, B.; Lindahl, E. GROMACS: High Performance Molecular Simulations through Multi-Level Parallelism from Laptops to Supercomputers. *SoftwareX* **2015**, *1–2*, 19–25. [CrossRef]
52. Malde, A.K.; Zuo, L.; Breeze, M.; Stroet, M.; Poger, D.; Nair, P.C.; Oostenbrink, C.; Mark, A.E. An Automated Force Field Topology Builder (ATB) and Repository: Version 1.0. *J. Chem. Theory Comput.* **2011**, *7*, 4026–4037. [CrossRef] [PubMed]
53. Schmid, N.; Christ, C.D.; Christen, M.; Eichenberger, A.P.; van Gunsteren, W.F. Architecture, Implementation and Parallelisation of the GROMOS Software for Biomolecular Simulation. *Comp. Phys. Commun.* **2012**, *183*, 890–903. [CrossRef]
54. Sharp, K.A.; Honig, B. Calculating Total Electrostatic Energies with the Nonlinear Pois-son-Boltzmann Equation. *J. Phys. Chem* **1990**, *94*, 7684–7692. [CrossRef]
55. Paissoni, C.; Spiliotopoulos, D.; Musco, G.; Spitaleri, A. GMXPBSA 2.1: A GROMACS Tool to Perform MM/PBSA and Computational Alanine Scanning. *Comput. Phys. Commun.* **2015**, *186*, 105–107. [CrossRef]
56. Daina, A.; Michielin, O.; Zoete, V. SwissADME: A free web tool to evaluate pharmacokinetics, drug-likeness and medicinal chemistry friendliness of small molecules. *Sci. Rep.* **2017**, *7*, 42717. [CrossRef] [PubMed]
57. Seul, South Corea: Bioinformatics and Molecular Design Research Center. Pre-ADMET Program. Available online: http//preadmet.bmdrc.org (accessed on 6 June 2022).

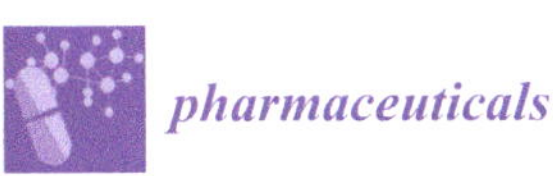

pharmaceuticals

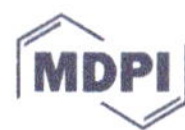

Article

Dipeptidyl Peptidase IV Inhibitory Peptides from Chickpea Proteins (*Cicer arietinum* L.): Pharmacokinetics, Molecular Interactions, and Multi-Bioactivities

José Antonio Mora-Melgem [1], Jesús Gilberto Arámburo-Gálvez [1], Feliznando Isidro Cárdenas-Torres [1], Jhonatan Gonzalez-Santamaria [1,2], Giovanni Isaí Ramírez-Torres [1,3], Aldo Alejandro Arvizu-Flores [4], Oscar Gerardo Figueroa-Salcido [1,5,*] and Noé Ontiveros [6,*]

[1]   Nutrition Sciences Postgraduate Program, Faculty of Nutrition Sciences, Autonomous University of Sinaloa, Culiacan 80010, Mexico; joseantoniomoramelgem@gmail.com (J.A.M.-M.); gilberto.aramburo@uas.edu.mx (J.G.A.-G.); feliznando@uas.edu.mx (F.I.C.-T.); jgonzalez@utp.edu.co (J.G.-S.); giovanni.ramirez@uas.edu.mx (G.I.R.-T.)
[2]   Faculty of Health and Sports Sciences, University Foundation of the Andean Area, Pereira 66001, Colombia
[3]   Faculty of Physical Education and Sports, Autonomous University of Sinaloa, Culiacan 80013, Mexico
[4]   Postgraduate Program in Health Sciences, Faculty of Biological and Health Sciences, University of Sonora, Hermosillo 83000, Mexico; aldo.arvizu@unison.mx
[5]   Integral Postgraduate Program in Biotechnology, Faculty of Chemical and Biological Sciences, Autonomous University of Sinaloa, Ciudad Universitaria, Culiacan 80010, Mexico
[6]   Clinical and Research Laboratory (LACIUS, CN), Department of Chemical, Biological, and Agricultural Sciences (DCQBA), Faculty of Biological and Health Sciences, University of Sonora, Navojoa 85880, Mexico
*   Correspondence: oscar.figueroa@uas.edu.mx (O.G.F.-S.); noe.ontiveros@unison.mx (N.O.)

Citation: Mora-Melgem, J.A.; Arámburo-Gálvez, J.G.; Cárdenas-Torres, F.I.; Gonzalez-Santamaria, J.; Ramírez-Torres, G.I.; Arvizu-Flores, A.A.; Figueroa-Salcido, O.G.; Ontiveros, N. Dipeptidyl Peptidase IV Inhibitory Peptides from Chickpea Proteins (*Cicer arietinum* L.): Pharmacokinetics, Molecular Interactions, and Multi-Bioactivities. *Pharmaceuticals* **2023**, *16*, 1109. https://doi.org/10.3390/ph16081109

Academic Editors: Roberta Rocca, Hasan Demirci, Halil İbrahim Ciftci and Belgin Sever

Received: 10 July 2023
Revised: 1 August 2023
Accepted: 1 August 2023
Published: 4 August 2023

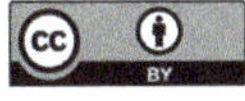

Abstract: Chickpea (*Cicer arietinum* L.) peptides can inhibit dipeptidyl peptidase IV (DPP-IV), an important type 2 diabetes mellitus therapeutic target. The molecular interactions between the inhibitory peptides and the active site of DPP-IV have not been thoroughly examined, nor have their pharmacokinetic properties. Therefore, the predictions of legumin- and provicilin-derived DPP-IV inhibitory peptides, their molecular interactions with the active site of DPP-IV, and their pharmacokinetic properties were carried out. Ninety-two unique DPP-IV inhibitory peptides were identified. Papain and trypsin were the enzymes with the highest A_E (0.0927) and lowest B_E (6.8625×10^{-7}) values, respectively. Peptide binding energy values ranged from -5.2 to -7.9 kcal/mol. HIS-PHE was the most potent DPP-IV inhibitory peptide and interacts with residues of the active sites S1 (TYR662) and S2 (GLU205/ARG125 (hydrogen bonds: <3.0 Å)), S2 (GLU205/GLU206 (electrostatic interactions: <3.0 Å)), and S2′ pocket (PHE357 (hydrophobic interaction: 4.36 Å)). Most peptides showed optimal absorption (76.09%), bioavailability (89.13%), and were non-toxic (97.8%) stable for gastrointestinal digestion (73.9%). Some peptides (60.86%) could also inhibit ACE-I. Chickpea is a source of non-toxic and bioavailable DPP-IV-inhibitory peptides with dual bioactivity. Studies addressing the potential of chickpea peptides as therapeutic or adjunct agents for treating type 2 diabetes are warranted.

Keywords: chickpea; bioactive peptides; DPP-IV inhibitors; in silico; molecular docking; ADMET

1. Introduction

Insufficient production of and resistance to insulin are characteristics of type 2 diabetes mellitus (DM2) [1]. There are therapeutic agents available for treating approximately 537 million adults with DM2 (around 10.5% of the adult population aged 20 to 79 years) [2], but their long-term usage could develop adverse effects such as headaches, urinary tract infections, arthralgia, hypersensitivity to gliptins, and pancreatitis [3,4]. Dipeptidyl peptidase IV (DPP-IV) is a ubiquitous proteolytic enzyme involved in the degradation of incretin hormones such as glucagon-like peptide 1 (GLP-1) and glucose-dependent insulinotropic polypeptide (GIP) [5]. These hormones assist in diverse biological processes, such as reducing postprandial plasma glucose levels, enhancing insulin synthesis, preserving pancreatic beta-cell function, facilitating peripheral glucose uptake and elimination, moderating gastric emptying rate, bolstering glucose metabolism, and promoting satiety [6]. Therefore, since DPP-IV inhibition increases the incretin system, DPP-IV inhibitors have been recognized as crucial therapeutic agents for managing DM2.

Because of their anticipated low or null toxicity [7] and potential antihypertensive, antioxidant, antitumor, and antidiabetic effects [8,9], interest in food-derived bioactive peptides (BPs) has increased. In this context, the identification of BPs from different sources can potentiate the production of ingredients for functional food development or lay the groundwork for peptide-based therapies. Bioinformatic tools have facilitated the identification of BPs, saving time working on the laboratory bench and, consequently, saving human and economic resources. Particularly, chickpea protein hydrolysates can inhibit DPP-IV in vitro [10,11], highlighting the potential use of chickpea peptides for treating DM2. However, the prediction of chickpea antidiabetic peptides and their pharmacokinetics remain largely unexplored, as do the molecular interactions between these peptides and DPP-IV. Therefore, to expand our knowledge about the predicted DPP-IV inhibitory peptides, in silico enzymatic hydrolyses of chickpea legumin and provicilin, as well as ADMET pharmacokinetic and molecular docking analyses of the identified antidiabetic peptides, were carried out in the present study.

2. Results and Discussion

2.1. Profile of Peptides Released after Enzymatic Hydrolysis

Enzymatic hydrolysis of dietary sources can produce DPP-IV inhibitory peptides [12]. In fact, antidiabetic peptides can be produced through alcalase or papain digestion [13]. Additionally, bromelain and ficin are inexpensive proteolytic enzymes with high specificity for hydrolysis, and can be used to produce bioactive peptides [14,15]. On the one hand, ficin is an enzyme extract composed of sulfhydryl proteases obtained from the latex of *Ficus carica*. This enzyme hydrolyzes diverse peptide bonds, but those following an aromatic residue are preferentially hydrolyzed by ficin [14]. The bioactivity of ficin hydrolysates and peptides has been evaluated in different in vitro models. For instance, ficin hydrolysates have shown the potential to inhibit the proliferation of breast cancer cell lines, such as MCF-7 and MDA-MB-231, and peptides released after the hydrolysis of proteins from different food matrices with ficin have shown antimicrobial, antioxidant, antihypertensive, and antidiabetic potential [16]. Supported by these and other findings, ficin is one of the most widely utilized vegetable enzymes for producing bioactive hydrolysates or peptides [14]. On the other hand, bromelain is a protease found in generous quantities in pineapple, and many reagent suppliers offer this enzyme for sale [15]. Both angiotensin-converting enzyme I (ACE-I) and DPP-IV inhibitory peptides can be released after the hydrolysis of proteins with bromelain. Abadía-García et al. [17] reported that whey protein hydrolysates obtained after hydrolysis with bromelain can inhibit ACE-I in vitro. Although the authors stated that ultrasound treatment of whey proteins before hydrolysis improves the ACE-I inhibitory activity of the peptides released, inhibitory peptides are released without the need for such a treatment [17]. Others reported that DPP-IV inhibitory peptides could be released after the hydrolysis of chickpea proteins with bromelain, but also stated that peptides released after pepsin and pancreatin digestion could have greater potential for inhibiting DPP-IV than those released after hydrolysis with bromelain [11]. Therefore, the present study included in silico alcalase, papain, bromelain, and ficin hydrolysis. Pepsin, trypsin, and chymotrypsin hydrolysis were also carried out, and to mimic gastrointestinal digestion, sequential hydrolysis with these three enzymes was performed. The likelihood of discovering DPP-IV inhibitory peptides increases when proteins are broken down by the aforementioned enzymes because a wide variety of peptides can be produced.

In this study, 290 and 275 DPP-IV inhibitory peptides from chickpea encrypted in the whole legumin and provicilin protein sequences were identified using the BIOPEP-UWM platform, respectively. After in silico enzymatic hydrolysis, a total of 191 legumin and 190 provicilin DPP-IV inhibitory peptides were released (Supplementary Materials Tables S1–S8). Among the 381 peptides identified, 376 were dipeptides and 5 were tripeptides. However, only 92 of them were unique. Notably, peptides of up to 10 amino acids have been reported to have low IC_{50} values and low binding energy in docking analyses [17,18]. These peptides were released after proteolysis of donkey blood, proteins from Brassica napus seeds, and chickpea proteins. These substrates were hydrolyzed with protease K, alcalase and trypsin, and pepsin and pancreatin, respectively [17–19]. It should be noted that the DPP-IV inhibitory peptides were identified using liquid chromatography with MS/MS detection, and in silico analyses were further carried out. Notably, a thirteen-amino acid peptide with a high energy of affinity with DDP-IV was released after the hydrolysis of chickpea protein with bromelain [19]. However, tetrapeptides or larger peptides could be hydrolyzed by digestive proteases, potentially losing their bioactivity in an in vivo model [20]. Contrarily, dipeptides and tripeptides are generally more resistant to gastrointestinal digestion than larger peptides, allowing for their bioavailability [12]. Certainly, ingested peptides are exposed to a variety of gastric and pancreatic proteases, as well as brush border peptidases such as pepsin, trypsin, chymotrypsin, and carboxypeptidases, among others. The peptide transport from the intestine to systemic circulation can occur through different mechanisms, such as the paracellular and transcellular routes and through peptide transporter 1 (a transmembrane protein found in the brush border) [21]. The paracellular route has a preference for di- and tripeptides with neutral or positive charges. Due to the lipidic composition of cell membranes, the transcellular route preferentially permeates hydrophobic peptides with estimated molecular weights of up to 700 Da. Regarding peptide transporter 1, this transport system is independent of the physicochemical properties of the di- and tripeptides that can be transported into the enterocyte [22]. Previous research highlights that peptide size could be more relevant than their net charge, hydrophobicity, or lipophilicity for becoming bioavailable, and that two-to-five amino acid peptides are most likely to reach the bloodstream [22]. In fact, in vitro studies show that DPP-IV inhibitory di- and tripeptides have lower binding energy in molecular docking analysis, and lower IC_{50} values than larger peptides, indicating their high potential to inhibit DPP-IV [5]. It should be noted that peptides that resist gastrointestinal digestion and become bioavailable are exposed to plasma peptidases, potentially limiting their half-life.

The frequency and potential of chickpea DPP-IV inhibitory peptides identified are shown in Table 1. Both chickpea proteins assessed are sources of DPP-IV inhibitory peptides and have similar A values, but legumin has sequences with higher DPP-IV inhibitory potential than provilicin (Table 1). After the enzymatic hydrolysis of provicilin, trypsin digestion releases peptides with the highest DPP-IV inhibitory potential. However, a higher quantity of DPP-IV inhibitory peptides is more likely to occur after bromelain or papain hydrolysis of provicilin (Table 1). Regarding legumin, the most abundant protein in chickpea seed [23], hydrolysis with papain or bromelain was more efficient in producing DPP-IV inhibitory peptides than hydrolysis performed with other enzymes evaluated in the present study (Table 1). The hydrolysis performed with alcalase or pepsin released peptides with the highest DPP-IV inhibitory potential (Table 1). Notably, pepsin hydrolyze peptide bonds with aromatic amino acids in the C-terminal region [24] and DPP-IV inhibitory peptides frequently have a hydrophobic or aromatic amino acid [25]. Overall, the results show that the interplay between peptidase and protein is relevant in the search for health-promoting food-derived hydrolysates and bioactive peptides.

Table 1. Occurrence and potential of DPP-IV inhibitory peptides in the sequence and hydrolysates of chickpea provicilin and legumin.

Protein	A	B	Enzyme	A_E	B_E
Provicilin	0.6093	0.0003526629028523	Pepsin	0.022	$4.7635643240156 \times 10^{-5}$
			Chymotrypsin	0.0287	$3.2429337219228 \times 10^{-5}$

Table 1. *Cont.*

Protein	A	B	Enzyme	A_E	B_E
			Trypsin	0.0088	$6.8625336714504 \times 10^{-7}$
			Gastrointestinal	0.0596	$6.7698735295912 \times 10^{-5}$
			Papain	0.0795	$8.271490429923 \times 10^{-5}$
			Ficin	0.0728	$6.4223543298536 \times 10^{-5}$
			Stem bromelain	0.0817	$6.0467750947608 \times 10^{-5}$
			Subtilisin (Alcalase)	0.0662	0.000165417
			Pepsin	0.0141	$5.3720267147866 \times 10^{-6}$
			Chymotrypsin	0.0423	$1.302957714179 \times 10^{-5}$
			Trypsin	0.0040	0
Legumin	0.5847	0.0002483186581999	Gastrointestinal	0.0585	$1.8401603856577 \times 10^{-5}$
			Papain	0.0927	$2.5172135076017 \times 10^{-5}$
			Ficin	0.0484	$4.2932403610376 \times 10^{-5}$
			Stem bromelain	0.0867	0
			Subtilisin (Alcalase)	0.0383	$9.1420948488684 \times 10^{-6}$

A = Frequency of DPP-IV inhibitory peptide occurrence in protein sequence; B = Potential DPP-IV activity of the protein; A_E = frequency of DPP-IV inhibitory peptide release by selected enzymes; B_E = Potential activity of DPP-IV inhibitory peptides released by enzymes. Higher values of A and A_E equal a higher frequency of DPP-IV inhibitory peptides. Lower values of B and B_E equal higher-potential DPP-IV inhibitory activity of the protein sequence and the peptides released by selected enzymes, respectively.

2.2. Molecular Interactions between DPP-IV and Their Inhibitory Peptides

The molecular docking analysis was validated by performing a redocking of the crystallographic structures of the ligand Omarigliptin (PDB ID: 4PNZ) with the DPP-IV. The RMSD between the best-docked conformation and the original ligand was 0.972 Å. Most molecular interactions of the predicted ligand with the active site of DPP-IV were shared with the crystallographic ligand (Supplementary Material Figure S1). Of the 92 DPP-IV inhibitory peptides, 46 had a tridimensional structure available in PubChem. Table 2 shows the binding energy of these inhibitory peptides with the DPP-IV active site. The binding energy values ranged from -5.2 kcal/mol to -7.9 kcal/mol, a range similar to the one reported for peptides from other food sources (-6.57 to -8.037 kcal/mol) [25–27]. The lower binding energy value indicates a higher affinity for the DPP-IV active site [5]. Interestingly, the binding energy values of some chickpea peptides are comparable to the values reported for DPP-IV inhibitor drugs, such as saxagliptin (-8.4 kcal/mol) and vildagliptin (-8.84 kcal/mol) [28,29], highlighting that DPP-IV inhibitory chickpea peptides have a high affinity for the DPP-IV active site, and suggesting that they could be effective competitive DPP-IV inhibitors. Analyses of molecular docking for all the peptides examined in the present study can be found in a freely accessible repository (https://doi.org/10.6084/m9.figshare.23652000.v1 (accessed on 10 July 2023)).

The DPP-IV active site has four pockets (S1, catalytic site, S2, and S2′): the S1 active site, which contains hydrophobic residues (Tyr 547, Tyr 631, Val 656, Trp 659, Tyr 662, Val 711), the catalytic site (CS) (Ser 630, Asp 708, Asn 710, His 740), S2 (Glu 205, Glu 206, Arg 125), and S2′ (Val 207, Ser 209, Arg 358, Phe 357) active sites [30]. Of the 46 peptides (65.2%), 30 could form hydrophobic interactions with the active site of DPP-IV. Of those, 21 (45.65%) and 17 (36.96%) had a hydrophobic amino acid or tyrosine in the N-terminal or C-terminal positions, respectively. DPP-IV inhibitory peptides usually have a hydrophobic or aromatic amino acid at the N-terminal (Ile, Leu, Val, Phe, Trp, or Tyr) [5], which is crucial for forming hydrophobic interactions with the S1 active site [31]. These peptide characteristics can explain the similar binding energy values between the peptides identified in the present study (Table 2) and the drugs saxagliptin (-8.4 kcal/mol) and vildagliptin (-8.84 kcal/mol) [28,29].

Table 2. DPP-IV inhibitory peptides, binding energy, and enzyme-releasing peptides.

Peptide	BIOPEP ID	Binding Energy (Kcal/Mol)	Protein	Location	Released by	Pubchem ID
HF	8791	-7.9	Provicilin	426–427	Stem bromelain; Subtilisin	152198
			Legumin	473–474	Stem bromelain; Subtilisin; Pepsin; Papain	
IW	8807	-7.8	Legumin	457–458	Subtilisin	7019084
YF	8935	-7.8	Provicilin	95–96	Stem bromelain	7009600
			Legumin	99–100	Stem bromelain; Papain	
QF	8870	-7.7	Provicilin	153–154	Gastrointestinal; Papain; Ficin	57288566
			Legumin	61–62	Gastrointestinal; Papain; Ficin	
YL	8940	-7.6	Legumin	182–183	Pepsin; Papain; Stem bromelain	87071
FR	8780	-7.5	Legumin	135–136	Trypsin	150903
KF	8809	-7.1	Legumin	124–125	Stem bromelain; Subtilisin	151410
VF	8917	-7.1	Provicilin	58–59 122–123	Papain; Subtilisin	6993120
			Legumin	103–104 148–149 403–404	Chymotrypsin; Gastrointestinal; Ficin; Subtilisin	
YA	8932	-7.1	Legumin	384–385 394–395	Stem bromelain	7020632
HL	8557	-7	Provicilin	72–73	Pepsin; Papain; Stem bromelain; Subtilisin	189008
NR	8849	-7	Provicilin	162–163	Papain; Ficin; Stem bromelain	14299174
			Legumin	133–134 225–226	Stem bromelain	
PH	8856	-7	Provicilin	295–296	Chymotrypsin; Gastrointestinal; Ficin	9856353
GF	8782	-6.9	Provicilin	63–64 375–376 377–378	Chymotrypsin; Pepsin; Gastrointestinal; Subtilisin	92953
			Legumin	212–213 312–313	Chymotrypsin; Gastrointestinal; Subtilisin	
GY	8788	-6.9	Legumin	98–99	Chymotrypsin; Gastrointestinal	92829
PF	8854	-6.9	Provicilin	362–363	Chymotrypsin; Gastrointestinal; Ficin	6351946
			Legumin	471–472	Stem bromelain	

Table 2. *Cont.*

Peptide	BIOPEP ID	Binding Energy (Kcal/Mol)	Protein	Location	Released by	Pubchem ID
SF	8891	−6.9	Provicilin	176–177	Chymotrypsin; Pepsin; Gastrointestinal; Papain	7009597
			Legumin	10–11 347–348	Chymotrypsin; Pepsin; Gastrointestinal; Papain	
TF	8900	−6.9	Provicilin	110–111	Gastrointestinal; Ficin	7010580
IPA	8304	−6.7	Provicilin	357–359	Stem bromelain	10040393
YV	8946	−6.7	Legumin	433–434	Stem bromelain	7009560
DR	8769	−6.6	Provicilin	203–204 416–417	Trypsin; Gastrointestinal; Ficin; Stem bromelain	16122509
			Legumin	440–441 429–430	Gastrointestinal; Ficin; Stem bromelain	
IR	8806	−6.6	Provicilin	442–443	Trypsin; Gastrointestinal; Ficin	7021814
ET	8774	−6.5	Legumin	109–110	Stem bromelain	6998031
PT	8863	−6.5	Legumin	144–145	Stem bromelain	53860028
IL	8802	−6.3	Provicilin	139–140 168–169 304–305 449–450	Gastrointestinal; Papain; Ficin; Stem bromelain; Subtilisin	7019083
			Legumin	382–383	Ficin; Stem bromelain; Subtilisin	
QP	8532	−6.3	Provicilin	431–432	Papain	11736661
			Legumin	25–26		
VE	8916	−6.3	Provicilin	56–57	Subtilisin	7009623
VN	8924	−6.3	Legumin	132–133 224–225	Chymotrypsin; Gastrointestinal	7020201
VQ	8925	−6.3	Provicilin	340–341	Subtilisin	7016045
EG	8770	−6.1	Legumin	48–49 121–122 137–138	Papain; Ficin; Stem bromelain	6427052
ES	8773	−6.1	Provicilin	244–245	Ficin; Subtilisin; Stem bromelain	6995653
			Legumin	116–117	Ficin; Stem bromelain	
HP	8520	−6	Legumin	477–478	Papain	152322
VL	8922	−6	Provicilin	92–93 101–102 104–105 124–125 186–187	Chymotrypsin; Pepsin; Gastrointestinal; Papain; Ficin; Subtilisin	6993117
IN	8804	−5.9	Provicilin	378–379	Papain	7016080
			Legumin	444–445	Chymotrypsin; Gastrointestinal; Subtilisin	
KG	8810	−5.9	Provicilin	311–312	Papain; Stem bromelain	7022320
			Legumin	248–249 387–388	Papain; Stem bromelain	
PK	8858	−5.9	Provicilin	195–196	Trypsin; Gastrointestinal; Ficin	9209431

Table 2. *Cont.*

Peptide	BIOPEP ID	Binding Energy (Kcal/Mol)	Protein	Location	Released by	Pubchem ID
SL	8560	−5.9	Provicilin	6–7 61–62 128–129 291–292	Chymotrypsin; Pepsin; Gastrointestinal; Papain	7015694
			Legumin	8–9 78–79 364–365 426–427	Chymotrypsin; Pepsin; Gastrointestinal; Papain	
VI	8920	−5.9	Provicilin	217–218	Subtilisin	7010531
VS	8926	−5.9	Provicilin	37–38 67–68 241–242	Ficin; Subtilisin	6992640
			Legumin	162–163	Subtilisin	
IA	8525	−5.8	Provicilin	69–70 166–167	Stem bromelain	7009577
			Legumin	160–161 422–423		
VK	8921	−5.8	Legumin	245–246 247–248	Trypsin; Gastrointestinal; Ficin; Subtilisin	168058
VT	8927	−5.8	Provicilin	120–121	Subtilisin	9815826
			Legumin	345–346	Papain	
GL	8561	−5.7	Provicilin	74–75	Chymotrypsin; Pepsin; Gastrointestinal; Subtilisin	1548899
SK	8894	−5.7	Provicilin	230–231	Gastrointestinal	16122513
PG	8855	−5.6	Provicilin	409–410	Papain; Ficin; Stem bromelain	6426709
			Legumin	105–106 463–464	Papain; Ficin; Stem bromelain	
VG	8918	−5.5	Provicilin	317–318	Papain; Ficin	6993110
MA	3173	−5.2	Legumin	1–2	Stem bromelain	7009581

Figure 1 shows the interactions of chickpea peptides with the active sites of DPP-IV (for more details see Supplementary Materials Table S9). Seventeen peptides (36.9%) form hydrophobic interactions with pocket S1 and thirty-two (69.5%) interact with the catalytic pocket through hydrogen bonds. Regarding pockets S2 and S2′, 35 (76.08%) and 21 (45.6%) peptides established electrostatic or hydrophobic interactions, respectively. Pocket S1 is the narrowest and tends to bind small hydrophobic compounds, while pocket S2 accommodates larger compounds through salt bridges [31]. Notably, hydrogen bonds contribute to stabilizing the complex peptide/active site of DPP-IV [32], highlighting an enhanced affinity of the peptides for the active site of DPP-IV.

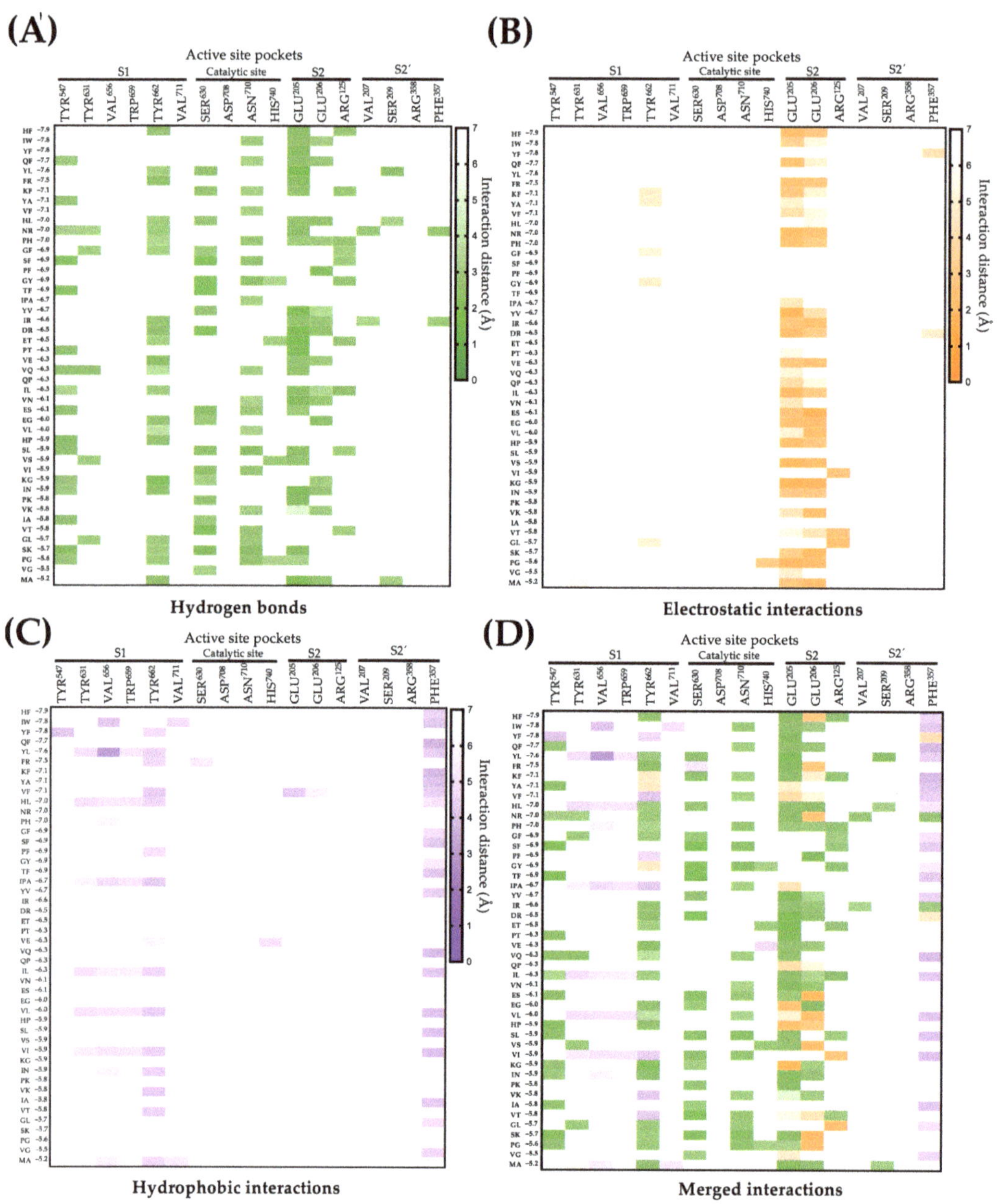

Figure 1. Interactions between chickpea peptides and the active site of DPP-IV. (**A**) Interactions by hydrogen bonds of peptides with the active site of DPP-IV. (**B**) Electrostatic interactions of peptides with the active site of DPP-IV. (**C**) Hydrophobic interactions of peptides with the active site of DPP-IV. (**D**) Merged interactions of peptides with the active site of DPP-IV.

The overlapping His–Phe peptide (−7.9 kcal/mol binding energy) in the 3D structure of the complex DPP-IV (PDB: 4PNZ)/omarigliptin is shown in Figure 2A. His–Phe could establish four electrostatic interactions with the residues Glu 205 and Glu 206 of the S2 pocket (Figure 2B). Furthermore, His could interact with the active site residues Arg 125 and Tyr 662 of S2 pocket through strong hydrogen bonds (<3 Å) (Figure 2B). On the other hand, Phe can foster hydrophobic interactions with other non-polar amino acids, enhancing the stability of the complex peptide/active site of DPP-IV. These overall interactions could explain the low binding energy of the complex His–Phe/active site of DPP-IV (−7.9 kcal/mol). Xu et al. [17,18] identified three promising peptides from *Brassica napus* seed proteins using HPLC Triple-TOF MS/MS. The authors stated that the peptides showed prominent inhibitory activity with the energy of affinity values with DPP-IV ranging from −2.21 to −1.76 kcal/mol (−9.27 to −7.38 kJ/mol) and IC50 values from 52.16 to 135.7 µM [17,18]. Others reported a thirteen-amino acid peptide from chickpea proteins, which was identified using liquid chromatography–electrospray ionization–MS/MS [19]. The peptide has an energy of affinity value with the DPP-IV of −7.3 kcal/mol, and according to the authors, chickpea peptides could be used as an ingredient for designing functional foods, or treating or preventing DM2.

2.3. ADMET Properties

ADMET helps predict the pharmacokinetics of BPs. Ideally, therapeutic compounds should be bioavailable, adequately distributed, non-toxic, and persist in the organism for enough time to perform their biological effect [33]. Table 3 presents the ADMET values of the 10 DPP-IV inhibitory peptides that have a 3D structure available in PubChem and show the lowest binding energy with the active site of DPP-IV. The specific ADMET values of all the peptides are detailed in the Supplementary Materials (Table S10). The 46 peptides passed the Lipinski rule, suggesting that they could reach systemic circulation (Table 3). Human intestinal absorption and oral bioavailability are relevant factors for novel therapeutic agents. In the present study, 35 (76.09%) and 41 (89.13%) chickpea DPP-IV inhibitory peptides showed optimal human intestinal absorption and bioavailability values, respectively (Table 3).

Table 3. ADMET pharmacokinetic properties of gliptins and chickpea-derived DPP-IV inhibitory peptides.

Peptide/Drug	Lipinski Rules	HIA	F 20%	F 30%	VD (L/kg)	T 1/2 (h)	ROAT
Omarigliptin	Accepted	Green	Green	Green	Green	0.151	Yellow
Saxagliptin	Accepted	Green	Green	Green	Green	0.309	Red
Vildagliptin	Accepted	Green	Green	Green	Green	0.37	Red
HF	Accepted	Green	Green	Green	Green	0.92	Green
IW	Accepted	Green	Green	Green	Green	0.91	Red
YF	Accepted	Green	Green	Green	Green	0.921	Yellow
QF	Accepted	Green	Green	Green	Green	0.61	Green
YL	Accepted	Green	Green	Green	Green	0.909	Green
FR	Accepted	Yellow	Green	Red	Green	0.826	Green
KF	Accepted	Red	Green	Green	Green	0.835	Green
VF	Accepted	Green	Green	Green	Green	0.872	Yellow
YA	Accepted	Green	Green	Green	Green	0.894	Green
HL	Accepted	Green	Green	Green	Green	0.919	Green
NR	Accepted	Yellow	Red	Red	Green	0.422	Green
PH	Accepted	Green	Yellow	Red	Green	0.887	Green

HIA: Human intestinal absorption, F20%: Bioavailability 20%, F30%: Bioavailability 30%, VD: Volume distribution, ROAT: Rat oral acute toxicity. Empirical decision: Green: Excellent, Yellow: Medium, Red: Poor, T1/2: probability to >3H (0–1.0).

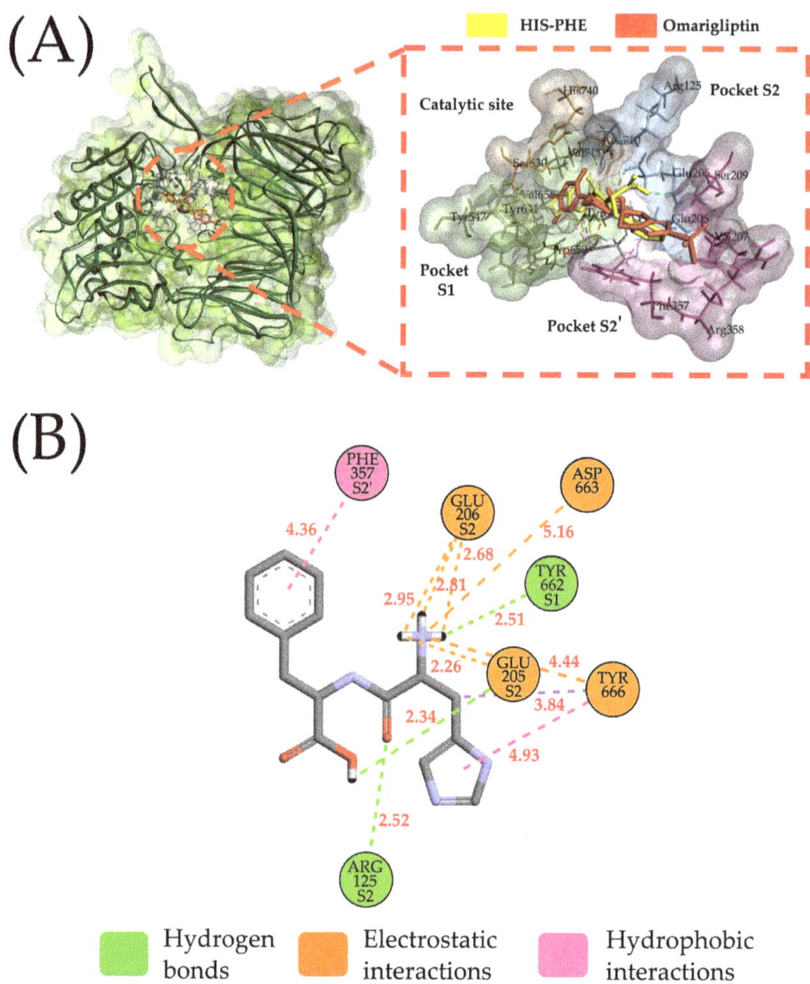

Figure 2. Molecular docking and interactions of the His–Phe peptide with DPP-IV. (**A**) Three-dimensional visualization of the molecular docking of the His–Phe peptide and the reference drug omarigliptin in the active site of DPP-IV (Red dashed lines show a close-up of the active site of DPP-IV). (**B**) Two-dimensional interactions of the His–Phe peptide with the active site of DPP-IV.

A high distribution volume suggests that therapeutic peptides can reach the target tissues, potentially increasing their effectiveness [34]. In this context, the 46 identified peptides showed optimal distribution values (Table 3). Furthermore, the peptides' likelihood of having an extended half-life (>3 h) is promising (Table 3). Contrary, vildagliptin has a half-life of approximately 90 min and saxagliptin of 2.5–3 h. Omarigliptin has a long half-life, mainly due to its strong affinity for plasma proteins such as albumin [35–37].

Of the 46 peptides, 45 (97.8%)were non-toxic. The Ile–Trp peptide was the only potentially toxic peptide identified, but it is a potent ACE-I inhibitor that has been reported as a potential therapeutic peptide [38,39]. These facts highlight that ADMET prediction should be considered as a guideline for designing in vitro and in vivo studies.

2.4. Multi-Bioactivities and Stability for Gastrointestinal Digestion

Biological activities other than DPP-IV inhibition were evaluated for the 46 identified peptides. Twenty-eight (60.86%) peptides showed ACE-I inhibitory potential and 7 (15.21%) the potential to inhibit renin. DPP-IV inhibitory peptides and ACE-I inhibitory ones share similar characteristics, such as low molecular weight, and usually contain aromatic and/or hydrophobic amino acids [12,25]. This is of relevance since approximately 70% of individuals with diabetes also suffer from hypertension [40]. Additionally, the 46 peptides were subjected to sequential pepsin, chymotrypsin, and trypsin hydrolysis to evaluate their gastrointestinal digestion stability. Thirty-four (73.9%) peptides were stable for such hydrolysis. These results are in line with the fact that di- and tripeptides tend to resist gastrointestinal digestion [12]. Notably, 24 out of 34 peptides showed multi-bioactivity in addition to stability for in silico gastrointestinal digestion.

3. Materials and Methods

3.1. Protein Sequence, Enzymatic Hydrolyses, and Analyses of DPP-IV Inhibitory Peptides

Figure 3 outlines the overall methodology employed in this study. The primary structures of chickpea legumin (UniProt ID: Q9SMJ4) and provicilin, (UniProt ID: Q304D4) were obtained (UniProtKB). These proteins are found in high proportion in the globulin fraction of chickpea seed proteins, which account for about 52% of the total chickpea protein content [41]. Hydrolyses were carried out using alcalase (EC 3.4.21.62), papain (3.4.22.2), bromelain (3.4.22.32), ficin (EC 3.4.22.3), pepsin (EC 3.4.23.1), trypsin (EC 3.4.21.4), and chymotrypsin (EC 3.4.21.1) (BIOPEP-UWM) [42]. Gastrointestinal digestion was also carried out (pepsin (EC 3.4.23.1), trypsin (EC 3.4.21.4), and chymotrypsin (EC 3.4.21.1)) (BIOPEP-UWM). The peptides released were screened for DPP-IV inhibitory activity. The frequency of occurrence values ('A' (in the proteins) and 'A_E' (in the hydrolysates)) and inhibitory potentials ('B' and 'B_E') of each DPP-IV inhibitory peptide were calculated (BIOPEP-UWM). A higher 'A_E' value indicated a larger number of DPP-IV inhibitory peptides released, and the lower the 'B_E' value, the higher the peptide's DPP-IV inhibitory potential. ADMET (absorption, distribution, metabolism, excretion, and toxicity) pharmacokinetic property prediction and molecular docking analyses [33] were carried out for peptides with a PubChem structure, as described below.

3.2. ADMET Predictions

The following pharmacokinetic properties were calculated for each DPP-IV inhibitory peptide using the ADMETLab2.0 platform [33]: (1) Lipinski's rule; (2) human intestinal absorption (HIA; optimal range (OR): 20–30%); (3) volume of distribution (VD; OR: 0.04–20 L/kg); (4) half-life (t1/2; OR: $\geq$ 3.0 h); (5) acute oral toxicity in rats (LD50; OR > 500 mg/kg). The results were interpreted following the ADMETLab2.0 platform criteria. Analyses were carried out as described previously [43].

3.3. Molecular Docking

The human DPP-IV crystallographic structure, complexed with the inhibitor Omarigliptin (PDB ID: 4PNZ), was obtained from the Protein Data Bank. Since DPP-IV is a homologous dimer, subunit B was utilized for carrying out in silico analyses. The accuracy and reliability of docking analysis were assessed by performing a re-docking of the original crystallographic ligand Omarigliptin (extracted from the exact coordinates of PDB ID: 4PNZ) with the human DPP-IV crystallographic structure. The root mean square deviation (RMSD) between the predicted ligand and the crystallographic ligand (as found in the crystallographic structure) was calculated using the validated DockingRMSD platform (University of Michigan, Ann Arbor, MI, USA.) [44]. An RMSD < 2 Å grid spacing between the best prediction of the docked ligand and the crystallographic ligand was considered acceptable.

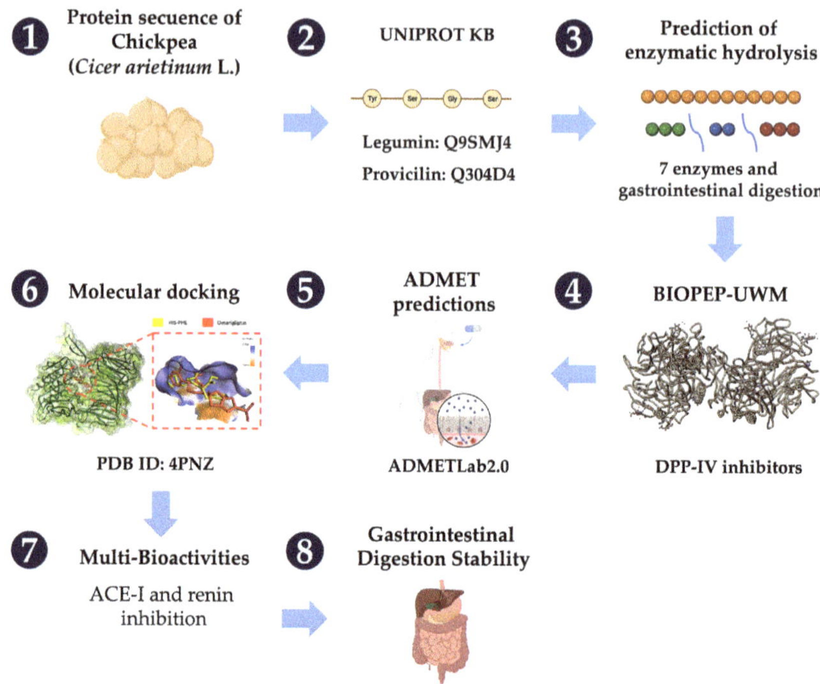

Figure 3. General outline of the methodology (Numbers indicate the order of the analyses performed, red dashed lines show a close-up of the active site of DPP-IV).

DPP-IV inhibitory peptides' 3D structures were obtained from the PubChem database. Peptides without 3D structures available were excluded. Polar hydrogens and charges were added to the peptides and DPP-IV for performing molecular docking [45]. Additionally, water molecules and the complexed inhibitor were removed from the DPP-IV structure (UCSF Chimera). For determining the coordinates including the DPP-IV active site, a redocking analysis was carried out (AutoDock Vina 1.1.2 flexible docking tool (Scripps Research Institute, San Diego, CA, USA.)) [46]. The coordinates were as follows: x: −6.733, y: 62.839; z: 35.416, with a radius of 20 Å. Molecular docking parameters were set as follows: the number of binding modes per (ligand was 10, the exhaustiveness was 8, and the maximum energy difference between the modes was 2 kcal/mol. The peptides that interact with the DPP-IV active site (visualized using Discovery Studio v21.1.0 (BIOVIA, Dassault Systèmes, San Diego, CA, USA.) in molecular docking were selected based on their binding energy, the lowest binding energy, and the best pose of each inhibitory peptide. Molecular dockings with unfavorable interactions were excluded.

3.4. Multi-Bioactivities and Stability to Gastrointestinal Digestion

For each peptide subjected to molecular docking, bioactivities other than DPP-IV inhibition were assessed, as well as their susceptibility to gastrointestinal digestion (pepsin (EC 3.4.23.1), trypsin (EC 3.4.21.4), and chymotrypsin (EC 3.4.21.1)) (BIOPEP-UWM).

4. Conclusions

Chickpea legumin and provicilin are promising sources of DPP-IV inhibitory peptides. Ninety-two unique peptides can be obtained after the hydrolysis of these chickpea proteins with commonly utilized proteolytic enzymes. The peptides released are di- and tripeptides, and most of them show favorable pharmacokinetic parameters, such as optimal human intestinal absorption and bioavailability values, high distribution volume, extended half-life, and reduced or lack of toxicity. Particularly, the peptides HF and IW showed promising energies of affinity with DPP-IV (-7.9 and -7.8, respectively). The HF peptide interacts with the residues of active sites S1 (TYR662) and S2 (GLU205/ARG125) of DPP-IV through hydrogen bonds (distances < 3.0 Å) and electrostatic interactions with residues of S2 (GLU205/GLU206) (distances < 3.0 Å). Furthermore, HF interacts with the PHE357 residue of the S2' pocket (4.36 Å) through a hydrophobic interaction. IW interacts with S1 (VAL656/VAL711) and S2' through hydrophobic interactions (distances < 5.0 A), with the catalytic site (ASN710) and S2 (GLU205/GLU206) through hydrogen bonds (distances < 3 Å), and with S2 (GLU205/GLU206) through electrostatic interactions (distance < 5.5 Å). Additionally, the peptides have the capacity to inhibit ACE-I, showing their antihypertensive potential. Due to the promising pharmacokinetics of the peptides and their energy of affinity with DPP-IV, studies to evaluate the peptides' DPP-IV inhibitory potential and their impact on insulin and glucose serum levels are warranted.

Supplementary Materials: The following supporting information can be downloaded at: https://www.mdpi.com/article/10.3390/ph16081109/s1, Table S1: Peptide release from legumin and provicilin proteins after trypsin hydrolysis; Table S2: Peptide release from legumin and provicilin proteins after pepsin hydrolysis; Table S3: Peptide release from legumin and provicilin proteins after chymotrypsin hydrolysis; Table S4: Peptide release from legumin and provicilin proteins after simulated gastrointestinal digestion; Table S5: Peptide release from legumin and provicilin proteins after papain hydrolysis; Table S6: Peptide release from legumin and provicilin proteins after alcalase hydrolysis; Table S7: Peptide release from legumin and provicilin proteins after ficin hydrolysis; Table S8: Peptide release from legumin and provicilin proteins after stem bromelain hydrolysis; Table S9. Interactions of chickpea peptides with the active site of DPP-IV; Table S10. Predictions of ADMET pharmacokinetics properties of 46 chickpea peptides; Figure S1: Docking validation of the crystallographic structures of Omarigliptin (PDB: 4PNZ) with the human DPP-IV.

Author Contributions: Conceptualization, O.G.F.-S. and N.O.; methodology, F.I.C.-T., J.G.A.-G. and A.A.A.-F.; software, J.A.M.-M. and J.G.-S.; formal analysis, J.A.M.-M.; writing—original draft preparation, J.A.M.-M., O.G.F.-S. and N.O.; writing—review and editing, G.I.R.-T., J.G.A.-G., F.I.C.-T. and A.A.A.-F. All authors have read and agreed to the published version of the manuscript.

Funding: This research received no external funding.

Institutional Review Board Statement: Not applicable.

Informed Consent Statement: Not applicable.

Data Availability Statement: Data are contained within the article and the Supplementary Materials.

Acknowledgments: In memory of Francisco Cabrera-Chávez, who encouraged the writing of the manuscript and contributed to its design and conceptualization.

Conflicts of Interest: The authors declare no conflict of interest.

References

1. Chatterjee, S.; Khunti, K.; Davies, M.J. Type 2 Diabetes. *Lancet* **2017**, *389*, 2239–2251. [CrossRef] [PubMed]
2. Magliano, D.J.; Boyko, E.J. *IDF Diabetes Atlas 10th Edition Scientific Committee. IDF Diabetes Atlas*, 10th ed.; International Diabetes Federation: Brussels, Belgium, 2021; ISBN 9782930229980.
3. Kasina, S.V.S.K.; Baradhi, K.M. *Dipeptidyl Peptidase IV (DPP IV) Inhibitors*; StatPearls Publishing: Treasure Island, FL, USA, 2019.
4. Sterrett, J.J.; Bragg, S.; Weart, C.W. Type 2 Diabetes Medication Review. *Am. J. Med. Sci.* **2016**, *351*, 342–355. [CrossRef] [PubMed]
5. Nongonierma, A.B.; FitzGerald, R.J. An in Silico Model to Predict the Potential of Dietary Proteins as Sources of Dipeptidyl Peptidase IV (DPP-IV) Inhibitory Peptides. *Food Chem.* **2014**, *165*, 489–498. [CrossRef] [PubMed]
6. Boer, G.A.; Holst, J.J. Incretin Hormones and Type 2 Diabetes—Mechanistic Insights and Therapeutic Approaches. *Biology* **2020**, *9*, 473. [CrossRef]
7. Jia, L.; Wang, L.; Liu, C.; Liang, Y.; Lin, Q. Bioactive Peptides from Foods: Production, Function, and Application. *Food Funct.* **2021**, *12*, 7108–7712. [CrossRef]
8. Daliri, E.B.-M.; Oh, D.H.; Lee, B.H. Bioactive Peptides. *Foods* **2017**, *6*, 32. [CrossRef]
9. El-Sayed, M.; Awad, S. Milk Bioactive Peptides: Antioxidant, Antimicrobial and Anti-Diabetic Activities. *Adv Biochem.* **2019**, *7*, 22–33. [CrossRef]

10. Acevedo Martínez, K.A.; Gonzalezde Mejia, E. Comparison of Five Chickpea Varieties, Optimization of Hydrolysates Production and Evaluation of Biomarkers for Type 2 Diabetes. *Food Res. Int.* **2021**, *147*, 110572. [CrossRef]
11. Chandrasekaran, S.; de Mejia, E.G. Optimization, Identification, and Comparison of Peptides from Germinated Chickpea (*Cicer rietinum*) Protein Hydrolysates Using Either Papain or Ficin and Their Relationship with Markers of Type 2 Diabetes. *Food Chem.* **2022**, *374*, 131717. [CrossRef]
12. Farias, T.C.; de Souza, T.S.P.; Fai, A.E.C.; Koblitz, M.G.B. Critical Review for the Production of Antidiabetic Peptides by a Bibliometric Approach. *Nutrients.* **2022**, *14*, 4275. [CrossRef]
13. Real Hernandez, L.M.; Gonzalez de Mejia, E. Enzymatic Production, Bioactivity, and Bitterness of Chickpea (*Cicer arietinum*) Peptides. *Compr. Rev. Food Sci. Food Saf.* **2019**, *18*, 1913–1946. [CrossRef] [PubMed]
14. Morellon-Sterling, R.; El-Siar, H.; Tavano, O.L.; Berenguer-Murcia, Á.; Fernández-Lafuente, R. Ficin: A Protease Extract with Relevance in Biotechnology and Biocatalysis. *Int. J. Biol. Macromol.* **2020**, *162*, 394–404. [CrossRef] [PubMed]
15. Nanda, R.F.; Bahar, R.; Syukri, D.; Thu, N.N.A.; Kasim, A. A Review: Application of Bromelain Enzymes in Animal Food Products. *Int. J. Agric. Nat. Sci. AIJANS* **2020**, *1*, 33–44. [CrossRef]
16. Dziuba, J.; Niklewicz, M.; Iwaniak, A.; Darewicz, M.; Minkiewicz, P. Bioinformatic-Aided Prediction for Release Possibilities of Bioactive Peptides from Plant Proteins. *Acta Aliment.* **2004**, *33*, 227–235. [CrossRef]
17. Ma, C.; Liu, D.; Hao, H.; Wu, X. Identification of the DPP-IV Inhibitory Peptides from Donkey Blood and Regulatory Effect on the Gut Microbiota of Type 2 Diabetic Mice. *Foods* **2022**, *11*, 2148. [CrossRef]
18. Xu, F.; Yao, Y.; Xu, X.; Wang, M.; Pan, M.; Ji, S.; Wu, J.; Jiang, D.; Ju, X.; Wang, L. Identification and Quantification of DPP-IV-Inhibitory Peptides from Hydrolyzed-Rapeseed-Protein-Derived Napin with Analysis of the Interactions between Key Residues and Protein Domains. *J. Agric. Food Chem.* **2019**, *67*, 3679–3690. [CrossRef]
19. Chandrasekaran, S.; Luna-Vital, D.; de Mejia, E.G. Identification and Comparison of Peptides from Chickpea Protein Hydrolysates Using Either Bromelain or Gastrointestinal Enzymes and Their Relationship with Markers of Type 2 Diabetes and Bitterness. *Nutrients* **2020**, *12*, 3843. [CrossRef]
20. Ahmed, T.; Sun, X.; Udenigwe, C.C. Role of Structural Properties of Bioactive Peptides in Their Stability during Simulated Gastrointestinal Digestion: A Systematic Review. *Trends Food Sci. Technol.* **2022**, *120*, 265–273. [CrossRef]
21. Amigo, L.; Hernández-Ledesma, B. Current Evidence on the Bioavailability of Food Bioactive Peptides. *Molecules* **2020**, *25*, 4479. [CrossRef]
22. Ramírez-Torres, G.I.; Ontiveros, N.; López-Teros, V.; Suarez-Jiménez, G.M.; Cabrera-Chávez, F. Food Matrices for the Delivery of Antihypertensive Peptides in Functional Foods. *Biotecnia* **2018**, *20*, 165–169. [CrossRef]
23. Grasso, N.; Lynch, N.L.; Arendt, E.K.; O'Mahony, J.A. Chickpea Protein Ingredients: A Review of Composition, Functionality, and Applications. *Compr. Rev. Food Sci. Food Saf.* **2022**, *21*, 435–452. [CrossRef] [PubMed]
24. Ahn, J.; Cao, M.-J.; Yu, Y.Q.; Engen, J.R. Accessing the Reproducibility and Specificity of Pepsin and Other Aspartic Proteases. *Biochim. Biophys. Acta BBA Proteins Proteom.* **2013**, *1834*, 1222–1229. [CrossRef] [PubMed]
25. Jin, R.; Teng, X.; Shang, J.; Wang, D.; Liu, N. Identification of Novel DPP–IV Inhibitory Peptides from Atlantic Salmon (*Salmo salar*) Skin. *Food Res. Int.* **2020**, *133*, 109161. [CrossRef] [PubMed]
26. Gao, J.; Gong, H.; Mao, X. Dipeptidyl Peptidase-IV Inhibitory Activity and Related Molecular Mechanism of Bovine α-Lactalbumin-Derived Peptides. *Molecules* **2020**, *25*, 3009. [CrossRef]
27. Gu, H.; Gao, J.; Shen, Q.; Gao, D.; Wang, Q.; Tangyu, M.; Mao, X. Dipeptidyl Peptidase-IV Inhibitory Activity of Millet Protein Peptides and the Related Mechanisms Revealed by Molecular Docking. *LWT* **2021**, *138*, 110587. [CrossRef]
28. Gupta, A.; Jacobson, G.A.; Burgess, J.R.; Jelinek, H.F.; Nichols, D.S.; Narkowicz, C.K.; Al-Aubaidy, H.A. Citrus Bioflavonoids Dipeptidyl Peptidase-4 Inhibition Compared with Gliptin Antidiabetic Medications. *Biochem. Biophys. Res. Commun.* **2018**, *503*, 21–25. [CrossRef]
29. Sneha, P.; Doss, C.G.P. Gliptins in Managing Diabetes-Reviewing Computational Strategy. *Life Sci.* **2016**, *166*, 108–120. [CrossRef]
30. Juillerat-Jeanneret, L. Dipeptidyl Peptidase IV and Its Inhibitors: Therapeutics for Type 2 Diabetes and What Else? *J. Med. Chem.* **2014**, *57*, 2197–2212. [CrossRef]
31. Nongonierma, A.B.; FitzGerald, R.J. Features of Dipeptidyl Peptidase IV (DPP-IV) Inhibitory Peptides from Dietary Proteins. *J. Food Biochem.* **2019**, *43*, e12451. [CrossRef]
32. Wang, W.; Liu, X.; Li, Y.; You, H.; Yu, Z.; Wang, L.; Liu, X.; Ding, L. Identification and Characterization of Dipeptidyl Peptidase-IV Inhibitory Peptides from Oat Proteins. *Foods* **2022**, *11*, 1406. [CrossRef] [PubMed]
33. Xiong, G.; Wu, Z.; Yi, J.; Fu, L.; Yang, Z.; Hsieh, C.; Yin, M.; Zeng, X.; Wu, C.; Lu, A. ADMETlab 2.0: An Integrated Online Platform for Accurate and Comprehensive Predictions of ADMET Properties. *Nucleic Acids Res.* **2021**, *49*, W5–W14. [CrossRef] [PubMed]
34. Smith, D.A.; Beaumont, K.; Maurer, T.S.; Di, L. Volume of Distribution in Drug Design: Miniperspective. *J. Med. Chem.* **2015**, *58*, 5691–5698. [CrossRef] [PubMed]
35. Dhillon, S.; Weber, J. Saxagliptin. *Drugs* **2009**, *69*, 2103–2114. [CrossRef] [PubMed]
36. Galloway, I.; McKay, G.; Fisher, M. Omarigliptin. *Pract. Diabetes* **2017**, *34*, 70–71. [CrossRef]
37. Lauster, C.D.; McKaveney, T.P.; Muench, S.V. Vildagliptin: A Novel Oral Therapy for Type 2 Diabetes Mellitus. *Am. J. Health Syst. Pharm.* **2007**, *64*, 1265–1273. [CrossRef]

38. Han, R.; Hernández Álvarez, A.J.; Maycock, J.; Murray, B.S.; Boesch, C. Comparison of Alcalase- and Pepsin-Treated Oilseed Protein Hydrolysates—Experimental Validation of Predicted Antioxidant, Antihypertensive and Antidiabetic Properties. *Curr. Res. Food Sci.* **2021**, *4*, 141–149. [CrossRef]

39. Michelke, L.; Deussen, A.; Dieterich, P.; Martin, M. Effects of Bioactive Peptides Encrypted in Whey-, Soy- and Rice Protein on Local and Systemic Angiotensin-Converting Enzyme Activity. *J. Funct. Foods* **2017**, *28*, 299–305. [CrossRef]

40. Naha, S.; Gardner, M.J.; Khangura, D.; Kurukulasuriya, L.R.; Sowers, J.R. Hypertension in Diabetes. *Eur. PMC* **2015**.

41. Chang, Y.-W.; Alli, I.; Molina, A.T.; Konishi, Y.; Boye, J.I. Isolation and Characterization of Chickpea (*Cicer arietinum* L.) Seed Protein Fractions. *Food Bioprocess Technol.* **2012**, *5*, 618–625. [CrossRef]

42. Minkiewicz, P.; Iwaniak, A.; Darewicz, M. BIOPEP-UWM Database of Bioactive Peptides: Current Opportunities. *Int. J. Mol. Sci.* **2019**, *20*, 5978. [CrossRef]

43. Arámburo-Gálvez, J.G.; Arvizu-Flores, A.A.; Cárdenas-Torres, F.I.; Cabrera-Chávez, F.; Ramírez-Torres, G.I.; Flores-Mendoza, L.K.; Gastelum-Acosta, P.E.; Figueroa-Salcido, O.G.; Ontiveros, N. Prediction of ACE-I Inhibitory Peptides Derived from Chickpea (*Cicer arietinum* L.): In Silico Assessments Using Simulated Enzymatic Hydrolysis, Molecular Docking and ADMET Evaluation. *Foods* **2022**, *11*, 1576. [CrossRef]

44. Bell, E.W.; Zhang, Y. DockRMSD: An Open-Source Tool for Atom Mapping and RMSD Calculation of Symmetric Molecules through Graph Isomorphism. *J. Cheminform.* **2019**, *11*, 40. [CrossRef] [PubMed]

45. Pettersen, E.F.; Goddard, T.D.; Huang, C.C.; Couch, G.S.; Greenblatt, D.M.; Meng, E.C.; Ferrin, T.E. UCSF Chimera—A Visualization System for Exploratory Research and Analysis. *J. Comput. Chem.* **2004**, *25*, 1605–1612. [CrossRef] [PubMed]

46. Eberhardt, J.; Santos-Martins, D.; Tillack, A.F.; Forli, S. AutoDock Vina 1.2. 0: New Docking Methods, Expanded Force Field, and Python Bindings. *J. Chem. Inf. Model.* **2021**, *61*, 3891–3898. [CrossRef] [PubMed]

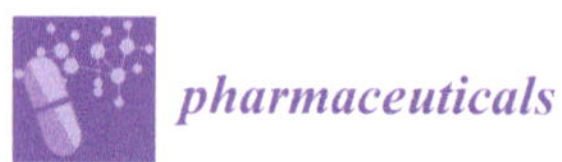 *pharmaceuticals*

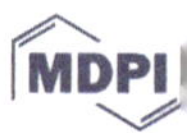

Article

Galactoside-Based Molecule Enhanced Antimicrobial Activity through Acyl Moiety Incorporation: Synthesis and In Silico Exploration for Therapeutic Target

Faez Ahmmed [1], Samiah Hamad Al-Mijalli [2], Emad M. Abdallah [3], Ibrahim H. Eissa [4], Ferdausi Ali [5], Ajmal R. Bhat [6], Joazaizulfazli Jamalis [7], Taibi Ben Hadda [8] and Sarkar M. A. Kawsar [1,*]

[1] Laboratory of Carbohydrate and Nucleoside Chemistry, Department of Chemistry, Faculty of Science, University of Chittagong, Chittagong 4331, Bangladesh; faezahmed8@gmail.com
[2] Department of Biology, College of Sciences, Princess Nourah Bint Abdulrahman University, Riyadh 11671, Saudi Arabia; shalmejale@pnu.edu.sa
[3] Department of Science Laboratories, College of Science and Arts, Qassim University, Ar Rass 51921, Saudi Arabia; 140208@qu.edu.sa
[4] Pharmaceutical Medicinal Chemistry & Drug Design Department, Faculty of Pharmacy (Boys), Al-Azhar University, Cairo 116884, Egypt; ibrahimeissa@azhar.edu.eg
[5] Department of Microbiology, Faculty of Biological Science, University of Chittagong, Chittagong 4331, Bangladesh; seema@cu.ac.bd
[6] Department of Chemistry, RTM Nagpur University, Nagpur 440033, India; bhatajmal@gmail.com
[7] Department of Chemistry, Universiti Teknologi Malaysia, Johor Bahru 81100, Malaysia; joazaizulfazli@utm.my
[8] Laboratory of Applied Chemistry & Environment, Faculty of Sciences, Mohammed Premier University, Oujda 60000, Morocco; taibi.ben.hadda@gmail.com
* Correspondence: akawsarabe@yahoo.com; Tel.: +88-017-6271-7081

Citation: Ahmmed, F.; Al-Mijalli, S.H.; Abdallah, E.M.; Eissa, I.H.; Ali, F.; Bhat, A.R.; Jamalis, J.; Ben Hadda, T.; Kawsar, S.M.A. Galactoside-Based Molecule Enhanced Antimicrobial Activity through Acyl Moiety Incorporation: Synthesis and In Silico Exploration for Therapeutic Target. *Pharmaceuticals* **2023**, *16*, 998. https://doi.org/10.3390/ph16070998

Academic Editors: Halil İbrahim Ciftci, Belgin Sever and Hasan Demirci

Received: 16 June 2023
Revised: 6 July 2023
Accepted: 10 July 2023
Published: 13 July 2023

Abstract: In this study, a series of galactoside-based molecules, compounds of methyl β-D-galactopyranoside (MDGP, **1**), were selectively acylated using 2-bromobenzoyl chloride to obtain 6-*O*-(2-bromobenzoyl) substitution products, which were then transformed into 2,3,4-tri-*O*-6-(2-bromobenzoyl) compounds (**2–7**) with various nontraditional acyl substituents. The chemical structures of the synthesized analogs were characterized by spectroscopic methods and physicochemical and elemental data analyses. The antimicrobial activities of the compounds against five human pathogenic bacteria and two phyto-fungi were evaluated in vitro and it was found that the acyl moiety-induced synthesized analogs exhibited varying levels of antibacterial activity against different bacteria, with compounds **3** and **6** exhibiting broad-spectrum activity and compounds **2** and **5** exhibiting activity against specific bacteria. Compounds **3** and **6** were tested for MIC (minimum inhibitory concentration) and MBC (minimum bactericidal concentration) based on their activity. The synthesized analogs were also found to have potential as a source of new antibacterial agents particularly against gram-positive bacteria. The antifungal results suggested that the synthesized analogs could be a potential source of novel antifungal agents. Moreover, cytotoxicity testing revealed that the compounds are less toxic. A structure-activity relationship (SAR) investigation revealed that the lauroyl chain [CH$_3$(CH$_2$)$_{10}$CO-] and the halo-aromatic chain [3(/4)-Cl.C$_6$H$_4$CO-] in combination with sugar, had the most potent activity against bacterial and fungal pathogens. Density functional theory (DFT)-calculated thermodynamic and physicochemical parameters, and molecular docking, showed that the synthesized molecule may block dengue virus 1 NS2B/NS3 protease (3L6P). A 150 ns molecular dynamic simulation indicated stable conformation and binding patterns in a stimulating environment. In silico ADMET calculations suggested that the designed (MDGP, **1**) had good drug-likeness values. In summary, the newly synthesized MDGP analogs exhibit potential antiviral activity and could serve as a therapeutic target for dengue virus 1 NS2B/NS3 protease.

Keywords: galactosides; dengue virus; antimicrobial; molecular docking; dynamics; ADMET

1. Introduction

There is a pressing need for the development of new antimicrobial drugs to combat the growing threat of antimicrobial resistance. New drugs are needed to target resistant bacteria, as well as to provide alternative treatments for common infections. However, the development of new antimicrobial drugs is challenging and the pipeline for new drugs is limited [1,2]. Organic chemistry plays a critical role in the innovation of new antimicrobial drugs. Most antimicrobial drugs are organic molecules that are intended to target specific parts of microbial cells, such as cell walls or enzymes [3]. Chemical synthesis is used to make and change these molecules, which improves their pharmacokinetic qualities, makes them more effective, and makes them less harmful. Additionally, chemical biology is a key part of finding new drug targets and making lead compounds work better. Using methods from chemical science to design and make new scaffolds can lead to the production of entirely new classes of antimicrobial drugs. In general, organic synthesis is a very important part of finding and making new antibacterial drugs [4].

Carbohydrates, the most available organic biomolecules, remain an attractive research subject for scientists due to their vital role in biological systems. The roles of carbohydrates comprise cell proliferation, communication between cells, and the immune response [5]. It is also the main source of metabolic energy and fine-tunes cell–cell connections and other key biological processes [6,7]. Carbohydrates also suppress harmful bacteria, viruses, protozoa, and fungi [8]. Due to their antimicrobial properties, carbohydrates have also been used to treat infectious disorders [9]. To synthesize novel antimicrobial agents with enhanced activity, a deep understanding of the antimicrobial action mechanism is best. The dengue virus (DENV), a member of the *Flaviviridae* family, is the most common arthropod-transmitted virus in humans. It causes self-limiting dengue fever, potentially fatal dengue hemorrhagic fever (DHF), and dengue shock syndrome (DSS) [10,11]. Within the genus Flavivirus, four closely related viral serotypes are associated with other human disease-causing viruses such as West Nile virus (WNV), yellow fever virus (YFV), and Japanese encephalitis virus (JEV).

MDGP derivatives can form a large group of natural proteins and synthetic agents that can strongly interact with glycosylated proteins. MDGP derivatives can be synthesized and isolated from different organisms. Each carbohydrate binding agent interacts in a specific way with monosaccharides, such as mannose, glucose, and galactose, residues present in the backbone of *N*-glycan structures. Since many enveloped viruses are glycosylated at the viral surface, such as HIV, HCV, and DENV, MDGP derivatives can interact with the glycosylated envelope of the virus and subsequently prevent viral entry into the host cell. Previously, antiviral activity against HIV and HCV was demonstrated for several carbohydrate binding agents isolated from plants and algae specifically binding mannose and *N*-acetylglucoosamine.

A literature survey suggested that biologically active molecules consist of aromatic ring substituents [12,13]. Benzene and its homologs, as well as nitrogen, sulfur, and halogen, act as a group and are known to enhance the biological activity of the parent molecule [14–16]. Moreover, it was reported that merging two active nuclei to form a molecule also increased the biological efficacy of the molecule [17,18]. The combination of two or more heteroaromatic rings and acyl groups can also increase the biological activity of the parent nucleus [19,20]. Monosaccharide derivatives have broad-spectrum antibacterial action against gram-negative and gram-positive pathogens, such as *Escherichia coli, Bacillus subtilis, Salmonella typhi*, and *Staphylococcus aureus* [21]. Monosaccharide analogs inhibited cancer cells in a recent study [22]. Isosteric changes at the hydroxyl group of nucleoside and monosaccharide structures were used to produce powerful antiviral [23–25] and antibacterial drugs [26]. Based on the above findings, we sought novel antimicrobial agents [27,28]. The current study aimed to synthesize a panel of (MDGP, **1**) analogs (**2–7**) and evaluate their in vitro antimicrobial activity against eight pathogens. Additionally, the study aimed to perform molecular docking studies against dengue virus 1 NS2B/NS3 protease (3L6P) and report the prediction of activity spectra for substances (PASS). To confirm the stability of the docked complexes, molecular dynamic simulations were performed for 150 ns. Furthermore, the study focused on optimizing the synthesized (MDGP, **1**) compounds and investigating their physicochemical behavior through density functional theory (DFT) studies. The overall objective of the study was to evaluate the potential of the synthesized analogs as antimicrobial and antiviral agents.

2. Results and Discussion

2.1. Chemistry

The main objective of this research work is to achieve the selective bromobenzoylation (Scheme 1) of MDGP (**1**) with 2-bromobenzoyl chloride using a direct acylation method. The resulting 2-bromobenzoylation product was transformed into a number of compounds employing various aliphatic and aromatic agents (Table 1). Figure 1 shows a schematic flow of the work plan.

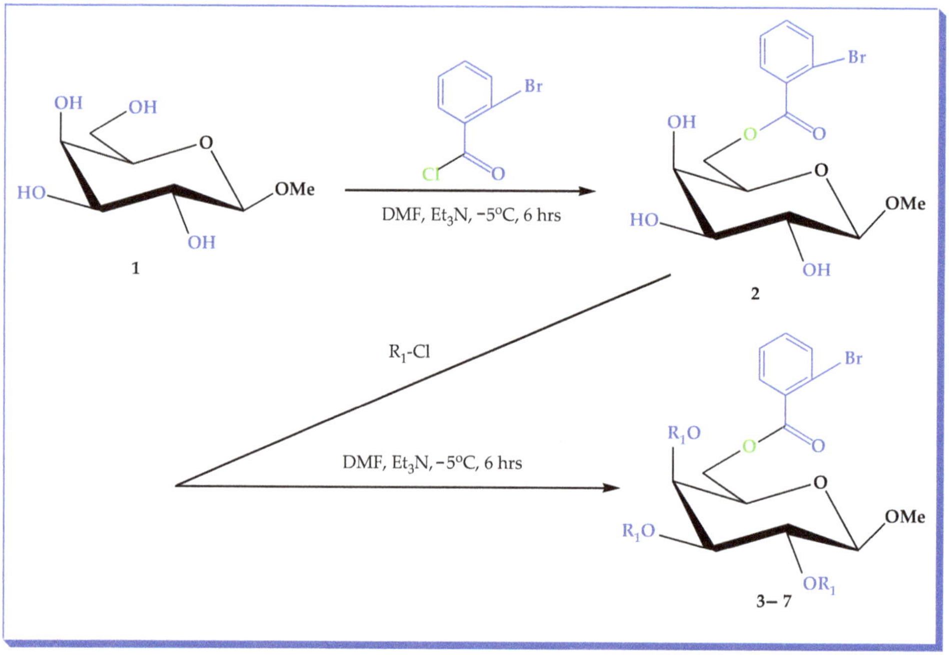

Scheme 1. General procedure for synthesizing compounds **2** to **7** of (MDGP, **1**).

Table 1. Structures of synthesized (MDGP, **1**) analogs **2–7**.

Entry	Chemical Structure	Mol. Formula
2	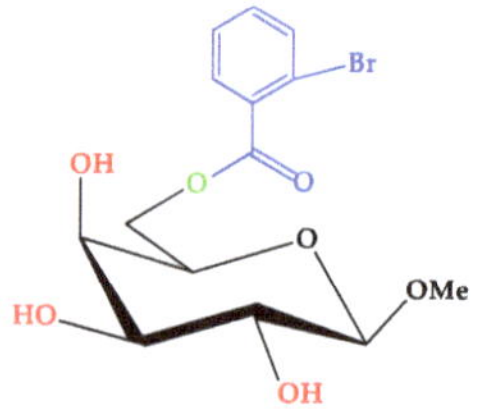	$C_{14}H_{17}O_7Br$

Table 1. *Cont.*

Entry	Chemical Structure	Mol. Formula
3	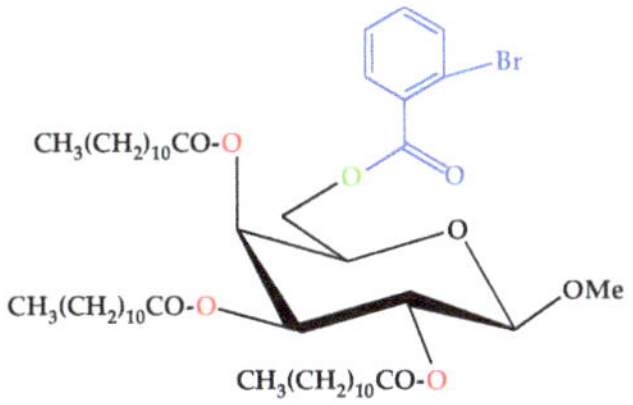 $CH_3(CH_2)_{10}CO\text{-}O$, $CH_3(CH_2)_{10}CO\text{-}O$, $CH_3(CH_2)_{10}CO\text{-}O$, Br, O, OMe	$C_{50}H_{83}O_{10}Br$
4	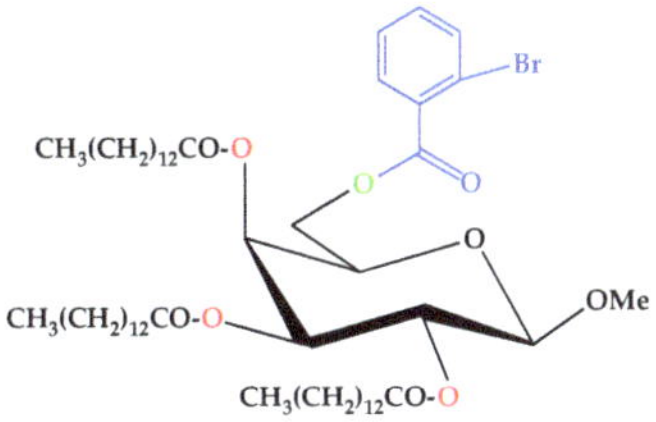 $CH_3(CH_2)_{12}CO\text{-}O$, $CH_3(CH_2)_{12}CO\text{-}O$, $CH_3(CH_2)_{12}CO\text{-}O$, Br, O, OMe	$C_{56}H_{95}O_{10}Br$
5	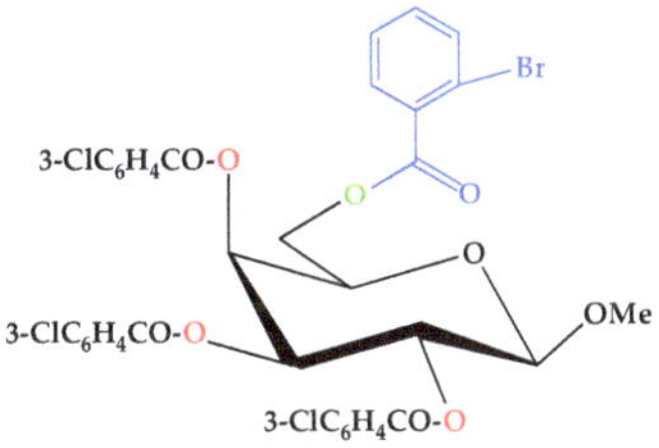 $3\text{-}ClC_6H_4CO\text{-}O$, $3\text{-}ClC_6H_4CO\text{-}O$, $3\text{-}ClC_6H_4CO\text{-}O$, Br, O, OMe	$C_{35}H_{26}O_{10}Br.Cl$
6	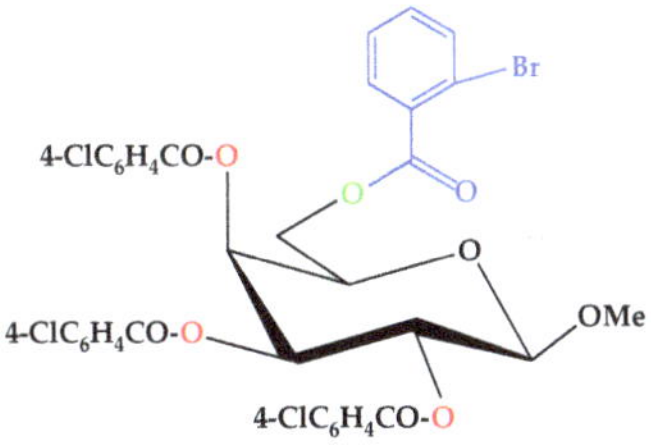 $4\text{-}ClC_6H_4CO\text{-}O$, $4\text{-}ClC_6H_4CO\text{-}O$, $4\text{-}ClC_6H_4CO\text{-}O$, Br, O, OMe	$C_{35}H_{26}O_{10}Br.Cl$
7	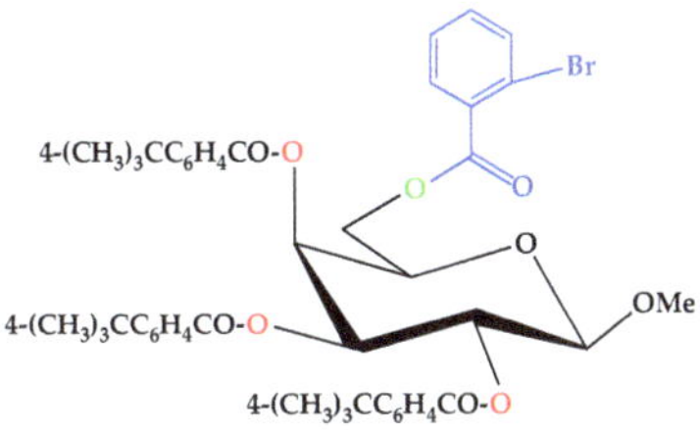 $4\text{-}(CH_3)_3CC_6H_4CO\text{-}O$, $4\text{-}(CH_3)_3CC_6H_4CO\text{-}O$, $4\text{-}(CH_3)_3CC_6H_4CO\text{-}O$, Br, O, OMe	$C_{47}H_{53}O_{10}Br$

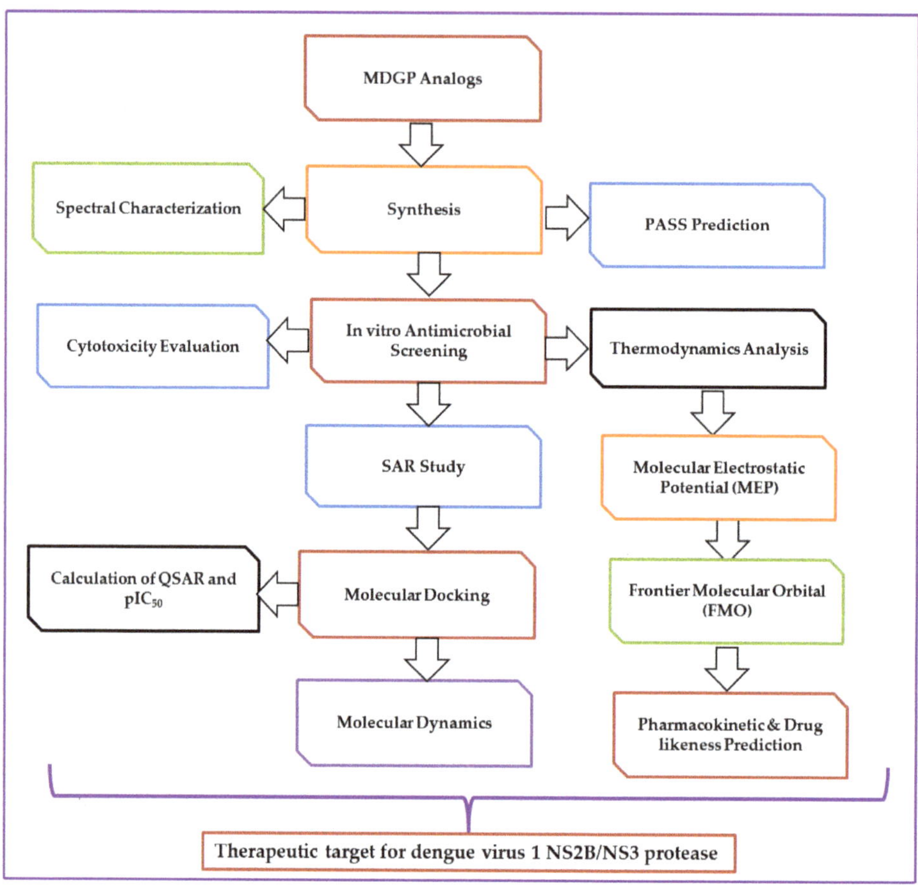

Figure 1. Illustrates the workflow of the present study.

2.2. Characterization

Regioselective 2-bromobenzoylation of methyl β-D-galactopyranoside (**1**) with 2-bromobenzoyl chloride utilizing the direct method was the initial goal of this work. A series of derivatives of the 2-bromobenzoylation product were acylated with six different acylating agents. Compound **2** was obtained as needles at 101–102 °C in 92% yield after conventional work-up and purification. The 2-bromobenzoyl derivative (**2**)'s structure was determined by ^{1}H NMR and ^{13}C NMR and mass spectra; (C=O) and (br, –OH) stretching absorption peaks were observed in this compound's FTIR (Figure S1). In its ^{1}H NMR spectrum (Figure S2), the presence of one 2-bromobenzoyl group in the molecule was confirmed by observing the following peaks: two one-proton doublets at δ 7.81 (as d, Ar-H) and δ 7.63 (as d, Ar-H) and a two-proton multiplet at δ 7.31 (1H, Ar-H) corresponding to the aromatic ring protons of the molecule. The 2-bromobenzoyl group was introduced at position 6 when C-6 deshielded from its usual value (~4.00 ppm) to 4.52 (as dd, J = 11.0, 6.4 Hz, 6a) and 4.50 (as dd, J = 11.0, 6.6 Hz, 6b) [29]. Derivative (**2**) may arise because of the increased reactivity of the sterically less hindered primary -OH group, 1-OH > 2-OH > 3-OH. The ^{13}C NMR spectra showed all the telltale peaks of a palmitoyl group. The chemical formula of compound (**3**) was $C_{14}H_{17}O_{7}Br$ and its mass spectrum featured a molecular ion peak at m/z $[M + 1]^{+}$ 378.14.

2.3. Two-Dimensional NMR

Attribution of the signals by analyzing its COSY, HSQC, and HMBC spectral experiments (Table 2 and Figure 2), along with the ^{13}C NMR spectrum, ascertained the structure as methyl 6-*O*-(2-bromobenzoyl)-*β*-D-galactopyranoside (**2**).

Table 2. ^{1}H NMR and ^{13}C NMR assignments were obtained from HSQC and HMBC experiments.

Position	δ_H (ppm) (*J* Hz)	(HSQC) δ_C (ppm)	HMBC
Ar-H	7.81 (d, *J* = 7.6)	136.3	H : Ar
Ar-H	7.63 (d, *J* = 7.4)	132.4	H : Ar
H-1	5.10 (d, *J* = 8.1)	104.1	H : 2, OCH$_3$
H-6a	4.52 (dd, *J* = 11.0 and 6.4)	63.1	H : 5, CO
H-6b	4.50 (dd, *J* = 11.0 and 6.6)	63.0	H : 5, CO
H-4	4.19 (d, *J* = 3.6)	77.0	H : 3, 5
H-3	4.00 (dd, *J* = 3.1 and 10.2)	75.2	H : 2, 4
H-2	3.87 (dd, *J* = 8.1 and 10.3)	77.2	H : 1, 3
H-5	3.76 (m)	69.1	H : 4, 6a, 6b
1-OCH$_3$	3.16 (s)	57.0	H : 1
2-Br.C$_6$H$_4$CO-		179.0	H : 6a, 6b

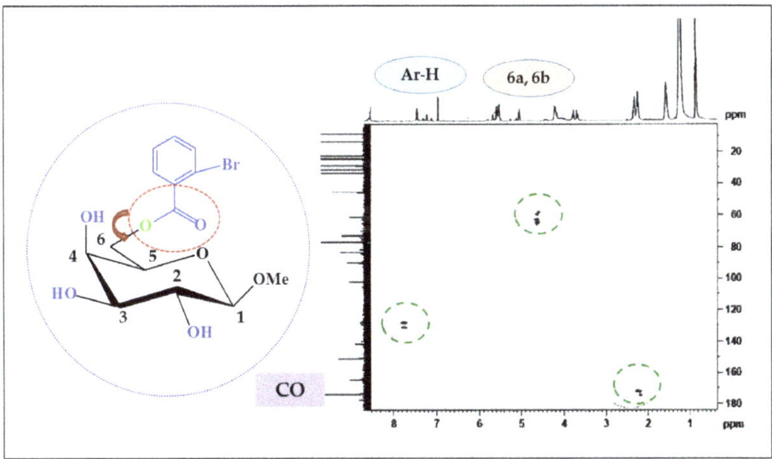

Figure 2. The HMBC correlations of analog **2**; -CO with Ar-H, H-6b, and H-6b protons.

The 2,3,4-tri-*O*-lauroyl compound (**3**) was prepared to support the structure of the 6-*O*-(2-bromobenzoyl) compound (**2**). Thus, treatment of the 2-bromobenzoate (**2**) with lauroyl chloride in pyridine yielded the laurate (**3**) in 90% yield. Two six-proton multiplets at δ 2.36 and δ 1.65 {3 × CH$_3$(CH$_2$)$_9$CH$_2$CO-}, a forty-eight-proton multiplet at δ 1.27, and a nine-proton multiplet at δ 0.89 were due to the three lauroyl groups. The three lauroyl groups were introduced at positions 2, 3, and 4 because the C-2, C-3, and C-4 protons were deshielded to δ 4.96 (as m), δ 4.91, and δ 4.51 from their predecessor (compound **2**) values of δ 3.87, δ 4.00, and δ 4.19. The structure of this molecule was determined by analyzing the FTIR, ^{1}H NMR, ^{13}C NMR, and mass spectra (Table 3) [30].

Table 3. FTIR, LC–MS, and physicochemical properties of the tested (MDGP, **1**) compounds (**2–7**).

Entry	Solvent and R_f	FTIR (KBr, v_{max}) cm^{-1}	LC–MS [M + 1]$^+$	mp. (°C)	Yield (%)	Found (Calculated)	
						%C	%H
2	CH$_3$OH-CHCl$_3$ (1:6) (R_f = 0.51)	1724 (C=O), 3404~3507 cm^{-1} (br) (-OH)	378.14	101–102	92	44.56 (44.55)	4.56 (4.54)
3	CH$_3$OH-CHCl$_3$ (1:7) (R_f = 0.52)	1715 (C=O)	924.93	107–108	90	64.93 (64.94)	9.08 (9.06)
4	CH$_3$OH-CHCl$_3$ (1:6) (R_f = 0.53)	1700 (C=O)	1009.08	154–155	70	66.67 (66.66)	9.52 (9.50)
5	CH$_3$OH-CHCl$_3$ (1:5) (R_f = 0.51)	1707 (-CO)	793.65	136–137	77	52.98 (52.99)	3.32 (3.31)
6	CH$_3$OH-CHCl$_3$ (1:5) (R_f = 0.54)	1711 (-CO)	793.65	184–185	77	52.98 (52.99)	3.33 (3.31)
7	CH$_3$OH-CHCl$_3$ (1:6) (R_f = 0.50)	1718 (-CO)	858.66	122–123	53	65.77 (65.76)	6.22 (6.23)

Again, the reaction of compound **2** with an excess of myristoyl chloride in pyridine, followed by aqueous work-up and chromatographic purification, yielded the myristoyl derivative (**4**) as needles, mp. 154–155 °C. After spectroscopic examination, we determined this compound's structure as methyl 6-*O*-(2-bromobenzoyl)-2,3,4-tri-*O*-myristoyl-*β*-D-galactopyranoside (**4**). 3-Chlorobenzoyl chloride was utilized to directly acylate molecule **2**. We obtained the 3-chlorobenzoyl derivative (**5**) after the typical work-up and purification. The structures of these compounds were confidently assigned as methyl 6-*O*-(2-bromobenzoyl)-2,3,4-tri-*O*-(3-chlorobenzoyl)-*β*-D-galactopyranoside (**5**) based on their spectra, which showed characteristic peaks at δ 8.01 (3H, m, Ar-H), δ 7.82 (3H, m, Ar-H), δ 7.47 (3H, m, Ar-H), and δ 7.34 (3H, m, Ar-H). Similar techniques were used to isolate compound **6**. In its ^{1}H NMR spectra, p-substituted benzoyl groups have two six-aromatic proton multiplets at δ 8.01 (as Ar-H) and δ 7.81 (as Ar-H). Conversion to 4-*t*-butylbenzoate (**7**) confirmed the structure of 6-*O*-2-bromobenzoate (**2**). The molecule's ^{1}H NMR spectra showed three 4-*t*-butylbenzoyl groups as two six-proton multiplets at δ 8.04 and δ 7.59 (3 × Ar-H) and three singlets at δ 1.25, δ 123, and δ 122 {27H, 3 × s, 3 × (CH$_3$)$_3$C-}. The rest of the spectra were consistent with the structure reported as methyl 6-*O*-(2-bromobenzoyl)-2,3,4-tri-*O*-(4-*t*-butylbenzoyl)-*β*-D-galactopyranoside (**7**).

2.4. Antibacterial Susceptibility

The results of the antibacterial screening of the tested synthesized compounds are shown in Table 4 and Figures S2 and S3. In general, the antibacterial activity of the compound is divided into three categories: weak activity at 10 mm or less, moderate activity at 10 to 15 mm, and high activity at 15 mm or more [31–33]. Accordingly, the results presented in this study demonstrate the antibacterial activity of seven synthesized analogs against a range of bacteria. Among the tested analogs, compounds **3** and **6** exhibited wide-spectrum antibacterial activity against all tested bacteria, with compound **3** showing particularly high activity against *B. cereus*. Compound **2** also showed antibacterial activity against most bacteria tested, except for *B. subtilis* but it demonstrated high activity against *P. aeruginosa*. Compound **5** showed no activity against any tested bacteria except for *P. aeruginosa*. On the other hand, compounds **1** and **4** did not exhibit any antibacterial activity and compound **7** showed weak or no activity against all tested bacteria. These results are consistent with previous studies that have reported the antibacterial activity of similar compounds against different bacterial strains. For example, compounds **3** and **6** have structural similarities to known antibacterial agents, such as macrolides and ketolides, which have been shown to have wide-spectrum activity against both gram-positive and gram-negative bacteria [34,35]. Compound **2**, which showed high activity against *P. aeruginosa*, has a structure similar to tetracyclines, which are known to be effective against this bacterial strain. Compound **5**, which showed no activity against most bacteria tested except for *P. aeruginosa*, may have a specific mechanism of action that targets this bacterial strain. Previous studies have shown that *P. aeruginosa* is resistant to many antibiotics due to its ability to form biofilms, which can protect it from antimicrobial agents [36]. Therefore, the high activity of compound **5** against *P. aeruginosa* suggests that it may have a unique mode of action that can overcome the resistance mechanisms of this bacterial strain. The observation that the synthesized compounds showed superior activity against gram-positive bacteria compared to gram-negative bacteria is consistent with previous studies that have reported similar findings [37]. This may be due to the differences in the cell-wall structure between gram-positive and gram-negative bacteria, which can affect the penetration and efficacy of antibacterial agents [38] (Figure S4). By inhibiting these fundamental pathways, glucopyranoside analogs are often efficient antibacterial agents [39].

Table 4. Antibacterial susceptibility by the tested analogs.

Entry	Diameter of Inhibition Zones (In mm)				
	B. subtilis (G + ve) (ATCC 6633)	*S. aureus* (G + ve) (BTCC 19)	*E. coli* (G − ve) (ATCC 8739)	*S. typhi* (G − ve) (AE 14612)	*P. aeruginosa* (G − ve) (ATCC 9027)
1	NI	NI	NI	NI	NI
2	NI	10.50 ± 0.2	NI	11.25 ± 0.2	* 15.00 ± 0.1
3	* 13.00 ± 0.1	* 15.50 ± 0.3	11.00 ± 0.2	* 12.25 ± 0.1	11.25 ± 0.3
4	NI	NI	NI	NI	NI
5	NI	NI	NI	NI	* 18.25 ± 0.3
6	* 12.75 ± 0.1	11.50 ± 0.3	11.25 ± 0.2	* 13.00 ± 0.3	11.50 ± 0.1
7	7.75 ± 0.1	NI	8.50 ± 0.1	9.00 ± 0.3	7.50 ± 0.3
Azithromycin	** 18.25 ± 0.2	** 17.50 ± 0.2	** 17.25 ± 0.2	** 18.0 ± 0.1	** 18.5 ± 0.3

All experimental triplicate values are shown. Asterisks (*) and double asterisks (**) indicate significant inhibition ($p < 0.05$). NI = No inhibition.

2.5. MIC and MBC Measurement

In this study, the antibacterial activity of two methyl β-D-galactopyranoside analogs (**3** and **6**) was tested using MIC and MBC assays (Figures 3 and 4 and Table S1). The disc-diffusion test indicated that these analogs had strong antibacterial activity, which prompted further investigation. The MIC values (Figure 3) revealed that lower MIC values corresponded to greater antimicrobial activity, indicating that drugs with lower MIC scores are more effective against bacterial growth [40]. Compound **3** showed the lowest MIC value with *S. typhi* (0.125 mg/mL), followed by *P. aeruginosa* (0.25 mg/mL) and *E. coli* (2.0 mg/mL), and the highest MIC values (less susceptibility) with *B. subtilis* and *B. cereus* (8.0 mg/mL). Compound **6** showed the lowest MIC values (the most susceptible) with *B. subtilis* (0.5 mg/mL), followed by *E. coli* (1.0 mg/mL), *B. cereus*, and *S. typhi* (2.0 mg/mL), while the highest MIC value (low susceptibility) was recorded by *P. aeruginosa* (8.0 mg/mL). Previous studies have also investigated the antibacterial activity of β-galactoside analogs. For example, it was found that *ortho*-nitrophenyl-β-galactoside analogs had remarkable antibacterial activity [41].

Similarly, a published study [42,43] reported that a methyl-(3-(1-(3,4-dichlorophenyl)-1H-1,2,3-triazol-4-yl)methoxy)phenyl)-β-carboline-3-car-boxylate analog exhibited antibacterial activity against various pathogenic bacteria with low MIC values (ranging between 64 and >128 µg/mL). These findings suggest that β-galactoside analogs are promising antimicrobial agents with low MIC values and the results of the present study further support this notion.

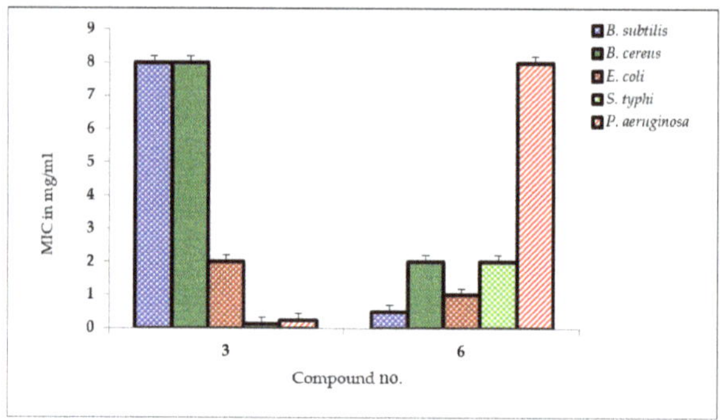

Figure 3. MIC values of compounds **3** and **6** against the tested organisms.

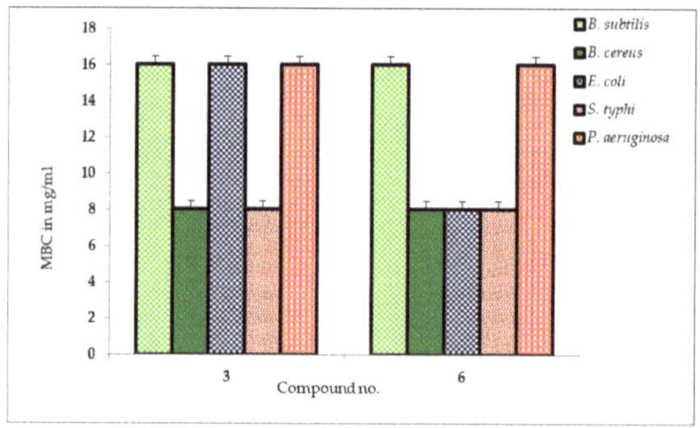

Figure 4. MBC values of analogs **3** and **6** against the tested organisms.

On the other hand, the results of the MBC test, which indicated the minimal antibacterial chemical concentration required to eradicate 99.9% of the test organisms from the original inoculum, are shown in Figure 4. The results of the MBC test revealed that *B. cereus* and *S. typhi* were the most susceptible bacteria to both analogs (methyl β-D-galactopyranoside compounds **3** and **6**), requiring only 8.0 mg/mL to eradicate 99.9% of the test organisms from the original inoculum. On the other hand, *B. subtilis*, *E. coli*, and *P. aeruginosa* required 16.0 mg/mL of the analogs to achieve the same level of antibacterial activity, according to the MBC test. The findings of this study are consistent with previous studies that have demonstrated the antibacterial potential of methyl β-D-galactopyranoside analogs against various bacterial species. For example, previous studies have investigated the antibacterial activity of a series of methyl β-D-galactopyranoside analogs against methicillin-resistant *S. aureus* (MRSA) and found that some analogs showed potent activity against MRSA, with low MBC values [44,45]. Moreover, the antibacterial activity of a methyl β-D-galactopyranoside derivative against *E. coli* was studied, and the compound exhibited a dose-dependent bactericidal effect against bacteria with MBC values ranging from 0.704 to 1.408 mg/mL [27]. In conclusion, the results of this study indicate that methyl β-D-galactopyranoside compounds **3** and **6** possess antibacterial activity against a range of bacterial species, with *B. cereus* and *S. typhi* being the most susceptible strains. Further research is warranted to investigate the potential clinical applications of these analogs in treating bacterial infections in vivo using experimental animals.

2.6. Antifungal Potential

Antifungal activity is an essential feature of a compound, especially in the treatment of fungal infections in agricultural activities and disease after harvest [46]. In this study, the antifungal activity of methyl β-D-galactopyranoside compounds was investigated against two phyto-fungal strains and the results were compared with those of the standard antibiotic nystatin. Table 5 presents the percent inhibition of the growth of the test fungal organisms by the tested methyl β-D-galactopyranoside compounds and the standard antibiotic nystatin. The results indicate that all the test compounds were sensitive toward the mycelial growth of fungi at different levels. Notably, three test compounds (**2**, **3**, and **6**) exhibited very high effectiveness against all the fungal strains used and, in most cases, the inhibition was higher than that of the standard antibiotic nystatin (Figure S5). This finding suggests that the tested analogs could be potential antifungal agents. In addition, compound **7** showed high inhibition against *A. niger*, while no inhibition was observed against *A. flavus*. This result suggests that the antifungal activity of the analogs varies depending on the fungal strain. This observation is consistent with previous studies that have reported the differential susceptibility of fungal strains to antifungal agents [47]. Moreover, the acylation of methyl β-D-galactopyranoside improves antifungal activity. This finding is consistent with previous studies that have reported the modification of sugar moieties as a strategy to improve the antifungal activity of compounds [48]. Therefore, the results of this study suggest that methyl β-D-galactopyranoside analogs could be a potential source of novel antifungal agents. Comparing the results of this study with those of previous studies, it is worth noting that the tested analogs exhibited high effectiveness against all the fungal strains used, which is a promising finding. However, further studies are necessary to investigate the mechanism of action of these analogs and their potential toxicity in vivo. Additionally, future studies could explore the potential of combining these analogs with other antifungal agents to improve their efficacy.

Table 5. Antifungal potentiality of the synthesized analogs in (%) of inhibition.

Entry	% Inhibition of Fungal Mycelial Growth in mm	
	Aspergillus niger (ATCC 16404)	*Aspergillus flavus* (ATCC 204304)
1	NI	NI
2	* 72.88 ± 1.0	* 85.66 ± 0.9
3	* 64.83 ± 1.1	* 84.02 ± 1.3
4	* 71.19 ± 1.0	NI
5	48.73 ± 1.1	* 81.97 ± 1.0
6	* 78.81 ± 1.0	* 81.97 ± 1.2
7	46.61 ± 0.7	NI
Nystatin	** 66.7 ± 1.1	** 65.2 ± 1.2

* Significant inhibition; ** Reference antibiotic, NI: no inhibition.

2.7. Cytotoxic Activity of MDGP Compounds

Figure 5 displays the cytotoxicity of synthesized MDGP compounds (**2–7**) as assessed by the brine shrimp lethality bioassay method [49]. The figure depicts the mortality percentage of shrimp at 24 and 48 h. The hydrophobicity and cytotoxicity were enhanced by long alkyl chains and phenyl rings, as reported in [44]. MDGP compound **3** (methyl 6-*O*-(2-bromobenzoyl)-2,3,4-tri-*O*-lauroyl-β-D-galactopyranoside) exhibited the least toxicity, resulting in a mortality rate of 30.09%, as per the data analysis. Compounds **4** (methyl 6-*O*-(2-bromobenzoyl)-2,3,4-tri-*O*-myristoyl-β-D-galactopyranoside) and **5** (methyl 6-*O*-(2-bromobenzoyl)-2,3,4-tri-*O*-(3-chlorobenzoyl)-β-D-galactopyranoside) exhibited the highest toxicity levels, resulting in increased mortality of 37.11% to 38.17%. This observation indicates that benzoyl derivatives exhibit lower cytotoxicity than alkyl chain derivatives. Furthermore, the cytotoxicity of alkyl chain derivatives exhibits a positive correlation with concentration.

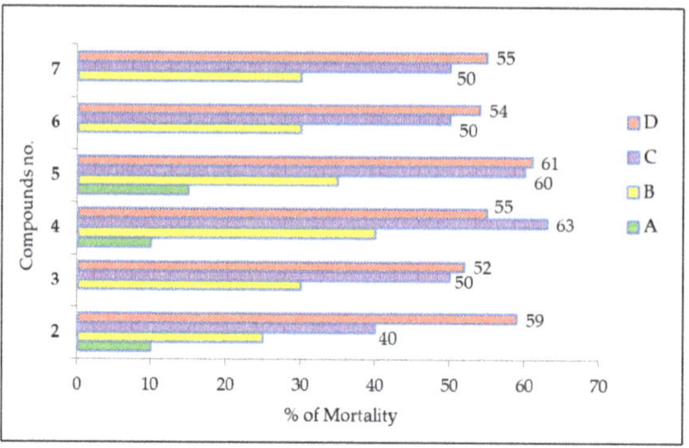

Figure 5. Cytotoxic activity of uridine derivatives (**2–7**).

2.8. Structure–Activity Relationship

Antimicrobial agents are used to prevent infections and diseases caused by pathogens and are heterocyclic molecules that play a vital role in the metabolism of living cells [50,51]. Structure–activity relationship (SAR) scanning is important for understanding the mechanisms of antibacterial activity for MDGP analogs (Figure 6). The SAR of MDGP analogs can be seen from the results of the antimicrobial activities displayed in Tables 4 and 5. Starting molecule **1** itself showed no activity against infective bacteria, so a swap in the **1** skeleton greatly affected the antibacterial activity. For most of the tested bacteria, fused lauroyl, 4-chlorobenzoyl moieties were more active than the 2-bromobenzoyl moiety. In contrast, the lauroyl containing compound (**3**) was stronger than the myristoyl compound (**4**). When aromatic-, alkyl- or electron-withdrawing groups are attached to the parent molecule, the antimicrobial activities are increased. In addition, hydrophobicity also contributes to increasing the antimicrobial activity. When hydrophobic interactions might occur between acyl chains of MDGP, **1** accumulates in the lipid-like nature of the bacterial membranes. Due to their hydrophobic interactions, bacteria lose their membrane permeability and, consequently, die [52].

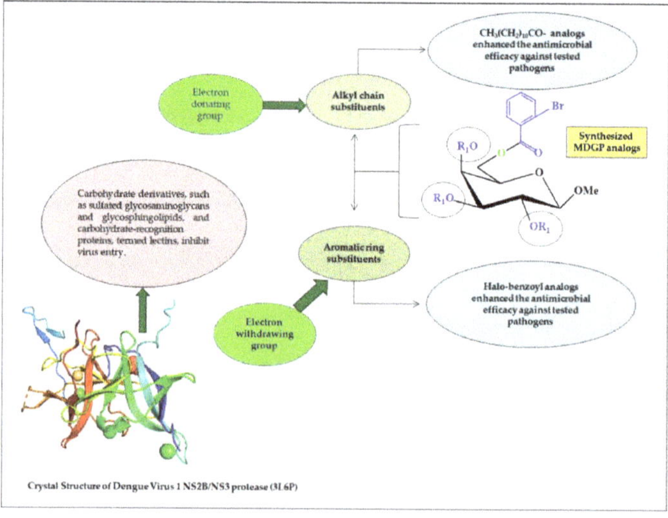

Figure 6. Structure–activity relationship of the synthesized (MDGP, **1**) compounds.

The acyl chains of MDGP accumulated in the lipid-like structure of bacterial membranes are hypothesized to engage in analogous hydrophobic interactions. Hydrophobic contact causes bacteria to lose membrane permeability, which leads to organism death. The structure–activity relationship (SAR) of the synthesized MDGP compounds was attempted based on the results. It was also shown that the antibacterial activity of MDGP (**1**) was enhanced by the addition of 2-Br.C_6H_5CO- and $CH_3(CH_2)_{10}$CO-groups to either the C-6 position or the C-2, C-3, and C-4 positions of compounds **1** or **2** (Figure 7). In addition, a computational study of the synthesized MDGP analogs revealed promising binding affinity against the membrane and NS2B/NS3 protease. Carbohydrate derivatives resemble natural glucoside/galactoside and incorporate into DNA and RNA to facilitate cellular metabolism. Most antibiotic carbohydrate derivatives work by obstructing viral DNA or RNA polymerase during the chain extension step of replication.

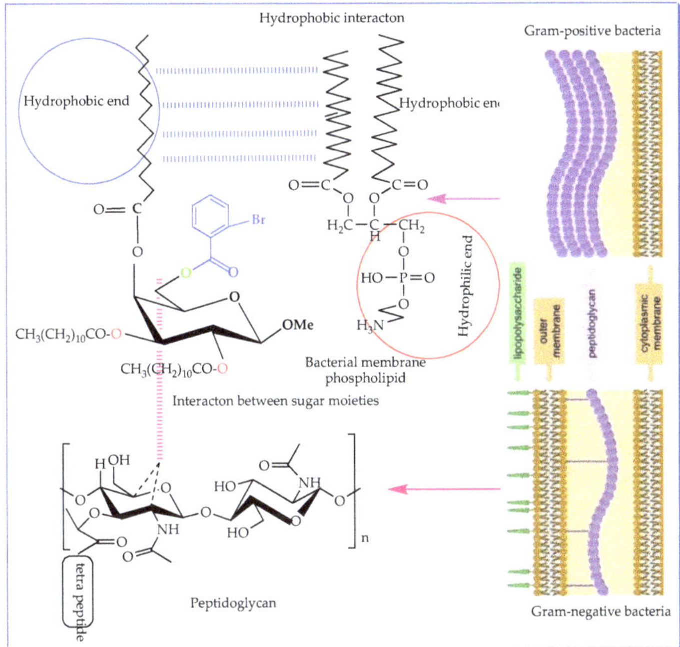

Figure 7. SAR study of the MDGP compounds with bacterial pathogens.

2.9. In Silico Studies

In silico studies are very popular and informative and are frequently used to predict how a compound will react with targeted proteins with ligands. In silico studies were performed by the following parameters.

2.10. Assessment of Antimicrobial Activity by PASS and Bioactivity

PASS predicted the antibacterial spectrum of compounds **2–7** (MDGP, **1**). The PASS results are shown in Table 6 as Pa and Pi. The results showed that (MDGP, **1**) compounds **2–7** have 0.48 < Pa < 0.55 antibacterial, 0.44 < Pa < 0.56 antifungal, and 0.39 < Pa < 0.60 antiviral activity. These compounds were more effective against bacterial and viral infections than fungal species. The insertion of lauroyl and myristoyl substituted groups decreased the antibacterial activity of (MDGP, **1**) (Pa = 0.414), while the addition of the *t*-butylbenzoyl group boosted it (Pa = 0.551). The most antifungal was compound **6**, which had a halobenzoyl aromatic group.

Table 6. Prediction of antimicrobial activity of the (MDGP, **1**) compounds.

Entry	Diameter of Inhibition Zone In mm					
	Antiviral		Antibacterial		Antifungal	
	Pa	Pi	Pa	Pi	Pa	Pi
1	0.511	0.021	0.414	0.036	0.374	0.091
2	0.607	0.011	0.502	0.024	0.440	0.032
3	0.411	0.107	0.487	0.022	0.473	0.024
4	0.393	0.131	0.487	0.022	0.473	0.024
5	0.571	0.045	0.533	0.024	0.504	0.048
6	0.554	0.129	0.539	0.062	0.567	0.048
7	0.548	0.066	0.551	0.039	0.536	0.21

The bioactivity score of molecules is greater than 0.00 if they have promising biological activity, 0.50 to 0.00 if they are moderately active, and −0.50 if they are inactive. Table 7 shows the bioactivity scores of all designed (MDGP, **1**) compounds. The bioactivity score showed promising efficacy for compounds **2**, **3**, and **5–7**.

Table 7. Determination of the drug-likeness score of (MDGP, **1**) compounds through the molinspiration cheminformatics online server.

Entry	GPCR Ligand	Ion Channel Modulator	Kinase Inhibitor	Nuclear Receptor Ligand	Protease Inhibitor	Enzyme Inhibitor
1	−0.13	−0.24	−0.17	−1.19	−0.71	0.88
2	0.04	0.23	0.09	0.47	0.21	0.55
3	0.19	−0.46	−0.23	−0.58	−0.23	0.11
4	−0.21	−0.91	−0.49	−0.77	−0.19	−0.06
5	−0.05	−1.09	0.63	−1.11	0.27	0.24
6	0.27	0.42	0.14	0.51	0.27	0.24
7	0.36	0.40	−0.11	0.34	0.26	0.23

2.11. Thermodynamic Analysis

Compound **5** has the greatest free energy (−6025.426 Hartree). The maximum enthalpy (−6025.296 Hartree) and electronic energy (−6025.295 Hartree) were also found in it. A high dipole moment value indicates polarity [53,54]. As demonstrated in Table S2, three compounds (**3**, **4**, and **6**) have an elevated dipole moment, which makes them more polar and promotes nonbonding interactions with the receptor protein. Compound (**6**)'s bulky group gave it the largest dipole moment (8.200 Debye), suggesting greater binding affinity. As the number of carbon atoms grew and the substituents had aromatic rings (**2–7**), all criteria scored higher. Thus, the MDGP compounds' thermodynamic characteristics are greatly enhanced by the acylation of their (-OH) groups.

2.12. Frontier Molecular Orbital (FMO)

Electronic absorption is the transition from the ground to the first excited state and is generally defined by one electron excitation from the HOMO to LUMO [55]. Table 8 shows the frontier molecular orbital (FMO) index of all tested compounds.

Table 8. Energy (eV) of HOMO, LUMO, Gap (Δ), hardness (η), softness (S), chemical potential (μ), and electronegativity (χ) and electrophilicity (ω) of (MDGP, **1**) compounds.

Entry	HOMO	LUMO	Gap (Δ_ζ)	η	S	μ	χ	ω
1	−6.021	−0.391	5.630	2.815	0.355	3.206	−3.206	2.317
2	−6.100	−0.863	5.237	2.618	0.381	3.481	−3.481	2.314
3	−6.233	−0.925	5.308	2.654	0.376	3.579	−3.579	2.413

Table 8. *Cont.*

Entry	HOMO	LUMO	Gap (Δ_ζ)	η	S	μ	χ	ω
4	−6.589	−0.897	5.692	2.846	0.351	3.743	−3.743	2.461
5	−5.148	−0.203	4.945	2.472	0.404	2.675	−2.675	1.447
6	−6.236	−0.758	5.478	2.739	0.365	3.497	−3.497	2.232
7	−5.850	−0.726	5.124	2.562	0.390	3.288	−3.288	2.019

As indicated in Table 8 and Figure 8, compound **4** had a higher energy-gap value (5.692 eV) than the other analogs, whereas compound **5** had a somewhat lower value (4.945 eV). Compound **5** has the lowest gap (4.945 eV) and maximum softness (0.404 eV) (Figure 8).

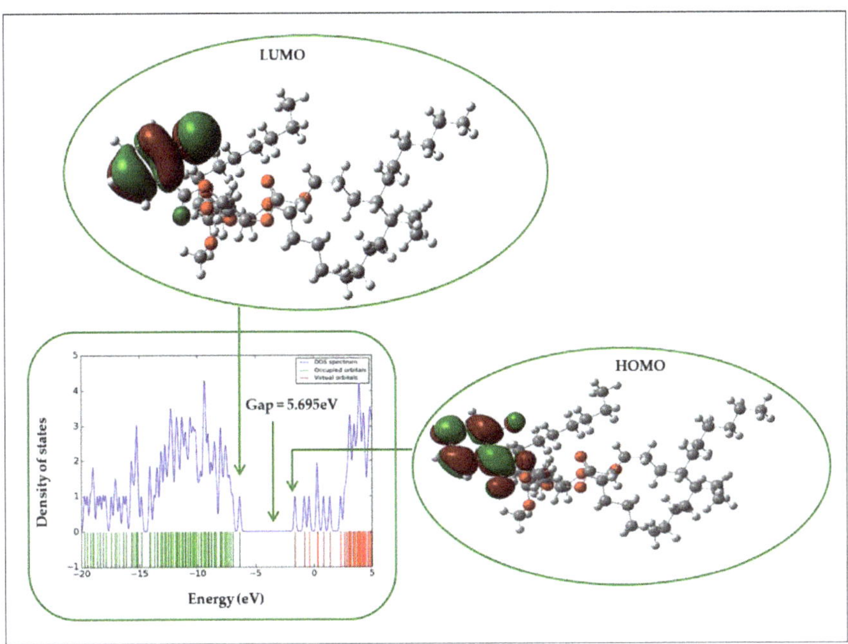

Figure 8. DOS plot and HOMO-LUMO energy gap of compound **4**.

2.13. Molecular Electrostatic Potential (MEP)

The molecular electrostatic potential (MEP) predicted reactive sites for the electrophilic and nucleophilic assault of all organic compounds [56,57]. Color-grading MEPs show molecular size, shape, and positive, negative, and neutral electrostatic potential areas. The MEP predicted electrophilic and nucleophilic reactive sites of MDGP, **1**, and its derivatives (**2–7**). Red is the maximum negative area, which is good for electrophilic assault, blue is the maximum positive area, good for a nucleophilic attack, and green is the zero potential region (Figure 9).

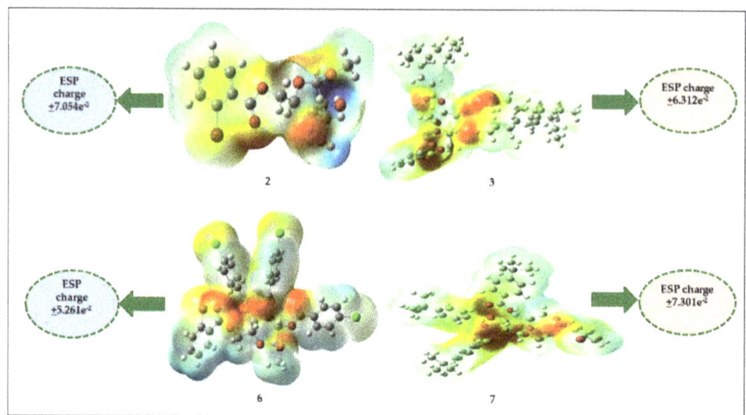

Figure 9. Molecular electrostatic potential (MESP) map of (MDGP, **1**) compounds (**2–7**).

2.14. Molecular Docking

In this study, AutoDock Vina software was used to study the binding energy and interaction modes of a series of compounds (MDGP, **1**) with the dengue virus-1 NS2B/NS3 protease (3L6P) active site (Tables 9 and 10). Docking screening revealed six compounds (**2–7**) with the highest binding energies to define the probable (MDGP, **1**) compound binding behavior. Aromatic compounds have superior binding scores than aliphatic analogs, as indicated in Table 9. Figure 8 depicts the docked conformation of the most active molecules (**6** and **7**) based on docking studies. The results (Figure 10) showed that (MDGP, **1**) compounds (**2–7**) are the most promising ligands with binding energies of −6.6, −6.1, −5.1, −8.1, −8.0, and −8.3 kcal/moL, respectively. These compounds are bound with both proteins via many hydrophobic bonding and hydrogen interactions. The binding sites were mainly located in a hydrophobic cleft bordered by the amino acid residues Ile215, Ile30, Val204, Val173, Ala141, Ala214, Lys43, Lys123, Lys124, Lys219, Phe166, Asp125, Trp17, Arg192, Leu31, and His23. There are twelve prominent hydrogen bond contacts with four different amino acids: Gln217, Lys124, Lys123, Thr168, Gly171, Glu20, Glu144, Leu31, Gln160, Arg192, Val212, and Lys43. The (MDGP, **1**) compounds (**5–7**) have a high electron density due to the additional benzene ring in the molecule, resulting in the highest binding scores. These data reveal that adding hetero groups such as –Cl, –Br, and –C(CH$_3$)$_3$ induced binding affinity fluctuations while adding an aromatic ring molecule and a –OH group boosted binding affinity. The docked pose demonstrated that drug molecules bind in the microbial macromolecular structure's active region.

Table 9. Binding energy of the (MDGP, **1**) compounds against dengue virus-1 NS2B/NS3 protease (3L6P).

Entry	3L6P (kcal/mol)
1	−5.5
2	−6.6
3	−6.1
4	−5.1
5	−8.1
6	−8.0
7	−8.3

Table 10. Nonbonding interaction data of (MDGP, **1**) compounds against dengue virus-1 NS2B/NS3 protease (3L6P).

Entry	Bond Category	Residues in Contact	Interaction Type	Distance (Å)
1	H	Gly201	CH	2.4942
	H	Phe180	CH	2.4973
	H	Gly183	CH	2.0541
	H	Thr184	CH	2.5129
	H	Tyr211	CH	1.9715
	H	Lys181	C	3.6387
	H	Gln217	CH	2.0536
2	H	Gln217	CH	2.1626
	H	Gln217	CH	2.3156
	H	Lys124	C	3.5204
	H	Thr168	C	3.5964
	Hydrophobic	Ile215	PA	5.2676
	H	Lys123	CH	2.1638
	H	Gly171	C	3.4559
3	Hydrophobic	Val204	A	5.0692
	Hydrophobic	Ala141	A	3.8337
	Hydrophobic	Lys123	PA	4.0691
	Hydrophobic	Phe166	PA	4.5004
	H	Gly171	C	3.73352
4	Hydrophobic	Lys219	A	3.7839
	Hydrophobic	Val173	A	5.4094
	Hydrophobic	Lys124	A	4.8909
	H	Glu20	CH	2.6152
	H	Leu31	CH	2.1156
	H	Gln160	CH	2.0824
	H	Arg192	CH	1.9956
	H	Arg192	CH	2.5099
	H	Arg192	CH	2.0967
5	Electrostatic	Glu19	PAn	4.1395
	Hydrophobic	Trp17	PPT	5.2745
	Hydrophobic	Arg192	A	3.9082
	Hydrophobic	Leu31	A	4.4797
	Hydrophobic	Arg192	PA	4.0916
	Hydrophobic	Leu31	PA	4.5535
	H	Glu144	CH	2.1561
	H	Gln160	CH	2.9897
	H	Gln160	CH	2.9917
	H	Arg192	CH	2.7495
	H	Lys43	C	3.7800
	H	Lys43	C	3.6630
6	Electrostatic	Glu19	PAn	3.6453
	Hydrophobic	Leu31	PS	3.4595
	Hydrophobic	Lys43	PS	3.7162
	Hydrophobic	Leu31	A	4.2217
	Hydrophobic	Ile30	A	4.7386
	Hydrophobic	His23	PA	4.2129
	Hydrophobic	Ile30	PA	3.8409

Table 10. *Cont.*

Entry	Bond Category	Residues in Contact	Interaction Type	Distance (Å)
	H	Val212	C	3.2112
	Electrostatic	Asp125	PAn	4.3311
	Hydrophobic	Val173	PS	3.9352
	Hydrophobic	Val204	PS	3.8277
	Hydrophobic	Phe166	PPS	4.8680
7	Hydrophobic	Ala214	A	4.3635
	Hydrophobic	Val173	A	5.0337
	Hydrophobic	Val204	A	5.0532
	Hydrophobic	Phe166	PA	5.0407
	Hydrophobic	Lys124	PA	4.7050
	Hydrophobic	Ala214	PA	5.1764
	Hydrophobic	Lys123	PA	5.3628

CH = Conventional Hydrogen Bond; C = Carbon Hydrogen Bond; A = Alkyl; PA = Pi-Alkyl; PS = Pi-sigma; PAn = Pi-anion; PPS = Pi-Pi stacked; PPT = Pi-Pi T-shaped.

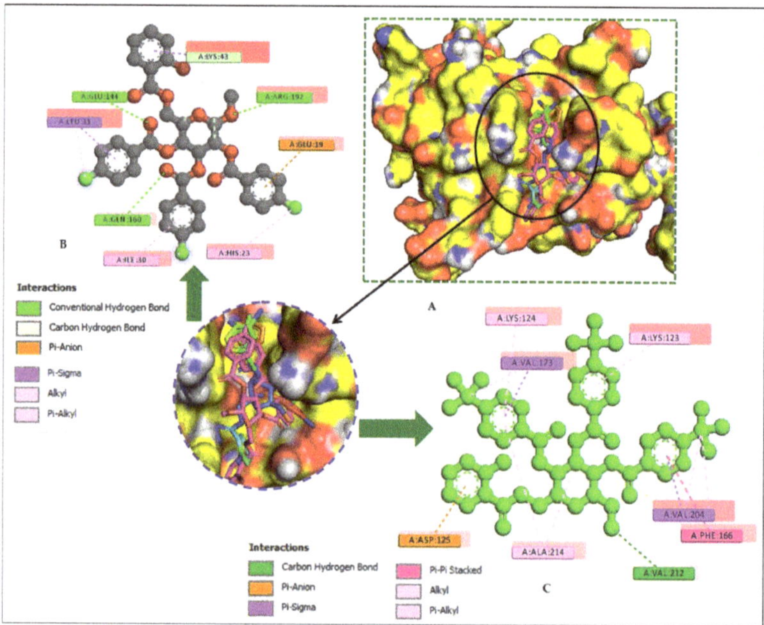

Figure 10. (**A**) Docking pose (space-filling model) and 2D interaction map of compounds **6** and **7** with dengue virus-1 NS2B/NS3 protease, (**B**) Nonbonding interactions of compound **6** with the active site of dengue virus-1 NS2B/NS3 protease, (**C**) Nonbonding interactions of compound **7** with the active site of dengue virus-1 NS2B/NS3 protease.

Along with Phe166, all compounds had the highest π–π interactions with Trp17, Lys43, and Lys124, indicating strong binding with the active site. Some studies imply that Phe166 is the main component of PPS and PPT that makes small molecules accessible at the active site. Due to hydrogen bonding, some compounds (**5–7**) have higher binding energies and modes [58]. The modifications of the -OH group in MDGP, **1** strengthened the π–π interactions with the amino acid chain at the binding site while their polarity improvement caused hydrogen bond interactions. The maximum numbers of H-bonds were observed by compounds **5** and **6** with Glu20, Glu144, Gln160, and Arg192 residues. The H-bond and hydrophobic surfaces of compound (**5**) with dengue virus-1 NS2B/NS3 protease are represented in Figure 9. It was observed from the docking study of all the

(MDGP, **1**) compounds with both targets that the molecules are generally surrounded by the abovementioned residues, suggesting that molecules may prevent the microbial activities of the target. The hydrogen bond surface and the hydrophobic bond surface of dengue virus-1 NS2B/NS3 protease with compound **5** are presented in Figure 11.

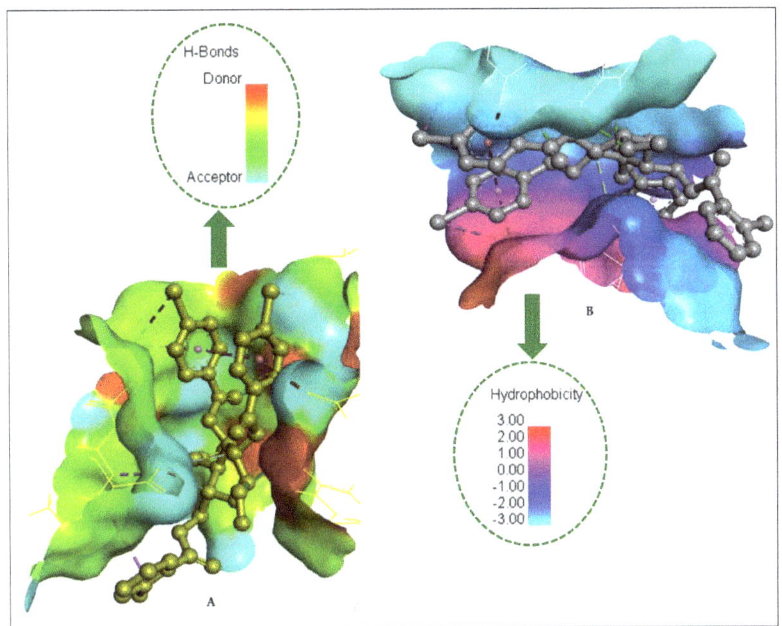

Figure 11. (**A**) Hydrogen bond surface of dengue virus−1 NS2B/NS3 protease compound **5**. (**B**) Hydrophobic bond surface of dengue virus−1 NS2B/NS3 protease with compound **5**.

2.15. Molecular-Dynamics (MD) Simulations

A molecular-dynamics simulation examined the docked complex's binding stability. To determine the docked complex binding rigidity, root mean square deviations from the C-alpha atoms of simulated complexes were studied. Figure 12A indicates that compounds **5**, **6**, and **7** had an initial upward trend, which indicates initial flexibility. All three complexes reached the stable state and did not fluctuate after 60 ns until the rest of the simulation periods, which indicated the overall stability of the complexes. The solvent-accessible surface area (SASA) of the simulated complexes was also analyzed. It is known that a higher SASA value defines higher flexibility and a lower SASA value indicates the truncated nature of the complexes. Figure 12B indicates that compound **7** possesses a reduced surface area after 60 ns upon ligand binding. The other two complexes exhibit similar binding patterns after 60 ns to the rest of the simulation time. The radius of gyration (Rg) profile of the simulated complexes defines the labile nature of the complexes, where a higher Rg value is related to a more mobile nature, whereas a lower Rg value is related to the stable conformations of the complexes. Figure 12C indicates that the three complexes have stable and steady trends in Rg and do not overfluctuate [59]. The hydrogen bond of the simulated complexes defines the stability of the drug–protein complexes, whereas all three complexes showed a steady hydrogen bond trend in the simulations (Figure 12D). The root mean square fluctuations (RMSF) of the complexes determine amino acid residue flexibility. Figure 12E shows that the complexes are stable because their maximal residues have lower RMSF.

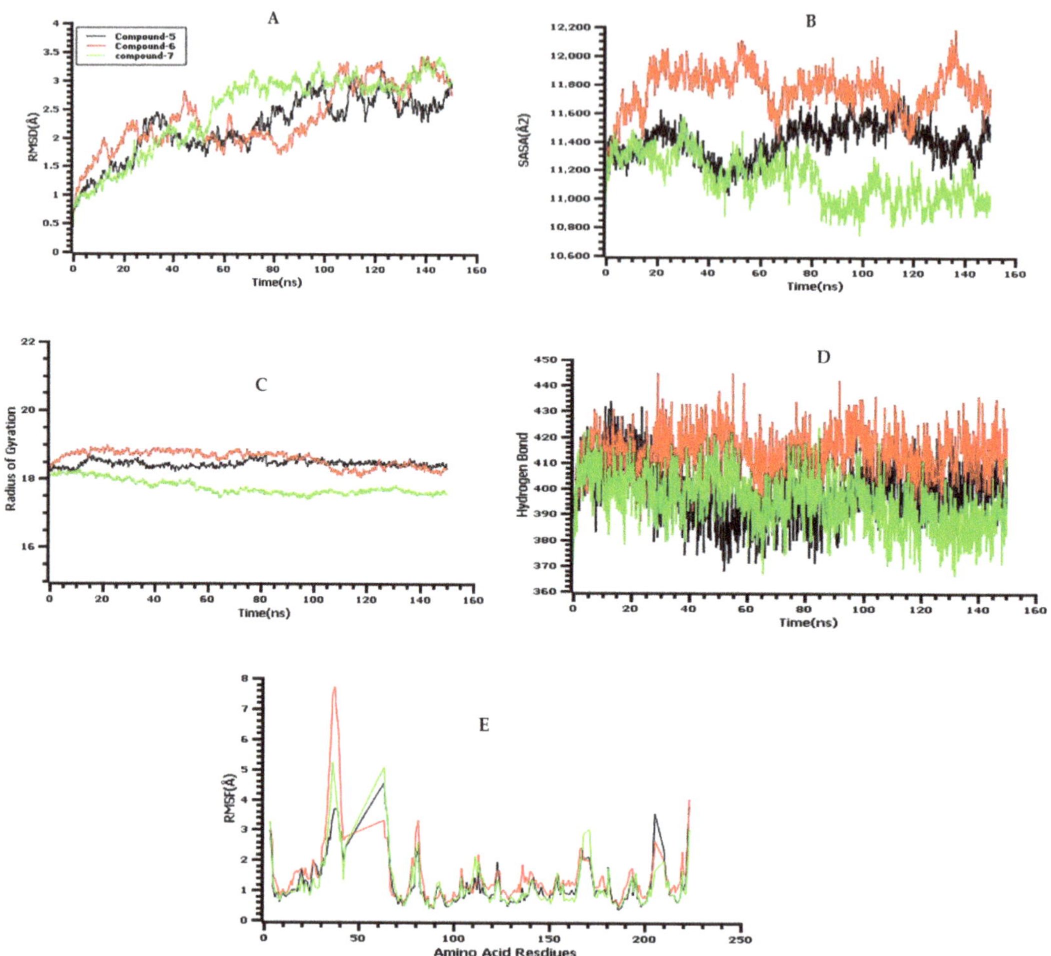

Figure 12. The molecular-dynamics simulation trajectories from 150 ns simulation time, here (**A**) root mean square deviation of the C-alpha atoms; (**B**) solvent accessible surface area of the docked complex; (**C**) radius of the gyration of the complexes; (**D**) hydrogen bond of the complexes and (**E**) root mean square fluctuation.

2.16. ADMET Profile and Drug Likeness

ADMET computations compared the absorption, metabolism, and toxicity of all MDGP, **1** molecule. Table 11 shows that all drugs had excellent absorption. If log Kp exceeds −2.5 cm/h, a molecule scarcely penetrates the skin. Skin permeability (Kp) of (MDGP, **1**) compounds ranges from −2.032 to −2.811 cm/h (<−2.5) from Table 11. Thus, all analogs penetrated the skin well. The pkCSM predicts log Papp values > 0.90 cm/s for high Caco-2 permeability. As shown in Table 11, the (MDGP, 1) compounds have poor Caco-2 permeability (log Papp). Table 11 shows that (MDGP, **1**) molecules are soluble [60].

Table 11. Prediction of in silico absorption of (MDGP, **1**) compounds.

Entry	Water Solubility (log mol/L)	Caco-2 Permeability	Intestinal Absorption	Skin Permeability
1	−3.01	−0.658	59.069	−3.118
2	−4.450	0.360	77.541	−2.032
3	−4.759	0.407	81.201	−2.237
4	−5.151	0.593	86.001	−2.370
5	−5.257	0.421	91.379	−2.561
6	−5.369	0.664	93.907	−2.791
7	−5.857	0.487	96.325	−2.811

As per the findings of Pires et al. [61], VDss is categorized as low if it falls below 0.71 L/kg (log VDss < −0.15) and high if it exceeds 2.81 L/kg (log VDss > 0.45). The results revealed that the (MDGP, **1**) compounds have VDss values ranging from −0.473 to 0.223, except for two compounds (**6** and **7**), which showed a VDss value < −0.15. Central nervous system medications require blood–brain partitioning and brain distribution. LogBB < −1 molecules are brain poor. From Table 12, MDGP analog logPS (central nervous system (CNS) permeability) ranges from −3.344 to −3.036, which is less than −3. Thus, compounds (**2–7**) cannot enter the CNS. From Table 12, (MDGP, **1**) substances had log(CLtot) values from 0.057 to 1.874 mL/min/kg. These values predict compound excretion.

Table 12. Prediction in silico of distribution and execution of (MDGP, **1**) compounds.

Entry	Distribution			Execration	
	Vdss	BBB Permeabilty	CNS Permeability	Total Clearance	Renal OCT2 Substrate
1	−0.204	−0.877	−4.087	0.321	No
2	−0.315	−1.114	−3.324	1.874	No
3	−0.473	−1.137	−3.344	1.850	No
4	0.223	−1.265	−3.231	1.379	No
5	−0.417	−1.301	−3.122	1.198	No
6	−0.079	−1.210	−3.036	0.057	No
7	−0.055	−1.354	−3.047	0.089	No

In addition, Table S3 shows that all the analogs do not affect or inhibit all the enzymes, except CYP3A4 for compounds **3**, **6**, and **7**. Therefore, it may be predicted that the other analogs may be metabolized by the P450 enzyme. Table S4 shows that MDGP compounds are fatal only at very large doses due to their high LD50 values (2.04 to 2.30).

2.17. Calculation of QSAR and pIC$_{50}$

QSAR and pIC50 were calculated using MLR (multiple linear regression) equations [62]. Our research shows that the total QSAR and pIC50 inquiry value meets all standards and different substances have different values. The QSAR and pIC50 ranged from 3.91 (compound **4**) to 6.25 (compound **6**) (Table 13). The approximate pIC50 value suggests that these newly identified compounds may be physiologically effective against gram-positive and gram-negative bacteria and pathogenic fungi.

Table 13. Data of QSAR.

Entry	Chiv5	(bcutm1)	(MRVSA9)	(MRVSA6)	(PEOEVSA5)	GATSv4	PIC50
1	0.494	2.343	0.000	0.00	0.00	0.92	4.78
2	1.112	2.884	7.299	0.00	58.270	0.99	4.25
3	1.710	4.917	15.109	73.32	68.807	1.07	4.24
4	2.873	4.816	28.237	81.41	77.896	1.15	3.91
5	4.027	3.201	35.342	93.71	80.100	1.21	5.66
6	5.630	4.663	55.317	98.22	107.636	1.23	6.25
7	6.449	4.371	39.441	107.11	144.675	1.37	6.07

3. Materials and Methods

3.1. Reagents and Instrumentation

Unless otherwise stated, Aldrich reagents were used as supplied. Uncorrected electrothermal melting points were measured in England. A Buchi rotary evaporator (W Germany) with a bath temperature below 40 °C evaporated under decreased pressure. A Bruker spectrospin spectrometer (Germany) at the BCSIR Laboratories in Dhaka acquired 400 MHz and 100 MHz ^{1}H NMR and ^{13}C NMR spectra for solutions in deuteriochloroform (CDCl$_3$) unless specified (internal Me4Si). Thin layer chromatography (t.l.c) on Kieselgel GF254-detected spots by spraying the plates with 1% H$_2$SO$_4$ and heating at 150–200 °C until coloration occurred. Column chromatography used silica gel G$_{60}$.

3.2. Synthesis of (MDGP, 1) Analogs

A solution of methyl β-D-galactopyranoside (**1**) (100 mg, 0.515 mmol) in dry dimethylformamide (DMF) (3 mL)/TEA (0.15 mL) was cooled to −5 °C and treated with 1.1 molar equivalents of 2-bromobenzoyl chloride (121.8 mg) with continuous stirring by maintaining 0 °C for 6–7 h. Stirring was continued overnight at room temperature. The reaction mixture was continuously stirred at the same temperature for 6 h. The progress of the reaction was monitored by TLC (CH$_3$OH-CHCl$_3$, 1:6). After stirring at room temperature overnight, the solvent was removed to give a semisolid mass, which was then applied to column chromatography. Initial elution with n-C$_6$H$_{14}$ removed the contaminated compounds, and further elution with CH$_3$OH-CHCl$_3$ (1:6) furnished the title compound, 2-bromobenzoyl derivative (**2**) (180 mg), as a crystalline solid.

Methyl 6-*O*-(2-bromobenzoyl)-β-D-galactopyranoside (**2**): Color white crysttaline solid, Yield 92%; m.p. 101–102 °C; (R_f = 0.52); FTIR: 1724 (C=O), 3404~3507 cm^{-1} (br) (-OH); ^{1}H NMR (400 MHz, CDCl$_3$): δ_H 7.81 (1H, d, J = 7.6 Hz, Ar-H), 7.63 (1H, d, J = 7.4 Hz, Ar-H), 7.31 (2H, m, Ar-H), 5.10 (1H, d, J = 8.1 Hz, H-1), 4.52 (1H, dd, J = 11.0 and 6.4 Hz, H-6a), 4.50 (1H, dd, J = 11.0 and 6.6 Hz, H-6b), 4.19 (1H, d, J = 3.6 Hz, H-4), 4.00 (1H, dd, J = 3.1 and 10.2 Hz, H-3), 3.87 (1H, dd, J = 8.1 and 10.3 Hz, H-2), 3.76 (1H, m, H-5), 3.16 (3H, s, 1-O*CH$_3$*); ^{13}C NMR (100 MHz, CDCl$_3$): δ_C 179.0 (2-Br.C$_6$H$_4$CO-), 136.3, 132.4, 130.9, 129.9, 126.5, 125.5 (2-Br.C$_6$H$_4$CO-), 104.1 (C-1), 77.2 (C-2), 77.0 (C-4), 75.2 (C-3), 69.1 (C-5), 63.0 (C-6), 57.0 (1-O*CH$_3$*); LC–MS [M + 1]$^{+}$ 378.14; Calcd. For C$_{14}$H$_{17}$O$_7$Br: C, 44.55%, H, 4.54%, Found: C, 44.56%, H, 4.56%.

3.3. General Procedure for the Synthesis of (2-Bromobenzoyl) Analogs 3–7

Compound **2** (111.3 mg, 0.30 mmoL) in dry DMF (3 mL) and TEA (0.15 mL) was stirred and cooled to 0 °C. It was then mixed with lauroyl chloride (0.33 mL, 5.0 molar eq.) and stirred for 6 h. Traditional work-up, as described earlier for compound **2**, followed by chromatographic purification (CH$_3$OH-CHCl$_3$, 1:6, as an eluent), gave lauroate **3** (247.21 mg).

Methyl 6-*O*-(2-bromobenzoyl)-2,3,4-tri-*O*-lauroyl-β-D-galactopyranoside (**3**): Color light white; Yield 90%; m.p. 107–108 °C; (R_f = 0.51); FTIR: ν_{max} 1715 (C=O) cm^{-1}. ^{1}H NMR (400 MHz, CDCl$_3$): δ_H 7.82 (1H, d, J = 7.6 Hz, Ar-H), 7.65 (1H, d, J = 7.4 Hz, Ar-H), 7.35 (2H, m, Ar-H), 5.01 (1H, d, J = 3.5 Hz, H-1), 4.96 (1H, m, H-2), 4.91 (1H, t, J = 9.6 Hz, H-3),

4.51 (1H, t, J = 9.4 Hz, H-4), 4.31 (1H, dd, J = 2.2 and 12.2 Hz, H-6b), 4.0 (1H, dd, J = 4.7 and 10.1 Hz, H-6a), 3.84 (1H, m, H-5), 3.19 (3H, s, 1-OCH_3), 2.36 (6H, m, 3 × $CH_3(CH_2)_9CH_2CO$-), 1.65 (6H, m, 3 × $CH_3(CH_2)_8CH_2CH_2CO$-), 1.27 (48H, m, 3 × $CH_3(CH_2)_8CH_2CH_2CO$-), 0.89 (9H, m, 3 × $CH_3(CH_2)_{10}CO$-); ^{13}C NMR (100 MHz, CDCl$_3$): δ_C 179.0 (2-Br.C$_6$H$_4$CO-), 172.5, 172.4, 172.3 {3 × $CH_3(CH_2)_{10}CO$-}, 135.5, 132.4, 130.9, 129.9, 126.5, 125.5 (2-Br.C$_6$H$_4$CO-), 104.1 (C-1), 77.2 (C-2), 77.1 (C-4), 75.2 (C-3), 69.4 (C-5), 63.0 (C-6), 57.4 (1-OCH_3), 34.3, 34.1 (×2), 31.9 (×3), 29.5 (×3), 29.4, 29.3 (×2), 29.2 (×3), 29.1, 25.0 (×2), 24.3, 22.6 (×3), 22.6, 22.5 (×3), 21.7, 21.6, 20.0 (×2) {3 × $CH_3(CH_2)_{10}CO$-}, 14.1, 14.0, 13.9 {3 × $CH_3(CH_2)_{10}CO$-}; LC–MS [M + 1]$^+$ 924.93; Calcd. For $C_{50}H_{83}O_{10}$Br: C, 64.94%, H, 9.06%; Found: C, 64.93%, H, 9.08%.

A similar reaction and purification procedure was applied to prepare compound **4** (myristoyl derivative, 339.4 mg), compound **5** (3-chlorobenzoyl derivative, 161.3 mg), compound **6** (4-chlorobenzoyl derivative, 190. 0 mg), and compound **7** (4-*t*-butylbenzoyl derivative, 167.5 mg).

Methyl 6-*O*-(2-bromobenzoyl)-2,3,4-tri-*O*-myristoyl-*β*-D-galactopyranoside (**4**): Color light white crystalline solid; Yield 70%, m.p. 154–155 °C; (R_f = 0.50); FTIR: ν_{max} 1700 cm^{-1} (C=O); ^{1}H NMR (400 MHz, CDCl$_3$): δ_H 7.81 (1H, d, J = 7.6 Hz, Ar-H), 7.63 (1H, d, J = 7.4 Hz, Ar-H), 7.31 (2H, m, Ar-H), 5.18 (1H, d, J = 3.4 Hz, H-1), 5.08 (1H, dd, J = 3.5 and 10.1 Hz, H-2), 4.93 (1H, m, H-3), 4. 88 (1H, t, J = 9.7 Hz, H-4), 4.11 (1H, dd, J = 4.6 and 11.4 Hz, H-6a), 4.0 (1H, m, H-6b), 3.95 (1H, m, H-5), 3.27 (3H, s, 1-OCH_3), 2.24 {6H, m, 3 × $CH_3(CH_2)_{11}CH_2CO$-}, 1.23 {66H, m, 3 × $CH_3(CH_2)_{11}CH_2CO$-}, 0.88 {9H, m, 3 × $CH_3(CH_2)_{12}CO$-}; ^{13}C NMR (100 MHz, CDCl$_3$): δ_C 179.0 (2-Br.C$_6$H$_4$CO-), 172.5, 172.4, 172.4 {3 × $CH_3(CH_2)_{12}CO$-}, 136.3, 132.4, 130.9, 129.9, 126.5, 125.5 (2-Br.C$_6$H$_4$CO-), 104.1 (C-1), 77.2 (C-2), 77.1 (C-4), 75.0 (C-3), 69.3 (C-5), 63.1 (C-6), 57.0 (1-OCH_3), 34.3, 34.3, 34.1 (×2), 31.8, 31.9 (×2), 29.5 (×2), 29.4, 29.3, 29.3 (×2), 29.2 (×3), 29.1, 25.0 (×2), 24.9, 24.9, 22.6 (×3), 22.6, 22.6 (×3), 22.6 (×3), 21.7, 21.6, 20.0 (×2), 20.0 {3 × $CH_3(CH_2)_{12}CO$-}, 14.1, 14.0, 13.9 {3 × $CH_3(CH_2)_{12}CO$-}; LC–MS [M + 1]$^+$ 1009.08; Calcd. For $C_{56}H_{95}O_{10}$Br: C, 66.66%, H, 9.50%; Found: C, 66.67%, H, 9.52%.

Methyl 6-*O*-(2-bromobenzoyl)-2,3,4-tri-*O*-(3-chlorobenzoyl)-*β*-D-galactopyranoside (**5**): Color white needles; Yield 77%; m.p. 136–137 °C; (R_f = 0.51); FTIR: ν_{max} 1707 (-CO) cm^{-1}. ^{1}H NMR (400 MHz, CDCl$_3$): δ_H 8.01 (3H, m, Ar-H), 7.85 (1H, d, J = 7.5 Hz, Ar-H), 7.82 (3H, m, Ar-H), 7.60 (1H, d, J = 7.2 Hz, Ar-H), 7.47 (3H, m, Ar-H), 7.37 (2H, m, Ar-H), 7.34 (3H, m, Ar -H), 5.32 (1H, d, J = 8.0 Hz, H-1), 5.21 (1H, dd, J = 8.0 and 10.2 Hz, H-2), 5.21 (1H, dd, J = 3.1 and 10.3 Hz, H-3), 4.72 (1H, d, J = 3.7 Hz, H-4), 4.51 (1H, dd, J = 11.1 and 6.6 Hz, H-6a), 4.22 (1H, dd, J = 11.2 and 6.8 Hz, H-6b), 4.03 (1H, m, H-5), 3.28 (3H, s, 1-OCH_3); ^{13}C NMR (100 MHz, CDCl$_3$): δ_C 179.1 (2-Br.C$_6$H$_4$CO-), 167.3, 165.2, 164.2 (3 × 3-Cl.C$_6$H$_4$.CO-), 136.3, 132.3, 130.3, 129.6, 126.5, 125.6 (2-Br.C$_6$H$_4$CO-), 131.9 (×3), 131.5 (×2), 131.1 (×3), 129.4 (×4), 129.0 (×4), 128.8 (×2) (3 × 3-Cl.C$_6$H$_4$.CO-), 104.3 (C-1), 77.1 (C-2), 77.1 (C-4), 75.2 (C-3), 69.1 (C-5), 63.3 (C-6), 57.1 (1-OCH_3); LC–MS [M + 1]$^+$ 793.65; Calcd. For $C_{35}H_{26}O_{10}$Br.Cl: C, 52.99%, H, 3.31%; Found: C, 52.98%, H, 3.32%.

Methyl 6-*O*-(2-bromobenzoyl)-2,3,4-tri-*O*-(4-chlorobenzoyl)-*β*-D-galactopyranoside (**6**): Color light white; Yield 77%, m.p. 184–185 °C; (R_f = 0.52); FTIR: ν_{max} 1711 (-CO) cm^{-1}. ^{1}H NMR (400 MHz, CDCl$_3$): δ_H 8.01 (6H, m, Ar-H), 7.81 (6H, m, Ar-H), 7.72 (1H, d, J = 7.6 Hz, Ar-H), 7.43 (1H, d, J = 7.4 Hz, Ar-H), 7.30 (2H, m, Ar-H), 5.79 (1H, d, J = 3.6 Hz, H-1), 5.53 (1H, dd, J = 3.6 and 10.0 Hz, H-2), 5.0 (1H, m, H-3), 4.76 (1H, t, J = 9.6 Hz, H-4), 4.22 (1H, m, H-6a), 4.0 (1H, t, J = 10.2 Hz, H-6b), 3.55 (1H, m, H-5), 3.18 (3H, s, 1-OCH_3); ^{13}C NMR (100 MHz, CDCl$_3$): δ_C 178.7 (2-Br.C$_6$H$_4$CO-), 167.2, 166.7, 164.2 (3 × 3-Cl.C$_6$H$_4$.CO-), 136.2, 132.3, 130.4, 129.5, 126.3, 125.6 (2-Br.C$_6$H$_4$CO-), 132.3 (×3), 131.4 (×2), 131.3 (×3), 129.3 (×4), 129.1 (×4), 128.2 (×2) (3 × 3-Cl.C$_6$H$_4$.CO-), 104.1 (C-1), 77.3 (C-2), 77.3 (C-4), 75.1 (C-3), 69.4 (C-5), 63.2 (C-6), 57.1 (1-OCH_3); LC–MS [M + 1]$^+$ 793.65; Calcd. For $C_{35}H_{26}O_{10}$Br.Cl: C, 52.99%, H, 3.31%; Found: C, 52.98%, H, 3.33%.

Methyl 6-*O*-(2-bromobenzoyl)-2,3,4-tri-*O*-(4-t-butylbenzoyl)-*β*-D-galactopyranoside (**7**): Color white; Yield 53%. m.p. 122–123 °C; (R_f = 0.53); FTIR: ν_{max} 1718 (-CO) cm^{-1}. ^{1}H NMR (400 MHz, CDCl$_3$): δ_H 8.04 (6H, m, 3 × Ar-H), 7.79 (1H, d, J = 7.4 Hz, Ar-H), 7.62 (1H, d, J = 7.4 Hz, Ar-H), 7.59 (6H, m, 3 × Ar-H), 7.31 (2H, m, Ar-H), 5.20 (1H, d,

$J = 8.2$ Hz, H-1), 5.71 (1H, dd, $J = 8.1$ and 10.5 Hz, H-2), 5.68 (1H, dd, $J = 3.1$ and 10.6 Hz, H-3), 5.12 (1H, d, $J = 3.5$ Hz, H-4), 5.0 (1H, dd, $J = 11.1$ and 6.2 Hz, H-6a), 4.81 (1H, dd, $J = 11.0$ and 6.3 Hz, H-6b), 4.08 (1H, m, H-5), 3.28 (3H, s, 1-OCH_3), 1.25, 123, 122{27H, 3 × s, 3×(CH_3)$_3$C-}; ^{13}C NMR (100 MHz, $CDCl_3$): δ_C 179.0 (2-Br.C_6H_4CO-), 174.4, 174.2, 174.1 {3×(CH_3)$_3$CC_6H_4CO-}, 135.8, 132.5, 130.4, 129.5, 126.5, 125.3 (2-Br.C_6H_4CO-), 132.4 (×3), 132.4 (×2), 132.4, 130.9 (×3), 129.9 (×3), 126.5 (×3), 125.5 (×3) {3×(CH_3)$_3$CC_6H_4CO-}, 104.3 (C-1), 77.3 (C-2), 77.1 (C-4), 75.3 (C-3), 69.3 (C-5), 63.2 (C-6), 57.1 (1-OCH_3), 35.6, 35.5, 35.4 {(×3)(CH_3)$_3$CC_6H_4CO-}, 13.6 (×3), 13.6 (×3), 13.4 (×3) {(×3)(CH_3)$_3$CC_6H_4CO-}; LC–MS [M+1]$^+$ 858.66; Calcd. For $C_{47}H_{53}O_{10}$Br: C, 65.76%, H, 6.23%; Found: C, 65.77%, H, 6.22%.

3.4. Microorganisms

Five human pathogenic bacteria and two plant pathogenic fungi were used in the current study. The details about these strains are shown in Table S5. All microorganisms were obtained from the Department of Microbiology, Faculty of Biological Science, University of Chittagong, Bangladesh. The isolates were kept frozen at a temperature of $-20\,^\circ$C until they were needed. When the bacterial strains were needed, they were grown on Mueller–Hinton agar medium for 18 h at a temperature between 30–37 $^\circ$C. Similarly, the fungal strains were grown on Sabouraud dextrose agar medium for a period of 5 to 7 days at 25 $^\circ$C [63].

3.5. Antibacterial Activity

The methodology employed to determine the antibacterial properties of the synthesized compounds (each compound dissolved in dimethyl sulfoxide 7% DMSO) involved the use of the disc diffusion approach. This was done following a previously described method with slight modifications [64]. First, an inoculum was obtained from a bacterial colony and diluted to a concentration of 0.5 McFarland standard in sterile saltwater containing 0.9% NaCl. The suspension was then transferred to a sterile tube and allowed to settle for 5 min, after which the top homogeneous solution was transferred to another sterile tube. The concentration of the solution was adjusted to a 0.5 McFarland turbidity standard to obtain an inoculum of approximately 10^6 CFU/mL.

3.6. Determination of MIC and MBC

To determine the minimum inhibitory concentration (MIC) of the synthesized compounds against the tested bacterial strains [63,64], a dilution method was employed. The objective was to establish the lowest concentration of the compound at which approximately 90% of bacterial growth was inhibited. To this end, a bacterial suspension of 300 μL at a concentration of 0.5 McFarland standard was seeded into individual tubes of 9 mL nutrient broth, with each tube receiving 1 mL of different concentrations of the synthesized compound at twofold serial dilutions and 7% DMSO, which served as the negative control. The tubes were then kept at 37 $^\circ$C for a whole night. The MIC and MBC values were determined by using the naked eye to compare the turbidity of the tube to that of a reference medium with a 0.5 McFarland value.

3.7. Antifungal Activity

The food poisoning method [65] with potato dextrose agar (PDA) as the culture medium was used to test the antifungal action. Twenty milliliters of 45 $^\circ$C sterilized, melted potato dextrose agar medium (PDA) was placed into sterile 70-mm glass Petri plates. The "poisoned food" method [64] was used to determine how the synthesized MDGP (1) derivatives affected the growth of the fungal mycelium.

3.8. Cytotoxic Activity Evaluation

The brine shrimp lethality assay (BSLA) was utilized to evaluate the toxicity of the MDGP analogs [66]. Each vial contained 5 mL of NaCl solution and 20 μL of MDGP analogs dissolved in DMSO. Vials A, B, C, and D had volumes of 4, 8, 16, and 32 μL, respectively.

Each vial was inoculated with 10 brine shrimp nauplii at three different concentrations. A control test was conducted using ten nauplii in 5 mL of saltwater. The vials were incubated at ambient temperature for 24–48 h. Following incubation, the vials were examined under magnification and enumerated to ascertain the number of viable specimens. Concentrations exhibit a mean nauplii mortality rate. There were no fatalities in the control group.

3.9. Structure–Activity Relationship (SAR)

A structure–activity relationship (SAR) analysis was performed to identify the active portion of the synthesized molecule. This popular technology is often used in drug design according to Hunt [67] and Kim's [68] membrane permeation concept.

3.10. PASS Prediction and Bioactivity

The online pass website (http://www.pharmaexpert.ru/passonline/) (accessed on 23 March 2023), which is the most accurate site for predicting the bioactivity of synthesized MDGP, **1** compound, was used to obtain the pass prediction data (Pa > Pi value) [69]. PASS outcomes are revealed by Pa (probability for active molecule) and Pi (probability for inactive molecule). With potentialities, the Pa and Pi scores vary in the range of 0.00 to 1.00 and, usually, Pa + Pi ≠ 1, as these potentialities are predicted freely. Biological actions with Pa > Pi are only thought of as probable for a selected drug molecule. In the present study, the Molinspiration online server (https://www.molinspiration.com/cgi-bin/properties) (accessed on 25 March 2023) was utilized to analyze the drug-like properties of lead compounds. The Molinspiration cheminformatics engine allows for the fast prediction of biological activity and virtual screening of large collections of molecules and the selection of molecules with the highest probability to show biological activity. Then, the compound structures were drawn and changed into their smile forms using the SwissADME free online weblink (http://www.swissadme.ch) (accessed on 26 March 2023) to find the antimicrobial spectrum using the PASS tool. In particular, the Pa > Pi value was examined for its antiviral, antifungal, and antibacterial effects.

3.11. Geometry DFT Optimization

In computer-aided drug design, quantum mechanical methods are often used to predict thermal, molecular orbital, and molecular electrostatic potential qualities. Using the Gaussian 09 tool [70], all structures' geometries were improved and changed further. Density functional theory (DFT) with Becke's three-parameter hybrid model (B) [71] and Lee, Yang, and Parr's (LYP) correlation functional [72]. The first optimization of all chemicals was performed in the gas phase. For each of the MDGP analogs, the HOMO-LUMO energy gap, hardness (η), and softness (S) were calculated from the energies of the frontier HOMO and LUMO as reported, considering Parr and Pearson's interpretation of DFT and Koopman's theorem [73] on the correlation of chemical potential (μ), electronegativity (χ), and electrophilicity (ω) with HOMO and LUMO energy (ε). The following equations were used to calculate global chemical reactivity by analyzing molecular orbital features [74].

$$\mathrm{Gap}(\Delta\varepsilon) = \varepsilon\mathrm{LUMO} - \varepsilon\mathrm{HOMO}$$

$$\eta = \frac{[\varepsilon\mathrm{LUMO} - \varepsilon\mathrm{HOMO}]}{2}$$

$$S = \frac{1}{\eta}$$

$$\mu = \frac{[\varepsilon\mathrm{LUMO} + \varepsilon\mathrm{HOMO}]}{2}$$

$$\chi = -\frac{[\varepsilon\mathrm{LUMO} + \varepsilon\mathrm{HOMO}]}{2}$$

$$\omega = \frac{\mu 2}{2\eta}$$

3.12. Protein Selection and Molecular Docking

The structure of the dengue virus 1 NS2B/NS3 protease (PDB ID: 3L6P) was found in the protein databank library [75]. Using PyMol (version 1.3) software packages [76] all heteroatoms and water molecules were removed. Using Swiss-PdbViewer (version 4.1.0), the protein's energy was minimized. Then, molecular docking modeling [77] was performed using the PyRx application (version 0.8), imagining the target protein as a macromolecule and the MDGP-1 compounds as ligands. The protein and ligands were input by converting the pdb format to pdbqt, and the AutoDock Tools of the MGL software package were used to perform this job. In AutoDockVina, the size of the grid box was maintained at (47.7033, 64.6084, and 51.6510 Å) along the X, Y, and Z axes and was centered using the following dimension, $-2.021 \times 2.164 \times 6.319$ and grid spacing 0.061×0.061 was used to cover the active site along with the essential residues within the binding pocket. After docking, the structures of both the macromolecule and ligand were saved in pdbqt format and Accelrys Discovery Studio (version 4.1) was employed to explore the results of docking and to predict the nonbonding interactions among the (MDGP, **1**) analogs and amino acid chains of the receptor protein [78,79]. Using a Lig plot and a Ramachandran plot (Figure S6) to check the validity of the target receptor, more than 90% of the residues were in the allowed area.

3.13. Molecular-Dynamics Simulation

The molecular-dynamics simulation study was performed with the help of the AMBER14 force field [80] and the YASARA dynamics [81] software package. The steepest gradient algorithms and the simulated annealing method (5000 cycles) were used to obtain starting energy levels as low as possible [82]. The simulations were run with a time step of 2.0 fs [83]. The simulation paths were saved every 100 ps and the end run was performed for 150 ns. Root mean square deviations (RMSD), root mean square fluctuations (RMSF), radius of gyrations (Rg), solvent accessible surface area (SASA), and hydrogen bonds were all calculated using the simulation paths [84,85].

3.14. Pharmacokinetic and Drug-Likeness Prediction

ADMET properties are one of the most significant aspects of drug molecules and are described as pharmacokinetic properties. For this reason, the best-identified analogs were evaluated using pkCSM [61] for their in silico pharmacokinetic parameters, including intestinal absorption, blood–brain barrier, metabolism, clearance, and toxicity.

4. Conclusions

In this research, a series of (MDGP, **1**) compounds were synthesized and analyzed for their in vitro antimicrobial, cytotoxicity, and in silico properties. The insertion of various aliphatic and aromatic groups into the (MDGP, **1**) structures can significantly improve their biological activity. The synthesized compounds were more effective against gram-positive bacteria than gram-negative bacteria. The examined compounds also showed potential efficacy against all fungal strains. In particular, the study showed that benzoyl compounds (**5–7**) had better pharmacokinetic and biological profiles and could be more effective against bacteria and fungi. Molecular docking was used to explain these findings because it showed that MDGP compounds have promising antimicrobial effects. With the dengue virus-1 NS2B/NS3 protease, MDGP compounds **2–7** had positive interactions and binding energies when they were bound to it. The ability of the compounds (**5–7**) to fight against the target was very effective in silico studies. The molecular electrostatic potential study showed where the ligand had the most negative and positive surface areas. This helped predict where the best places for hydrogen bonding sites would be. This finding was strongly supported by MD simulations at 150 ns, which showed that the docked complex was stable in its binding in the trajectory analysis. Additionally, most of the designed molecules had better kinetic factors and still followed all of the rules for drugs and therapeutics.

Supplementary Materials: The following supporting information can be downloaded at: https://www.mdpi.com/article/10.3390/ph16070998/s1, Figure S1: Spectra; Figure S2–S5: Antimicrobial; Figure S6: Alignment and Ramachandran plot of dengue virus 1 NS2B/NS3. Table S1: MIC and MBC values; Tables S2–S4: In silico; Table S5: Name of the pathogenic microorganisms.

Author Contributions: F.A. (Faez Ahmmed): synthetic experiments; S.H.A.-M. and E.M.A.: editing, validation, resources; I.H.E.: computation and interpretation of results; F.A. (Ferdausi Ali): microbial assay; A.R.B., J.J. and T.B.H.: validation and improvement of the article; S.M.A.K.: conceptualization, methodology, article writing, results monitoring, and supervision. All authors have read and agreed to the published version of the manuscript.

Funding: This work was supported by Princess Nourah Bint Abdulrahman University Researchers Supporting Project number (PNURSP2023R158) Princess Nourah Bint Abdulrahman University, Riyadh, Saudi Arabia. Additionally, this work was supported by the Research and Publication Cell (2022–2023), University of Chittagong, Bangladesh.

Institutional Review Board Statement: Not applicable.

Informed Consent Statement: Not applicable.

Data Availability Statement: Data are available in the article and the Supplementary Materials.

Acknowledgments: The authors are thankful to the Princess Nourah Bint Abdulrahman University Researchers for supporting this research [Project number (PNURSP2023R158)] Princess Nourah Bint Abdulrahman University, Riyadh, Saudi Arabia. In addition, this work was supported by the Research and Publication Cell (2022–2023), University of Chittagong, Bangladesh. We are very much indebted to the Director, Wazed Miah Science Research Centre, JU, and Dhaka, Bangladesh for recording the spectra.

Conflicts of Interest: The authors declare no conflict of interest.

References

1. Cowan, M.M. Plants Products as Antimicrobial Agents. *Clin. Microbiol Rev.* **1999**, *12*, 564–582. [CrossRef]
2. Coates, A.; Hu, Y.; Bax, R.; Page, C. The Future Challenges Facing the Development of New Antimicrobial Drugs. *Nat. Rev. Drug Discov.* **2002**, *1*, 895–910. [CrossRef]
3. Wright, P.M.; Seiple, I.B.; Myers, A.G. The Evolving Role of Chemical Synthesis in Antibacterial Drug Discovery. *Angew. Chem. Int. Edit.* **2014**, *53*, 8840–8869. [CrossRef]
4. Arshad, M.; Bhat, A.; Athar, F. Heterocyclic Azoles and their Biological Application as Antimicrobials. *J. Nat. Sci. Biol. Med.* **2011**, *2*, 131.
5. Kato, K.; Ishiwa, A. The Role of Carbohydrates in Infection Strategies of Enteric Pathogens. *Trop. Med. Health* **2015**, *43*, 41–52. [CrossRef] [PubMed]
6. Sears, P.; Wong, C.H. Intervention of Carbohydrate Recognition by Proteins and Nucleic Acids. *Proc. Natl. Acad. Sci. USA* **1996**, *93*, 12086–12093. [CrossRef]
7. Seeberger, P.H.; Werz, D.B. Synthesis and Medical Applications of Oligosaccharides. *Nature* **2007**, *446*, 1046–1051. [CrossRef]
8. Chen, S.; Fukuda, M. Cell Type-specific roles of carbohydrates in tumor metastasis. *Meth. Enzymol.* **2006**, *416*, 371–380.
9. Kabir, A.K.M.S.; Kawsar, S.M.A.; Bhuiyan, M.M.R.; Rahman, M.S.; Banu, B. Biological evaluation of some octanoyl derivatives of methyl 4,6-O-cyclohexylidene-α-D-glucopyranoside. *Chittagong Univ. J. Biol. Sci.* **2008**, *3*, 53–64. [CrossRef]
10. Gubler, D.J. Dengue and dengue hemorrhagic fever. *Clin. Microbiol. Rev.* **1998**, *11*, 480–496. [CrossRef] [PubMed]
11. Monath, T.P. Dengue: The risk to developed and developing countries. *Proc. Natl. Acad. Sci. USA* **1994**, *91*, 2395–2400. [CrossRef]
12. Shagir, A.C.; Bhuiyan, M.M.R.; Ozeki, Y.; Kawsar, S.M.A. Simple and rapid synthesis of some nucleoside derivatives: Structural and spectral characterization. *Curr. Chem. Lett.* **2016**, *5*, 83–92.
13. Meadows, D.C.; Sanchez, T.; Neamati, N.; North, T.W.; Gervay-Hague, J. Ring Substituents Effects on Biological Activity of Vinyl Sulfones as Inhibitors of HIV-1. *Bioorg. Med. Chem.* **2007**, *15*, 1127–1137. [CrossRef]
14. Bulbul, M.Z.H.; Chowdhury, T.S.; Misbah, M.M.H.; Ferdous, J.; Dey, S.; Hasan, I.; Fujii, Y.; Ozeki, Y.; Kawsar, S.M.A. Synthesis of new series of pyrimidine nucleoside derivatives bearing the acyl moieties as potential antimicrobial agents. *Pharmacia* **2021**, *68*, 23–34. [CrossRef]
15. Klekota, J.; Roth, F.P. Chemical Substructures that Enrich for Biological Activity. *Bioinformatics* **2008**, *24*, 2518–2525. [CrossRef]

16. Maowa, J.; Alam, A.; Rana, K.M.; Hosen, A.; Dey, S.; Hasan, I.; Fujii, Y.; Ozeki, Y.; Kawsar, S.M.A. Synthesis, characterization, synergistic antimicrobial properties and molecular docking of sugar modified uridine derivatives. *Ovidius. Univ. Ann. Chem.* **2021**, *32*, 6–21. [CrossRef]

17. Kabir, A.K.M.S.; Kawsar, S.M.A.; Bhuiyan, M.M.R.; Islam, M.R.; Rahman, M.S. Biological Evaluation of Some Mannopyranoside Derivatives. *Bull. Pure Appl. Sci.* **2004**, *23*, 83–91.

18. Alam, A.; Hosen, M.A.; Hosen, A.; Fujii, Y.; Ozeki, Y.; Kawsar, S.M.A. Synthesis, characterization, and molecular docking against a receptor protein FimH of *Escherichia coli* (4XO8) of thymidine derivatives. *J. Mex. Chem. Soc.* **2021**, *65*, 256–276. [CrossRef]

19. Islam, M.; Zzaman, A.; Rahman, M.; Rahman, M.A.; Kawsar, S.M.A. Novel methyl 4,6-O-benzylidene-α-D-glucopyranoside derivatives: Synthesis, structural characterization and evaluation of antibacterial activities. *Hacettepe J. Biol. Chem.* **2019**, *47*, 153–164. [CrossRef]

20. Insuasty, D.; Castillo, J.; Becerra, D.; Rojas, H.; Abonia, R. Synthesis of Biologically Active Molecules through Multicomponent Reactions. *Molecules* **2020**, *25*, 505. [CrossRef] [PubMed]

21. Odds, F.; Brown, A.J.P.; Gow, N.A.R. Antifungal Agents: Mechanism of Action. *Trends Microbiol.* **2003**, *6*, 272–279. [CrossRef] [PubMed]

22. Kawsar, S.M.A.; Hosen, M.A.; Fujii, Y.; Ozeki, Y. Thermochemical, DFT, molecular docking and pharmacokinetic studies of methyl β-D-galactopyranoside esters. *J. Comput. Chem. Mol. Model* **2020**, *4*, 452–462. [CrossRef]

23. Maowa, J.; Hosen, M.A.; Alam, A.; Rana, K.M.; Fujii, Y.; Ozeki, Y.; Kawsar, S.M.A. Pharmacokinetics and molecular docking studies of uridine derivatives as SARS- COV-2 M^{pro} inhibitors. *Phys. Chem. Res.* **2021**, *9*, 385–412.

24. Jumina, J.; Mutmainah, M.; Purwono, B.; Kuniawan, Y.S.; Syah, Y.M. Antibacterial and Antifungal Activity of Three Monosaccharide Monomyristate Derivatives. *Molecules* **2019**, *24*, 3692. [CrossRef] [PubMed]

25. Lucarini, S.; Fagioli, L.; Campana, R.; Cole, H.; Duranti, A.; Baffone, W.; Vllasaliu, D.; Casettari, L. Unsaturated fatty acids lactose esters: Cytotoxicity, permeability enhancement and antimicrobial activity. *Eur. J. Pharm. Biopharm.* **2016**, *107*, 88–96. [CrossRef]

26. Kawsar, S.M.A.; Hosen, M.A. An optimization and pharmacokinetic studies of some thymidine derivatives. *Turkish Comp. Theo. Chem.* **2020**, *4*, 59–66. [CrossRef]

27. Spriha, S.E.; Rahman, S.M.A. A Review on Biological Activities of Sugars and Sugar Derivatives. *Dhaka Univ. J. Pharm. Sci.* **2022**, *20*, 381–394. [CrossRef]

28. Wang, G.; Dyatkina, N.; Prhavc, M.; Williams, C.; Serebryany, V.; Hu, Y.; Huang, Y.; Wu, X.; Chen, T.; Huang, W.; et al. Synthesis and anti-HCV activity of sugar-modified guanosine analogues: Discovery of AL-611 as an HCV NS5B polymerase inhibitor for the treatment of chronic hepatitis C. *J. Med. Chem.* **2020**, *63*, 10380–10395. [CrossRef]

29. Frommer, J.; Karg, B.; Weisz, K.; Muller, S. Preparation and Characterization of Pyrene Modified Uridine Derivatives as Potential Electron Donors in RNA. *Org. Biomol. Chem.* **2018**, *16*, 7663–7673. [CrossRef]

30. Staro, J.; Dbrowski, J.M.; Guzik, M. Lactose esters: Synthesis and Biotechnological Applications. *Crit. Rev. Biotechnol.* **2018**, *38*, 1–14. [CrossRef]

31. ALrajhi, M.; Al-Rasheedi, M.; Eltom, S.E.M.; Alhazmi, Y.; Mustafa, M.M.; Ali, A.M. Antibacterial Activity of Date Palm Cake Extracts (Phoenix dactylifera). *Cogent Food Agric.* **2019**, *5*, 1625479. [CrossRef]

32. Alfindee, M.N.; Zhang, Q.; Subedi, Y.P.; Shrestha, J.P.; Kawasaki, Y.; Grilley, M.; Takemoto, J.Y.; Chang, C.T. One Step Synthesis of Carbohydrate Esters as Antibacterial and Antifungal Agent. *Bioorg. Med. Chem.* **2018**, *26*, 765–774. [CrossRef]

33. Mutmainah, J.; Purwono, B. Chemical synthesis of monosaccharide lauric acid esters as antibacterial and antifungal agents. *Mater. Sci. Forum.* **2019**, *948*, 63–68. [CrossRef]

34. LeTourneau, N.; Vimal, P.; Klepacki, D.; Mankin, A.; Melman, A. Synthesis and Antibacterial Activity of Desosamine-Modified Macrolide Derivatives. *Bioorg. Med. Chem. Lett.* **2012**, *22*, 4575–4578. [CrossRef]

35. Payne, D.J.; Gwynn, M.N.; Holmes, D.J.; Pompliano, D.L. Drugs for bad bugs: Confronting the challenges of antibacterial discovery. *Nat. Rev. Drug Discov.* **2007**, *6*, 29–40. [CrossRef]

36. Mulcahy, L.R.; Isabella, V.M.; Lewis, K. Pseudomonas aeruginosa biofilms in disease. *Micro. Ecol.* **2014**, *68*, 1–12. [CrossRef]

37. Martins, P.M.; Merfa, M.V.; Takita, M.A.; De Souza, A.A. Persistence in phytopathogenic bacteria: Do we know enough? *Front. Microbiol.* **2018**, *9*, 1099. [CrossRef]

38. Silhavy, T.J.; Kahne, D.; Walker, S. The bacterial cell envelope. *Cold Spring Harb. Perspect. Biol.* **2010**, *2*, a000414. [CrossRef] [PubMed]

39. Isono, K. Nucleoside antibiotics: Structure, biological activity, and biosynthesis. *J. Antibiot.* **1988**, *41*, 1711–1739. [CrossRef]

40. Aljeldah, M.M.; Yassin, M.T.; Mostafa, A.A.F.; Aboul-Soud, M.A.M. Synergistic Antibacterial Potential of Greenly Synthesized Silver Nanoparticles with Fosfomycin against some Nosocomial Bacterial Pathogens. *Infect. Drug Resist.* **2023**, *2023*, 125–142. [CrossRef]

41. Wang, Y.; Chen, J.; Zheng, X.; Yang, X.; Ma, P.; Cai, Y.; Chen, Y. Design of novel analogues of short antimicrobial peptide anoplin with improved antimicrobial activity. *J. Peptide Sci.* **2014**, *20*, 945–951. [CrossRef]

42. Salehi, P.; Babanezhad-Harikandei, K.; Bararjanian, M.; Al-Harrasi, A.; Esmaeili, M.-A.; Aliahmadi, A. Synthesis of novel 1, 2, 3-triazole tethered 1, 3-disubstituted β-carboline derivatives and their cytotoxic and antibacterial activities. *Med. Chem. Res.* **2016**, *25*, 1895–1907. [CrossRef]

43. Yoon, B.K.; Jackman, J.A.; Valle-Gonzalez, E.R.; Cho, N.J. Antibacterial free fatty acids and monoglycerides: Biological activities, experimental testing, and therapeutic applications. *Int. J. Mol. Sci.* **2018**, *19*, 1114. [CrossRef] [PubMed]

44. Kawsar, S.M.A.; Matsumoto, R.; Fujii, Y.; Matsuoka, H.; Masuda, N.; Iwahara, C.; Yasumitsu, H.; Kanaly, R.A.; Sugawara, S.; Hosono, M.; et al. Cytotoxicity and Glycan-Binding Profile of α-D-Galactose-Binding Lectin from the Eggs of a Japanese Sea Hare (*Aplysia kurodai*). *Protein J.* **2011**, *30*, 509–519. [CrossRef] [PubMed]
45. Almeida, R.D.; Han, N.; Perez, Y.; Kirkpatrick, J.; Wang, S.; Sheridan, Y.M.C. Design, synthesis, and nanostructure-dependent antibacterial activity of cationic peptide amphiphiles. *ACS Appl. Mat. Interfaces* **2018**, *11*, 2790–2801. [CrossRef] [PubMed]
46. Smith, A.; Nobmann, P.; Henehan, G.; Bourke, P.; Dunne, J. Synthesis and Antimicrobial Evaluation of Carbohydrate and Polyhydroxylated Non-Carbohydrate Fatty Acid Ester and Ether Derivatives. *Carbohydr. Res.* **2008**, *343*, 2557–2566. [CrossRef]
47. Martínez-Culebras, P.V.; Gandía, M.; Boronat, A.; Marcos, J.F.; Manzanares, P. Differential susceptibility of mycotoxin-producing fungi to distinct antifungal proteins (AFPs). *Food Microbiol.* **2021**, *97*, 103760. [CrossRef]
48. Perfect, J.R. The Antifungal Pipeline: A Reality Check. *Nat. Rev. Drug Discov.* **2017**, *16*, 603–616. [CrossRef]
49. de Souza, L.S.; Tosta, C.L.; Borlot, J.R.P.O.; Varricchio, M.C.B.N.; Kitagawa, R.R.; Filgueiras, P.R.; Kuster, R.M. Chemical Profile and Cytotoxic Evaluation of Aerial Parts of *Euphorbia tirucalli* L. on Gastric Adenocarcinoma (AGS Cells). *Nat. Prod. Res.* **2023**, *37*, 1–7. [CrossRef]
50. Saleh, S.S.; Salihi, S.S.A.; Mohammed, I.A. Biological activity Study for some heterocyclic compounds and their impact on the gram positive and negative bacteria. *Energy Procedia* **2019**, *157*, 296–306. [CrossRef]
51. Li, W.R.; Xie, X.B.; Shi, Q.S.; Zeng, H.Y.; Ou-Yang, Y.S.; Chen, Y.B. Antibacterial activity and mechanism of silver nanoparticles on *Escherichia coli*. *Appl. Microbiol. Biotechnol.* **2010**, *85*, 1115–1122. [CrossRef] [PubMed]
52. Judge, V.; Narasimhan, B.; Ahuja, M.; Sriram, D.; Yogeeswari, P.; Clercq, E.D.; Pannecouque, C.; Balzarini, J. Synthesis, antimycobacterial, antiviral, antimicrobial activities, and QSAR studies of isonicotinic acid-1-(substituted phenyl)-ethylidene/cycloheptylidene hydrazides. *Med. Chem. Res.* **2012**, *21*, 1935–1952. [CrossRef]
53. Cohen, N.; Benson, S.W. Estimation of heats of formation of organic compounds by additivity methods. *Chem. Rev.* **1993**, *93*, 2419–2438. [CrossRef]
54. Lien, E.J.; Guo, Z.R.; Li, R.L.; Su, C.T. Use of dipole moment as a parameter in drug-receptor interaction and quantitative structure-activity relationship studies. *J. Pharm. Sci.* **1982**, *71*, 641–655. [CrossRef] [PubMed]
55. Saravanan, S.; Balachandran, V. Quantum chemical studies, natural bond orbital analysis and thermodynamic function of 2,5-di-chlorophenylisocyanate. *Spectrochim. Acta Part A Mol. Biomol. Spectrosc.* **2014**, *120*, 351–364. [CrossRef]
56. Amin, M.L. P-glycoprotein inhibition for optimal drug delivery. *Drug Target Insight* **2013**, *7*, 27–34. [CrossRef]
57. Politzer, P.; Murray, J.S. Molecular electrostatic potentials and chemical reactivity. *Rev. Comput. Chem.* **1991**, *2*, 273–312.
58. Liu, X.; Wang, X.J. Potential inhibitors against 2019-nCoV coronavirus M protease from clinically approved medicines. *J. Genet. Genom.* **2020**, *7*, 119–121. [CrossRef]
59. Kawsar, S.M.A.; Mamun, S.M.A.; Rahman, M.S.; Yasumitsu, H.; Ozeki, Y. In Vitro Antibacterial and Antifungal Effects of a 30 kDa D-Galactoside-Specific Lectin from the Demosponge, *Halichondria okadai*. *Int. J. Biol. Life Sci.* **2011**, *6*, 31–37.
60. Hirata, K.; Uchida, T.; Nakajima, Y.; Maekawa, T.; Mizuki, T. Chemical Synthesis and Cytotoxicity of Neo-Glycolipids; Rare Sugar-Glycerol-Lipid Compounds. *Heliyon* **2018**, *4*, e00861. [CrossRef]
61. Pires, D.E.V.; Blundell, T.L.; Ascher, B.D. pkCSM: Predicting small-molecule pharmacokinetic and toxicity properties using graph-based signatures. *J. Med. Chem.* **2015**, *58*, 4066–4072. [CrossRef] [PubMed]
62. Oliveira, D.B.D.; Gaudio, A.C. BuildQSAR: A new computer program for QSAR analysis. *Mol. Inform.* **2001**, *19*, 599–601. [CrossRef]
63. Zhang, H.; Yang, J.; Zhao, Y. High Intensity Ultrasound Assisted Heating to Improve Solubility, Antioxidant and Antibacterial Properties of Chitosan-Fructose Maillard Reaction Products. *LWT Food Sci. Technol.* **2015**, *60*, 253–262. [CrossRef]
64. Jumina, N.A.; Fitria, A.; Pranowo, D.; Sholikhah, E.N.; Kurniawan, Y.S.; Kuswandi, B. Monomyristin and Monopalmitin Derivatives: Synthesis and Evaluation as Potential Antibacterial and Antifungal Agents. *Molecules* **2018**, *23*, 3141. [CrossRef]
65. Grover, R.K.; Moore, J.D. In-vitro efficacy of certain essential oils and plant extracts against three major pathogens of *Jatropha curcas* L. *Phytopathology* **1962**, *52*, 876–879.
66. McLaughlin, J.L. Crown-Gall Tumors in Potato Discs and Brine Shrimp Lethality: Two Simple Bioassays for Higher Plant Screening and Fractionation. In *Methods in Plant Biochemistry: Assays for Bioactivity*; Hostettmann, K., Ed.; Academic Press: Cambridge, MA, USA, 1991; Volume 6, pp. 1–32.
67. Hunt, W.A. The effects of aliphatic alcohols on the biophysical and biochemical correlates of membrane function. *Adv. Exp. Med. Biol.* **1975**, *56*, 195–210.
68. Kim, Y.M.; Farrah, S.; Baney, R.H. Structure–antimicrobial activity relationship for silanols, a new class of disinfectants, compared with alcohols and phenols. *Int. J. Antimicrob. Agents* **2007**, *29*, 217–222. [CrossRef]
69. Kumaresan, S.; Senthilkumar, V.; Stephen, A.; Balakumar, B.S. GC-MS analysis and pass-assisted prediction of biological activity spectra of extract of *Phomopsis* sp. isolated from *Andrographis paniculata*. *World J. Pharm. Res.* **2015**, *4*, 1035–1053.
70. Frisch, M.J.; Trucks, G.W.; Schlegel, H.B.; Scuseria, G.E.; Robb, A.; Cheeseman, J.R.; Scalmani, G.; Barone, V.; Mennucci, M.; Petersson, G.A.; et al. *Gaussian 09*; Gaussian Inc.: Wallingford, CT, USA, 2009.
71. Becke, A.D. Density-functional exchange-energy approximation with correct asymptotic behaviour. *Phys. Rev. A* **1988**, *38*, 3098–3100. [CrossRef]
72. Lee, C.; Yang, W.; Parr, R.G. Development of the colle-Salvetti correlation-energy formula into a functional of the electron density. *Phys. Rev. B* **1988**, *37*, 785–789. [CrossRef] [PubMed]

73. Pearson, R.G. Absolute electronegativity and hardness correlated with molecular orbital theory. *Proc. Nat. Acad. Sci. USA* **1986**, *83*, 8440–8441. [CrossRef] [PubMed]

74. Ouassaf, M.; Belaidi, S.; Khamouli, S.; Belaidi, H.; Chtita, S. Combined 3D-QSAR and Molecular Docking Analysis of Thienopyrimidine Derivatives as Staphylococcus aureus Inhibitors. *Acta. Chim. Slov.* **2021**, *68*, 289–303. [CrossRef]

75. Berman, H.M.; Westbrook, J.; Feng, Z.; Gilliland, G.; Bhat, T.N.; Weissig, H.; Shindyalov, I.N.; Bourne, P.E. The protein data bank. *Nucleic Acids Res.* **2000**, *28*, 235–242. [CrossRef] [PubMed]

76. Delano, W.I. *The PyMOL Molecular Graphics System*; De-Lano Scientific: San Carlos, CA, USA, 2002.

77. Guex, N.; Peitsch, M.C. SWISS-MODEL and the Swiss-PdbViewer: An environment for comparative protein modeling. *Electrophoresis* **1997**, *18*, 2714–2723. [CrossRef] [PubMed]

78. Aouidatea, A.; Ghaleba, A.; Ghamalia, M.; Chtitaa, S.; Choukrada, M.; Sbaia, A.; Bouachrineb, M.; Lakhlifi, M. Combined 3D-QSAR and Molecular Docking Study on 7,8-dialkyl-1,3-diaminopyrrolo-[3,2-f] Quinazoline Series Compounds to understand the binding mechanism of DHFR Inhibitors. *J. Mol. Strutc.* **2017**, *1139*, 319–327. [CrossRef]

79. Belhassana, A.; Chtita, S.; Zaki, H.; Alaqarbehd, M.; Alsakhene, N.; Almohtasebf, F.; Lakhlifia, T.; Bouachrinea, M. In silico detection of potential inhibitors from vitamins and their derivatives compounds against SARS-CoV-2 main protease by using molecular docking, molecular dynamic simulation and ADMET profiling. *J. Mol. Strutc.* **2022**, *1258*, 132652. [CrossRef]

80. Land, H.; Humble, M.S. YASARA: A tool to obtain structural guidance in biocatalytic investigations. *Methods Mol. Biol.* **2018**, *1685*, 43–67.

81. Wang, J.; Wolf, R.M.; Caldwell, J.W.; Kollman, P.A.; Case, D.A. Development and testing of a general Amber force field. *J. Comput. Chem.* **2004**, *25*, 1157–1174. [CrossRef]

82. Krieger, E.; Nielsen, J.E.; Spronk, C.A.E.M.; Vriend, G. Fast empirical pKa prediction by Ewald summation. *J. Mol. Graph. Model.* **2006**, *25*, 481–486. [CrossRef]

83. Krieger, E.; Vriend, G. New ways to boost molecular dynamics simulations. *J. Comput. Chem.* **2015**, *36*, 996–1007. [CrossRef]

84. Ouassaf, M.; Belaidi, S.; Al Mogren, M.M.; Chtita, S.; Khan, S.U.; Htar, T.T. Combined docking methods and molecular dynamics to identify effective antiviral 2, 5-diaminobenzophenonederivatives against SARS-CoV-2. *J. King Saud Univ. Sci.* **2021**, *33*, 101352. [CrossRef] [PubMed]

85. Ouassaf, M.; Belaidi, S.; Chtita, S.; Lanez, T.; Qais, F.A.; Amiruddin, H.M. Combined molecular docking and dynamics simulations studies of natural compounds as potent inhibitors against SARS-CoV-2 main protease. *J. Biomol. Struct. Dyn.* **2022**, *40*, 11264–11273. [CrossRef] [PubMed]

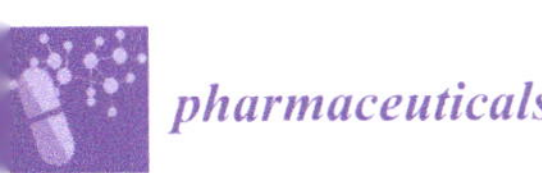

pharmaceuticals

MDPI

Review

The Role of AI in Drug Discovery: Challenges, Opportunities, and Strategies

Alexandre Blanco-González [1,2,3], Alfonso Cabezón [1,2], Alejandro Seco-González [1,2], Daniel Conde-Torres [1,2], Paula Antelo-Riveiro [1,2], Ángel Piñeiro [2,*] and Rebeca Garcia-Fandino [1,*]

[1] Department of Organic Chemistry, Center for Research in Biological Chemistry and Molecular Materials, University of Santiago de Compostela, CIQUS, 15705 Santiago de Compostela, Spain
[2] Soft Matter & Molecular Biophysics Group, Department of Applied Physics, Faculty of Physics, University of Santiago de Compostela, 15705 Santiago de Compostela, Spain
[3] MD.USE Innovations S.L., Edificio Emprendia, 15782 Santiago de Compostela, Spain
[*] Correspondence: Angel.Pineiro@usc.es (Á.P.); rebeca.garcia.fandino@usc.es (R.G.-F.)

Abstract: Artificial intelligence (AI) has the potential to revolutionize the drug discovery process, offering improved efficiency, accuracy, and speed. However, the successful application of AI is dependent on the availability of high-quality data, the addressing of ethical concerns, and the recognition of the limitations of AI-based approaches. In this article, the benefits, challenges, and drawbacks of AI in this field are reviewed, and possible strategies and approaches for overcoming the present obstacles are proposed. The use of data augmentation, explainable AI, and the integration of AI with traditional experimental methods, as well as the potential advantages of AI in pharmaceutical research, are also discussed. Overall, this review highlights the potential of AI in drug discovery and provides insights into the challenges and opportunities for realizing its potential in this field. *Note from the human authors*: This article was created to test the ability of ChatGPT, a chatbot based on the GPT-3.5 language model, in terms of assisting human authors in writing review articles. The text generated by the AI following our instructions (see Supporting Information) was used as a starting point, and its ability to automatically generate content was evaluated. After conducting a thorough review, the human authors practically rewrote the manuscript, striving to maintain a balance between the original proposal and the scientific criteria. The advantages and limitations of using AI for this purpose are discussed in the last section.

Keywords: artificial intelligence; drug discovery; AI-assisted content generation; AI-limitations

Citation: Blanco-González, A.; Cabezón, A.; Seco-González, A.; Conde-Torres, D.; Antelo-Riveiro, P.; Piñeiro, Á.; Garcia-Fandino, R. The Role of AI in Drug Discovery: Challenges, Opportunities, and Strategies. *Pharmaceuticals* 2023, 16, 891. https://doi.org/10.3390/ph16060891

Academic Editors: Halil İbrahim Ciftci, Belgin Sever and Hasan Demirci

Received: 22 May 2023
Revised: 14 June 2023
Accepted: 15 June 2023
Published: 18 June 2023

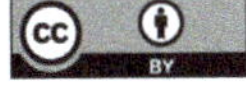

1. Methods for Writing this Paper

This paper was generated with the assistance of ChatGPT, a chatbot based on the GPT-3.5 language model, trained with a large corpus of text via OpenAI [1], which at that time did not have connection to the Internet. This tool is a natural language processing system, released on 30 November 2022, which is able to generate human-like text based on the inputs provided to it. For the purposes of this paper, the human authors provided the input, including the topic of the paper (the use of AI in drug discovery) and the number of sections to be considered, as well as the specific prompts and instructions for each section. The pieces of text generated by the AI were edited to correct and enrich the content, and to avoid repetitions and inconsistencies. All the references suggested by the AI were also revised. The final version of this work resulted from an iterative process of revisions by the human authors, assisted by the AI. The total percentage of similarity between the preliminary text, obtained directly from ChatGPT, and the current version of the manuscript is: identical 4.3%, minor changes 13.3%, and related meaning 16.3% [2]. The percentage of correct references in the preliminary text, obtained directly from ChatGPT, was just 6%. The original version generated by ChatGPT, along with the inputs used to create it, are included in the Supporting Information. The manuscript was first made public as a preprint on

8 December 2022 (https://doi.org/10.48550/arXiv.2212.08104). The image from the abstract was generated with DALL-E https://labs.openai.com/e/f9L5L4yGx1QFFeL5zHzHWNvI (Accessed on 6 December 2022)

2. Introduction to AI and Its Potential for Use in Drug Discovery

The use of artificial intelligence (AI) in medicinal chemistry has gained significant attention in recent years as a potential means of revolutionizing the pharmaceutical industry [3]. Drug discovery, the process of identifying and developing new medications, is a complex and time-consuming endeavor that traditionally relies on labor-intensive techniques, such as trial-and-error experimentation and high-throughput screening. However, AI techniques such as machine learning (ML) and natural language processing offer the potential to accelerate and improve this process by enabling more efficient and accurate analysis of large amounts of data [4]. The successful use of deep learning (DL) to predict the efficacy of drug compounds with high accuracy has been described recently by the authors of [5]. AI-based methods have also been able to predict the toxicity of drug candidates [6]. These and other research efforts have highlighted the capacity of AI to improve the efficiency and effectiveness of drug discovery processes. However, the use of AI in developing new bioactive compounds is not without challenges and limitations. Ethical considerations must be taken into account, and further research is needed to fully understand the advantages and limitations of AI in this area [7]. Despite these challenges, AI is expected to significantly contribute to the development of new medications and therapies in the next few years.

3. Limitations of the Current Methods in Drug Discovery

Currently, medicinal chemistry methods rely heavily on a hit-and-miss approach and large-scale testing techniques [8]. These techniques involve examining large numbers of potential drug compounds, in order to identify those with the desired properties. However, these methods can be slow, costly, and often yield results with low accuracy [6]. In addition, they can be limited by the availability of suitable test compounds and the difficulty of accurately predicting their behavior in the body [9].

Different algorithms based on AI, including supervised and unsupervised learning methods, reinforcement, and evolutionary or rule-based algorithms, can potentially contribute to solving these problems. These methods are typically based on the analysis of large amounts of data that can be exploited in different ways [9–11]. For instance, the efficacy and toxicity of new drug compounds can be predicted using these approaches, with greater accuracy and efficiency than when using traditional methods [12,13]. Furthermore, AI-based algorithms can also be employed to identify new targets for drug development, such as the specific proteins or genetic pathways involved in diseases [14]. This can expand the scope of drug discovery beyond the limitations of more conventional approaches and may eventually lead to the development of novel and more effective medications [15]. Thus, while traditional methods of pharmaceutical research have been relatively successful in the past, they are limited by their reliance on trial-and-error experimentation and their inability to accurately predict the behavior of new potential bioactive compounds [16]. AI-based approaches, on the other hand, have the ability to improve the efficiency and accuracy of drug discovery processes and can lead to the development of more effective medications.

4. The Role of ML in Predicting Drug Efficacy and Toxicity

One of the key applications of AI in medicinal chemistry is the prediction of the efficacy and toxicity of potential drug compounds. Classical protocols of drug discovery often rely on labor-intensive and time-consuming experimentation to assess the potential effects of a compound on the human body. This can be a slow and costly process, and the results are often uncertain and subject to a high degree of variability. AI techniques such as ML are able to overcome these limitations. Based on the analysis of a large amount of information, ML algorithms can identify patterns and trends that may not be apparent to human researchers.

This can enable the proposal of new bioactive compounds with minimum side effects in a much faster process than when using classical protocols. For instance, a DL algorithm has recently been trained using a dataset of known drug compounds, along with their corresponding biological activity [11]. The algorithm was then able to predict the activity of novel compounds with high accuracy. Significant contributions to prevent the toxicity of potential drug compounds, employing intensive training using large databases of known toxic and non-toxic compounds for ML, have also been published [17].

Another important application of AI in drug discovery is the identification of drug–drug interactions that take place when several drugs are combined for the same or different diseases in the same patient, resulting in altered effects or adverse reactions. This issue can be identified by AI-based approaches by analyzing large datasets of known drug interactions and recognizing the patterns and trends. This has been recently addressed by an ML algorithm used to accurately predict the interactions of novel drug pairs [18]. The role of AI to identify possible drug–drug interactions in the context of personalized medicine is also relevant, enabling the development of custom-made treatment plans that minimize the risk of adverse reactions. Personalized medicine aims to tailor treatment to the individual characteristics of each patient, including their genetic profile and response to medications.

The previous examples from the literature demonstrate that the use of AI in pharmaceutical research offers the ability to improve the prediction of the efficacy and toxicity of potential drug compounds. This can enable the development of more effective and safer medications and accelerate the drug discovery process.

5. The Impact of AI on the Drug Discovery Process and Potential Cost Savings

Another key application of AI in drug discovery is the design of novel compounds with specific properties and activities. Traditional methods often rely on the identification and modification of existing compounds, which can be a slow and labor-intensive process. AI-based approaches, on the other hand, can enable the rapid and efficient design of novel compounds with desirable properties and activities. For example, a deep learning (DL) algorithm has recently been trained on a dataset of known drug compounds and their corresponding properties, to propose new therapeutic molecules [10] with desirable characteristics such as solubility and activity, demonstrating the potential of these methods for the rapid and efficient design of new drug candidates.

Recently, DeepMind has made a significant contribution to the field of AI research with the development of AlphaFold, a revolutionary software platform for advancing our understanding of biology [19]. It is a powerful algorithm that uses protein sequence data and AI to predict the proteins' corresponding three-dimensional structures. This advance in structural biology is expected to revolutionize personalized medicine and drug discovery. AlphaFold represents a significant step forward in the use of AI in structural biology and life sciences in general.

ML techniques and molecular dynamics (MD) simulations are currently being used in the field of de novo drug design to improve efficiency and accuracy. The technique of combining these methodologies is being explored to take advantage of the synergies between them [20]. The use of interpretable machine learning (IML) and DL methods is also contributing to this effort. By leveraging the power of AI and MD, researchers are able to design drugs more effectively and efficiently than ever before.

6. Case Studies of Successful AI-Aided Drug Discovery Efforts

The potential of AI in the context of drug discovery has been demonstrated in several case studies. For example, the successful use of AI to identify novel compounds for the treatment of cancer has recently been reported by Gupta, R., et al. [21]. These authors trained a DL algorithm on a large dataset of known cancer-related compounds and their corresponding biological activity. As an output, novel compounds with high potential for future cancer treatment were obtained, demonstrating the ability of this method to discover new therapeutic candidates. The use of ML to identify small-molecule inhibitors of the protein MEK [22] has recently been described. MEK is also a possible target for the treatment of cancer, but the development of effective inhibitors has been challenging. The ML algorithm was able to identify novel inhibitors for this protein. Another example is the identification of novel inhibitors of beta-secretase (BACE1), a protein involved in the development of Alzheimer's disease [23] by using an ML algorithm. AI has also been successfully applied in the discovery of new antibiotics [24]. A pioneering ML approach has identified powerful types of antibiotic from a pool of more than 100 million molecules, including one that works against a wide range of bacteria, such as tuberculosis and untreatable bacterial strains [25]. The use of AI in the discovery of drugs to combat COVID-19 has been a promising area of research during the last two years. ML algorithms have been used to analyze large datasets of potential compounds and identify those with the most potential for treating the virus. In some cases, these AI-powered approaches have been able to identify promising drug candidates in a fraction of the time that it would take when using traditional methods [26–31].

Many more examples are available [3,32–37], showing that AI-based methods can accelerate the drug discovery process and enable the development of more effective medications.

7. The Role of Collaboration between AI Researchers and Pharmaceutical Scientists

The role of collaboration between AI researchers and pharmaceutical scientists is crucial in the development of innovative and effective treatments for various diseases. By combining their expertise and knowledge, they can create powerful algorithms and machine-learning models intended to predict the efficacy of potential drug candidates and speed up the drug discovery process. This collaboration can also help improve the accuracy and efficiency of clinical trials, as AI algorithms can be used to analyze the data collected during these trials to identify trends and the potential adverse effects of the drugs being tested. This can help pharmaceutical companies to make informed decisions about which drug candidates to pursue and can speed up the overall drug development process. Furthermore, collaboration between AI researchers and pharmaceutical scientists can also help to improve the accessibility and affordability of healthcare. By using AI algorithms to analyze data from large populations, they can be used to identify trends and patterns that can help predict the effectiveness of potential drug candidates for specific patient populations, which can help tailor treatments to the needs of individual patients. An illustrative example is the collaboration between the pharmaceutical company Merck and the AI company Numerate to develop AI-based approaches for medicinal chemistry [38]. Many new companies are currently arising around this area of research and their impact is expected to be significant in the short term [39]. By working together, they can help to identify new targets for drug development and improve the effectiveness of existing treatments, ultimately benefiting patients and improving their quality of life.

8. Challenges and Limitations of Using AI in Drug Discovery

Despite the potential benefits of AI in drug discovery, there are several challenges and limitations that must be considered. One of the key challenges is the availability of suitable data [40]. AI-based approaches typically require a large volume of information for training purposes [41]. In many cases, the amount of data that is accessible may be limited, or the data may be of low quality or inconsistent, which can affect the accuracy and reliability of the results [10]. Another challenge is presented by ethical considerations [42] since AI-based approaches may raise concerns about fairness and bias (see next section) [43]. For example, if the data used to train an ML algorithm are biased or unrepresentative, the resulting predictions may be inaccurate or unfair [44]. Ensuring the ethical and fair use of AI for the development of new therapeutic compounds is an important consideration that must be addressed [45]. Several strategies and approaches can be used to overcome the obstacles faced by AI in the context of chemical medicine. One approach is the use of data augmentation [46], which involves the generation of synthetic data to supplement existing datasets. This can increase the quantity and diversity of the data available for training ML algorithms, improving the accuracy and reliability of the results [47]. Another approach is the use of explainable AI (XAI) methods [48], which aim to provide interpretable and transparent explanations for the predictions made by ML algorithms. This can help to address concerns about bias and fairness in AI-based approaches [43] and provide a better understanding of the underlying mechanisms and assumptions behind the predictions [49].

Current AI-based approaches are not a substitute for traditional experimental methods, and they cannot replace the expertise and experience of human researchers [50,51]. AI can only provide predictions based on the data available, and the results must then be validated and interpreted by human researchers [52]. However, the integration of AI with traditional experimental methods can also enhance the drug discovery process [3]. By combining the predictive power of AI with the expertise and experience of human researchers [53], it is possible to optimize the drug discovery process and accelerate the development of new medications [54].

9. Ethical Considerations Regarding the Use of AI in the Pharmaceutical Industry

As discussed in the previous section, it is important to consider the ethical implications of using AI in this field [55,56]. One key issue is the potential for AI to be used to make decisions that affect people's health and well-being, such as decisions about which drugs to develop, which clinical trials to conduct, and how to market and distribute drugs. Another key concern is the potential for bias in AI algorithms, which could result in unequal access to medical treatment and the unfair treatment of certain groups of people. This could undermine the principles of equality and justice. The use of AI in the pharmaceutical industry also raises concerns about job losses due to automation. It is important to consider the potential impact on workers and provide support for those who may be affected. Additionally, the use of AI in the pharmaceutical industry raises questions about data privacy and security. As AI systems rely on large amounts of data to function, there is a risk that sensitive personal information could be accessed or misused. This could have serious consequences for individuals, as well as for the reputation of the companies involved. The collection and use of sensitive medical data must be performed in a way that respects the individuals' privacy and complies with the relevant regulations.

Overall, the ethical use of AI in the pharmaceutical industry requires careful consideration and the adoption of thoughtful approaches to addressing these concerns. This can include measures such as ensuring that AI systems are trained on diverse and representative data, regularly reviewing and auditing AI systems for bias, and implementing strong data privacy and security protocols. By addressing these issues, the pharmaceutical industry can use AI in a responsible and ethical manner.

10. Conclusions and Summary of the Potential of AI for Revolutionizing Drug Discovery

In conclusion, AI has the potential to revolutionize the drug discovery process, offering improved efficiency and accuracy, accelerated drug development, and the capacity for the development of more effective and personalized treatments (Figure 1). However, the successful application of AI in drug discovery is dependent on the availability of high-quality data, the addressing of ethical concerns, and the recognition of the limitations of AI-based approaches.

Recent developments in AI, including the use of data augmentation, explainable AI, and the integration of AI with traditional experimental methods, offer promising strategies for overcoming the challenges and limitations of AI in the context of drug discovery. The growing levels of interest and attention from researchers, pharmaceutical companies, and regulatory agencies, combined with the potential benefits of AI, make this an exciting and promising area of research, with the potential to transform the drug discovery process.

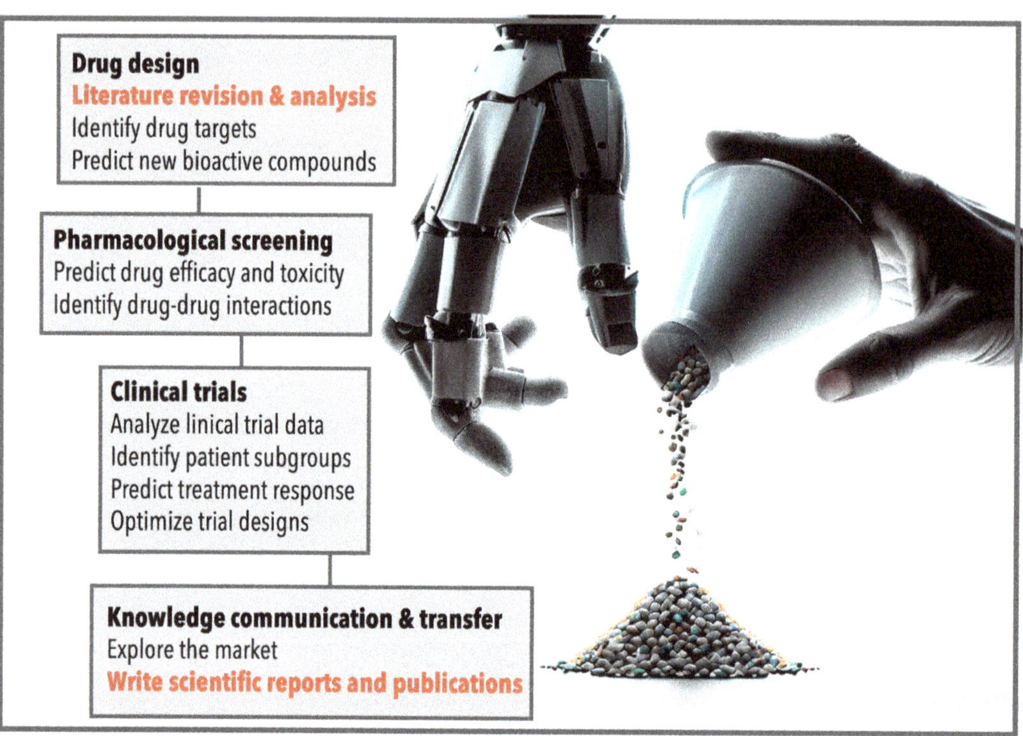

Figure 1. Graphical flowchart illustrating the development process of a pharmacologically active molecule, from design to knowledge communication and transfer. AI-based approaches complement traditional methods but still cannot replace human expertise. By combining the predictive power of AI with human researchers' knowledge, the drug discovery process can be optimized and accelerated. The present work examines the cutting-edge advancements in the stages of "Literature revision and analysis" and "Write scientific reports and publications" (highlighted in red) using ChatGPT, a chatbot based on the GPT-3.5 language model.

11. Expert Opinions from the Human Authors about ChatGPT and AI-Based Tools for Scientific Writing

As discussed in previous sections, AI has the potential to play a crucial role in the various stages of drug discovery, ranging from drug design to the final market introduction (Figure 1). However, the impact of AI extends beyond these areas and can greatly benefit the processing and analysis of scientific literature. Integrating AI into a literature review and article writing in the field of drug design holds immense promise. AI algorithms can expedite the review process, provide comprehensive insights from diverse data sources, and assist in identifying new research avenues. Additionally, AI-powered writing tools can enhance the quality and efficiency of scientific writing, enabling researchers to effectively communicate their findings. By embracing AI technologies in these domains, we not only save time and resources but also enhance the overall quality of drug design research, bringing us closer to the development of innovative and life-changing therapies.

The utilization of AI when composing literature reviews makes a significant contribution to drug discovery, which is the primary focus of this manuscript. Incorporating AI in the creation and evaluation of scientific literature offers several advantages that expedite the process of developing and approving new drugs. These advantages include efficient analysis of a large volume of articles, accurate extraction and summarization of information, access to up-to-date knowledge, the discovery of hidden insights, and integration across different disciplines. In the near future, the autonomous AI-assisted preparation of reviews is expected to become an integral part of the workflow of AI-assisted drug discovery. In the present review, we aimed to test the state-of-the-art AI tools for writing and revising the literature, contributing to the development of this research direction by establishing the initial foundations.

ChatGPT, a chatbot based on the GPT-3.5 language model (at the moment of preparation of this manuscript), has not been designed as an assistant for writing scientific papers. However, its ability to engage in coherent conversations with humans and provide new information on a wide range of topics, as well as its ability to correct and even generate pieces of computational code, has been a surprise to the scientific community. Therefore, we decided to test its potential to contribute to the preparation of a short review on the role of AI algorithms in drug discovery. As an AI assistant to write scientific papers, ChatGPT has several advantages, including its capacity to generate and optimize text quickly, as well as its ability to help users with several tasks, including the organization of information or even connecting ideas in some cases. However, this tool is in no way ideal as a technique to generate new content. Our revision of the text, which was generated by the AI following our instructions, required the application of major edits and corrections, including the replacement of nearly all the references since those provided by the software were clearly incorrect. This is a huge problem with ChatGPT, and it represents a key difference with respect to other computational tools such as typical web browsers, which are focused on providing reliable references for the required information. Another important problem of the employed AI-based tool is that it was trained in 2021 and so does not work with updated information. Most of these problems could be solved relatively quickly, which introduces new and urgent challenges regarding the control of apparently new content.

As a result of this experiment, we can state that ChatGPT is not a useful tool for writing reliable scientific texts without substantial human intervention. The program lacks the knowledge and expertise necessary to accurately and adequately convey complex scientific concepts and information. Additionally, the language and style used by ChatGPT may not be suitable for academic writing. In order to produce high-quality scientific texts, human input and human review are essential. One of the main reasons why this AI is not yet ready to be used in the production of scientific articles is its lack of ability to evaluate the veracity and reliability of the information that it processes. As a result, scientific text generated by ChatGPT will definitely contain errors or misleading information. It is also important to note that reviewers may find it not a trivial matter to distinguish between an article written by a human or by this AI. This makes it essential for the review processes to be thorough in order to prevent the publication of false or misleading information. A real risk is that predatory journals may exploit the opportunity for the quick production of scientific articles to generate large amounts of low-quality content. These journals, often motivated by profit rather than a commitment to scientific advancement, may use AI to rapidly produce articles, flooding the market with subpar research that undermines the credibility of the scientific community. One of the biggest dangers is the potential for the proliferation of false information in scientific articles, which could lead to a devaluation of the scientific enterprise itself. Losing trust in the accuracy and integrity of scientific research could have a detrimental impact on the progress of science.

There are several possible solutions for mitigating the risks associated with the use of AI in the production of scientific articles. One solution is to develop AI algorithms that are specifically designed for the production of scientific articles. These algorithms could be trained on large datasets of high-quality, peer-reviewed research, which would help to ensure the veracity of the information they generate. Additionally, these algorithms could be programmed to flag potentially problematic information, such as references to unreliable sources, which would alert researchers to the need for further review and verification. Another approach would be to develop AI systems that are better able to evaluate the authenticity and reliability of the information they process. This could involve training the AI on large datasets of high-quality scientific articles, as well as using techniques such as cross-validation and peer review to ensure that the AI produces accurate and trustworthy results. Another potential solution is to establish stricter guidelines and regulations for the use of AI in scientific research. This could include requiring researchers to disclose when they have used AI in the production of their articles, and implementing review processes to ensure that the AI-generated content meets certain standards of quality and accuracy. Additionally, it could also include requirements for researchers to thoroughly review and verify the exactitude of any information generated using AI before it is published, as well as penalties for those who fail to do so. It may also be useful to educate the public about the limitations of AI and the potential dangers of relying on it for scientific information. This could help to prevent the spread of misinformation and ensure that the public is better able to distinguish between reliable and unreliable sources of scientific information. Funding agencies and academic institutions could also play a role in promoting the responsible use of AI in scientific research by providing training and resources to help researchers understand the limitations of the technology.

Overall, addressing the risks associated with the use of AI in the production of scientific articles will require a combination of technical solutions, regulatory frameworks, and public education. By implementing these measures, we can ensure that AI is used responsibly and effectively in the world of science. It is important for researchers and policymakers to carefully consider the potential dangers of using AI in scientific research and to take steps to mitigate these risks. Until AI can be trusted to produce reliable and accurate information, it should be used with caution in the world of science. It is essential to carefully evaluate the information provided by AI tools and to validate it using reliable sources.

Supplementary Materials: The following supporting information can be downloaded at: https://www.mdpi.com/article/10.3390/ph16060891/s1. The Supplementary Information outlines the queries posed to ChatGPT on 6 December 2022, and the corresponding AI-generated responses. It offers insight into the AI's content generation process. Also, it provides an overview of the key AI algorithms and techniques mentioned in the manuscript, aiding readers' understanding of the AI methodologies used in the study.

Funding: This work was supported by the Spanish Agencia Estatal de Investigación (AEI) and the ERDF (RTI2018-098795-A-I00, PID2019-111327GB-I00, and PDC2022-133402-I00) by Xunta de Galicia and the ERDF (ED431F 2020/05, ED431B 2022/36, ED431F 2020/05, ED431B 2022/36, 06_IN606D_2021_2600276 and Centro Singular de Investigación de Galicia, accreditation 2016-2019, ED431G/09). R.G.-F. thanks the Ministerio de Ciencia, Innovación y Universidades for a "Ramón y Cajal" contract (RYC-2016-20335). D.C.-T. thanks Xunta de Galicia for a predoctoral contract (ED481A 2022/290).

Institutional Review Board Statement: Not applicable.

Informed Consent Statement: Not applicable.

Data Availability Statement: Data is contained within the article and Supplementary Material.

Acknowledgments: This work was funded by the Spanish Agencia Estatal de Investigación (AEI) and the ERDF (RTI2018-098795-A-I00, PID2019-111327GB-I00, and PDC2022-133402-I00) by Xunta de Galicia and the ERDF (ED431F 2020/05, ED431B 2022/36, and Centro Singular de Investigación de Galicia, accreditation 2016-2019, ED431G/09). R.G.-F. thanks the Ministerio de Ciencia, Innovación y Universidades for a "Ramón y Cajal" contract (RYC-2016-20335).

Conflicts of Interest: Author Alexandre Blanco-González was employed by the company MD.USE Innovations SL. The remaining authors declare that the research was conducted in the absence of any commercial or financial relationships that could be construed as a potential conflict of interest.

References

1. OpenAI. ChatGPT (Dec 6 Version) [Large Language Model]. 2022. Available online: https://chat.openai.com/chat (accessed on 6 December 2022).
2. Plagiarism Detector Software | Anti-Plagiarism Tools | Copyleaks. Available online: https://copyleaks.com (accessed on 6 December 2022).

3. Paul, D.; Sanap, G.; Shenoy, S.; Kalyane, D.; Kalia, K.; Tekade, R.K. Artificial intelligence in drug discovery and development. *Drug Discov. Today* **2021**, *26*, 80–93. [CrossRef] [PubMed]
4. Xu, Y.; Liu, X.; Cao, X.; Huang, C.; Liu, E.; Qian, S.; Liu, X.; Wu, Y.; Dong, F.; Qiu, C.W.; et al. Artificial intelligence: A powerful paradigm for scientific research. *Innovation* **2021**, *2*, 100179. [CrossRef] [PubMed]
5. Zhuang, D.; Ibrahim, A.K. Deep learning for drug discovery: A study of identifying high efficacy drug compounds using a cascade transfer learning approach. *Appl. Sci.* **2021**, *11*, 7772. [CrossRef]
6. Pu, L.; Naderi, M.; Liu, T.; Wu, H.C.; Mukhopadhyay, S.; Brylinski, M. EToxPred: A machine learning-based approach to estimate the toxicity of drug candidates. *BMC Pharmacol. Toxicol.* **2019**, *20*, 2. [CrossRef]
7. Rees, C. The Ethics of Artificial Intelligence. In *IFIP Advances in Information and Communication Technology*, 1st ed.; Chapman and Hall/CRC; CRC Press/Taylor & Francis Group: Boca Raton, FL, USA, 2020; Volume 555, pp. 55–69, ISBN 9781351251389.
8. Wess, G.; Urmann, M.; Sickenberger, B. Medicinal Chemistry: Challenges and Opportunities. *Angew. Chem. Int. Ed.* **2001**, *40*, 3341–3350. [CrossRef]
9. Chen, R.; Liu, X.; Jin, S.; Lin, J.; Liu, J. Machine learning for drug-target interaction prediction. *Molecules* **2018**, *23*, 2208. [CrossRef] [PubMed]
10. Gómez-Bombarelli, R.; Wei, J.N.; Duvenaud, D.; Hernández-Lobato, J.M.; Sánchez-Lengeling, B.; Sheberla, D.; Aguilera-Iparraguirre, J.; Hirzel, T.D.; Adams, R.P.; Aspuru-Guzik, A. Automatic Chemical Design Using a Data-Driven Continuous Representation of Molecules. *ACS Central Sci.* **2018**, *4*, 268–276. [CrossRef]
11. Hansen, K.; Biegler, F.; Ramakrishnan, R.; Pronobis, W.; Von Lilienfeld, O.A.; Müller, K.R.; Tkatchenko, A. Machine learning predictions of molecular properties: Accurate many-body potentials and nonlocality in chemical space. *J. Phys. Chem. Lett.* **2015**, *6*, 2326–2331. [CrossRef]
12. Gawehn, E.; Hiss, J.A.; Schneider, G. Deep Learning in Drug Discovery. *Mol. Inform.* **2016**, *35*, 3–14. [CrossRef]
13. Lysenko, A.; Sharma, A.; Boroevich, K.A.; Tsunoda, T. An integrative machine learning approach for prediction of toxicity-related drug safety. *Life Sci. Alliance* **2018**, *1*, e201800098. [CrossRef]
14. You, J.; McLeod, R.D.; Hu, P. Predicting drug-target interaction network using deep learning model. *Comput. Biol. Chem.* **2019**, *80*, 90–101. [CrossRef]
15. Liu, X.; IJzerman, A.P.; van Westen, G.J.P. Computational Approaches for De Novo Drug Design: Past, Present, and Future. In *Methods in Molecular Biology*; Humana Press Inc.: Totowa, NJ, USA, 2021; Volume 2190, pp. 139–165.
16. Bannigan, P.; Aldeghi, M.; Bao, Z.; Häse, F.; Aspuru-Guzik, A.; Allen, C. Machine learning directed drug formulation development. *Adv. Drug Deliv. Rev.* **2021**, *175*, 113806. [CrossRef]
17. Santín, E.P.; Solana, R.R.; García, M.G.; Suárez, M.D.M.G.; Díaz, G.D.B.; Cabal, M.D.C.; Rojas, J.M.M.; Sánchez, J.I.L. Toxicity prediction based on artificial intelligence: A multidisciplinary overview. *Wiley Interdiscip. Rev. Comput. Mol. Sci.* **2021**, *11*, e1516. [CrossRef]
18. Jang, H.Y.; Song, J.; Kim, J.H.; Lee, H.; Kim, I.W.; Moon, B.; Oh, J.M. Machine learning-based quantitative prediction of drug exposure in drug-drug interactions using drug label information. *npj Digit. Med.* **2022**, *5*, 100. [CrossRef] [PubMed]
19. Nussinov, R.; Zhang, M.; Liu, Y.; Jang, H. AlphaFold, Artificial Intelligence (AI), and Allostery. *J. Phys. Chem. B* **2022**, *126*, 6372–6383. [CrossRef] [PubMed]
20. Bai, Q.; Liu, S.; Tian, Y.; Xu, T.; Banegas-Luna, A.J.; Pérez-Sánchez, H.; Huang, J.; Liu, H.; Yao, X. Application advances of deep learning methods for de novo drug design and molecular dynamics simulation. *Wiley Interdiscip. Rev. Comput. Mol. Sci.* **2022**, *12*, e1581. [CrossRef]
21. Gupta, R.; Srivastava, D.; Sahu, M.; Tiwari, S.; Ambasta, R.K.; Kumar, P. Artificial intelligence to deep learning: Machine intelligence approach for drug discovery. *Mol. Divers.* **2021**, *25*, 1315–1360. [CrossRef] [PubMed]
22. Zhu, J.; Wang, J.; Wang, X.; Gao, M.; Guo, B.; Gao, M.; Liu, J.; Yu, Y.; Wang, L.; Kong, W.; et al. Prediction of drug efficacy from transcriptional profiles with deep learning. *Nat. Biotechnol.* **2021**, *39*, 1444–1452. [CrossRef]
23. Dhamodharan, G.; Mohan, C.G. Machine learning models for predicting the activity of AChE and BACE1 dual inhibitors for the treatment of Alzheimer's disease. *Mol. Divers.* **2022**, *26*, 1501–1517. [CrossRef]
24. Melo, M.C.R.; Maasch, J.R.M.A.; de la Fuente-Nunez, C. Accelerating antibiotic discovery through artificial intelligence. *Commun. Biol.* **2021**, *4*, 1050. [CrossRef]
25. Marchant, J. Powerful antibiotics discovered using AI. *Nature* **2020**. *Online ahead of print.* [CrossRef]
26. Lv, H.; Shi, L.; Berkenpas, J.W.; Dao, F.Y.; Zulfiqar, H.; Ding, H.; Zhang, Y.; Yang, L.; Cao, R. Application of artificial intelligence and machine learning for COVID-19 drug discovery and vaccine design. *Brief. Bioinform.* **2021**, *22*, bbab320. [CrossRef]
27. Monteleone, S.; Kellici, T.F.; Southey, M.; Bodkin, M.J.; Heifetz, A. Fighting COVID-19 with Artificial Intelligence. In *Methods in Molecular Biology*; Humana Press Inc.: Totowa, NJ, USA, 2022; Volume 2390, pp. 103–112.
28. Zhou, Y.; Wang, F.; Tang, J.; Nussinov, R.; Cheng, F. Artificial intelligence in COVID-19 drug repurposing. *Lancet Digit. Health* **2020**, *2*, e667–e676. [CrossRef] [PubMed]
29. Verma, N.; Qu, X.; Trozzi, F.; Elsaied, M.; Karki, N.; Tao, Y.; Zoltowski, B.; Larson, E.C.; Kraka, E. Predicting potential SARS-CoV-2 drugs-in depth drug database screening using deep neural network framework ssnet, classical virtual screening and docking. *Int. J. Mol. Sci.* **2021**, *22*, 1392. [CrossRef]
30. Bung, N.; Krishnan, S.R.; Bulusu, G.; Roy, A. De novo design of new chemical entities for SARS-CoV-2 using artificial intelligence. *Future Med. Chem.* **2021**, *13*, 575–585. [CrossRef]

31. Floresta, G.; Zagni, C.; Gentile, D.; Patamia, V.; Rescifina, A. Artificial Intelligence Technologies for COVID-19 De Novo Drug Design. *Int. J. Mol. Sci.* **2022**, *23*, 3261. [CrossRef] [PubMed]

32. Vatansever, S.; Schlessinger, A.; Wacker, D.; Kaniskan, H.Ü.; Jin, J.; Zhou, M.M.; Zhang, B. Artificial intelligence and machine learning-aided drug discovery in central nervous system diseases: State-of-the-arts and future directions. *Med. Res. Rev.* **2021**, *41*, 1427–1473. [CrossRef]

33. Farghali, H.; Canová, N.K.; Arora, M. The Potential Applications of Artificial Intelligence in Drug Discovery and Development. *Physiol. Res.* **2021**, *70* (Suppl. S4), S715–S722. [CrossRef]

34. Ganesh, G.S.; Kolusu, A.S.; Prasad, K.; Samudrala, P.K.; Nemmani, K.V.S. Advancing health care via artificial intelligence: From concept to clinic. *Eur. J. Pharmacol.* **2022**, *934*. [CrossRef]

35. Koromina, M.; Pandi, M.T.; Patrinos, G.P. Rethinking Drug Repositioning and Development with Artificial Intelligence, Machine Learning, and Omics. *OMICS A J. Integr. Biol.* **2019**, *23*, 539–548. [CrossRef]

36. Mak, K.K.; Pichika, M.R. Artificial intelligence in drug development: Present status and future prospects. *Drug Discov. Today* **2019**, *24*, 773–780. [CrossRef] [PubMed]

37. Fleming, N. How artificial intelligence is changing drug discovery spotlight. *Nature* **2018**, *557*, S55–S57. [CrossRef] [PubMed]

38. Available online: https://www.fiercebiotech.com/biotech/numerate-forms-drug-discovery-collaboration-merck-to-utilize-numerate-s-silico-drug-design (accessed on 6 December 2022).

39. 11 Companies Using Pharma AI to Stimulate Growth in the Industry. Available online: https://www.p360.com/data360/11-companies-using-pharma-ai-to-stimulate-growth-in-the-industry-1/ (accessed on 6 December 2022).

40. Vamathevan, J.; Clark, D.; Czodrowski, P.; Dunham, I.; Ferran, E.; Lee, G.; Li, B.; Madabhushi, A.; Shah, P.; Spitzer, M.; et al. Applications of machine learning in drug discovery and development. *Nat. Rev. Drug Discov.* **2019**, *18*, 463–477. [CrossRef] [PubMed]

41. Tsuji, S.; Hase, T.; Yachie-Kinoshita, A.; Nishino, T.; Ghosh, S.; Kikuchi, M.; Shimokawa, K.; Aburatani, H.; Kitano, H.; Tanaka, H. Artificial intelligence-based computational framework for drug-target prioritization and inference of novel repositionable drugs for Alzheimer's disease. *Alzheimer Res. Ther.* **2021**, *13*, 92. [CrossRef]

42. Basu, T.; Engel-Wolf, S.; Menzer, O. The ethics of machine learning in medical sciences: Where do we stand today? *Indian J. Dermatol.* **2020**, *65*, 358–364. [CrossRef] [PubMed]

43. Kleinberg, J. Inherent Trade-Offs in Algorithmic Fairness. In Proceedings of the Abstracts of the 2018 ACM International Conference on Measurement and Modeling of Computer Systems, Irvine, CA, USA, 18–22 June 2018; Association for Computing Machinery (ACM): New York, NY, USA, 2018; p. 40.

44. Silvia, H.; Carr, N. When Worlds Collide: Protecting Physical World Interests Against Virtual World Malfeasance. *Michigan Technol. Law Rev.* **2020**, *26*, 279. [CrossRef]

45. Shimao, H.; Khern-am-nuai, W.; Kannan, K.; Cohen, M.C. Strategic Best Response Fairness in Fair Machine Learning. In Proceedings of the 2022 AAAI/ACM Conference on AI, Ethics, and Society, New York, NY, USA, 7–9 February 2022; Association for Computing Machinery (ACM): New York, NY, USA, 2022; p. 664.

46. Kusam, L.; Mayank, D.; Nishanth, K.N. Data Augmentation Using Generative Adversarial Network. In Proceedings of the 2nd International Conference on Advanced Computing and Software Engineering (ICACSE) 2019, Sultanpur, India, 8 February 2019. [CrossRef]

47. Taylor, L.; Nitschke, G. Improving Deep Learning with Generic Data Augmentation. In Proceedings of the 2018 IEEE Symposium Series on Computational Intelligence, SSCI 2018, Piscataway, NJ, USA, 18–21 November 2018; Institute of Electrical and Electronics Engineers Inc.: Piscataway, NJ, USA, 2019; pp. 1542–1547.

48. Minh, D.; Wang, H.X.; Li, Y.F.; Nguyen, T.N. Explainable artificial intelligence: A comprehensive review. *Artif. Intell. Rev.* **2022**, *55*, 3503–3568. [CrossRef]

49. Arrieta, A.B.; Díaz-Rodríguez, N.; Del Ser, J.; Bennetot, A.; Tabik, S.; Barbado, A.; Garcia, S.; Gil-Lopez, S.; Molina, D.; Benjamins, R.; et al. Explainable Artificial Intelligence (XAI): Concepts, taxonomies, opportunities and challenges toward responsible AI. *Inf. Fusion* **2020**, *58*, 82–115. [CrossRef]

50. Grebner, C.; Matter, H.; Kofink, D.; Wenzel, J.; Schmidt, F.; Hessler, G. Application of Deep Neural Network Models in Drug Discovery Programs. *ChemMedChem* **2021**, *16*, 3772–3786. [CrossRef]

51. Schraagen, J.M.; van Diggelen, J. A Brief History of the Relationship Between Expertise and Artificial Intelligence. In *Expertise at Work*; Palgrave Macmillan: Cham, Switzerland, 2021; pp. 149–175.

52. Gilpin, L.H.; Bau, D.; Yuan, B.Z.; Bajwa, A.; Specter, M.; Kagal, L. Explaining explanations: An overview of interpretability of machine learning. In Proceedings of the 2018 IEEE 5th International Conference on Data Science and Advanced Analytics, DSAA Turin, Itali, 1–3 October 2018; Institute of Electrical and Electronics Engineers Inc.: Piscataway, NJ, USA, 2019; pp. 80–89.

53. Jarrahi, M.H. Artificial intelligence and the future of work: Human-AI symbiosis in organizational decision making. *Bus. Horiz.* **2018**, *61*, 577–586. [CrossRef]

54. Wang, L.; Ding, J.; Pan, L.; Cao, D.; Jiang, H.; Ding, X. Artificial intelligence facilitates drug design in the big data era. *Chemom. Intell. Lab. Syst.* **2019**, *194*, 103850. [CrossRef]

5. Naik, N.; Hameed, B.M.Z.; Shetty, D.K.; Swain, D.; Shah, M.; Paul, R.; Aggarwal, K.; Brahim, S.; Patil, V.; Smriti, K.; et al. Legal and Ethical Consideration in Artificial Intelligence in Healthcare: Who Takes Responsibility? *Front. Surg.* **2022**, *9*, 266. [CrossRef] [PubMed]

6. Karimian, G.; Petelos, E.; Evers, S.M.A.A. The ethical issues of the application of artificial intelligence in healthcare: A systematic scoping review. *AI Ethics* **2022**, *2*, 539–551. [CrossRef]

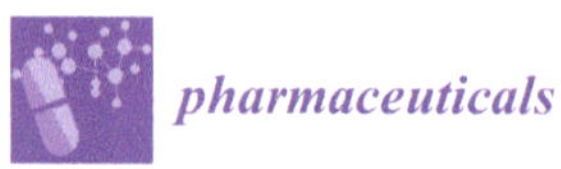

pharmaceuticals

MDPI

Article

In Silico Development of Novel Benzofuran-1,3,4-Oxadiazoles as Lead Inhibitors of *M. tuberculosis* Polyketide Synthase 13

Ali Irfan [1], Shah Faisal [2], Ameer Fawad Zahoor [1,*], Razia Noreen [3], Sami A. Al-Hussain [4,*], Burak Tuzun [5], Rakshanda Javaid [1], Ahmed A. Elhenawy [6,7], Magdi E. A. Zaki [4], Sajjad Ahmad [8] and Magda H. Abdellattif [9]

[1] Department of Chemistry, Government College University Faisalabad, Faisalabad 38000, Pakistan; raialiirfan@gmail.com (A.I.); rakshanda880@gmail.com (R.J.)
[2] Department of Chemistry, Islamia College University Peshawar, Peshawar 25120, Pakistan; faisalvbs@gmail.com
[3] Department of Biochemistry, Government College University Faisalabad, Faisalabad 38000, Pakistan; razianoreen@hotmail.com
[4] Department of Chemistry, College of Science, Imam Mohammad Ibn Saud Islamic University (IMSIU), Riyadh 13623, Saudi Arabia; mezaki@imamu.edu.sa
[5] Plant and Animal Production Department, Technical Sciences Vocational School of Sivas, Sivas Cumhuriyet University, Sivas 58140, Turkey; theburaktuzun@yahoo.com
[6] Chemistry Department, Faculty of Science, Al-Azhar University, Nasr City, Cairo 11884, Egypt; elhenawy_sci@hotmail.com
[7] Chemistry Department, Faculty of Science and Art, AlBaha University, Mukhwah, Al Bahah 65731, Saudi Arabia
[8] Department of Health and Biological Sciences, Abasyn University, Peshawar 25000, Pakistan; sajjad.ahmad@abasyn.edu.pk
[9] Department of Chemistry, College of Science, Taif University, Taif 21944, Saudi Arabia; m.hasan@tu.edu.sa
* Correspondence: fawad.zahoor@gcuf.edu.pk (A.F.Z.); sahussain@imamu.edu.sa (S.A.A.-H.); Tel.: +92-3336729186

Citation: Irfan, A.; Faisal, S.; Zahoor, A.F.; Noreen, R.; Al-Hussain, S.A.; Tuzun, B.; Javaid, R.; Elhenawy, A.A.; Zaki, M.E.A.; Ahmad, S.; et al. In Silico Development of Novel Benzofuran-1,3,4-Oxadiazoles as Lead Inhibitors of *M. tuberculosis* Polyketide Synthase 13. *Pharmaceuticals* **2023**, *16*, 829. https://doi.org/10.3390/ph16060829

Academic Editors: Halil İbrahim Ciftci, Belgin Sever and Hasan Demirci

Received: 26 April 2023
Revised: 24 May 2023
Accepted: 26 May 2023
Published: 1 June 2023

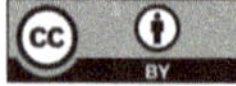

Abstract: Benzofuran and 1,3,4-oxadiazole are privileged and versatile heterocyclic pharmacophores which display a broad spectrum of biological and pharmacological therapeutic potential against a wide variety of diseases. This article reports in silico CADD (computer-aided drug design) and molecular hybridization approaches for the evaluation of the chemotherapeutic efficacy of 16 S-linked *N*-phenyl acetamide moiety containing benzofuran-1,3,4-oxadiazole scaffolds **BF1–BF16**. This virtual screening was carried out to discover and assess the chemotherapeutic efficacy of **BF1–BF16** structural motifs as *Mycobacterium tuberculosis* polyketide synthase 13 (Mtb Pks13) enzyme inhibitors. The CADD study results revealed that the benzofuran clubbed oxadiazole derivatives **BF3**, **BF4** and **BF8** showed excellent and remarkably significant binding energies against the Mtb Pks13 enzyme comparable with the standard benzofuran-based **TAM-16** inhibitor. The best binding affinity scores were displayed by 1,3,4-oxadiazoles-based benzofuran scaffolds **BF3** (−14.23 kcal/mol), **BF4** (−14.82 kcal/mol), and **BF8** (−14.11 kcal/mol), in comparison to the binding affinity score of the standard reference **TAM-16** drug (−14.61 kcal/mol). 2,5-Dimethoxy moiety-based bromobenzofuran-oxadiazole derivative **BF4** demonstrated the highest binding affinity score amongst the screened compounds, and was higher than the reference Pks13 inhibitor **TAM-16** drug. The bindings of these three leads **BF3**, **BF4**, and **BF8** were further confirmed by the MM-PBSA investigations in which they also exhibited strong bindings with the Pks13 of Mtb. Moreover, the stability analysis of these benzofuran-1,3,4-oxadiazoles in the active sites of the Pks13 enzyme was achieved through molecular dynamic (MD) simulations at 250 ns virtual simulation time, which indicated that these three in silico predicted bio-potent benzofuran tethered oxadiazole molecules **BF3**, **BF4**, and **BF8** demonstrated stability with the active site of the Pks13 enzyme.

Keywords: benzofuran-1,3,4-oxadiazole; tuberclosis; Pks13 inhibitor; molecular docking; MM-PBSA; MD simulations; ADMET study; SAR

---

1. Introduction

TB (tuberculosis) is among the deadliest transmittable infectious lung disease caused by *Mycobacterium tuberculosis* (Mtb). The global TB report 2018 described that Mtb is the leading cause of single infectious disease [1]. TB and its percentage are higher than human immunodeficiency virus (HIV) and AIDS. Amongst the infectious diseases after HIV, TB is a global health issue, being the second major cause of death across the world. In today's world, antibiotic resistance is a major global problem in curing contagious microbial diseases (CMD) caused by deadly microbes [2,3]. The drug-resistant TB is a major health concern of today's scientific community due to its resistance against the first-line drug rifampicin (RR-TB) [4,5]. To counter multi-drug resistance (MDR) and pan-drug resistance bacteria resulting from the development of mutagenicity [4–8], novel wide spectrum chemotherapeutic agents are urgently necessitated. It is imperative to discover novel anti-tuberculosis chemotherapeutic agents to stop resistance in Mtb strains, and ideally cure the disease in a shorter time [4–10]. There is an urgent demand and necessity for the designing, discovery, and development of novel curative candidates active against all forms of Mtb [8–13]. Heterocycles-based ring systems such as quinoxalines, coumarins, benzothiazoles, benzoxazoles, thiadiazoles, benzofurans, and oxadiazoles, etc., constitute a powerful backbone of different chemotherapeutic agents with a wide spectrum of biological activities in medicine, pharmacology, and pharmaceutics [14–21]. Benzofuran (Figure 1) is a five-membered oxygen containing a fused heterocyclic compound first synthesized by Perkin in 1870 [22]. Benzofuran moiety is an important structural unit of many of the natural and synthetic derivatives (Figure 1) displaying a versatile array of biological activities against a wide variety of diseases, such as anti-cancer, hemolytic, thrombolytic [23], anti-microbial [24], anti-tuberculosis [25,26], anti-Alzheimer's [27,28], inflammation inhibitory activity [29], anti-parasitic [30], anti-viral [31], analgesic, anti-pyretic [32], anti-bacterial [33], anti-hyperglycemic [34], and anti-oxidant activities [33,35]. On the other hand, 1,3,4-oxadiazole scaffolds showed a broad spectrum of pharmacological applications; for example, anti-Alzheimer's [36], anti-neoplastic [37], anti-viral [38], anti-cancer [39], FAK inhibitors [40], anti-fungal [41], anti-inflammatory [42], anti-bacterial [43] and anti-tubular activities [44]. The benzofuran-oxadiazoles also exhibited anti-lung cancer, human tyrosinase inhibitors, anti-HepG-2, anti-hemolytic, and anti-thrombotic activities [24,45]. The different marketed anti-TB drugs are listed in Figure 2, while potent anti-TB bioactive compounds with oxadiazole and furan cores are depicted in Figure 3 [46–52].

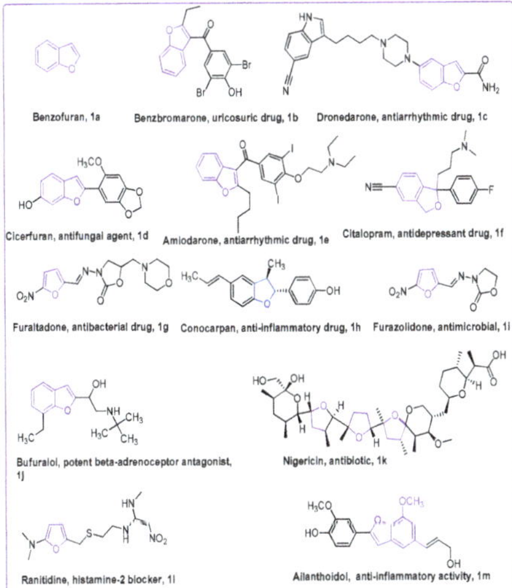

Figure 1. Structures of natural and synthetic furan scaffolds **1a–1m**.

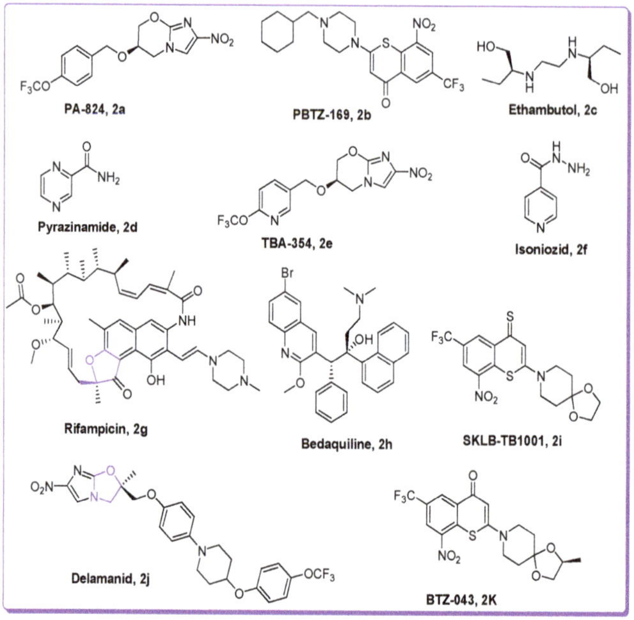

Figure 2. Structures of commercially available anti-TB drugs in market.

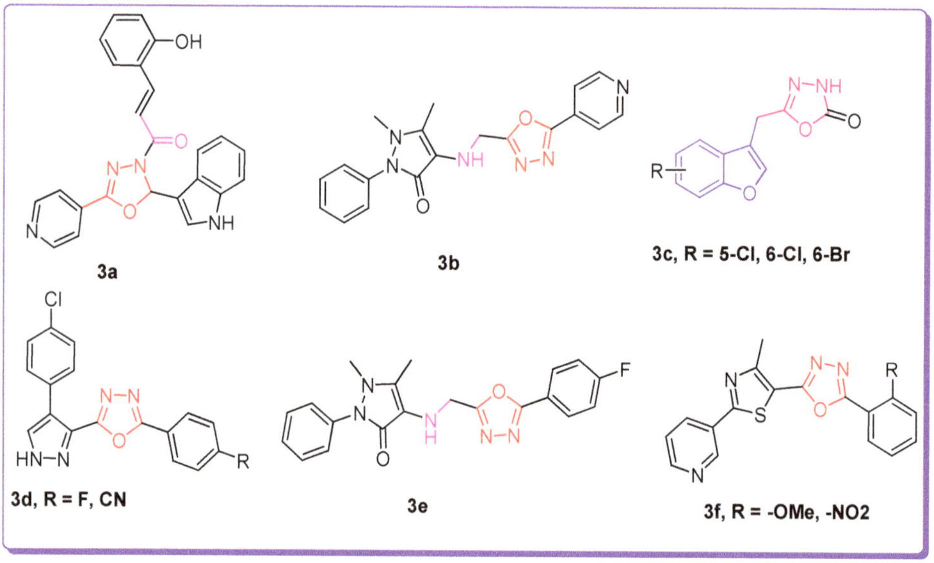

Figure 3. Structures of oxadiazole and benzofuran-based anti-TB scaffolds.

The previous work reported on benzofuran-oxadiazoles as anti-microbial agents by our research group and the current comprehensive literature study (Figure 4) [17,42–52] is the basis of the rationale to discover novel benzofuran-appended oxadiazole structural hybrids as anti-TB drug candidates with the help of different in silico techniques.

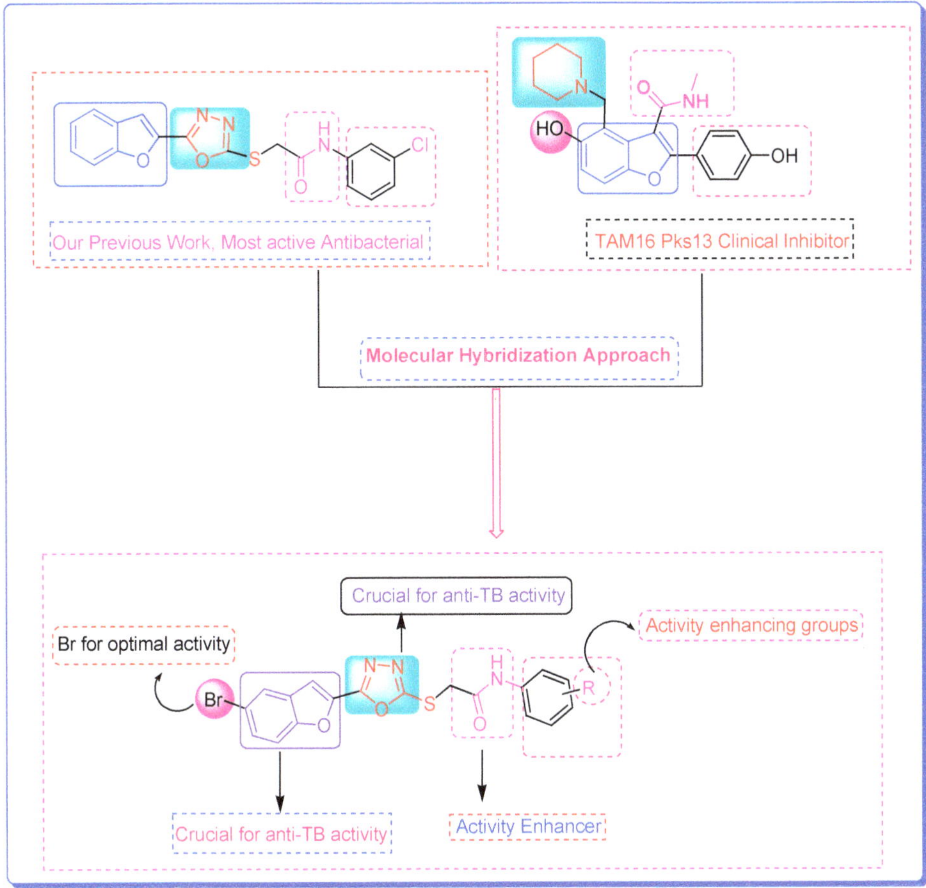

Figure 4. Rational design of benzofuran-1,3,4-oxadiazole derivatives **BF1–BF16** as anti-tuberculosis agents [24,46,47].

2. Results and Discussion

2.1. Evalaution of Anti-Mtb Potenial of Benzofurans-1,3,4-Oxadiazoles Using Computational Approaches

Mycobacterium Tuberculosis

Benzofuran-1,3,4-oxadiazoles **BF1–BF16** [23,45,52] were evaluated for their anti-Mtb potential using computational approaches. Tuberculosis is a bacterial disease that predominantly affects the lungs and is caused by *Mycobacterium tuberculosis* [53]. Even though macrophages are crucial to the host immune system because they identify and eliminate potential intruders (pathogens), Mtb has developed several tactics that allow it to live and proliferate inside these lung macrophages, which are the main host cells for Mtb infection [54]. It is one of the prevalent causes of death worldwide, particularly in people who have also been infected by other pathogenic viruses and have viral infections. The existing TB treatment regimens take between six and nine months to complete, which makes it difficult for patients to adhere to them, which causes multi-drug resistant TB, which is essentially resistant to antibacterial drug treatments [55]. Hence, new potential anti-TB chemotherapeutics need to be designed and developed to overcome the MDR problem by targeting novel pathways and enzymes involved in bacterial growth, with new modes of action to lessen the likelihood of a relapse of the TB infection when existing medications are no longer reliable [5,6,13].

Intensive research has been put into finding new Mtb targets and their inhibitors that can stop the spread of this bacterial pathogen and mitigate its drug resistance [6,13,56]. Similarly, an important class of enzymes known as polyketide synthases (Pks) has not been explored as a therapeutic target for microbial infection. The Pks are enzymes that produce mycolic acids, which are essential for the survival and pathogenicity of Mtb [57]. More than 20 (Pks) enzymes are a part of various multi-enzyme complexes that work together to produce mycolic acid in Mtb [58]. These Pks13-derived lipid metabolites (mycolic acids) are important constituents of Mtb's distinctively sophisticated and lipid-rich cell wall [59], which has been suggested as a way for it to live in hostile environments in host macrophages while also providing an inherent resistance to numerous anti-microbial medications [60]. As it is recognized that these mycolic acids, a feature of the genus mycobacterium, are essential for the survival of this pathogen, disruption of this important biosynthesis pathway is a promising drug target for TB mitigation [59,60].

One of the important enzymes of the Pks enzyme family is Pks13, which is responsible for the condensation of two fatty acid chains into α-alkyl β-ketoacyl, a primary precursor of the mycolates. Therefore, Pks13 is a crucial enzyme for mycobacterial survival, making it a desirable new target for the pursuit of possible anti-tuberculosis drug candidates [61]. Research has been going on to identify drugs targeting this Pks13 enzyme, and several benzofuran-based scaffold-carrying compounds have been identified as potent repressive agents of Pks13 using structure-based drug design techniques [17,42,43,62]. These novel benzofurans oxadiazoles **BF1–16** had strong anti-Pks13 activity in various investigational models [46,63]. Moreover, benzofuran-based compounds have also been identified to target other vital enzymes of Mtb [64]. Taking into account these potent inhibitory activities of benzofuran-based compounds against *Mycobacterium tuberculosis*, we will evaluate the potential anti-Mtb activities of our synthesized compounds (**BF1** to **BF16**) in this study by utilizing computer-aided drug discovery techniques (CADD) by targeting the important Pks13 enzyme of Mtb.

2.2. Molecular Docking Investigations of BF1–BF16 against the Pks13 Enzyme

The in silico molecular docking approach was utilized to screen the 1,3,4-oxadiazole based benzofuran compounds via MOE (molecular operating environment) against the Pks13 of Mtb, and these results were compared with the co-crystallized inhibitor (TAM-16) of Pks13. The standard reference benzofuran **TAM-16** inhibitor of anti-Mtb displayed an excellent binding affinity score (−14.61 kcal/mol) due to its strong binding interaction with the Pks13 enzyme active site (which is involved in the Mtb mycolic acid biosynthesis). The conformation analysis of the interaction of **TAM-16** inhibitor with the active site pocket of Pks13 indicated that the **TAM-16** inhibitor interacts with multiple amino acids residues (ASP1644, ASN1640, and GLN1633). The **TAM-16** inhibitor made different multiple conventional and carbon-hydrogen-type hydrogen bonds with different amino acids of the active site. In the analysis, the Pks13 and **TAM-16** protein-ligand complex demonstrated several other Pi-Pi and Amide-Pi Stacked-type molecular interactions. In addition, other types of molecular interactions—such as Alkyl, Pi-Alkyl, and Pi-Sigma interactions, which stabilize a compound inside a pocket—were also observed with the ILE1643, TYR1663, ALA1667, and TYR1674 between the Pks13 and the **TAM-16** inhibitor. Furthermore, researchers that first discovered **TAM-16** against Pks13 have stated that it exerts its inhibitory action by obstructing access to the Pks13 active site, which houses the catalytic triad (Ser1533, Asp1560, and His1699); in this study, it can be seen that **TAM-16** also occupied the active site pocket and blocked access to these residues, as seen in Figure 5

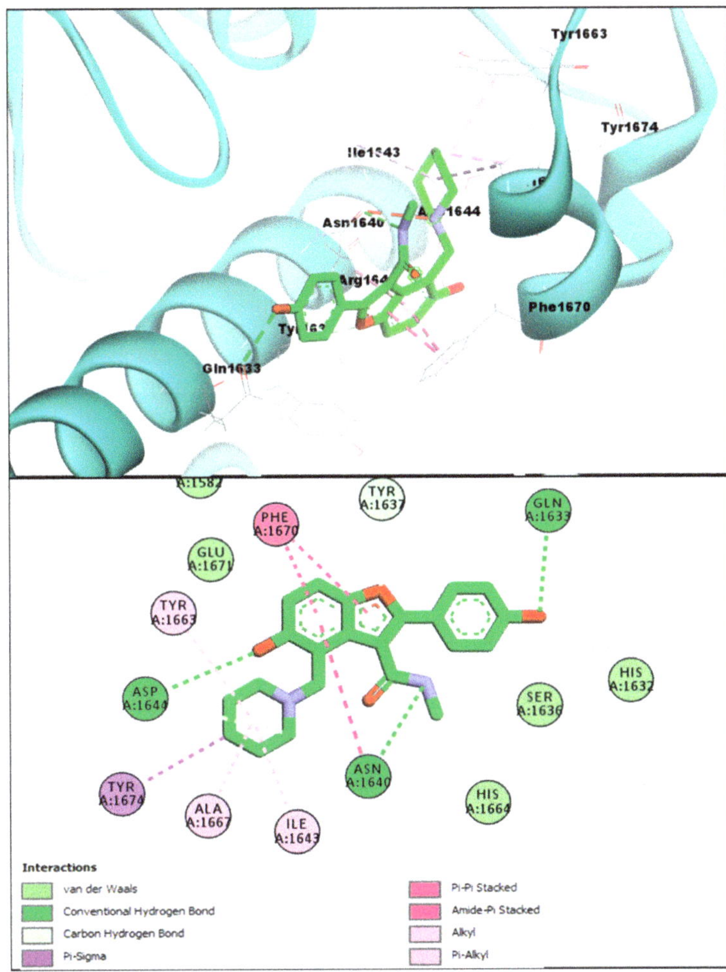

Figure 5. TAM-16 inhibitor (upper panel) 3D pose (obtained through molecular docking) with the Pks13 interacting residues labeled, and its 2D interactive pose (lower panel) with the Pks13 enzyme.

The afforded benzofuran molecules demonstrated strong binding affinities and robust interactions with the Pks13 enzyme active site in comparison to the benzofuran-based **TAM-16** reference standard inhibitor. Out of the 16 novel synthesized analogs **BF1** to **BF16**, three of them, **BF3**, **BF4**, and **BF8** showed similar affinities to that of **TAM-16** with the Mtb Pks13 enzyme. The conformation analysis of the pose and binding affinity of benzofuran-appended 1,3,4-oxadiazole derivative **BF3** showed the binding affinity score (−14.23 kcal/mol) with the Pks13 active site due to the multiple molecular interactions with the Pks13 receptor residues. The benzofuran ring of the derivative **BF3** demonstrated hydrogen bonds of conventional and carbon-hydrogen types with TYR1663, along with an H-bond between the HIS1664 and the sulphur atom. Moreover, other interactions such as Pi-Pi T-shaped (With the HIS1699 catalytic residue), Pi-Pi Stacked, Pi-Sigma and Alkyl were present, as were Pi-Alkyl interactions between the benzofuran ring and the Pks13. Several of the Pks13 receptor residues also made Van der Waals and Pi-Lone Pair molecular interactions with this compound; they are graphically presented in Figure 6.

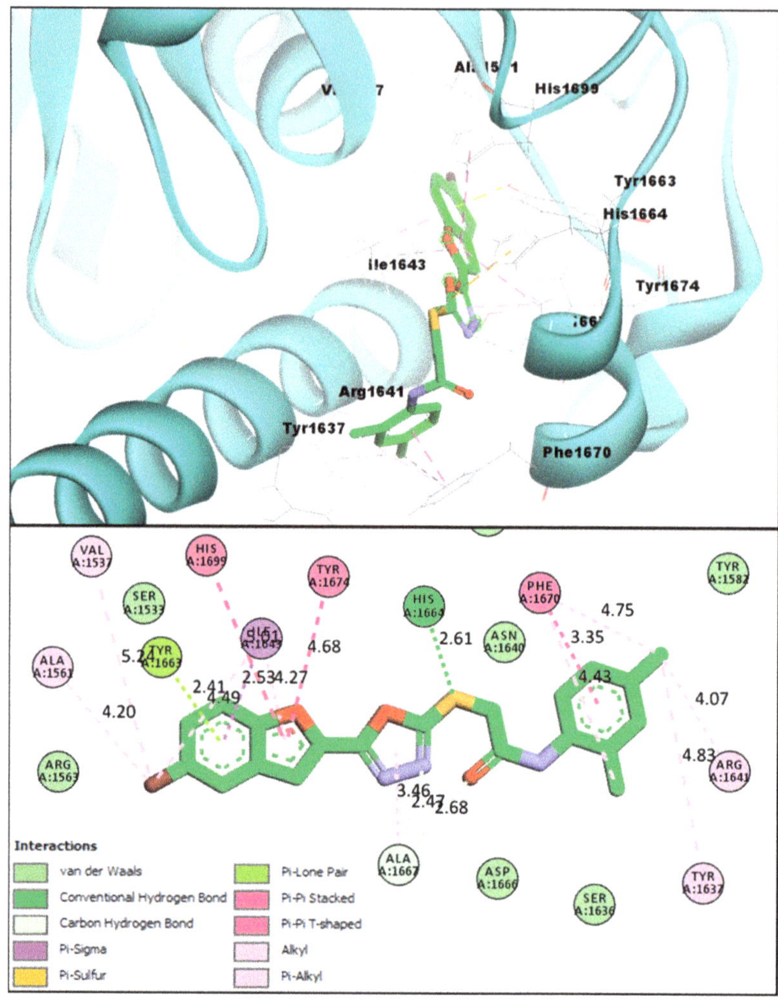

Figure 6. BF3 compound's 3D pose (upper panel) interacting receptor residues are labeled, and its 2D interactive pose (lower panel) with the Pks13 enzyme.

During the molecular docking studies, compound **BF4** also showed a strong binding affinity score with the Pks13 active site (−14.82 kcal/mol) as compared to the **TAM-16** binding affinity, which was (−14.61 kcal/mol) with the Pks13 enzyme; **BF4** showed relatively stronger binding to the active site of the target protein. Furthermore, the interaction analysis of **BF4** and the Pks13 protein complexes showed that **BF4** directly interacted with the catalytic residues (Ser1533 and His1699), which are directly involved in the mycolic acid synthesis and are essential to the Pks13 activity. The benzofuran **BF4** blocked access to these catalytic residues by interacting similarly to the **TAM-16** inhibitor, as mentioned in previous paragraphs. It can be seen in Figure 7 that **BF4** was able to engage the HIS1699 catalytic residue via a carbon-hydrogen-type hydrogen bonding with the oxygen atom of the oxadiazole ring. This oxadiazole ring's nitrogen atom also engaged the other important catalytic residue (SER1533) by forming a conventional hydrogen bond. Furthermore, the benzofuran moiety of **BF4** also made multiple molecular contacts, as was previously seen in the **BF3** and Pks13 complex, and formed a hydrogen bond with the TYR1663, a Pi-Sigma interaction with the ILE1643, and multiple stabilizing interactions with Alkyl, Pi-Alkyl, Pi-Pi T-shaped and Pi-Pi Stacked; these Pi-Sulfur and Pi-Sigma interactions were also present in **BF4** and the Pks13 complex.

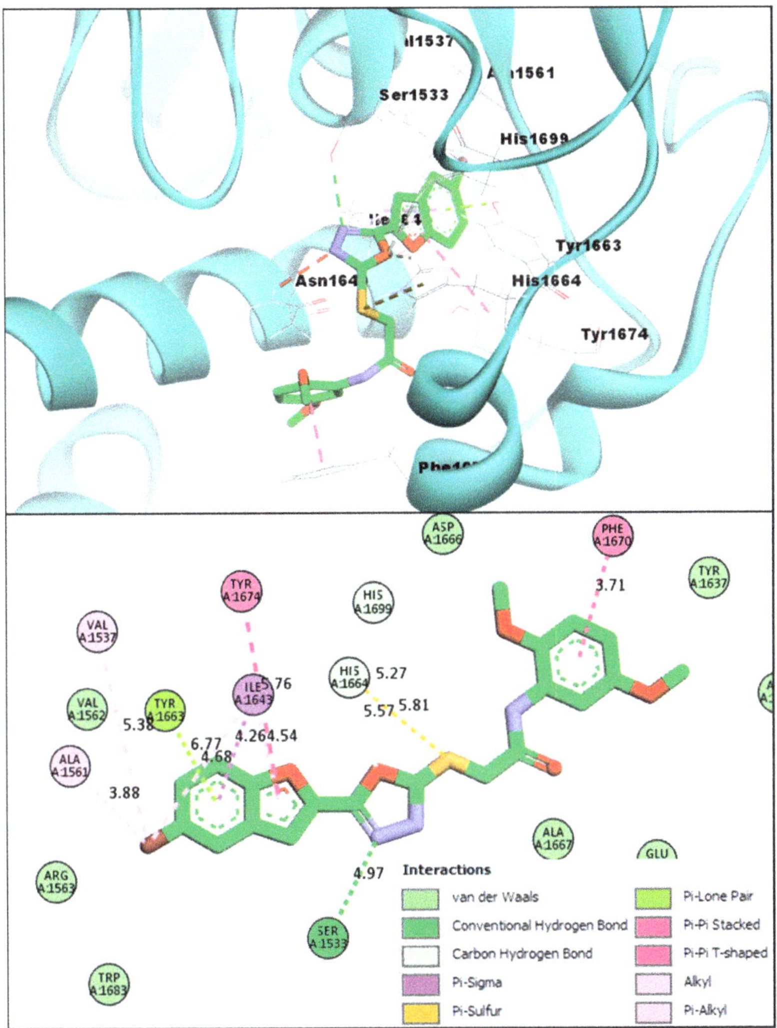

Figure 7. **BF4** compound's 3D pose (upper panel) interacting receptor residues are labeled, and its 2D interactive pose (lower panel) with the Pks13 enzyme.

The third novel benzofuran **BF8** also showed comparable binding affinity in comparison to that of **TAM-16**, and was able to bind to the Pks13 active site with a binding affinity score of −14.11 kcal/mol. It also directly engaged one of the crucial catalytic residues HIS1699 with its oxadiazole ring's nitrogen atom via a conventional H-bond. Moreover, the benzofuran moiety of **BF8** also showed stable molecular interactions of multiple types with the Pks13 receptor residues, and the TYR1663 made an H-bond with the bromine atom of this ring and made Alkyl and Pi-Alkyl interactions, as previously seen in the other benzofurans. In addition, other molecular interactions, i.e., Pi-Pi T-shaped, Pi-Pi Stacked-type, Amide-Pi Stacked, Pi-Sigma, and interactions of fluorine on the phenyl ring of **BF8** with the ASP1644 of Pks13 receptor were also seen in **BF8** and the Pks13 protein complex, as seen in Figure 8.

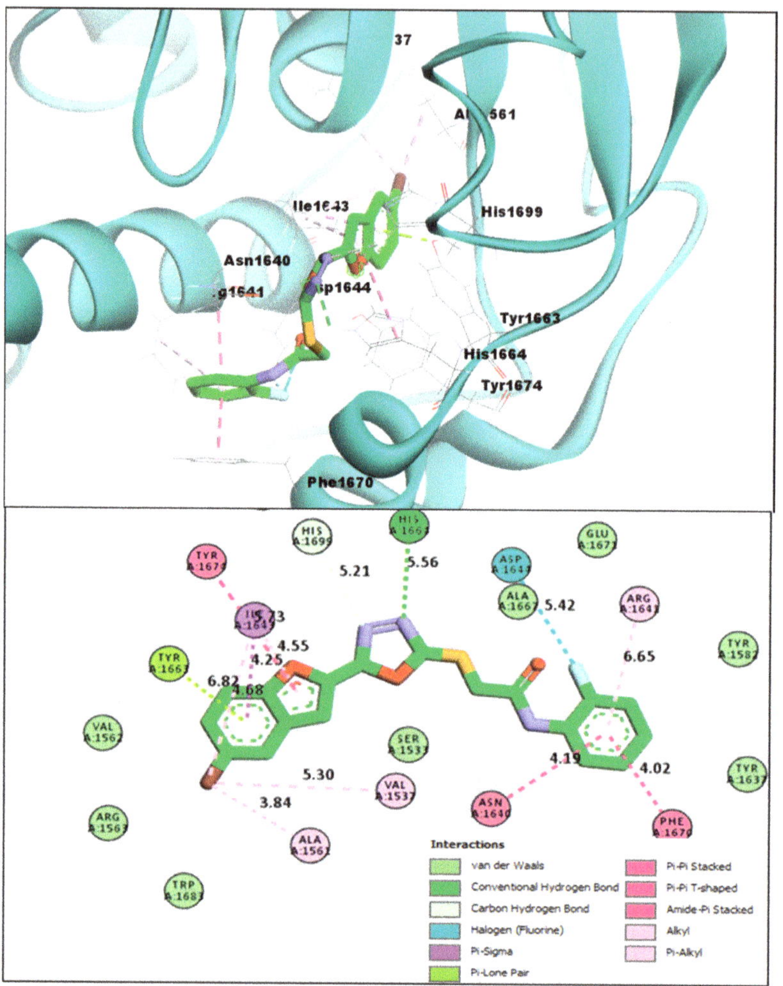

Figure 8. BF8 compound's 3D pose (upper panel), the interacting receptor residues are labeled, and its 2D interactive pose (lower panel) with the Pks13 enzyme.

An overview of the binding affinity scores of the studied bromo-substituted benzofuran 1,3,4-oxadiazoles **BF1–BF9** and the interactive residues engaged by these compounds in the active pocket of the Pks13 enzyme are presented in Table 1; while the bromo-unsubstituted benzofuran-1,3,4-oxadiazole structural hybrids **BF10–BF16** that showed less binding affinity scores with the Pks13 enzyme are presented in the Supplementary Table S1.

Table 1. The molecular docking profile of bromobenzofuran-oxadiazoles **BF1–BF9** against Pks13.

Compounds	Binding Affinities	Interacting Residues of Pks13	Interaction Types
BF1	−12.93 kcal/mol	ILE1643, TYR1663, HIS1632, HIS1699, ALA1667, TYR1674,	Carbon-Hydrogen Bond, Van der Waals, Pi-Pi T-Shaped, Pi-Alkyl, and Alkyl.
BF2	−12.71 kcal/mol	ASN1640, ILE1643, TYR1637, TYR1663, HIS1632, ALA1667, TYR1674, PHE1670	C-Hydrogen Bond, Van der Waals, Pi-Pi T-Shaped, Pi-Pi Stacked, and Alkyl.
BF3	−14.23 kcal/mol	VAL1537, ALA1561, PHE1637, ARG1641, ILE1643, TYR1663, HIS1664, ALA1667, PHE1670, TYR1674, HIS1699	Conventional H-bond, C-Hydrogen Bond, Van der Waals, Pi-Pi T-Shaped, Pi-Alkyl, Pi-Lone pair, Pi-Sulfur, Pi-Sigma, and Pi-Pi Stacked
BF4	−14.82 kcal/mol	VAL1537, SER1533, ALA1561, VAL1537, TYR1674, ILE1643, PHE1670, ALA1667	Conventional H-bond, C-Hydrogen Bond, Van der Waals, Pi-Pi T-Shaped, Pi-Alkyl, Pi-Lone pair, Pi-Sulfur, Pi-Sigma, and Pi-Pi Stacked
BF5	−12.31 kcal/mol	ALA1561, TYR1663, ILE1643, HIS1664, TYR1674, ALA1667	C-Hydrogen Bond, Van der Waals, Pi-Pi T-Shaped, Pi-Alkyl, Pi-Lone pair, and Alkyl.
BF6	−11.89 kcal/mol	SER1533, ALA1667, ALA1561, TYR1663, ILE1643, HIS1664, GLN1633, TYR1674	Conventional H-bond, C-Hydrogen Bond, Van der Waals, Pi-Pi T-Shaped, Pi-Alkyl, Pi-Lone pair, Halogen, and Alkyl.
BF7	−12.23 kcal/mol	HIS1632, TYR1637, ILE1643, TYR1663, ALA1667, PHE1670, TYR1674	Carbon-Hydrogen Bond, Van der Waals, Pi-Pi Stacked, Pi-Alkyl, and Alkyl.
BF8	−14.11 kcal/mol	VAL1537, ALA1561, TYR1663, ASN1640, ILE1643, PHE1670, ARG1641, ASP1644, HIS1664	Conventional H-bond, C-Hydrogen Bond, Van der Waals, Pi-Pi T-Shaped, Pi-Alkyl, Pi-Lone pair, Amide-Pi Stacked
BF9	−13.44 kcal/mol	ILE1643, ALA1667, PHE1670, VAL1562, HIS1699, TYR1674, TYR1637	Conventional H-bond, C-Hydrogen Bond, Van der Waals, Pi-Pi T-Shaped, Pi-Pi Stacked, Pi-Alkyl, and Alkyl
TAM-16 (Standard)	−14.61 kcal/mol	SER1533, GLN1633, ASN1640, ASP1644, ILE1643, TYR1663, ALA1667, PHE1670, TYR1674	Conventional H-bond, C-Hydrogen Bond, Van der Waals, Pi-Pi Stacked, Pi-Alkyl, Amide Pi-Stacked, Pi-Sigma, and Alkyl

2.3. Structure-Activity Relationship (SAR) of Bromobenzofuran-1,3,4-Oxadiazoles BF3, BF4, and BF8

The analysis of the structure-activity relationship (SAR) of the novel 5-bromobenzofuran-oxadiazole compounds **BF1–BF9** revealed that the simple benzofuran moiety containing oxadiazole molecules **BF10–BF16** showed less binding affinity towards the Pks13 enzyme active site as compared to the 5-bromo moiety-based benzofuran-oxadiazoles. Among the 5-bromobenzofuran-oxadiazole compounds, **BF3** and **BF8** compounds having methyl (-CH$_3$) and highly electronegative atom fluorine on the phenyl rings (Figure 9) displayed comparable binding affinities with reference to the benzofuran **TAM-16** standard Pks13 inhibitor. Meanwhile, the 2,5-dimehoxy functionality containing the **BF4** molecule demonstrated stronger binding affinities due to stable conformation, alignments, robust interactions, and direct bindings to the catalytic residues of Pks13 active site pocket compared to the standard **TAM-16** inhibitor, which only blocked access to the Pks13 of Mtb active site pocket residues. Overall, the SAR study of all **B1–BF9** predicted that phenyl position 2 of the *N*-phenyl acetamide fragment is more active in comparison to other positions in the S-alkylated 5-bromobenzofuran-oxadiazoles tethered *N*-phenyl acetamides **BF1–BF9**. These findings suggest that the in silico identified compounds can be effective novel anti-Mtb agents, and may help tackle the resistant strains of Mtb and reduce the treatment times if used in combinatorial therapy against *Mycobacterium tuberculosis* infections.

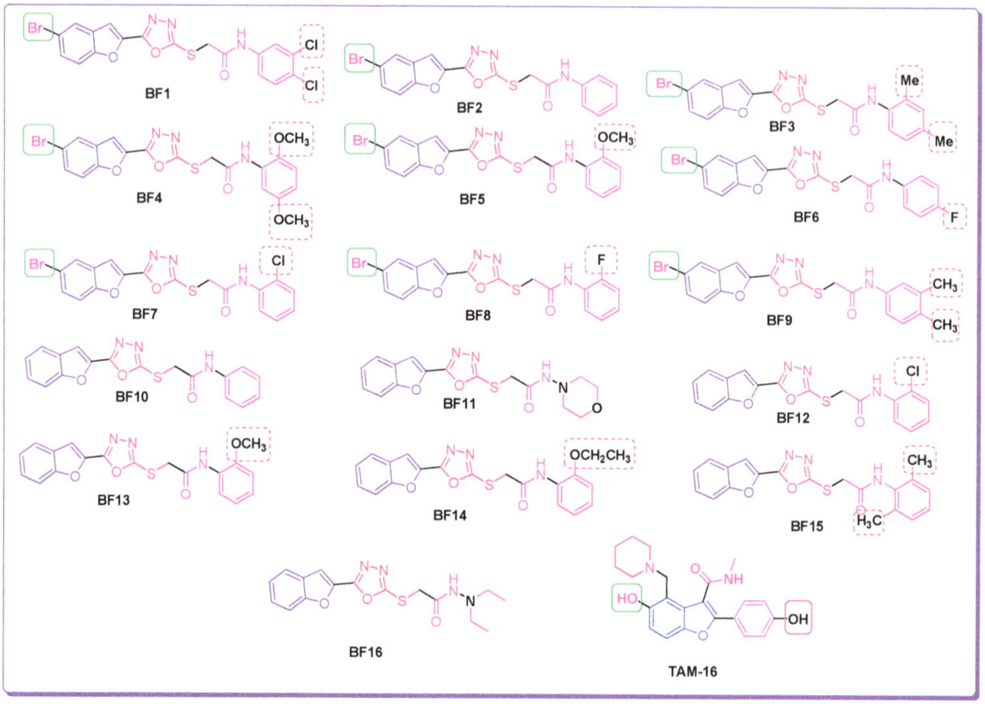

Figure 9. Structural data of benzofuran-1,3,4-oxadiazole derivatives **BF1–BF16 and TAM-16** inhibitor.

2.4. ADMET and Drug-Likeness Studies of Benzofuran-1,3,4-Oxadiazoles BF1–BF16

The ADMET and drug likeness studies of novel benzofuran clubbed 1,3,4-oxadiazole compounds **BF1–BF9** are already reported by Irfan et al. [23,45,52]). In this study, AD-MET and drug likeness studies of benzofuran oxadiazoles **BF10–BF16** (Supplementary Tables S2 and S3) were carried out in order to check their profile in comparison to previously reported derivatives **BF1–BF9**. In general, benzofuran oxadiazoles **BF1–BF16** showed good human intestinal absorptions and were classified as HIA+ based on pharmacokinetics and ADMET analysis. The novel benzofuran-appended 1,3,4-oxadiazoles demonstrated acceptable lipophilic (iLogP) characteristics and good Log S (ESOL) water solubility values. Additionally, they were not P-gp protein substrates (P-glycoprotein, or P-gp, is a transporter protein of cell membranes that controls the efflux of substances and medications from cells). Studies on metabolism have revealed that these substances are CYP450 3A4 substrates, which means that after these drug-like compounds have completed their task inside the body, the CYP450 3A4 can easily biotransform these substances inside the liver before sending them to the excretory organs for excretion from the body. These novel compounds were also non-inhibitors of the renal-OCT proteins (transporter proteins), which are crucial in the detoxifying/excretion of exogenous chemicals/drugs from the body. The toxicity investigations of these substances also revealed that they are not carcinogenic, non-AMES toxic, do not affect or inhibit the ThERG II ion channel that regulates cardiac action potential repolarization, and are non-interferers in its regular operation. According to these studies, just like **BF1–BF9**, the derivatives under study **BF10–BF16** had shown favorable ADMET properties compared to the standard **TAM-16**, which shows that these compounds, if utilized, would pose no significant health hazards to its subjects upon administration.

Moreover, the drug-likeness investigations involving identifying these compounds' physicochemical properties and medicinal chemistry showed that these **BF1–BF9** and **BF10–BF16** compounds had an excellent topological surface area (TPSA), acceptable molecular weight values, and good synthetic accessibility scores. These benzofuran **BF1–BF9** and **BF10–BF16** compounds followed the drug-likeness rules, such as Pfizer and Lipinski's drug rules. These compounds also showed no PAINS alerts, and along with this, they also followed the Golden Triangle rule and had good bioavailability scores (greater than 0.10). ADMET and drug-likeness data of **BF10–BF16** along with the reference compound **TAM-16** are presented in the Supplementary Tables S2 and S3, respectively.

2.5. MD Simulations Study of Benzofuran-1,3,4-oxadiazoles BF3, BF4, and BF8

The variation and stability of the in silico predicted bioactive benzofuran-1,3,4-oxadiazoles **BF3**, **BF4**, and **BF8** were studied by applying the C-alpha atoms root means square deviation (RMSD) approach. The three complexes displayed the initial upper phase, which resulted in the flexible behavior depicted in Figure 10. At the 25 ns simulation time, the complexes reached a steady state and the complexes retained stability until the simulations' last segment. On the other hand, **BF3** had fluctuations at 150 ns, 180 ns, and 230 ns. The higher RMSD for **BF3** than other compounds demonstrates how these complexes are more adaptable than the other molecules, **BF4** and **BF8**. The analyzed complexes were defined as having a stable comparative characteristic because their RMSD was below 2.5 during the simulation. The SASA simulation (solvent-accessible-surface-area) was carried out on complexes **BF3**, **BF4**, and **BF8**. The SASA simulation approach was utilized to study the variation of the complexes' topology, which showed that higher SASA reflected the extent of the surface volumes, while the elongated nature defined the lower SASA, as shown in Figure 9. Their stability was proved by the steady-state for **BF3**, **BF4**, and **BF8** after 48 ns and the low fluctuation degree for SASA profiles along the simulated trajectories. Additionally, each complex had SASA degrees that were roughly comparable, and the interaction over **BF3**, **BF4**, and **BF8** compounds described these protein complexes in their compact form. The **BF3**, **BF4**, and **BF8** complexes were analyzed for radius-gyration (RG) and trajectories. The trajectories demonstrated the flexibility and degree of mobility. The complexes **BF3**, **BF4**, and **BF8** RG steady degree appeared at 7 ns.

To assess the flexibility of the residues of amino acids, the root-means-square-fluctuations (RMSF) were likewise also explored (Figure 10). The high Firmness of **BF4** and **BF8** complexes was demonstrated by their low RMSF values of 2.5 Å, but the relative flexibility of the back-bone of amino acid residues in the **BF3** complex was demonstrated by its growing RMSF value of 6Å. Additionally, the small variations in the RMSD of **BF3**, **BF4**, and **BF8** systems demonstrated loops variations in Mtb Pks13, which are naturally flexible. These RMSD variations correspond to enzyme structure adaptations in order to strongly engage the compounds at the binding site, as suggested by the H-bonding pattern. [65,66].

The H-bond played an important role in identifying the stability of the interaction-strength in the ligand and protein. The in silico predicted bioactive **BF3**, **BF4**, and **BF8** have constant H-bonds range between 2 and 10 in the simulation process. The changing H-bond between the ligand-enzyme may suggest that the conformation around the ligands inside the binding site change through simulation. Overall, simulations supported the high stability of all protein-ligand complexes.

2.6. MM-PBSA Investigations of the Most In Silico Bioactive Benzofuran-1,3,4-oxadiazoles

Deciphering intermolecular interactions and energies at different nanoseconds are important to unveil microscopic information important for guiding stable docked complexes. This in turn ensures the selection of compounds that can inhibit the receptor enzyme. Although the ligand molecules are pretty flexible in the calculations, the Pks13 protein does not have this flexibility. In Molecular Mechanics-Poisson-Boltzmann surface area (MM-PSBA) calculations, the interaction between the ligand and Pks13 protein is done at the ns level. Both the ligand molecule and the Pks13 protein have flexibility in calculations of MM-PSBA. The interaction occurring in these calculations were examined every 10 ns, and the energy change is given in Figure 11.

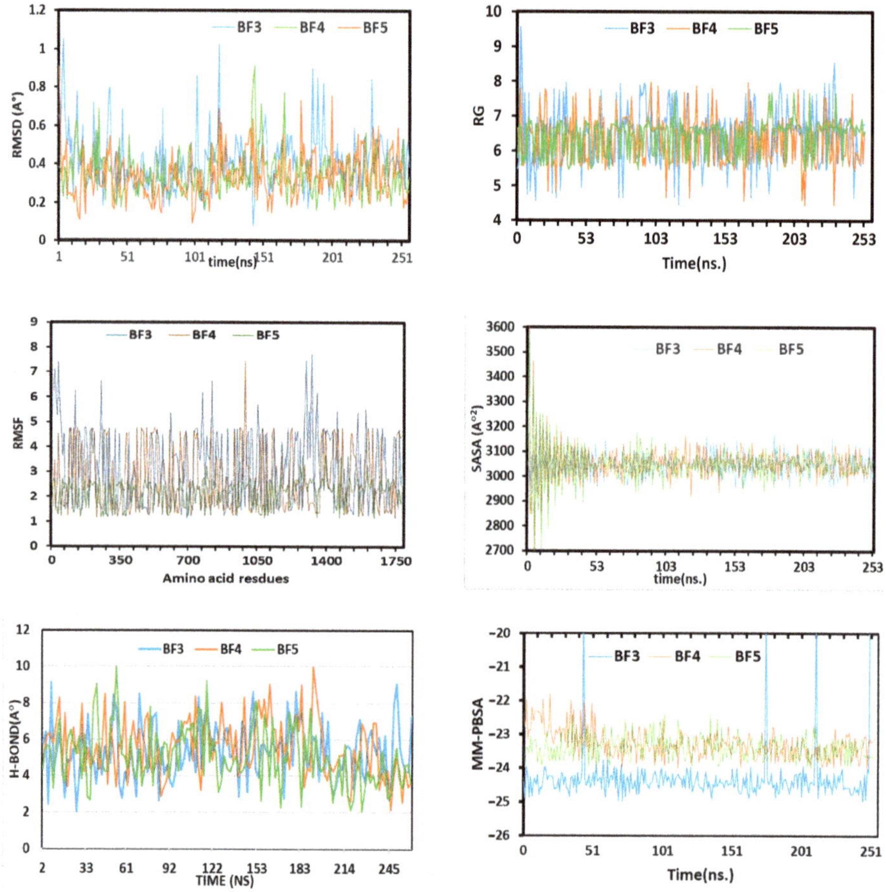

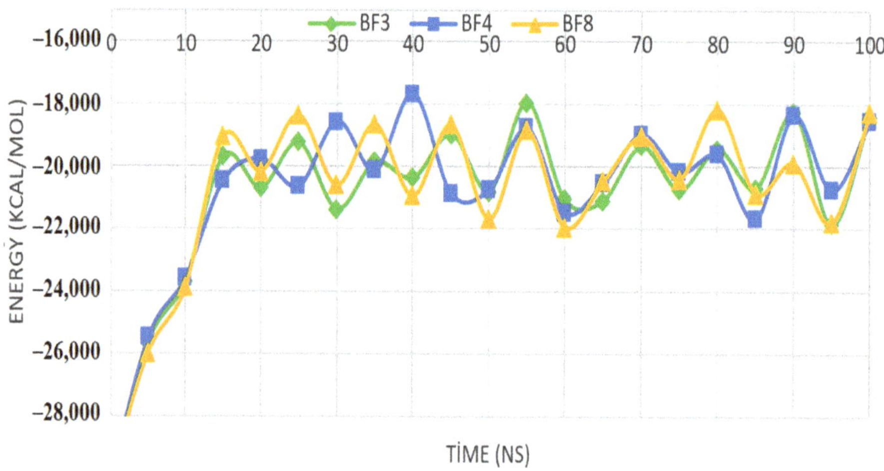

Figure 10. The molecular dynamics simulation trajectories from 250-ns simulation time.

Figure 11. Display of Gibbs free energy values of protein and ligand molecules at ten ns intervals.

The generated graph displays the binding free energy variations and changes for each interval of ten (ns), along with standard deviations (±) given in Table 2. The high affinity bromobenzofuran-1,3,4-oxadiazole binders to Mtb Pks13 were **BF3**, **BF4**, and **BF8** molecules, which were then compared to one another. Using this comparison, calculations were performed to support the (MM-PBSA) method's estimation of the bonding's free energies. The relevant parameters' negative values signify stronger binding [67]. According to calculations using equation-1, the average values of Gibbs free energies are −31.4 kcal/mol for Pks13+**BF3**, −48.8 for Pks13+**BF4**, and −41.5 for Pks13+**BF8**. It can be seen in Table 2 that at each ns, the compounds showed robust strong intermolecular interactions energy. This further demonstrates the formation of high stable complexes and the strong binding of the compounds to the Mtb Pks13 enzyme. However, as standard deviation values are moderate to high, further extensive calculations are needed to validate the energy values. In light of these results, it can be seen that the free energy values of these three molecules show that they may possess better repressive properties against the important Mtb Pks13 enzyme.

Table 2. The binding free energy changes and deviations in each ten (ns) interval. The energy values are presented in kcal/mol.

Nanoseconds	Pks13+BF3	Pks13+BF4	Pks13+BF8
10	−59.4 ± 149.6	−956.2 ± 586.2	−87.8 ± 235.6
20	−135.2 ± 235.5	−105.3 ± 387.4	−508.9 ± 245.1
30	−95.8 ± 269.3	−912.3 ± 189.3	−354.2 ± 245.3
40	−570.3 ± 684.2	−245.3 ± 245.6	−150.8 ± 250.4
50	−856.2 ± 345.6	−856.3 ± 409.8	−750.4 ± 150.6
60	−135.2 ± 248.6	−301.7 ± 204.8	−723.3 ± 523.6
70	−486.3 ± 367.3	−501.1 ± 193.5	−685.8 ± 351.2
80	−648.8 ± 385.2	−1101.3 ± 497.6	−289.7 ± 487.5
90	−329.2 ± 301.2	−687.5 ± 260.1	−350.4 ± 293.7
100	−300.8 ± 283.2	−423.4 ± 305.3	−145.8 ± 354.6

3. Materials and Methods

3.1. Chemistry

All the benzofuran-oxadiazole structural motifs **BF1–16** were afforded, and their characterization data were published by Irfan et al. [23,45,52]. The structures of benzofuran-1,3,4-oxadiazoles **BF1–BF16** along with the **TAM-16** standard reference inhibitor structure are given in Figure 11.

3.2. Molecular Docking of Benzofuran-1,3,4-oxadiazoles BF1–BF16

The protein PDB structure of the target enzyme Pks13 of *Mycobacterium tuberculosis* was achieved from the RCSB to carry out the molecular docking study (computational research) [68] website with the PDB Identifier (5V3Y) [62]. The molecular docking study of sixteen novel benzofuran-1,3,4-oxadiazoles was carried out with MOE (Ver-2009.10) software [69]. The first step was the preparation of protein structure of the Pks13 enzyme by removing water molecules and heteroatoms from the protein PDB structure with the help of Biovia DS [70] software for molecular docking study. The Chem-draw professional (Ver-16) software [71] (by PerkinElmer Informatics) was used to draw the structures of benzofuran-1,3,4-oxadiazole ligands **BF1–BF16** and saved in the mol format for further studies. Before docking, the ligand structures were loaded in the MOE, and their energy was minimized via the MMFF94x forcefield, and the partial charges were also added to the ligand structures. Using the Triangle Matcher placement strategies, the compounds were docked in the binding pocket and scored by the Dock module using the London-dG scoring function of MOE. The protein PDB was opened in MOE, and was 3D-protonated using the Amber99-ff. The active site of the Pks13 was located and selected using the Site

Finder function of MOE. The ligand-protein interaction was viewed using the software Biovia DS Studio (Ver-2017) [72].

3.3. ADMET and Drug-Likeness Investigations of Benzofuran-1,3,4-oxadiazoles

The ADME and drug-likeness studies of benzofuran-1,3,4-oxadiaole compounds were carried out by utilizing the Swissadme (Ver-1) [73] and ADMET lab (Ver-2.0) [74] online web-servers, while for the toxicity investigations, the ADMETSAR (Ver-1.0) [75,76] online server was utilized.

3.4. MD Simulation Study of the Most In Silico Bioactive BF3, BF4, and BF8 Derivatives

The MD Simulations of the most in silico predicted biologically active benzofuran-1,3,4-oxadiazole **BF3**, **BF4**, and **BF8** scaffolds were performed by GROMACS. Using GROMACS (Ver-2021) and the Linux 5.4 package, MD simulation of the protein-ligand complexes was carried out. The ligand topologies were created using the PRODRG server, and the GROMOS96 forcefield was used as the force field for proteins. Simple point charge (SPC) water molecules in a rectangular box were used to solvate each complex. Na + and Cl + ions were added to electrically make the simulation system neutral, whereas salt concentrations of 0.15 mol/L were set in each system. All solvated complexes underwent energy minimization for 5000 steps using the steepest descent method. Different productions were run in the MD simulation, including the constant number of particle, pressure, and temperature (NPT) series and the constant number of particle, volume, and temperature (NVT) series. For the simulation, a V-rescale thermostat and a Parrinello-Rahman barostat were chosen, and the NVT and NPT series were conducted at 300 K and 1 atm for 300 ps. Finally, the production run was completed after 250 ns at 300 K. [77,78].

3.5. MM-PBSA Binding Free Energy Calculations of the Most In Silico Bioactive BF3, BF4, and BF8 Derivatives

Molecular mechanics Poisson-Boltzmann surface area (MM-PBSA) calculations of molecules were made with molecular dynamic calculations. The different types of binding free energies, i.e., Van der Waals, electrostatic, kinetic, and potential energy changes of the studied **BF3**, **BF4**, and **BF8** molecules were determined for these calculations. In addition, this study examined the interactions between **BF3**, **BF4**, and **BF8** molecules and the 5V3Y protein, which is the Pks13 protein. These interaction energies were investigated at 100 ns. As a result of the interaction of the three molecules studied with the protein, the values of the binding free energy change were calculated. This calculation is given in Equation (1).

$$\Delta G_{Bind} = G_{complex} - (G_{res} + G_{lig}) \tag{1}$$

In the above equation, ΔG_{Bind} gives the total binding free energy value between the ligand and the Pks13 protein. G_{lig}, G_{res}, and $G_{complex}$ values in the equation are the values of the ligand molecule, Pks13 receptor protein, and complex molecule, respectively [79].

4. Conclusions

In conclusion, the novel series of sixteen benzofuran-1,3,4-oxadiazoles **BF1–BF16** was evaluated for their therapeutic inhibitory effect on Mtb Pks13 enzyme by applying various in silico approaches, such as molecular docking, MM-PBSA, pharmacokinetics, ADMET, and molecular dynamic simulations. The results of the CADD approach indicated that three in silico predicted lead compounds such as the 2,4-dimethyl moiety containing **BF3**, 2,5-dimethoxy moiety-based **BF4**, and 2-flouro moiety containing **BF8** displayed excellent in silico anti-TB chemotherapeutic potential due to the strong interaction with the active site of the Pks13 enzyme and the greater stability of these complexes in comparison to the standard reference benzofuran drug **TAM-16**. The conformational pose and binding affinity analysis of **BF3**, **BF4**, and **BF8** showed that these derivatives bind to the Pks13 active site with a binding affinity score of −14.23 kcal/mol, −14.82 kcal/mol, and of −14.11 kcal/mol, respectively, in comparison with the standard reference **TAM-16** (−14.61 kcal/mol). The

BF4 bromobenzofuran-1,3,4-oxadiazole showed higher binding affinity -14.82 kcal/mol than the reference Pks13 inhibitor **TAM-16** (-14.61 kcal/mol), which was further confirmed by the MM-PBSA calculations and the MD simulations studies. The ADMET studies of all the screened bromobenzofuran-oxadiazole structural hybrids demonstrated a high degree of drug-likeness profile. Overall, it is seen that the bromobenzofuran-1,3,4-oxadiazole **BF4** derivative has a more stable total binding free energy value against the 5V3Y protein. On the basis of different in silico techniques, 2,5-dimethoxy phenyl-substituted bromobenzofuran-1,3,4-oxdiazole **BF4** is a more in silico predicted effective reagent than **TAM-16**, so this in silico bioactive **BF4** can be a future lead anti-TB chemotherapeutic candidate after further in vitro and in vivo evaluations, which would be necessary to establish its chemotherapeutic efficacy against Mtb.

Supplementary Materials: The following supporting information can be downloaded at: https://www.mdpi.com/article/10.3390/ph16060829/s1. Binding affinities of benzofuran-1,3,4-oxadiazole **BF10–16** are present in the supplementary Table S1; ADMET and drug-likeness data is depicted in Tables S2 and S3, respectively.

Author Contributions: Conceptualization, A.F.Z. and A.I.; methodology, A.I.; software, S.F., B.T., M.H.A., A.A.E. and S.A.; validation, S.F., B.T. and M.H.A.; formal analysis, S.F., R.J. and M.H.A.; investigation, R.J. and A.I.; resources, S.A.A.-H.; data curation, S.A.A.-H. and R.J.; writing—original draft preparation, A.I.; writing—review and editing, A.I., S.F., R.N., A.F.Z. and M.E.A.Z.; Visualization, A.I. and S.F; supervision, A.F.Z.; project administration, A.F.Z. and M.E.A.Z. funding acquisition, S.A.A.-H. and M.E.A.Z. All authors have read and agreed to the published version of the manuscript.

Funding: This research was supported by the Deanship of Scientific Research, Imam Mohammad Ibn Saud Islamic University, Saudi Arabia.

Institutional Review Board Statement: Not applicable.

Informed Consent Statement: Not applicable.

Data Availability Statement: Data is contained within the article and Supplementary material.

Acknowledgments: Authors acknowledge the Government college university Faisalabad for research facilities provided to carry out this research work.

Conflicts of Interest: The authors declare no conflict of interest.

References

1. WHO. *Global Tuberculosis Report 2018*; WHO: Geneva, Switzerland, 2018; pp. 1–277. ISBN 978-92-4-156564-6. Available online: https://apps.who.int/iris/handle/10665/274453 (accessed on 8 May 2023).
2. Espinal, M.A. The Global Situation of MDR-TB. *Proc. Tuberc.* **2003**, *83*, 44–51. [CrossRef] [PubMed]
3. WHO. *Global Tuberculosis Report 2022*; WHO: Geneva, Switzerland, 2022; pp. 1–68. ISBN 978-92-4-006173-6.
4. Prasad, R.; Gupta, N.; Banka, A. Multidrug-resistant tuberculosis/rifampicin-resistant tuberculosis: Principles of management. *Lung India* **2018**, *35*, 78–81. [CrossRef] [PubMed]
5. Sotgiu, G.; Migliori, G.B. Facing Multi-Drug Resistant Tuberculosis. *Pulm. Pharmacol. Ther.* **2015**, *32*, 144–148. [CrossRef] [PubMed]
6. Aspatwar, A.; Kairys, V.; Rala, S.; Parikka, M.; Bozdag, M.; Carta, F.; Supuran, C.T.; Parkkila, S. Mycobacterium Tuberculosis β-Carbonic Anhydrases: Novel Targets for Developing Antituberculosis Drugs. *Int. J. Mol. Sci.* **2019**, *20*, 5153. [CrossRef]
7. Kaul, G.; Kapoor, E.; Dasgupta, A.; Chopra, S. Management of multidrug-resistant tuberculosis in the 21st century. *Drugs Today* **2019**, *55*, 215–224. [CrossRef]
8. Saxena, A.K.; Singh, A. Mycobacterial tuberculosis Enzyme Targets and their Inhibitors. *Curr. Top. Med. Chem.* **2019**, *19*, 337–355. [CrossRef]
9. Harding, E. WHO Global Progress Report on Tuberculosis Elimination. *Lancet. Respir. Med.* **2020**, *8*, 19. [CrossRef]
10. Tsai, Y.-P. Effectiveness of Tuberculosis Case Management. *J. Microbiol. Immunol. Infect.* **2015**, *48*, S121. [CrossRef]
11. Zumla, A.; Nahid, P.; Cole, S.T. Advances in the Development of New Tuberculosis Drugs and Treatment Regimens. *Nat. Rev. Drug Discov.* **2013**, *12*, 388–404. [CrossRef]
12. Chimeh, R.A.; Gafar, F.; Pradipta, I.S.; Akkerman, O.W.; Hak, E.; Alffenaar, J.W.C.; van Boven, J.F.M. Clinical and Economic Impact of Medication Non-Adherence in Drug-Susceptible Tuberculosis: A Systematic Review. *Int. J. Tuberc. Lung Dis.* **2020**, *24*, 811–819. [CrossRef]

13. Wang, X.; Dowd, C.S. The Methylerythritol Phosphate Pathway: Promising Drug Targets in the Fight against Tuberculosis. *ACS Infect. Dis.* **2018**, *4*, 278–290. [CrossRef]

14. Hiremathad, A.; Patil, M.R.; Chethana, K.R.; Chand, K.; Santos, M.A.; Keri, R.S. Benzofuran: An Emerging Scaffold for Anti-microbial Agents. *RSC Adv.* **2015**, *5*, 96809–96828. [CrossRef]

15. Xu, Z.; Zhao, S.; Lv, Z.; Feng, L.; Wang, Y.; Zhang, F.; Bai, L.; Deng, J. Benzofuran Derivatives and Their Anti-Tubercular, Antibacterial Activities. *Eur. J. Med. Chem.* **2019**, *162*, 266–276. [CrossRef]

16. Gill, C.; Jadhav, G.; Shaikh, M.; Kale, R.; Ghawalkar, A.; Nagargoje, D.; Shiradkar, M. Clubbed [1,2,3] Triazoles by Fluorine Benzimidazole: A Novel Approach to H37Rv Inhibitors as a Potential Treatment for Tuberculosis. *Bioorganic Med. Chem. Lett.* **2008**, *18*, 6244–6247. [CrossRef]

17. Irfan, A.; Sabeeh, I.; Umer, M.; Naqvi, A.Z.; Fatima, H.; Yousaf, S.; Fatima, Z. A Review On The Therapeutic Potential of Quinoxaline Derivatives. *World J. Pharm. Res.* **2017**, *6*, 47–68.

18. Rubab, L.; Afroz, S.; Ahmad, S.; Hussain, S.; Nawaz, I.; Irfan, A.; Batool, F.; Kotwica-Mojzych, K.; Mojzych, M. An Update on Synthesis of Coumarin Sulfonamides as Enzyme Inhibitors and Anticancer Agents. *Molecules* **2022**, *27*, 1604. [CrossRef]

19. Irfan, A.; Batool, F.; Irum, S.; Ullah, S.; Umer, M.; Shaheen, R.; Chand, A.J. A Therapeutic Journey Of Sulfonamide Derivatives As Potent Anti-Cancer Agents: A Review. *WJPR* **2018**, *7*, 257–270.

20. Aziz, H.; Zahoor, A.F.; Shahzadi, I.; Irfan, A. Recent Synthetic Methodologies Towards the Synthesis of Pyrazoles. *Polycycl. Aromat. Compd.* **2019**, *41*, 698–720. [CrossRef]

21. Irfan, A.; Batool, F.; Ahmad, S.; Ullah, R.; Sultan, A.; Sattar, R.; Nisar, B.; Rubab, L. Recent trends in the synthesis of 1,2,3-thiadiazoles. *Phosphorus Sulfur Silicon Relat. Elem.* **2019**, *194*, 1098–1115. [CrossRef]

22. Irfan, A.; Faisal, S.; Ahmad, S.; Al-Hussain, S.A.; Javed, S.; Zahoor, A.F.; Parveen, B.; Zaki, M.E.A. Structure-Based Virtual Screening of Furan-1,3,4-Oxadiazole Tethered *N*-phenylacetamide Derivatives as Novel Class of hTYR and hTYRP1 Inhibitors. *Pharmaceuticals* **2023**, *16*, 344. [CrossRef]

23. Irfan, A.; Faiz, S.; Rasul, A.; Zafar, R.; Zahoor, A.F.; Kotwica-Mojzych, K.; Mojzych, M. Exploring the Synergistic Anticancer Potential of Benzofuran–Oxadiazoles and Triazoles: Improved Ultrasound-and Microwave-Assisted Synthesis, Molecular Docking, Hemolytic, Thrombolytic and Anticancer Evaluation of Furan-Based Molecules. *Molecules* **2022**, *27*, 1023. [CrossRef] [PubMed]

24. Faiz, S.; Zahoor, A.F.; Ajmal, M.; Kamal, S.; Ahmad, S.; Abdelgawad, A.M.; Elnaggar, M.E. Design, Synthesis, Antimicrobial Evaluation, and Laccase Catalysis Effect of Novel Benzofuran–Oxadiazole and Benzofuran–Triazole Hybrids. *J. Heterocycl. Chem.* **2019**, *56*, 2839–2852. [CrossRef]

25. Bhargava, S.; Rathore, D. Synthetic Routes and Biological Activities of Benzofuran and Its Derivatives: A Review. *Lett. Org. Chem.* **2017**, *14*, 381–402. [CrossRef]

26. Nevagi, R.J.; Dighe, S.N.; Dighe, S.N. Biological and Medicinal Significance of Benzofuran. *Eur. J. Med. Chem.* **2015**, *97*, 561–581. [CrossRef] [PubMed]

27. Hiremathad, A.; Chand, K.; Tolayan, L.; Rajeshwari; Keri, R.S.; Esteves, A.R.; Cardoso, S.M.; Chaves, S.; Santos, M.A. Hydroxypyridinone-Benzofuran Hybrids with Potential Protective Roles for Alzheimer's Disease Therapy. *J. Inorg. Biochem.* **2018**, *179*, 82–96. [CrossRef]

28. Goyal, D.; Kaur, A.; Goyal, B. Benzofuran and Indole: Promising Scaffolds for Drug Development in Alzheimer's Disease. *ChemMedChem* **2018**, *13*, 1275–1299. [CrossRef]

29. Zeni, G.; Lüdtke, D.S.; Nogueira, C.W.; Panatieri, R.B.; Braga, A.L.; Silveira, C.C.; Stefani, H.A.; Rocha, J.B.T. New Acetylenic Furan Derivatives: Synthesis and Anti-Inflammatory Activity. *Tetrahedron Lett.* **2001**, *42*, 8927–8930. [CrossRef]

30. Thévenin, M.; Thoret, S.; Grellier, P.; Dubois, J. Synthesis of Polysubstituted Benzofuran Derivatives as Novel Inhibitors of Parasitic Growth. *Bioorganic Med. Chem.* **2013**, *21*, 4885–4892. [CrossRef]

31. Zhong, M.; Peng, E.; Huang, N.; Huang, Q.; Huq, A.; Lau, M.; Colonno, R.; Li, L. Discovery of Novel Potent HCV NS5B Polymerase Non-Nucleoside Inhibitors Bearing a Fused Benzofuran Scaffold. *Bioorganic Med. Chem. Lett.* **2018**, *28*, 963–968. [CrossRef]

32. Xie, Y.S.; Kumar, D.; Bodduri, V.D.V.; Tarani, P.S.; Zhao, B.X.; Miao, J.Y.; Jang, K.; Shin, D.S. Microwave-Assisted Parallel Synthesis of Benzofuran-2-Carboxamide Derivatives Bearing Anti-Inflammatory, Analgesic and Antipyretic Agents. *Tetrahedron Lett.* **2014**, *55*, 2796–2800. [CrossRef]

33. Rangaswamy, J.; Kumar, H.V.; Harini, S.T.; Naik, N. Functionalized 3-(Benzofuran-2-Yl)-5-(4-Methoxyphenyl)-4,5-Dihydro-1H-Pyrazole Scaffolds: A New Class of Antimicrobials and Antioxidants. *Arab. J. Chem.* **2017**, *10*, S2685–S2696. [CrossRef]

34. Singh, F.V.; Chaurasia, S.; Joshi, M.D.; Srivastava, A.K.; Goel, A. Synthesis and in Vivo Antihyperglycemic Activity of Nature-Mimicking Furanyl-2-Pyranones in STZ-S Model. *Bioorganic Med. Chem. Lett.* **2007**, *17*, 2425–2429. [CrossRef]

35. Simonetti, S.O.; Larghi, E.L.; Bracca, A.B.J.; Kaufman, T.S. Angular Tricyclic Benzofurans and Related Natural Products of Fungal Origin. Isolation, Biological Activity and Synthesis. *Nat. Prod. Rep.* **2013**, *30*, 941–969. [CrossRef]

36. Mei, W.; Ji, S.; Xiao, W.; Wang, X.; Jiang, C.; Ma, W.; Zhang, H.; Gong, J.; Guo, Y. Synthesis and Biological Evaluation of Benzothiazol-Based 1,3,4-Oxadiazole Derivatives as Amyloid β-Targeted Compounds against Alzheimer's Disease. *Mon. für Chem.* **2017**, *148*, 1807–1815. [CrossRef]

37. Nieddu, V.; Pinna, G.; Marchesi, I.; Sanna, L.; Asproni, B.; Pinna, G.A.; Bagella, L.; Murineddu, G. Synthesis and Antineoplastic Evaluation of Novel Unsymmetrical 1,3,4-Oxadiazoles. *J. Med. Chem.* **2016**, *59*, 10451–10469. [CrossRef]

38. Calcagno, A.; D'Avolio, A.; Bonora, S. Pharmacokinetic and Pharmacodynamic Evaluation of Raltegravir and Experience from Clinical Trials in HIV-Positive Patients. *Expert Opin. Drug Metab. Toxicol.* **2015**, *11*, 1167–1176. [CrossRef]

39. Bondock, S.; Adel, S.; Etman, H.A.; Badria, F.A. Synthesis and Antitumor Evaluation of Some New 1,3,4-Oxadiazole-Based Heterocycles. *Eur. J. Med. Chem.* **2012**, *48*, 192–199. [CrossRef]

40. Sun, J.; Ren, S.Z.; Lu, X.Y.; Li, J.J.; Shen, F.Q.; Xu, C.; Zhu, H.L. Discovery of a Series of 1,3,4-Oxadiazole-2(3H)-Thione Derivatives Containing Piperazine Skeleton as Potential FAK Inhibitors. *Bioorganic Med. Chem.* **2017**, *25*, 2593–2600. [CrossRef]

41. Prakash, O.; Kumar, M.; Kumar, R.; Sharma, C.; Aneja, K.R. Hypervalent Iodine(III) Mediated Synthesis of Novel Unsymmetrical 2,5-Disubstituted 1,3,4-Oxadiazoles as Antibacterial and Antifungal Agents. *Eur. J. Med. Chem.* **2010**, *45*, 4252–4257. [CrossRef]

42. Akhter, M.; Husain, A.; Azad, B.; Ajmal, M. Aroylpropionic Acid Based 2,5-Disubstituted-1,3,4-Oxadiazoles: Synthesis and Their Anti-Inflammatory and Analgesic Activities. *Eur. J. Med. Chem.* **2009**, *44*, 2372–2378. [CrossRef]

43. Janardhanan, J.; Chang, M.; Mobashery, S. The Oxadiazole Antibacterials. *Curr. Opin. Microbiol.* **2016**, *33*, 13–17. [CrossRef] [PubMed]

44. Ahsan, M.J.; Samy, J.G.; Khalilullah, H.; Nomani, M.S.; Saraswat, P.; Gaur, R.; Singh, A. Molecular Properties Prediction and Synthesis of Novel 1,3,4-Oxadiazole Analogues as Potent Antimicrobial and Antitubercular Agents. *Bioorg. Med. Chem. Lett.* **2011**, *21*, 7246–7250. [CrossRef] [PubMed]

45. Irfan, A.; Zahoor, A.F.; Rasul, A.; Al-Hussain, S.A.; Faisal, S.; Ahmad, S.; Noor, R.; Muhammed, M.T.; Zaki, M.E.A. BTEAC Catalyzed Ultrasonic-Assisted Synthesis of Bromobenzofuran-Oxadiazoles: Unravelling Anti-HepG-2 Cancer Therapeutic Potential through In Vitro and In Silico Studies. *Int. J. Mol. Sci.* **2023**, *24*, 3008. [CrossRef] [PubMed]

46. Wilson, C.; Ray, P.; Zuccotto, F.; Hernandez, J.; Aggarwal, A.; Mackenzie, C.; Caldwell, N.; Taylor, M.; Huggett, M.; Mathieson, M.; et al. Optimization of TAM16, a Benzofuran That Inhibits the Thioesterase Activity of Pks13; Evaluation toward a Preclinical Candidate for a Novel Antituberculosis Clinical Target. *J. Med. Chem.* **2022**, *65*, 409–423. [CrossRef] [PubMed]

47. Verma, S.K.; Verma, R.; Verma, S.; Vaishnav, Y.; Tiwari, S.P.; Rakesh, K.P. Anti-Tuberculosis Activity and Its Structure-Activity Relationship (SAR) Studies of Oxadiazole Derivatives: A Key Review. *Eur. J. Med. Chem.* **2021**, *209*, 112886. [CrossRef]

48. Makane, V.B.; Krishna, V.S.; Krishna, E.V.; Shukla, M.; Mahizhaveni, B.; Misra, S.; Chopra, S.; Sriram, D.; Azger Dusthackeer, V.N.; Rode, H.B. Novel 1,3,4-Oxadiazoles as Antitubercular Agents with Limited Activity against Drug-Resistant Tuberculosis. *Future Med. Chem.* **2019**, *11*, 499–510. [CrossRef]

49. Desai, N.C.; Somani, H.; Trivedi, A.; Bhatt, K.; Nawale, L.; Khedkar, V.M.; Jha, P.C.; Sarkar, D. Synthesis, Biological Evaluation and Molecular Docking Study of Some Novel Indole and Pyridine Based 1,3,4-Oxadiazole Derivatives as Potential Antitubercular Agents. *Bioorgan. Med. Chem. Lett.* **2016**, *26*, 1776–1783. [CrossRef]

50. Chobe, S.S.; Kamble, R.D.; Patil, S.D.; Acharya, A.P.; Hese, S.V.; Yemul, O.S.; Dawane, B.S. Green Approach towards Synthesis of Substituted Pyrazole-1,4-Dihydro,9-Oxa, 1,2,6,8-Tetrazacyclopentano[b]Naphthalene-5-One Derivatives as Antimycobacterial Agents. *Med. Chem. Res.* **2013**, *22*, 5197–5203. [CrossRef]

51. Dhumal, S.T.; Deshmukh, A.R.; Bhosle, M.R.; Khedkar, V.M.; Nawale, L.U.; Sarkar, D.; Mane, R.A. Synthesis and Antitubercular Activity of New 1,3,4-Oxadiazoles Bearing Pyridyl and Thiazolyl Scaffolds. *Bioorganic Med. Chem. Lett.* **2016**, *26*, 3646–3651. [CrossRef]

52. Irfan, A.; Zahoor, A.F.; Kamal, S.; Hassan, M.; Kloczkowski, A. Ultrasonic-Assisted Synthesis of Benzofuran Appended Oxadiazole Molecules as Tyrosinase Inhibitors: Mechanistic Approach through Enzyme Inhibition, Molecular Docking, Chemoinformatics, ADMET and Drug-Likeness Studies. *Int. J. Mol. Sci.* **2022**, *23*, 10979. [CrossRef]

53. Marimani, M.; Ahmad, A.; Duse, A. The Role of Epigenetics, Bacterial and Host Factors in Progression of Mycobacterium Tuberculosis Infection. *Tuberculosis* **2018**, *113*, 200–214. [CrossRef]

54. Ryndak, M.B.; Laal, S. *Mycobacterium tuberculosis* Primary Infection and Dissemination: A Critical Role for Alveolar Epithelial Cells. *Front. Cell. Infect. Microbiol.* **2019**, *9*, 299. [CrossRef]

55. Abdoli, A.; Falahi, S.; Kenarkoohi, A. COVID-19-Associated Opportunistic Infections: A Snapshot on the Current Reports. *Clin. Exp. Med.* **2022**, *22*, 327–346. [CrossRef]

56. Oh, S.; Park, Y.; Engelhart, C.A.; Wallach, J.B.; Schnappinger, D.; Arora, K.; Manikkam, M.; Gac, B.; Wang, H.; Murgolo, N.; et al. Discovery and Structure-Activity-Relationship Study of N-Alkyl-5-Hydroxypyrimidinone Carboxamides as Novel Antitubercular Agents Targeting Decaprenylphosphoryl-β-D-Ribose 2′-Oxidase. *J. Med. Chem.* **2018**, *61*, 9952–9965. [CrossRef]

57. Mohanty, D.; Sankaranarayanan, R.; Gokhale, R.S. Fatty Acyl-AMP Ligases and Polyketide Synthases Are Unique Enzymes of Lipid Biosynthetic Machinery in *Mycobacterium tuberculosis*. *Tuberculosis* **2011**, *91*, 448–455. [CrossRef]

58. Singh, S.; Singh, D.; Hameed, S.; Fatima, Z. An Overview of Mycolic Acids. Structure–function–classification, biosynthesis, and beyond. In *Biology of Mycobacterial Lipids*; Academic Press: Cambridge, MA, USA, 2022; pp. 1–25. [CrossRef]

59. Maitra, A.; Munshi, T.; Healy, J.; Martin, L.T.; Vollmer, W.; Keep, N.H.; Bhakta, S. Cell Wall Peptidoglycan in *Mycobacterium tuberculosis*: An Achilles' Heel for the TB-Causing Pathogen. *FEMS Microbiol. Rev.* **2019**, *43*, 548–575. [CrossRef]

60. Howard, N.C.; Marin, N.D.; Ahmed, M.; Rosa, B.A.; Martin, J.; Bambouskova, M.; Sergushichev, A.; Loginicheva, E.; Kurepina, N.; Rangel-Moreno, J.; et al. *Mycobacterium tuberculosis* Carrying a Rifampicin Drug Resistance Mutation Reprograms Macrophage Metabolism through Cell Wall Lipid Changes. *Nat. Microbiol.* **2018**, *3*, 1099–1108. [CrossRef]

61. Wellington, S.; Hung, D.T. The Expanding Diversity of *Mycobacterium tuberculosis* Drug Targets. *ACS Infect. Dis.* **2018**, *4*, 696–714. [CrossRef]

62. Aggarwal, A.; Parai, M.K.; Shetty, N.; Wallis, D.; Woolhiser, L.; Hastings, C.; Dutta, N.K.; Galaviz, S.; Dhakal, R.C.; Shrestha, R.; et al. Development of a Novel Lead That Targets M. Tuberculosis Polyketide Synthase 13. *Cell* **2017**, *170*, 249–259.e25. [CrossRef]
63. Çınaroğlu, S.S.; Timuçin, E. Insights into an Alternative Benzofuran Binding Mode and Novel Scaffolds of Polyketide Synthase 13 Inhibitors. *J. Mol. Model.* **2019**, *25*, 130. [CrossRef]
64. He, Y.; Xu, J.; Yu, Z.H.; Gunawan, A.M.; Wu, L.; Wang, L.; Zhang, Z.Y. Discovery and Evaluation of Novel Inhibitors of Mycobacterium Protein Tyrosine Phosphatase B from the 6-Hydroxy-Benzofuran-5-Carboxylic Acid Scaffold. *J. Med. Chem.* **2013**, *56*, 832–842. [CrossRef] [PubMed]
65. Lokhande, K.B.; Shrivastava, A.; Singh, A. In silico discovery of potent inhibitors against monkeypox's major structural proteins. *J. Biomol. Struct. Dyn.* **2023**, *25*, 1–16. [CrossRef] [PubMed]
66. Nagare, S.; Lokhande, K.B.; Swamy, K.V. Docking and simulation studies on cyclin D/CDK4 complex for targeting cell cycle arrest in cancer using flavanone and its congener. *J. Mol. Model.* **2023**, *29*, 90. [CrossRef] [PubMed]
67. Gupta, M.K.; Vemula, S.; Donde, R.; Gouda, G.; Behera, L.; Vadde, R. In-Silico Approaches to Detect Inhibitors of the Human Severe Acute Respiratory Syndrome Coronavirus Envelope Protein Ion Channel. *J. Biomol. Struct. Dyn.* **2021**, *39*, 2617–2627. [CrossRef] [PubMed]
68. Burley, S.K.; Berman, H.M.; Bhikadiya, C.; Bi, C.; Chen, L.; Di Costanzo, L.; Christie, C.; Dalenberg, K.; Duarte, J.M.; Dutta, S.; et al. RCSB Protein Data Bank: Biological Macromolecular Structures Enabling Research and Education in Fundamental Biology, Biomedicine, Biotechnology and Energy. *Nucleic Acids Res.* **2019**, *47*, D464–D474. [CrossRef]
69. Vilar, S.; Cozza, G.; Moro, S. Medicinal Chemistry and the Molecular Operating Environment (MOE): Application of QSAR and Molecular Docking to Drug Discovery. *Curr. Top. Med. Chem.* **2008**, *8*, 1555–1572. [CrossRef]
70. Faisal, S.; Lal Badshah, S.; Kubra, B.; Sharaf, M.; Emwas, A.H.; Jaremko, M.; Abdalla, M. Computational Study of SARS-CoV-2 Rna Dependent Rna Polymerase Allosteric Site Inhibition. *Molecules* **2022**, *27*, 223. [CrossRef]
71. Accelrys Software Inc. *Discovery Studio Modeling Environment, Release 3.5*; Accelrys Software Inc.: San Diego, CA, USA, 2012.
72. Mills, N. ChemDraw Ultra 10.0 CambridgeSoft, 100 CambridgePark Drive, Cambridge, MA 02140. Www.Cambridgesoft.Com. Commercial Price: $1910 for Download, $2150 for CD-ROM; Academic Price: $710 for Download, $800 for CD-ROM. *J. Am. Chem. Soc.* **2006**, *128*, 13649–13650. [CrossRef]
73. Daina, A.; Michielin, O.; Zoete, V. SwissADME: A Free Web Tool to Evaluate Pharmacokinetics, Drug-Likeness and Medicinal Chemistry Friendliness of Small Molecules. *Sci. Rep.* **2017**, *7*, 42717. [CrossRef]
74. Xiong, G.; Wu, Z.; Yi, J.; Fu, L.; Yang, Z.; Hsieh, C.; Yin, M.; Zeng, X.; Wu, C.; Lu, A.; et al. ADMETlab 2.0: An Integrated Online Platform for Accurate and Comprehensive Predictions of ADMET Properties. *Nucleic Acids Res.* **2021**, *49*, W5–W14. [CrossRef]
75. GFYang, H.; Lou, C.; Sun, L.; Li, J.; Cai, Y.; Wang, Z.; Li, W.; Liu, G.; Tang, Y. AdmetSAR 2.0: Web-Service for Prediction and Optimization of Chemical ADMET Properties. *Bioinformatics* **2019**, *35*, 1067–1069. [CrossRef]
76. Cheng, F.; Li, W.; Zhou, Y.; Shen, J.; Wu, Z.; Liu, G.; Lee, P.W.; Tang, Y. AdmetSAR: A Comprehensive Source and Free Tool for Assessment of Chemical ADMET Properties. *J. Chem. Inf. Model.* **2012**, *52*, 3099–3105. [CrossRef]
77. Jo, S.; Kim, T.; Iyer, V.G.; Im, W. CHARMM-GUI: A web-based graphical user interface for CHARMM. *J. Comput. Chem.* **2008**, *29*, 1859–1865. [CrossRef]
78. Lee, J.; Cheng, X.; Swails, J.M.; Yeom, M.S.; Eastman, P.K.; Lemkul, J.A.; Wei, S.; Buckner, J.; Jeong, J.C.; Qi, Y.; et al. CHARMM-GUIInput Generator for NAMD, GROMACS, AMBER, OpenMM, and CHARMM/OpenMM Simulations Using the CHARMM36Additive Force Field. *J. Chem. Theory Comput.* **2016**, *12*, 405–413. [CrossRef]
79. Aktaş, A.; Tüzün, B.; Aslan, R.; Sayin, K.; Ataseven, H. New Anti-Viral Drugs for the Treatment of COVID-19 Instead of Favipiravir. *J. Biomol. Struct. Dyn.* **2021**, *39*, 7263–7273. [CrossRef]

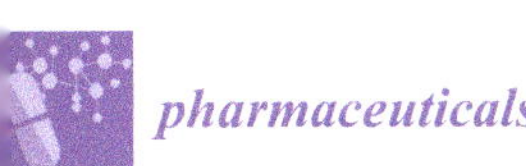 *pharmaceuticals*

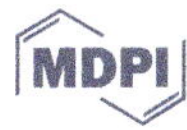

Article

Synthesis, Physicochemical Characterization, Biological Evaluation, In Silico and Molecular Docking Studies of Pd(II) Complexes with P, S-Donor Ligands

Hizbullah Khan [1,*], Muhammad Sirajuddin [1,*], Amin Badshah [2], Sajjad Ahmad [3], Muhammad Bilal [4], Syed Muhammad Salman [5], Ian S. Butler [6], Tanveer A. Wani [7] and Seema Zargar [8]

[1] Department of Chemistry, University of Science and Technology, Bannu 28100, Pakistan
[2] Department of Chemistry, Quaid-i-Azam University, Islamabad 45320, Pakistan; aminbadshah@qau.edu.pk
[3] Department of Health and Biological Sciences, Abasyn University, Peshawar 25000, Pakistan; sajjademman8@gmail.com
[4] Department of Chemistry, Kohat University of Science and Technology, Kohat 26000, Pakistan; mbilal@kust.edu.pk
[5] Department of Chemistry, Islamia College University, Peshawar 25120, Pakistan; salman@icp.edu.pk
[6] Department of Chemistry, University of McGill, Montreal, QC H3A 0B8, Canada; ian.butler@mcgill.ca
[7] Department of Pharmaceutical Chemistry, College of Pharmacy, King Saud University, P.O. Box 2457, Riyadh 11451, Saudi Arabia; twani@ksu.edu.sa
[8] Department of Biochemistry, College of Science, King Saud University, P.O. Box 22452, Riyadh 11451, Saudi Arabia; szargar@ksu.edu.sa
* Correspondence: dr.hizbullah@ustb.edu.pk (H.K.); dr.sirajuddin@ustb.edu.pk (M.S.)

Citation: Khan, H.; Sirajuddin, M.; Badshah, A.; Ahmad, S.; Bilal, M.; Salman, S.M.; Butler, I.S.; Wani, T.A.; Zargar, S. Synthesis, Physicochemical Characterization, Biological Evaluation, In Silico and Molecular Docking Studies of Pd(II) Complexes with P, S-Donor Ligands. *Pharmaceuticals* **2023**, *16*, 806. https://doi.org/10.3390/ph16060806

Academic Editors: Halil Ibrahim Ciftci, Belgin Sever and Hasan Demirci

Received: 12 May 2023
Revised: 25 May 2023
Accepted: 26 May 2023
Published: 29 May 2023

Abstract: One homoleptic (**1**) and three heteroleptic (**2–4**) palladium(II) complexes were synthesized and characterized by various physicochemical techniques, i.e., elemental analysis, FTIR, Raman spectroscopy, ^{1}H, ^{13}C, and ^{31}P NMR. Compound **1** was also confirmed by single crystal XRD, showing a slightly distorted square planar geometry. The antibacterial results obtained via the agar-well diffusion method for compound **1** were maximum among the screen compounds. All the compounds have shown good to significant antibacterial results against the tested bacterial strains, *Escherichia coli*, *Klebsiella pneumonia*, and *Staphylococcus aureus*, except **2** against *Klebsiella pneumonia*. Similarly, the molecular docking study of compound **3** has shown the best affinity with binding energy scores of −8.6569, −6.5716, and −7.6966 kcal/mol against *Escherichia coli*, *Klebsiella pneumonia*, and *Staphylococcus aureus*, respectively. Compound **2** has exhibited the highest activity (3.67 µM), followed by compound **3** (4.57 µM), **1** (6.94 µM), and **4** (21.7 µM) against the DU145 human prostate cancer cell line using the sulforhodamine B (SRB) method as compared to cisplatin (>200 µM). The highest docking score was obtained for compounds **2** (−7.5148 kcal/mol) and **3** (−7.0343 kcal/mol). Compound **2** shows that the Cl atom of the compound acts as a chain side acceptor for the DR5 receptor residue *Asp B218* and the pyridine ring is involved in interaction with the *Tyr A50* residue via arene-H, while Compound **3** interacts with the *Asp B218* residue via the Cl atom. The physicochemical parameters determined by the SwissADME webserver revealed that no blood-brain barrier (BBB) permeation is predicted for all four compounds, while gastrointestinal absorption is low for compound **1** and high for the rest of the compounds (**2–4**). As concluding remarks based on the obtained in vitro biological results, the evaluated compounds after in vivo studies might be a good choice for future antibiotics and anticancer agents.

Keywords: Pd(II) complexes; X-ray structure; antibacterial activity; antitumor activity; in silico study; molecular docking

1. Introduction

Cancer is a devastating disease, yet many types can be entirely treated if discovered early on, and for many others, patients' lives can be greatly prolonged. Surgery, radiation therapy, and chemotherapy [1] are three common cancer treatment modalities that are usually used in conjunction. The form of treatment is determined by the nature of the disease and the stage at which it has progressed [2]. Chemotherapy is one of the most common treatments for numerous forms of malignancies. Localized tumors can be efficiently treated with surgery and radiotherapy; however, their success is hampered by cancer cells spreading to other parts of the body [2]. Although radiotherapy and surgery can cure 40% of cancer patients (mostly those with tiny tumors), the spread of cancer cells may result in the death of the remaining 60% [3–5]. Surgery and radiation therapy cannot be utilized to treat metastasized tumors; hence, chemotherapy offers this advantage [6,7]. An ideal antitumor medication would be one that destroys only malignant cells while leaving healthy cells alone.

In actuality, all anticancer medications also impact healthy cells, resulting in a variety of side effects, including nausea, vomiting, and exhaustion [2,4]. Since anticancer medicines can harm blood cells, patients may develop anemia and a reduced white blood cell count [8]. The side effects are normally treatable and diminish once the treatment is completed. Combination chemotherapy combines medications with diverse methods to overcome resistance, reduce adverse effects, and kill as many malignant cells as possible [9]. Therapeutic medications cause DNA damage either directly or indirectly by interfering with biomolecules that are utilized to manufacture DNA, such as enzymes and proteins [10].

Many efforts have been made to clarify cisplatin's biological targets since its discovery as an anticancer medication [11]. Cisplatin has the potential to target DNA, RNA, and glutathione, although DNA is likely to be the most significant target [12]. We now have a fairly thorough grasp of how cisplatin and its analogues interact with DNA and what structural alterations take place as a result of this interaction after decades of research [13,14]. Although only around 1% of cisplatin molecules attach to DNA [15], the anticancer action of cisplatin is thought to be predominantly due to DNA binding [16]. With the N7 of guanine and adenine, Pt^{2+} produces both nonfunctional and bifunctional adducts.

Khan et al. [17–19] prepared palladium(II) complexes using three antibiotics: tetracycline, doxycycline, and chlortetracycline. Elemental studies, conductivity analyses, thermogravimetry, and infrared spectroscopy were used to properly describe the complexes. ^{1}H NMR was used to explore the mechanism of interaction between Pd(II) ions and tetracycline. Through the amide and hydroxyl groups at ring A, all three antibiotics create 1:1 compounds with Pd(II). Tetracycline's Pd(II) complex was 16 times more efficient than tetracycline at slowing down the growth of *E. coli* HB101/pBR322, a bacterial strain that is resistant to tetracycline, and it was just as successful at stifling the growth of two *E. coli* susceptible bacterial strains. In the resistant strain, the palladium(II) combination with doxycycline increased its activity by a factor of two [20]. At concentrations of $(4.6–9.1) \times 10^{-4}$ mol/L, several palladium (II) compounds showed broad-spectrum antibacterial action against a variety of human diseases [21,22]. Dithiocrabamates are highly versatile ligands that form stable complexes with transition elements and with the majority of the main group elements, lanthanides and actinides [23,24]. The orgaotin(IV) dithiocarbamate complexes have good coordination chemistry, stability, and diverse molecular structures, which make them suitable for diverse biological activities [25,26].

Palladium(II) and platinum(II) complexes have structural and thermodynamic similarities [27–30]. As a result, creating palladium medications with the highest level of pharmacological action is of great importance. In this investigation, several mixed-ligand palladium(II) complexes have proven to be quite promising [29,31,32]. Palladium(II) metallodrugs are suitable models for studying how biological molecules interact with one another in vivo due to their greater liability (103 times quicker on average than platinum) and ease of hydration in vitro [33]. It is hypothesized that palladium complexes are more successful in treating cisplatin-resistant gastrointestinal malignancies [17,34]. Dithiocarbamates have shown medicinal importance in various fields such as agriculture, pharmaceuticals, and medicine, especially in anticancer, antioxidant, and antimicrobial activities. So keeping in view their biological importance, we have selected dithiocarbamate-based ligands to synthesize Pd(II) complexes with phosphorus donor ligands.

2. Results and Discussion

The physical data of the reported compounds, including molecular formula, yield, melting point, and elemental analysis, is given in the Section 3. The sharp melting points and close matching of the elemental analysis data confirm the purity of the prepared compounds. The compounds were soluble in common organic solvents and stable at room temperature.

2.1. FT-IR and Raman Results

The FT-IR and Raman data of the prepared compounds are given in the Section 3. A peak in the range of 2852–2935 cm^{-1} and 3040–3052 cm^{-1} was attributed to the sp^3 hybridized aliphatic C-H and the sp^2 hybridized aromatic C-H, respectively. The Raman peaks for Pd-Cl, Pd-P, and Pd-S bonds appeared at 298–308 cm^{-1}, 210–221 cm^{-1} and 380–395 cm^{-1}, respectively. The appearance of the formation of the Pd-S verifies the Pd dithiocarbamate bond formation. The peak at 1092–1097 cm^{-1} was assigned to the SCS group, while that at 1520–1530 cm^{-1} was ascribed to the C $=\!=\!=$ N moiety. The partial double bond character in the C-N bond for dithiocarbamate complexes was confirmed from the appearance of the peak in the range of 1520–1530 cm^{-1} as the single C-N bond appears at 1251–1361 cm^{-1} while the C=N shift value is reported at 1640–1690 cm^{-1} [17]. The presence of a single asymmetric SCS peak in the range of 1092–1097 cm^{-1} indicates the bidentate bonding mode of the dithiocarbamate ligand with palladium moiety; for monodentate bonding, two peaks are to be observed in this region if the dithiocarbamate [35]. Figure S1 of the Supplementary Materials shows the FTIR spectrum of Complex **2**.

2.2. Multinuclear NMR (^1H, ^{13}C and ^{31}P)

The NMR data of the ligands and their palladium complexes is given in the Section 3. The ^1H NMR data is almost similar, with no conspicuous differentiation. The ^{13}C NMR of the characteristic SCS fragment is observed in the range of 207.3–208.2 ppm and provides an important indication for the complex's formation. A slight up field from the ligand due to the accumulation of electronic density over the carbon atom in SCS after the complexation with palladium metal was observed. The ^{31}P NMR of the synthesized compounds is observed in the range of 20.3–27.5 ppm, and it also depicts a slight up field from the ligand as a result of the transfer of electron density from the ligand to the Pd^{2+} center. Figures S2–S4 of the Supplementary Materials show the ^1H, ^{13}C, and ^{31}P NMR spectra of complex **1**.

2.3. Structural Study of Complex **1**

Complex **1** single crystal XRD data was collected at 200 K using a STOE IPDS image plate detector using MoK_α radiation, as depicted in Table 1. The STOE X-AREA application was used to get cell parameters, gather data, and integrate data. With hydrogen atoms in optimal locations, all non-H atoms were refined anisotropically after the structure was solved and refined using SHELXT [36] and SHELXL-2015 [37].

The ORTEP view of complex **1** in a monoclynic crystla system with the P21 space group is given in Figure 1. The dimensions of the unit cell are: a = 16.3128(4)Å, b = 10.2144(2)Å, and c = 18.7283(4)Å, while the α and $\gamma = 90°$ and $\beta = 115.793(1)°$. The crystal unit contains two independent molecules. The environment around the palladium atom is square planar with slight distortion, having bond angles of Cl1-Pd1-Cl2 = 178.40° and P(2)-Pd1-P(1) = 179.39°, as given in Table 2. Similarly, the geometry around the P1 atom is distorted tetrahedral, with bond angles of C(21)-P(1)-C(31) = 102.4°, C(21)-P(1)-C(11) = 106.8°, and C(21)-P(1)-Pd1 = 117.5°. The geometrical arrangement around the P2 atom is also distorted tetrahedral, with the largest distortion being caused by the palladium atom due to its large size, and the bond angles are: C(51)-P(2)-Pd1 = 118.7°, C(51)-P(2)-C(61) = 101.0°, and C(51)-P(2)-C(41) = 105.9°. The hydrogen bonding and other short contacts in a molecule affect the phyiscochemical properties of the molecule. The synthesized compound of palladium shows no hydrogen bonding, but it exhibits short contacts around some outer hydrogen and carbon atoms present in the propyl and benzene rings. The torsion angle for the atoms Cl1-Pd1-P(1)-C(21) is −30.7(5)°, which is synclinal; Cl2-Pd1-P(1)-C(21) is 147.7(5)°, which is anticlinal; and P(2)-Pd1-P(1)-C(21) is −74(11)°, which is also anticlinal.

Table 1. Single crystal XRD data of complex **1**.

Parameter	Data
Molecular formula and weigth	$C_{30}H_{34}Cl_2P_2Pd$ & 633.81
Temperature and λ	200 K & 1.54178 Å
Crystal system and Space group	Monoclinic and $P2_1$
dimensions of unit cell	a = 16.3128(4) Å, b = 10.2144(2) Å, c = 18.7283(4)α, γ = 90°, β = 115.793(1)°
Volume and Z	2809.71(11)Å^3 & 4
ρ, μ & F(000)	1.498 g/cm^3, 8.280 mm^{-1} & 1296
θ range	2.62 to 72.50°
Index	$-19 \leq h \leq 20, -12 \leq k \leq 12, -23 \leq l \leq 23$
Collec. Ref.	37,079
Indep. Ref.	5866 [Rint = 0.045]
Max. and min. transmission	0.5601 and 0.3968
Data/restraints/parameters	5866/1/636
S on F^2	1.144
Final R indices [I > 2sigma(I)]	R_1 = 0.0584, wR$_2$ = 0.1387
R indices (all data)	R_1 = 0.0586, wR$_2$ = 0.1389
Largest diff. peak and hole	5.871 and −1.371 e/Å^3
CCDC#	2,218,216

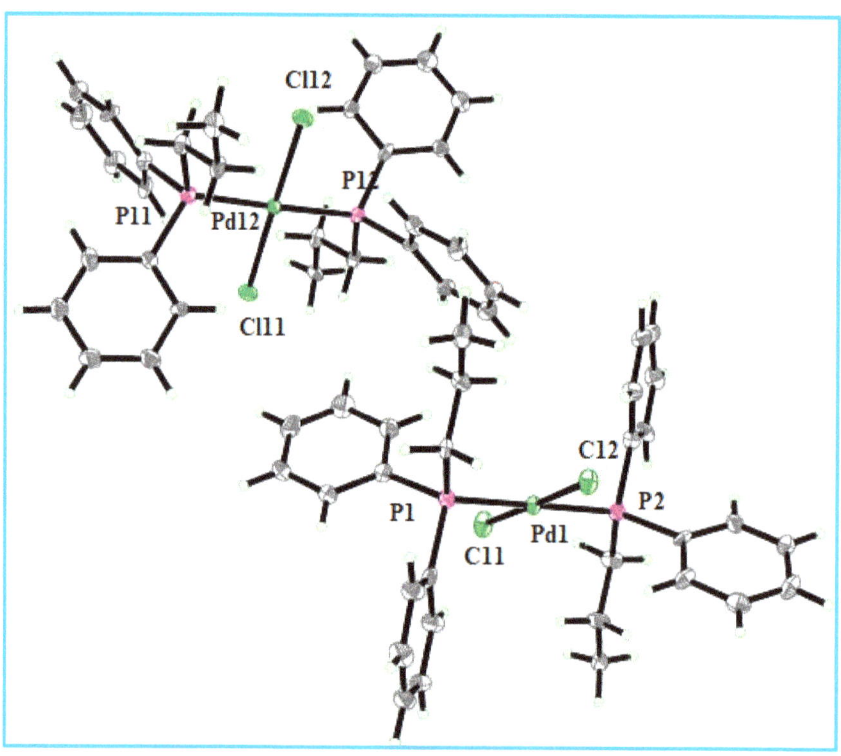

Figure 1. ORTEP view of **1**, with non-H, C atom numbering.

Table 2. Selected bond lengths and angles for complex **1**.

Selected Bond Length/Å			
Atom–Atom	**Length**	**Atom–Atom**	**Length**
Pd1–Cl1	2.301(2)	Pd12–Cl11	2.301(2)
Pd1–Cl2	2.302(2)	Pd12–Cl12	2.300(2)
Pd1–P1	2.328(3)	Pd12–P11	2.318(3)
Pd1–P2	2.326(3)	Pd12–P12	2.328(3)
P1–C11	1.853(13)	P11–C111	1.833(11)
P1–C21	1.822(11)	P11–C121	1.846(13)
P1–C31	1.829(10)	P11–C131	1.841(11)
P2–C41	1.858(12)	P12–C141	1.807(12)
P2–C51	1.814(10)	P12–C151	1.824(11)
P2–C61	1.825(12)	P12–C161	1.841(12)

Selected Bond Length/°			
Atom–Atom–Atom	**Angle**	**Atom–Atom–Atom**	**Angle**
Cl1–Pd1–Cl2	178.40(11)	Cl11–Pd12–P11	90.56(10)
Cl1–d1–P1	90.46(10)	Cl11–Pd12–P12	90.25(10)
Cl1–Pd1–P2	89.09(10)	Cl12–Pd12–Cl11	178.86(11)
Cl2–Pd1–P1	89.68(10)	Cl12–Pd12–P11	89.45(10)
Cl2–Pd1–P2	90.77(10)	Cl12–Pd12–P12	89.77(10)
P2–Pd1–P1	179.39(13)	P11–Pd12–P12	178.11(11)
C11–P1–Pd1	106.6(4)	C111–P11–Pd12	119.3(4)
C21–P1–Pd1	117.5(4)	C121–P11–Pd12	105.9(4)
C31–P1–Pd1	116.4(3)	C131–P11–Pd12	117.9(4)
C41–P2–Pd1	108.0(4)	C141–P12–Pd12	117.2(4)
C51–P2–Pd1	118.7(4)	C151–P12–Pd12	109.9(4)
C61–P2–Pd1	115.8(4)	C161–P12–Pd12	114.6(4)

2.4. Biological Investigation Results

2.4.1. Antitumor Results

Table 3 describes the anticancer efficacy of the Pd(II) complexes against cisplatin-resistant DU145 human prostate carcinoma cells. The screened compounds have shown activity in the order of **2** > **3** > **4** > **1**. The higher activity of the heteroleptic compounds **2**, **3**, and **4** containing different organophosphine ligands despite sharing a dithiocarbamate group is due to the electronegative nitrogen atom included in the organophosphine ligand, which can interact with the DNA strands of the carcinoma cells in a variety of ways'. This may be responsible for the greater activity of compound **2**.

Table 3. IC$_{50}$ (µM) values of the synthesized compounds (**1–4**).

Compound #	IC$_{50}$ (µM)
1	6.94 ± 0.58
2	3.67 ± 0.17
3	4.57 ± 0.57
4	21.7 ± 1.15
cisplatin	>200 [38]

2.4.2. Antibacterial Results

Table 4 describes the antibacterial potentials of the Pd(II) complexes against various Gram-positive and negative bacterial strains. Compound **1** is the most active, while complex **3** is the least active compound. The higher activity of complex **1** may be attributed to the fact that it has no dithiocarbamate ligand, while the other three complexes (**2–4**) have dithiocarbamate ligands, which can react with other active compounds inside the cell, so they may not have reached the target moiety.

Table 4. Antibacterial activity (inhibition zone in mm) of Pd(II) complexes [a].

Sample	*E. coli*	*K. pneumoniae*	*S. aureus*	*B. subtilis*	*S. epidermidis*
1	19 ± 0.33	17 ± 0.31	21 ± 0.41	17 ± 0.31	16 ± 0.15
2	18 ± 0.30	14 ± 0.24	17 ± 0.31	18 ± 0.30	16 ± 0.15
3	19 ± 0.33	2 ± 0.11	18 ± 0.30	18 ± 0.30	20 ± 0.31
4	20 ± 0.34	16 ± 0.15	17 ± 0.31	16 ± 0.15	19 ± 0.33
SD	26 ± 0.21	26 ± 0.23	35 ± 0.11	35 ± 0.11	35 ± 0.11
DMSO	0	0	0	0	0

[a] Criteria for determining antibacterial assay: no activity: <9 mm; non-significant: 9–12 mm; good activity: 16–18 mm; significant activity: >18 mm. SD: standard drug (Streptomycin with concentration of 2 mg/mL).

2.5. In Silico Assessment

In order to make a crucial decision on a daily basis about which compound should be synthesized, tested, and promoted as a drug candidate, the study of pharmacokinetics has utmost importance. Not only the efficacy and toxicity but also other parameters such as absorption, distribution, metabolism, and excretion are thoroughly studied before the processing of a molecule to be marketed as medicine for the benefit of patients.

The pharmacokinetic parameters of the synthesized complexes were studied by *SwissADME* webserver. The physicochemical properties show that the complexes **1**, **2**, **3**, and **4** have 10, 5, 7, and 5 rotatable bonds, respectively, as shown in Table 5. The lipophilicity $LogP_{o/w}$ (*iLOGP*) is zero for all four complexes, while $LogP_{o/w}$ (*XLOGP3*) is 9.49, 6.46, 7.54 and 7.56 for complexes 1, 2, 3, and 4, respectively. Poor solubility in water is predicted, which is in agreement with the experimental observation. No blood-brain barrier (*BBB*) permeation is predicted for all four complexes, while gastrointestinal (*GI*) absorption is low for complex 1 and high for the rest of the three complexes. No drug likeness for complexes 1, 3, and 4 and yes for complex 2 is predicted by the *Lipinsky* model, while the *Veber* model has predicted positive drug likeness for all four complexes. The medicinal chemistry parameter has predicted zero alerts for all four complexes by *PAINS*, one alert for complexes 1, 2, and 4, and two alerts for complex 3 by *Brenk*.

Table 5. ADMET and drug-like parameters of synthesized compounds predicted by SwissADME web server [a].

Comp. #	Physicochemical Properties		Lipophilicity		Water Solubility (mg/mL)		Pharmacokinetics		Drug Likeness			Medicinal Chemistry	
	M. W.	RT	$LogP_{o/w}$ (iLOGP)	$LogP_{o/w}$ (XLOGP)	S	Class	BBB P	GI A	Lipinsky	Veber	PAINS	Brenk
1	633.4	10	0.00	9.49	1.61×10^{-7}	PS	No	Low	No; 2 vio: MW > 500, MLOGP > 4.15	Yes	0 alert	1 alert: phosphor
2	526.4	5	0.00	6.46	2.42×10^{-5}	PS	No	High	Yes; 1 vio: MW > 500	Yes	0 alert	1 alert: phosphor
3	568.4	7	0.00	7.54	4.55×10^{-6}	PS	No	High	No; 2 vio: MW > 500, MLOGP > 4.15	Yes	0 alert	2 alerts: phosphor, thiocarbonyl group
4	539.4	5	0.00	7.56	4.36×10^{-6}	PS	No	High	No; 2 vio: MW > 500,	Yes	0 alert	1 alert: phosphor

[a] MW: molecular weight; RT: rotatable bonds; S: solubility; PS: poorly soluble; GI A: gastrointestinal absorption; vio: violation; BBB P: blood brain barrier permeant.

2.6. Molecular Docking Results

The compounds docking results with the selected antibacterial targets are provided in Table 6. Lower binding energies indicate a stronger binding affinity of the complexes with the target proteins. Among the screened compounds, **3** have shown the highest binding affinity of −8.6569, −6.5716, and −7.6966 kcal/mol against *E. coli*, *K. pneumonia*, and *S. aureus*, respectively. The next highest binding energy is shown by compound **4** against all three bacterial strains, which is evident from the binding energy value given in Table 6. The docking confirmation and 2D interaction diagram of complex **3** against the three bacterial proteins are given in Figures 2–4. Figure 2 shows that the Cl atoms of Compound 3 interact with the *His 203* and *Lys 162* residues of *E. coli*. Figure 3 shows that the benzene ring of Compound **3** interacts with the *Asn B220* residues of *K. pneumonia* via arene–H.

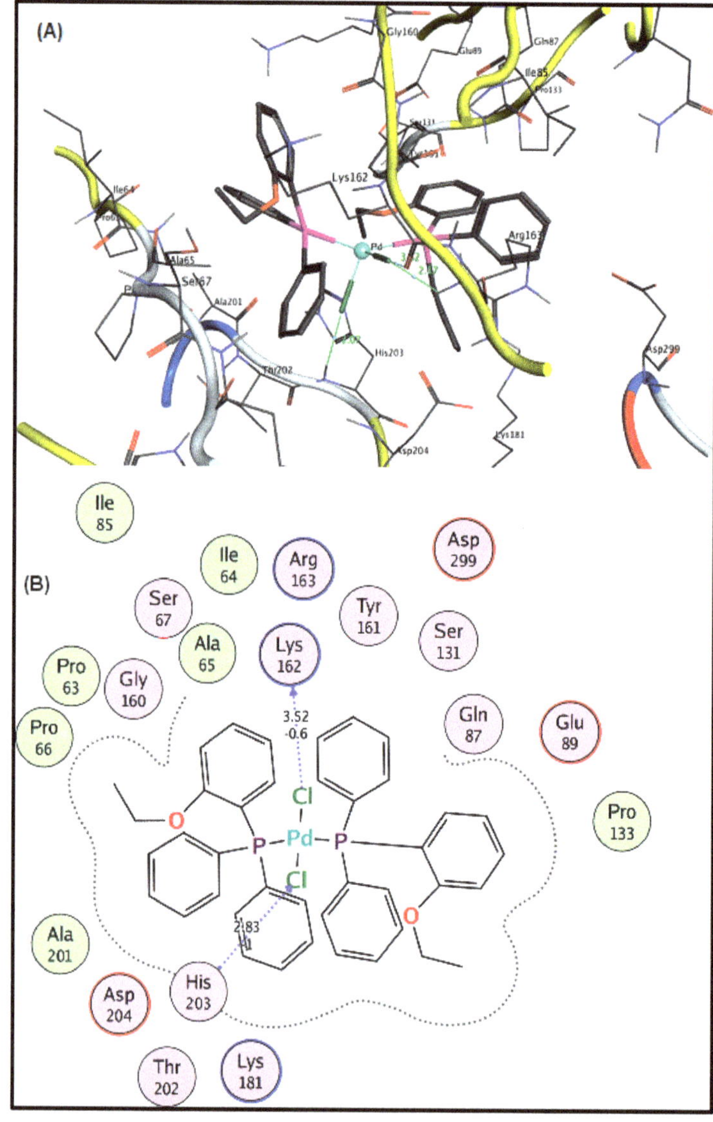

Figure 2. (**A**) Computed and (**B**) 2D interaction of complex **3** with *E. Coli*.

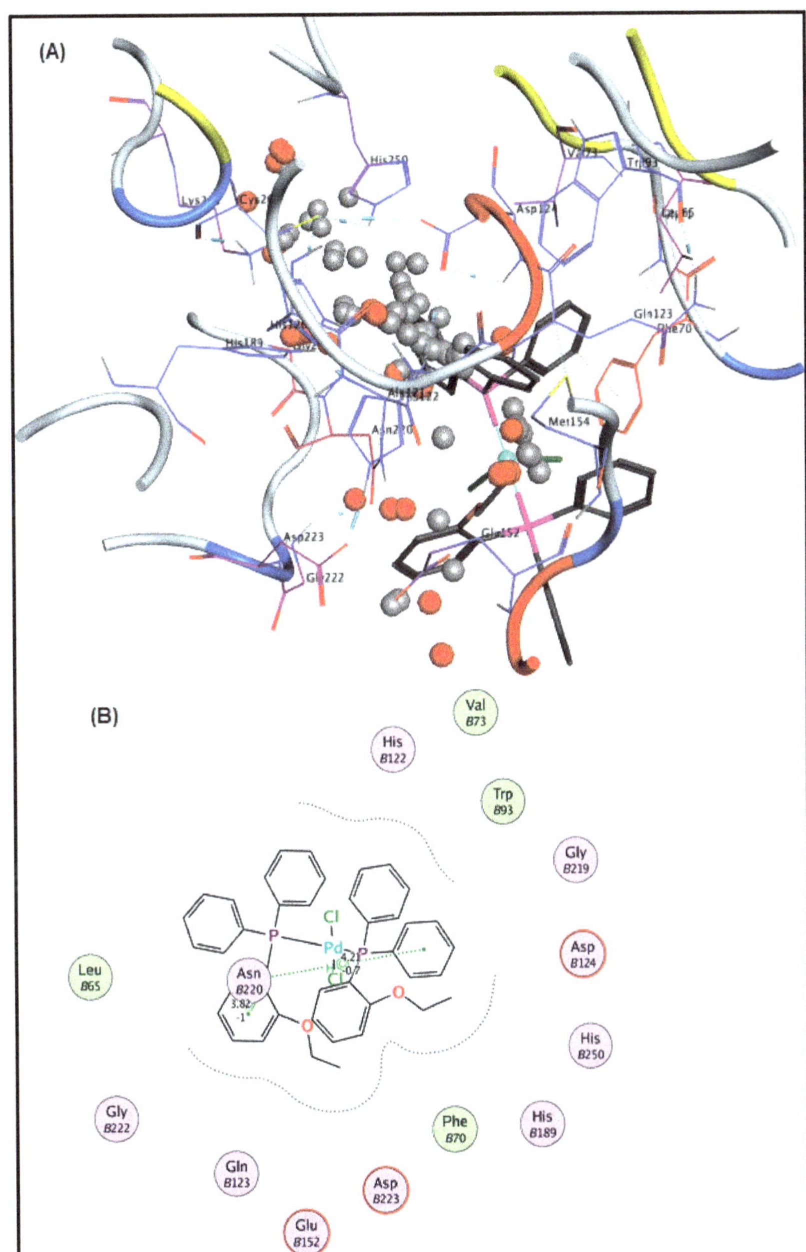

Figure 3. (**A**) Docked conformation and (**B**) 2D interaction of complex **3** with *K. pneumonia*.

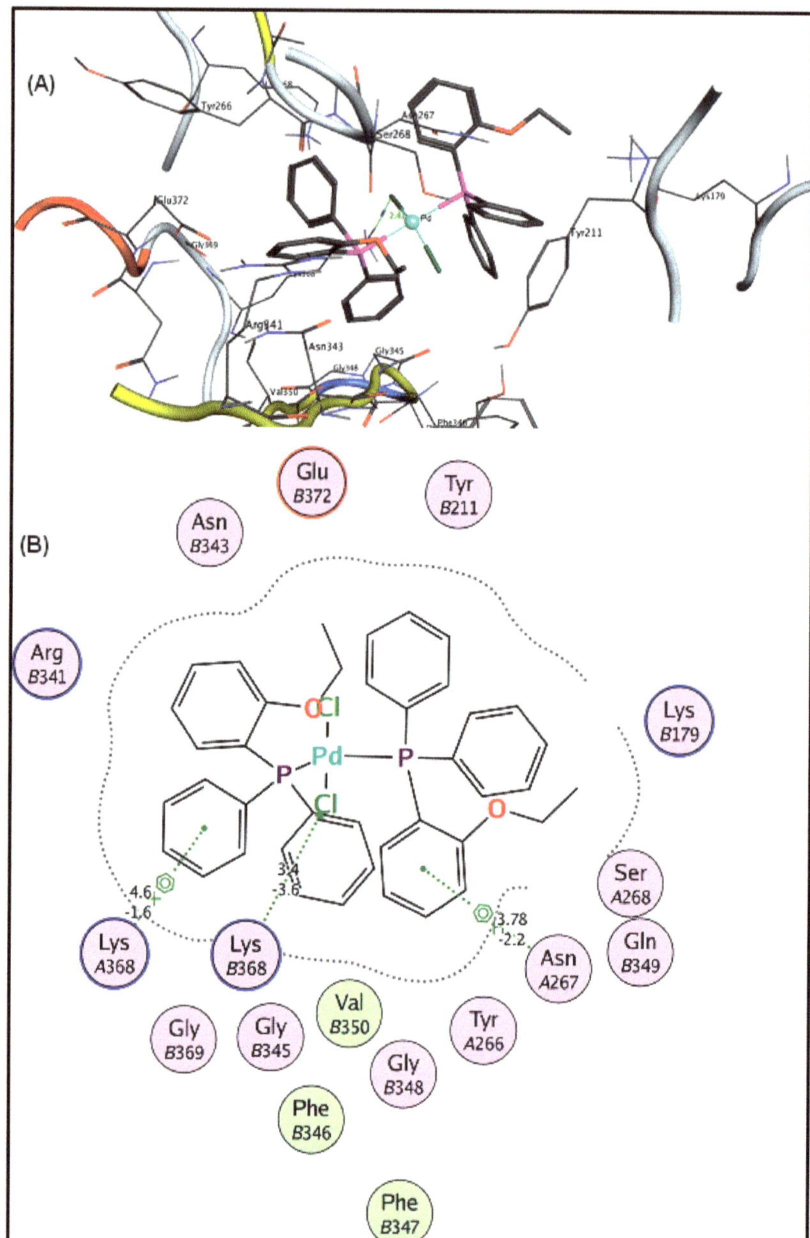

Figure 4. (**A**) Docked conformation and (**B**) 2D interaction of complex **3** with *S. aureus*.

The interaction of the compounds **1–4** with DR5 (1BU3) shows that the maximum binding affinity was observed for compounds **2** (−7.5148 kcal/mol) and then for compound **3** (−7.0343 kcal/mol). The maximum in vitro antitumor activity was also observed for compound **2**. The docking results reinforced the in vitro results. The interaction with the DR5 receptor of representative compounds **2** and **3** is given in Figures 5 and 6, respectively. The 2D diagram of compound **2** shows that the Cl atom of the compound acts as a chain side acceptor for the DR5 receptor residue *Asp B218* while the pyridine ring is involved in interaction with the *Tyr A50* residue via arene–H. Similarly, compound **3** interacts with the *Asp B218* residue via the Cl atom.

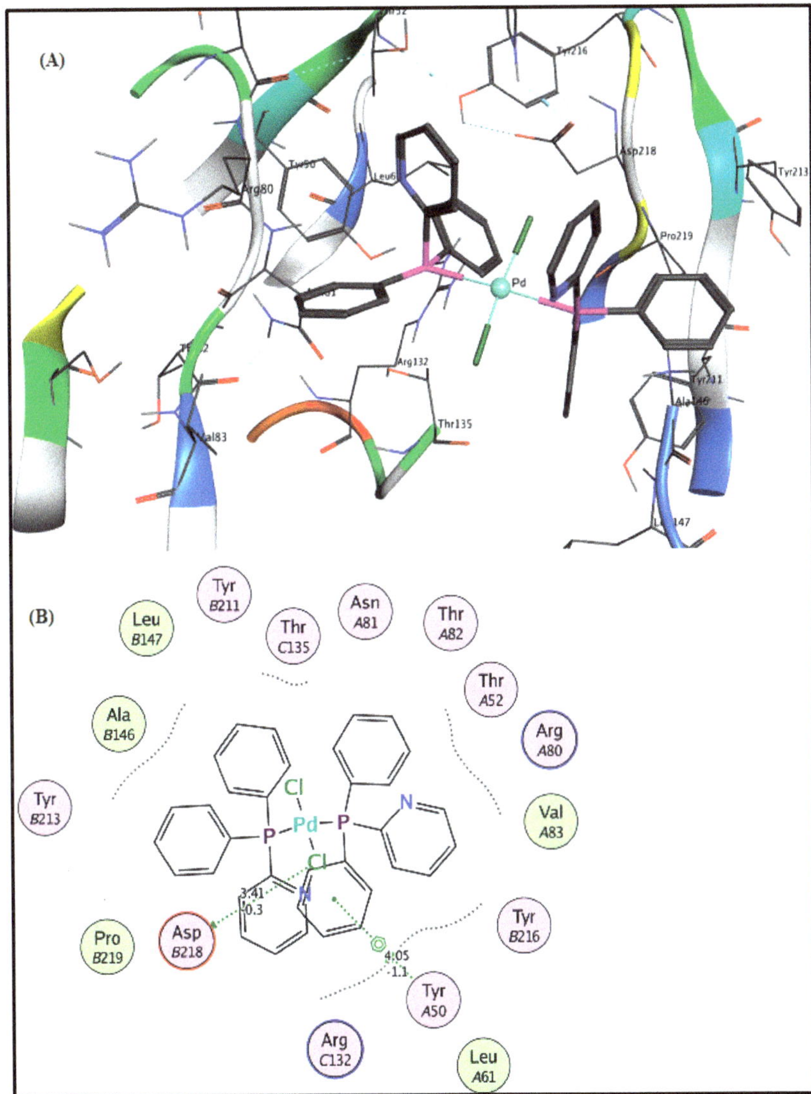

Figure 5. (**A**) Computed and (**B**) 2D interaction of complex **2** with DR5 (1DU3).

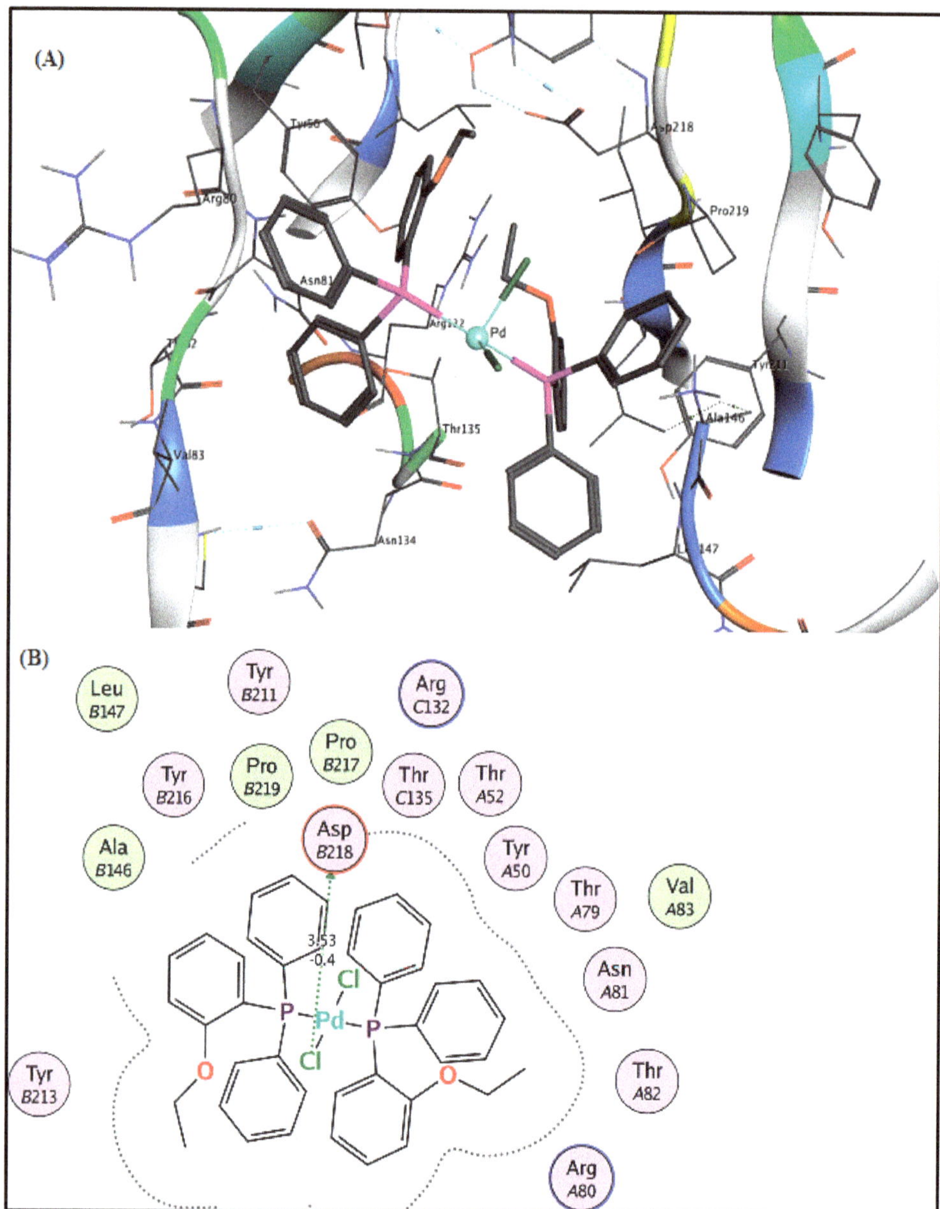

Figure 6. (**A**) Computed and (**B**) 2D interaction of complex **3** with DR5 (1DU3).

The interaction of the starting precursors (potassium dimethylcarbamodithioate and $(PR_3)_2PdCl_2$, where PR_3 = diphenyl–2–pyridylphosphine, diphenyl–2–ethoxyphenyl phosphine, and diphenyl–*p*–tolylphosphine) was checked against the three bacteria receptors: *E. coli* (PDB_ID: 6G9S), *K. pneumonia* (PDB_ID: 4EXS), and *S. aureus* (PDB_ID: 5ZH8), as well as DR5 (1DU3).

Against *E. coli*, the best affinity was shown by the Pd(II) organophosphine precursor having a diphenyl–*p*–tolylphosphine moiety (−6.8335 kcal/mol), followed by a diphenyl-2-

pyridylphosphine moiety (−6.3463 kcal/mol). Similarly, against *K. pneumonia* and *S. aureus*, the maximum binding affinity was observed for the Pd(II) organophosphine precursor having a diphenyl–2–ethoxyphenyl phosphine moiety (−5.3247, −6.1572 kcal/mol), followed by a diphenyl–*p*–tolylphosphine moiety (−5.0306, −6.0522 kcal/mol), respectively.

The best binding affinity against DR5 (1DU3) was observed for the Pd(II) organophosphine precursor having a diphenyl–2–ethoxyphenyl phosphine moiety (−7.1002 kcal/mol), followed by a diphenyl–*p*–tolylphosphine moiety (−6.9220 kcal/mol). From the comparison of binding energy, we can say that the starting Pd(II) organophosphine precursors have low binding affinity as compared to their corresponding Pd dithiocarbamate complexes. The results are shown in Table S1 and Figures S5–S8 of the Supplementary Materials.

Table 6. Binding energy score of compounds (**1–4**) with the receptor.

Receptor	Ligand	Binding Affinity (kcal/mol)
E. coli (PDB_ID: 6G9S)	1	−5.3894
	2	−6.1962
	3	−8.6569
	4	−6.8761
K. pneumonia (PDB_ID: 4EXS)	1	−5.5038
	2	−5.9045
	3	−6.5716
	4	−6.4517
S. aureus (PDB_ID: 5ZH8)	1	−6.1450
	2	−7.5425
	3	−7.6966
	4	−7.4745
DR5 (PDB_ID: 1DU3)	1	−6.4104
	2	−7.5148
	3	−7.0343
	4	−6.6559
	Cisplatin	−3.5666

3. Experimental

3.1. Materials and Methods

$PdCl_2$ was obtained from Alfa-Aesar, whilst organophosphines, diphenyl-*n*-propylphosphine, diphenyl–2–pyridylphosphine, diphenyl–*p*–tolylphosphine, diphenyl-2–ethoxyphenyl phosphine, potassium hydroxide, hydrochloric acid, methanol, and dichloromethane were acquired from Sigma–Aldrich and put to use directly without further purification.

NMR spectra were recorded on Mercury 200 MHz and Bruker 300 MHz spectrometers. ^{1}H NMR (300.13 MHz): $CDCl_3$ (7.26 from SiMe4). ^{13}C NMR (75.47 MHz), internal standard TMS; ^{31}P NMR (121.49 MHz): $CDCl_3$. IR spectra were recorded on a Nicolet 6700 FT-IR instrument in the range of 400–4000 cm^{-1} and Raman spectra (±1 cm^{-1}) were measured with an InVia Renishaw spectrometer, using argon ion (514.5 nm) and near infrared diode (785 nm) lasers. Wire 2.0 software was used for the Raman data acquisition and spectra manipulations. The elemental analyses were conducted on a LECO-183 CHNS analyzer. Melting points were measured on the Stuart SMP10 apparatus and are uncorrected. GraphPad Prism was applied for statistical analysis.

3.2. Synthesis

The synthesized compounds were prepared in three steps. In step-1, dithiocarbamate was prepared; in step-2, palladium(II) organophosphine complexes were prepared;

and in step-3, heteroleptic palladium complexes containing both organophosphine and dithiocarbamate ligands were prepared [17,18].

A carbon disulfide solution (30 mL) in dry methanol was added dropwise to dimethyl amine and potassium hydroxide dissolved in methanol (30 mL) in an equimolar ratio. The reaction mixture was stirred for 4 h at 0 °C (Scheme 1). A white-colored product was precipitated, followed by filtration and washing with methanol, and finally dried in an open atmosphere.

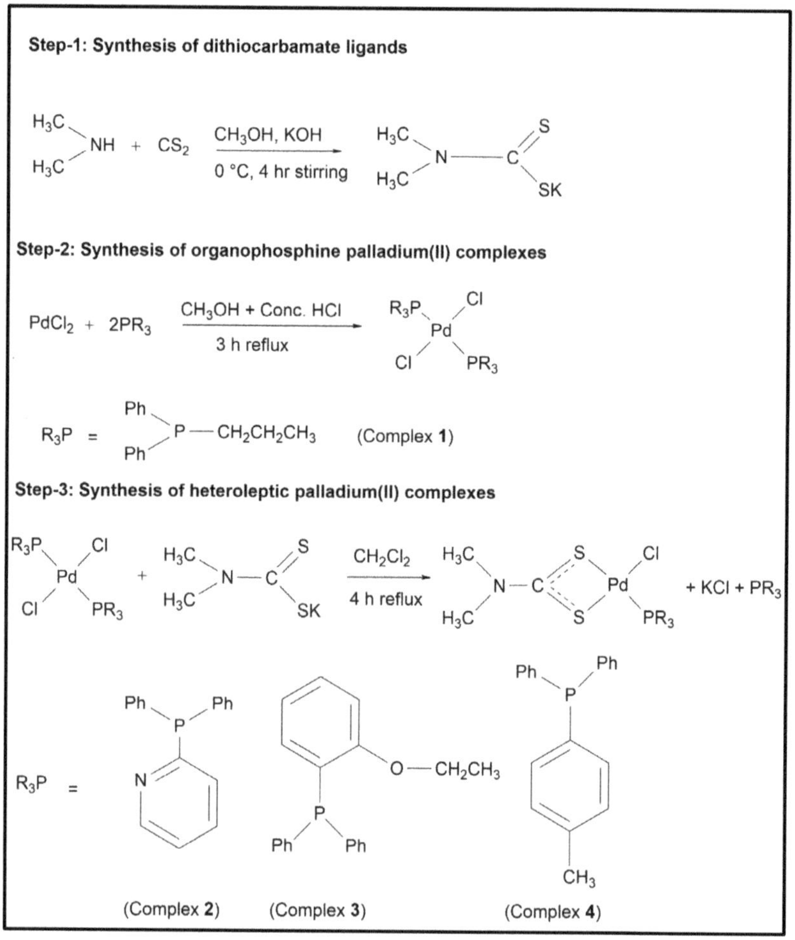

Scheme 1. Schematic representation of dithiocarbamate ligands, organophosphine Pd(II) complexes (**1**) and heteroleptic palladium(II) complexes (**2–4**).

Palladium(II) organophosphine complex (**1**) was prepared by reacting $PdCl_2$ dissolved in methanol (30 mL) along with 4 drops of concentrated HCl with organophosphine dissolved in acetone (25 mL) in 1:2. The reaction mixture was refluxed and stirred for 3 h (Scheme 1). The product was filtered, washed with methanol several times, and dried in a vacuum.

Heteroleptic or mixed ligand palladium(II) complexes (**2–4**) were prepared by the reaction of potassium salt of dithiocarbamate dissolved in dichloromethane (25 mL) with palladium phosphine complex dissolved in dichloromethane (30 mL), Scheme 1. The reaction mixture was kept on reflux with vigorous stirring until the completion of the reaction. Thin-layer chromatography was used to monitor the development of the reaction.

Upon the completion of the reaction, the solid by-product was filtered, the solvent was evaporated by a rotary evaporator, and the product was dissolved in a suitable mixture of solvents for recrystallization.

3.2.1. Dichlorido(diphenyl–*n*–propylphosphine)palladium(II) (1)

An amount of 0.08 g (0.45 mmol) of $PdCl_2$ was reacted with 0.20 mL (0.90 mmol) of diphenyl–*n*–propylphosphine. Yield: 79% (0.23 g). Melting point: 161–162 °C. Elemental analysis for complex **1** having a molecular formula $C_{30}H_{34}Cl_2P_2Pd$: % Calculated (found): H, 5.41 (5.39); C, 56.85 (56.71). **FT-IR** (cm^{-1}): 2922, 2854 υ(C–H, aliphatic), 3052 υ(C–H, aromatic). **Raman** (cm^{-1}): 298 υ(Pd–Cl), 221 υ(Pd–P). **^{1}H NMR** (ppm): 0.96 (t, ^3J: 7.2 Hz) $CH_3CH_2CH_2$-, 1.49–1.55 (m) $CH_3CH_2CH_2$-, 2.39–2.44 (t, ^3J: 7.2) $CH_3CH_2CH_2$-, 7.25–7.71 (m) Ar-*H*. **^{13}C NMR** (ppm): 14.7 ($CH_3CH_2CH_2$-), 23.0 ($CH_3CH_2CH_2$-), 28.9 ($CH_3CH_2CH_2$-), 128.3, 128.4, 134.5, 134.6 (Ar-*C*). **^{31}P NMR** (ppm): 17.1.

3.2.2. Chlorido–(dimethyldithiocarbamato–κ^2S,S′)(diphenyl-2-pyridylphosphine) palladium(II) (2)

A total of 0.05 g (0.41 mmol) of potassium salt of dimethyldithiocarbamate was reacted with 0.29 g (0.41 mmol) of Pd-phosphine complex. Yield: 78% (0.23 g). Melting point: 197–198 °C. Elemental analysis for complex **2** having a molecular formula $C_{20}H_{20}ClN_2PPdS_2$: % Calculated (Found) S, 12.21 (12.26); N, 5.33 (5.30); H, 3.84 (3.87); C, 45.72 (45.80). **FT-IR** (cm^{-1}) analysis: 1096 υ(SCS), 1548 υC ═ N, 2925, 2861, υ(C-H, aliphatic), 3056 υ(C-H, aromatic). **Raman** (cm^{-1}): 380 υ(Pd–S), 300 υ(Pd–Cl), 218 υ(Pd–P). **^{1}H NMR** (ppm): 2.80 (s), 3.58 (s) (CH_3), 7.37–8.73 (m) (Ar-*H*). **^{13}C NMR** (ppm): 35.5, 38.6 (CH_3), 125.0, 128.9, 130.0, 130.8, 131.3, 134.7, 134.6, 134.9, 149.3, 157.6 (Ar-*C*) 207.5 (S*C*S). **^{31}P NMR** (ppm): 27.5.

3.2.3. Chlorido–(dimethyldithiocarbamato–κ^2S,S′)(diphenyl–2–ethoxyphenyl phosphine)palladium(II) (3)

A total of 0.03 g (0.25 mmol) of potassium salt of dimethyldithiocarbamate was reacted with 0.19 g (0.25 mmol) of Pd-phosphine complex. Yield: 85% (0.17 g). Melting point: 223–224 °C. The elemental analysis for complex **3** has a molecular formula. $C_{22}H_{23}ClNOPPdS_2$: % Calculated (found) for: S, 11.57 (11.60); N, 2.53 (2.57); C, 47.66 (47.70). **FT-IR** (cm^{-1}): 1097 υ(SCS), 1528 υ(C═N), 2930, 2850 υ(C–H, aliphatic), 3052 υ(C–H, aromatic). **Raman** (cm^{-1}): 390 υ(Pd–S), 301 υ(Pd–Cl), 215 υ(Pd–P). **^{1}H NMR** (ppm): 3.14 (s), 3.26 (s) (CH_3), 3.98 (q, –CH_2), 1.33 (s, CH_3), 6.90–7.76 (m, Ar-*H*). **^{13}C NMR** (ppm): 14.3 (-CH_2CH_3), 65.2 (-CH_2CH_3), 120.1, 126.3, 128.2, 130.4, 131.7, 133.2, 164.0 (Ar-*C*), 208.2 (S*C*S). **^{31}P NMR** (ppm): 20.3.

3.2.4. Chlorido–(dimethyldithiocarbamato–κ^2S,S′)(diphenyl–*p*–tolylphosphine) palladium(II) (4)

A total of 0.04 g (0.33 mmol) of potassium salt of dimethyldithiocarbamate was reacted with 0.24 g (0.33 mmol) of Pd-phosphine complex. Yield: 77% (0.19 g). Melting point: 216–217 °C. Elemental analysis for complex **4** having a molecular formula $C_{22}H_{23}ClNPPdS$: % Calculated (found) for: S, 11.91 (11.87); N, 2.60 (2.64); H, 4.31 (4.40); C, 49.08 (49.00). **FT-IR** (cm^{-1}) analysis: 1092 υ(SCS); 1530 υ(C═N) 2935, 2852, υ(C–H, aliphatic), 3040 υ(C–H, aromatic). **Raman** (cm^{-1}): 395 υ(Pd–S), 308 υ(Pd–Cl), 210 υ(Pd–P). **^{1}H NMR** (ppm): 3.09 (s), 3.27 (s) (CH_3), 2.38 (s) (Ph–CH_3), 7.43–7.92 (m) (Ar-*H*). **^{13}C NMR** (ppm): 36.4, 39.1 (CH_3), 128.3, 129.5, 134.0, 136.5, 136.8, 137.1, 137.6, 141.7 (Ar-*C*), 22.5 (Ph–CH_3), 207.3 (S*C*S). **^{31}P NMR** (ppm): 22.8.

3.3. Biological Activity Assays

3.3.1. Antibacterial Activity Assay

The antimicrobial potential of the prepared compounds was evaluated using the agar-well diffusion method against five bacterial strains: two Gram-negative and three Gram-positive strains: *E. coli*, *K. pneumoniae*, *S. epidermidis*, *S. aureus*, and *B. subtilis* [39]. Using a sterile cotton swab, about 10^4–10^6 colony-forming units (CFU)/mL of bacterial inoculums were dispersed on top of nutritional agar. The tested compounds having a concentration of 2 mg/mL in DMSO were transferred to each well, and then the plates were incubated for 20 h at 37 °C, and finally the inhibition zone (in mm) was measured to determine the antibacterial activity. Streptomycin was used as the standard drug and DMSO as a positive control for the determination of growth inhibition, and the experiment was performed three times [39].

3.3.2. Antitumor Activity

Using the technique described in the referred articles, the anticancer activity of the synthesized compounds was assessed against DU145 human prostate cancer (HTB-81) cells [40–42]. Cisplatin was used as a reference drug. Compounds with a concentration of 50 mmol were dissolved in DMSO and diluted into nine consecutive concentrations, with the final concentration of DMSO on the cells not exceeding 0.05 percent. In 96-well flat-bottom microtiter plates, DU145 prostate cancer cells were planted at a density of 5000 cells per well for the growth inhibition test. Following a 24-h incubation period, cells were treated for four days with varying doses of each treatment. The remaining viable cells were fixed with 50% cold trichloroacetic acid for 60 min at 4 °C, stained with 0.4% sulforhodamine B (SRB) for four hours at 25 °C, washed with 1% acetic acid, and allowed to dry overnight. After dissolving the colored residue in 10 mM Tris base (pH = 10) and at 490 nm using an ELx808 microplate reader, the optical density was recorded. Graph Pad Prism was applied for data analysis, and the sigmoidal dose response curve was used to compute the IC_{50}. The test for growth inhibition was repeated three times [40–42].

3.4. In Silico Studies

The attrition rate for clinical trials used to develop new drugs has increased to 90% during the last ten years. Over a five-year period, on average, 26.8 small molecules were approved as FDA drugs. Only 12 innovative small-molecule medicines were approved by the FDA in 2016—the fewest such approvals over the previous fifty years [43,44]. Pharmaceutical firms invest millions of dollars to push a new treatment through clinical trials; therefore, failure in the latter stages of drug development often results in large financial losses [45]. The major reasons why drug candidates fail in clinical trials are undesirable pharmacokinetic characteristics and unacceptable toxicity [46]. Therefore, it is crucial for science to select candidates with the right balance of potency along with absorption, distribution, metabolism, excretion, and toxicity (ADMET). Parameters for ADMET and drug-like properties are given in Table 5.

3.5. Molecular Docking Analysis

The binding mode and affinity of a small molecule or ligand with a macromolecule, such as a protein or DNA, can be predicted using molecular docking. In the case of drug discovery, molecular docking is used to identify potential drug candidates that can bind to a target protein with high affinity and specificity. Here we have treated Palladium (II) complexes against three bacterial strains: *K. pneumoniae*, *S. aureus*, and *E. coli*, as well as trial receptor DR5, for which the PDB files were obtained from the RCSB PDB homepage.

MOE-Dock software version 2015 was used to perform docking studies so as to identify the binding interactions of the screened compounds in the active site of three antibacterial targets, such as PDB_ID: 4EXS from *Klebsiella pneumonia* [47], PDB_ID: 5ZH8 from *Staphylococcus aureus* [48,49], and PDB_ID: 6G9S from *Escherichia coli* [50], as well as death receptor (DR5) PDB_ID: 1DU3. The compounds were built in MOE, and energy was minimized by using the MOE's default settings parameters, Placement: Triangle Matcher and Rescoring: London dG, for the docking study [51]. Two conformations were generated for each ligand. For further molecular interaction analysis, the highest-ranked conformation of each compound with the lowest binding energy score was used. The interactions between receptor–solvent and ligand–solvent were excluded during the generation of the 2D interaction diagram.

4. Conclusions

A total of four Pd(II) complexes, including one homoleptic and three heteroleptic, have been prepared quantitatively. The single crystal analysis of complex **1** shows that the geometry around the palladium atom is square planar with slight distortion. The synthesized compounds have shown significant antibacterial activity against the selected targets. Compound **2** has shown the maximum antitumor activity against DU145 human prostate carcinoma cells. The lower binding energy or higher inhibition values indicate a stronger binding affinity of complex **3** with the target proteins. The molecular docking study of the evaluated compounds with DR5 (1BU3) shows the highest binding affinity for compound **2** (-7.5148 kcal/mol) and then for compound **3** (-7.0343 kcal/mol). In silico studies have been performed by the SwissADME webserver, and the compounds generally have shown one or two violations of Lipinski's rule of five.

Supplementary Materials: The following supporting information can be downloaded at: https://www.mdpi.com/article/10.3390/ph16060806/s1, Figure S1: FTIR spectrum of complex **2**; Figure S2: ^{1}H NMR of complex **1**; **Figure S3**: ^{13}C NMR of complex **1**; Figure S4: ^{31}P NMR of complex **1**; Figure S5: (A) Computed and (B) 2D interaction of $(PR_3)_2PdCl_2$ where PR_3 = diphenyl-p-tolylphosphine precursor with *E. coli* (PDB_ID: 6G9S); Figure S6: (A) Computed and (B) 2D interaction of $(PR_3)_2PdCl_2$ where PR_3 = diphenyl-p-tolylphosphine precursor with S. aureus (PDB_ID: 5ZH8); Figure S7:; Figure S8: (A) Computed and (B) 2D interaction of $(PR_3)_2PdCl_2$ where PR_3 = diphenyl-p-tolylphosphine precursor with DR5 (1DU3). **Table S1**: Binding energy score of starting organophosphorous Pd precursors with the receptor.

Author Contributions: Conceptualization, methodology, investigation, writing—original draft preparation, H.K.; M.S.; supervision, writing—review and editing, validation, data curation, project administration, A.B.; software, formal analysis, data curation, S.A.; M.B.; S.M.S.; I.S.B.; project administration, funding acquisition, writing—review and editing, T.A.W.; S.Z. All authors have read and agreed to the published version of the manuscript.

Funding: Researchers Supporting Project number (RSP2023R357), King Saud University, Riyadh, Saudi Arabia.

Institutional Review Board Statement: Not applicable.

Informed Consent Statement: Not applicable.

Data Availability Statement: Data will be available on request to corresponding authors.

Acknowledgments: The authors are thankful to the Higher Education Commission of Islamabad, Pakistan (Project # 20-10669). The authors extend their appreciation to the Researchers Supporting Project number (RSP2023R357), King Saud University, Riyadh, Saudi Arabia, for funding this work.

Conflicts of Interest: There are no conflict of interest.

References

1. Parvez, T. Cancer treatment: What's ahead? *J. Coll. Physicians Surg. Pak.* **2005**, *15*, 738–745. [PubMed]
2. Huq, F. Molecular modelling analysis of the metabolism of benzene. *Int. J. Pure Appl. Chem.* **2006**, *1*, 461–467.
3. Meyskens, F.L., Jr.; Tully, P. Principles of cancer prevention. *Semin. Oncol. Nurs.* **2005**, *21*, 229–235. [CrossRef] [PubMed]
4. Saeed, M.A.; Khan, H.; Sirajuddin, M.; Salman, S.M. DNA Interaction and Biological Activities of Heteroleptic Palladium (II) Complexes. *J. Chem. Soc. Pak.* **2021**, *43*, 227–243.
5. Verweij, J.; De Jonge, M. Achievements and future of chemotherapy. *Eur. J. Cancer* **2000**, *36*, 1479–1487. [CrossRef]
6. Galanski, M.; Arion, V.; Jakupec, M.; Keppler, B. Recent developments in the field of tumor-inhibiting metal complexes. *Curr. Pharm. Des.* **2003**, *9*, 2078–2089. [CrossRef]
7. Loehrer, P.J.; Einhorn, L.H. Cisplatin. *Ann. Intern. Med.* **1984**, *100*, 704–713. [CrossRef]
8. Goyns, M.H. *Cancer and You: How to Stack the Odds in Your Favour*; CRC Press: Boca Raton, FL, USA, 1999.
9. Stern, T.A.; Sekeres, M.A. *Facing Cancer: A Complete Guide for People with Cancer, Their Families, and Caregivers*; McGraw Hill Professional: New York City, NY, USA, 2004.
10. Mehdi, I. Second Malignancy-A Rare Phenomenon. *J. Pak. Med. Assoc.* **1998**, *48*, 345–346.
11. Fichtinger-Schepman, A.; Veer, J.; Lohman, P.; Reedijk, J. A simple method for the inactivation of monofunctionally DNA-bound cis-diamminedichloroplatinum (II). *J. Inorg. Biochem.* **1984**, *21*, 103–111. [CrossRef]

12. Lippard, S.J. New chemistry of an old molecule: Cis-[Pt(NH3)2Cl2]. *Science* **1982**, *218*, 1075–1082. [CrossRef]

13. Imran, M.; ur Rehman, Z.; Hogarth, G.; Tocher, D.A.; Butler, I.S.; Bélanger-Gariepy, F.; Kondratyuk, T. Two new monofunctional platinum (ii) dithiocarbamate complexes: Phenanthriplatin-type axial protection, equatorial-axial conformational isomerism, and anticancer and DNA binding studies. *Dalton Trans.* **2020**, *49*, 15385–15396. [CrossRef] [PubMed]

14. Martinho, N.; Marquês, J.M.; Todoriko, I.; Prieto, M.; de Almeida, R.F.; Silva, L.C. Effect of Cisplatin and Its Cationic Analogues in the Phase Behavior and Permeability of Model Lipid Bilayers. *Mol. Pharm.* **2023**, *20*, 918–928. [CrossRef]

15. Abbotto, A.; Beverina, L.; Bradamante, S.; Facchetti, A.; Klein, C.; Pagani, G.A.; Redi-Abshiro, M.; Wortmann, R. A distinctive example of the cooperative interplay of structure and environment in tuning of intramolecular charge transfer in second-order nonlinear optical chromophores. *Chem. A Eur. J.* **2003**, *9*, 1991–2007. [CrossRef] [PubMed]

16. Gonzalez, V.M.; Fuertes, M.A.; Alonso, C.; Perez, J.M. Is cisplatin-induced cell death always produced by apoptosis? *Mol. Pharmacol.* **2001**, *59*, 657–663. [CrossRef] [PubMed]

17. Khan, H.; Badshah, A.; Murtaz, G.; Said, M.; Neuhausen, C.; Todorova, M.; Jean-Claude, B.J.; Butler, I.S. Synthesis, characterization and anticancer studies of mixed ligand dithiocarbamate palladium (II) complexes. *Eur. J. Med. Chem.* **2011**, *46*, 4071–4077. [CrossRef] [PubMed]

18. Khan, H.; Badshah, A.; Said, M.; Murtaza, G.; Ahmad, J.; Jean-Claude, B.J.; Todorova, M.; Butler, I.S. Anticancer metallopharmaceutical agents based on mixed-ligand palladium (II) complexes with dithiocarbamates and tertiary organophosphine ligands. *Appl. Organomet. Chem.* **2013**, *27*, 387–395. [CrossRef]

19. Khan, H.; Badshah, A.; Said, M.; Murtaza, G.; Shah, A.; Butler, I.S.; Ahmed, S.; Fontaine, F.-G. New dimeric and supramolecular mixed ligand Palladium (II) dithiocarbamates as potent DNA binders. *Polyhedron* **2012**, *39*, 1–8. [CrossRef]

20. Guerra, W.; de Andrade Azevedo, E.; de Souza Monteiro, A.R.; Bucciarelli-Rodriguez, M.; Chartone-Souza, E.; Nascimento, A.M.A.; Fontes, A.P.S.; Le Moyec, L.; Pereira-Maia, E.C. Synthesis, characterization, and antibacterial activity of three palladium (II) complexes of tetracyclines. *J. Inorg. Biochem.* **2005**, *99*, 2348–2354. [CrossRef]

21. Khan, B.T.; Najmuddin, K.; Shamsuddin, S.; Annapoorna, K.; Bhatt, J. Synthesis, antimicrobial, and antitumor activity of a series of palladium (II) mixed ligand complexes. *J. Inorg. Biochem.* **1991**, *44*, 55–63. [CrossRef]

22. Khan, H.; Badshah, A.; Said, M.; Murtaza, G.; Sirajuddin, M.; Ahmad, J.; Butler, I.S. Synthesis, structural characterization and biological screening of heteroleptic palladium (II) complexes. *Inorg. Chim. Acta* **2016**, *447*, 176–182. [CrossRef]

23. Hogarth, G. Metal-dithiocarbamate complexes: Chemistry and biological activity. *Mini Rev. Med. Chem.* **2012**, *12*, 1202–1215. [CrossRef]

24. Marta Nagy, E.; Ronconi, L.; Nardon, C.; Fregona, D. Noble metal-dithiocarbamates precious allies in the fight against cancer. *Mini Rev. Med. Chem.* **2012**, *12*, 1216–1229. [CrossRef]

25. Adeyemi, J.O.; Onwudiwe, D.C. Organotin (IV) dithiocarbamate complexes: Chemistry and biological activity. *Molecules* **2018**, *23*, 2571. [CrossRef]

26. Sirajuddin, M.; Ali, S.; Tahir, M.N. Pharmacological investigation of mono-, di-and tri-organotin (IV) derivatives of carbodithioates: Design, spectroscopic characterization, interaction with SS-DNA and POM analyses. *Inorg. Chim. Acta* **2016**, *439*, 145–158. [CrossRef]

27. Micklitz, W.; Sheldrick, W.S.; Lippert, B. Mono-and dinuclear palladium (II) complexes of uracil and thymine model nucleobases and the x-ray structure of [(bpy) Pd (1-MeT) 2Pd (bpy)](NO$_3$) 2. cntdot. 5.5 H$_2$O (head-head). *Inorg. Chem.* **1990**, *29*, 211–216. [CrossRef]

28. Barnham, K.J.; Bauer, C.J.; Djuran, M.I.; Mazid, M.A.; Rau, T.; Sadler, P.J. Outer-Sphere Macrochelation in [Pd (en)(5′-GMP-N7) 2]. cntdot. 9H$_2$O and [Pt (en)(5′-GMP-N7) 2]. cntdot. 9H$_2$O: X-ray Crystallography and NMR Spectroscopy in Solution. *Inorg. Chem.* **1995**, *34*, 2826–2832. [CrossRef]

29. Shen, W.-Z.; Gupta, D.; Lippert, B. Cyclic Trimer versus Head—Tail Dimer in Metal—Nucleobase Complexes: Importance of Relative Orientation (Syn, Anti) of the Metal Entities and Relevance as a Metallaazacrown Compound. *Inorg. Chem.* **2005**, *44*, 8249–8258. [CrossRef]

30. Rau, T.; Van Eldik, R. Mechanistic insight from kinetic studies on the interaction of model palladium (II) complexes with nucleic acid components. *Met. Ions Biol. Syst.* **1996**, *32*, 339. [PubMed]

31. Gao, E.-J.; Wang, L.; Zhu, M.-C.; Liu, L.; Zhang, W.-Z. Synthesis, characterization, interaction with DNA and cytotoxicity in vitro of the complexes [M (dmphen)(CO$_3$)]· H$_2$O [M = Pt (II), Pd (II)]. *Eur. J. Med. Chem.* **2010**, *45*, 311–316. [CrossRef] [PubMed]

32. Budzisz, E.; Małecka, M.; Lorenz, I.-P.; Mayer, P.; Kwiecień, R.A.; Paneth, P.; Krajewska, U.; Rózalski, M. Synthesis, cytotoxic effect, and structure—Activity relationship of Pd (II) complexes with coumarin derivatives. *Inorg. Chem.* **2006**, *45*, 9688–9695. [CrossRef] [PubMed]

33. Ewais, H.A.; Taha, M.; Salm, H.N. Palladium (II) Complexes Containing Dipicolinic Acid (DPA), Iminodiacetic Acid (IDA), and Various Biologically Important Ligands. *J. Chem. Eng. Data* **2010**, *55*, 754–758. [CrossRef]

34. Imran, M.; Kondratyuk, T.; Bélanger-Gariepy, F. New ternary platinum (II) dithiocarbamates: Synthesis, characterization, anticancer, DNA binding and DNA denaturing studies. *Inorg. Chem. Commun.* **2019**, *103*, 12–20. [CrossRef]

35. Shaheen, F.; Badshah, A.; Gielen, M.; Croce, G.; Florke, U.; de Vos, D.; Ali, S. In vitro assessment of cytotoxicity, anti-inflammatory, antifungal properties and crystal structures of metallacyclic palladium (II) complexes. *J. Organomet. Chem.* **2010**, *695*, 315–322. [CrossRef]

36. Sheldrick, G.M. SHELXT–Integrated space-group and crystal-structure determination. *Acta Crystallogr. A* **2015**, *71*, 3–8. [CrossRef]

37. Sheldrick, G.M. Crystal structure refinement with SHELXL. *Acta Crystallogr. C Struct. Chem.* **2015**, *71*, 3–8. [CrossRef]
38. Zhu, W.; Li, Y.; Gao, L. Cisplatin in combination with programmed cell death protein 5 increases antitumor activity in prostate cancer cells by promoting apoptosis. *Mol. Med. Rep.* **2015**, *11*, 4561–4566. [CrossRef]
39. Chohan, Z.H.; Sumrra, S.H.; Youssoufi, M.H.; Hadda, T.B. Metal based biologically active compounds: Design, synthesis, and antibacterial/antifungal/cytotoxic properties of triazole-derived Schiff bases and their oxovanadium (IV) complexes. *Eur. J. Med. Chem.* **2010**, *45*, 2739–2747. [CrossRef]
40. Skehan, P.; Storeng, R.; Scudiero, D.; Monks, A.; McMahon, J.; Vistica, D.; Warren, J.T.; Bokesch, H.; Kenney, S.; Boyd, M.R. New colorimetric cytotoxicity assay for anticancer-drug screening. *J. Natl. Cancer Inst.* **1990**, *82*, 1107–1112. [CrossRef]
41. Valente, C.; Ferreira, M.J.; Abreu, P.M.; Pedro, M.; Cerqueira, F.; Nascimento, M.S.J. Three new jatrophane-type diterpenes from Euphorbia pubescens. *Planta Med.* **2003**, *69*, 361–366. [CrossRef]
42. Kim, Y.; Bang, S.-C.; Lee, J.-H.; Ahn, B.-Z. Pulsatilla saponin D: The antitumor principle from Pulsatilla koreana. *Arch. Pharmacal Res.* **2004**, *27*, 915–918. [CrossRef]
43. Fleming, N. How artificial intelligence is changing drug discovery. *Nature* **2018**, *557*, S55. [CrossRef] [PubMed]
44. Kinch, M.S.; Griesenauer, R.H. 2017 in review: FDA approvals of new molecular entities. *Drug Discov. Today* **2018**, *23*, 1469–1473. [CrossRef] [PubMed]
45. Sertkaya, A.; Wong, H.-H.; Jessup, A.; Beleche, T. Key cost drivers of pharmaceutical clinical trials in the United States. *Clin. Trials* **2016**, *13*, 117–126. [CrossRef]
46. M Honorio, K.; L Moda, T.; Andricopulo, A.D. Pharmacokinetic properties and in silico ADME modeling in drug discovery. *Med. Chem.* **2013**, *9*, 163–176. [CrossRef] [PubMed]
47. King, D.T.; Worrall, L.J.; Gruninger, R.; Strynadka, N.C. New Delhi metallo-β-lactamase: Structural insights into β-lactam recognition and inhibition. *J. Am. Chem. Soc.* **2012**, *134*, 11362–11365. [CrossRef] [PubMed]
48. Dalal, V.; Kumar, P.; Rakhaminov, G.; Qamar, A.; Fan, X.; Hunter, H.; Tomar, S.; Golemi-Kotra, D.; Kumar, P. Repurposing an ancient protein core structure: Structural studies on FmtA, a novel esterase of Staphylococcus aureus. *J. Mol. Biol.* **2019**, *431*, 3107–3123. [CrossRef] [PubMed]
49. Dalal, V.; Kumar, P.; Rakhaminov, G.; Qamar, A.; Fan, X.; Hunter, H.; Tomar, S.; Kotra, D.; Kumar, P. Repurposing an ancient protein core structure: Structural studies on FmtA, a novel esterase of Staphylococcus aureus. *Acta Crystallogr. Sect. A* **2021**, *77*, C706. [CrossRef]
50. Levy, N.; Bruneau, J.-M.; Le Rouzic, E.; Bonnard, D.; Le Strat, F.; Caravano, A.; Chevreuil, F.; Barbion, J.; Chasset, S.; Ledoussal, B. Structural basis for E. coli penicillin binding protein (PBP) 2 inhibition, a platform for drug design. *J. Med. Chem.* **2019**, *62*, 4742–4754. [CrossRef]
51. Naz, N.; Sirajuddin, M.; Haider, A.; Abbas, S.M.; Ali, S.; Wadood, A.; Ghufran, M.; Rehman, G.; Mirza, B. Synthesis, characterization, biological screenings and molecular docking study of Organotin (IV) derivatives of 2, 4-dichlorophenoxyacetic acid. *J. Mol. Struct.* **2019**, *1179*, 662–671. [CrossRef]

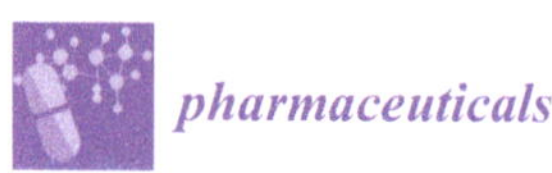

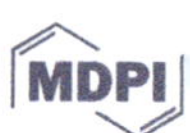

Article

Diosgenin and Monohydroxy Spirostanol from *Prunus amygdalus var amara* Seeds as Potential Suppressors of EGFR and HER2 Tyrosine Kinases: A Computational Approach

Mohammed Helmy Faris Shalayel [1], Ghassab M. Al-Mazaideh [2,*], Abdulkareem A. Alanezi [3], Afaf F. Almuqati [2] and Meshal Alotaibi [1]

[1] Department of Pharmacy Practice, College of Pharmacy, University of Hafr Al Batin, Hafr Al Batin 31991, Saudi Arabia

[2] Department of Pharmaceutical Chemistry, College of Pharmacy, University of Hafr Al Batin, Hafr Al Batin 31991, Saudi Arabia

[3] Department of Pharmaceutics, College of Pharmacy, University of Hafr Al Batin, Hafr Al Batin 31991, Saudi Arabia

* Correspondence: gmazaideh@uhb.edu.sa

Citation: Shalayel, M.H.F.; Al-Mazaideh, G.M.; Alanezi, A.A.; Almuqati, A.F.; Alotaibi, M. Diosgenin and Monohydroxy Spirostanol from *Prunus amygdalus var amara* Seeds as Potential Suppressors of EGFR and HER2 Tyrosine Kinases: A Computational Approach. *Pharmaceuticals* **2023**, *16*, 704. https://doi.org/10.3390/ph16050704

Academic Editors: Halil İbrahim Ciftci, Belgin Sever, Hasan Demirci and Anna Artese

Received: 8 March 2023
Revised: 20 April 2023
Accepted: 24 April 2023
Published: 6 May 2023

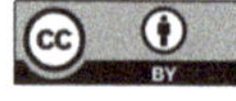

Abstract: Cancer continues to be leading cause of death globally, with nearly 7 million deaths per year. Despite significant progress in cancer research and treatment, there remain several challenges to overcome, including drug resistance, the presence of cancer stem cells, and high interstitial fluid pressure in tumors. To tackle these challenges, targeted therapy, specifically targeting HER2 (Human Epidermal Growth Factor Receptor 2) as well as EGFR (Epidermal Growth Factor Receptor), is considered a promising approach in cancer treatment. In recent years, phytocompounds have gained recognition as a potential source of chemopreventive and chemotherapeutic agents in tumor cancer treatment. Phytocompounds are compounds derived from medicinal plants that have the potential to treat and prevent cancer. This study aimed to investigate phytocompounds from *Prunus amygdalus var amara* seeds as inhibitors against EGFR and HER2 enzymes using in silico methods. In this study, fourteen phytocompounds were isolated from *Prunus amygdalus var amara* seeds and subjected to molecular docking studies to determine their ability to bind to EGFR and HER2 enzymes. The results showed that diosgenin and monohydroxy spirostanol exhibited binding energies comparable to those of the reference drugs, tak-285, and lapatinib. Furthermore, the drug-likeness and ADMET predictions, performed using the admetSAR 2.0 web-server tool, suggested that diosgenin and monohydroxy spirostanol have similar safety and ADMET properties as the reference drugs. To get deeper insight into the structural steadiness and flexibility of the complexes formed between these compounds and theEGFR and HER2 proteins, molecular dynamics simulations were performed for 100 ns. The results showed that the hit phytocompounds did not significantly affect the stability of the EGFR and HER2 proteins and were able to form stable interactions with the catalytic binding sites of the proteins. Additionally, the MM-PBSA analysis revealed that the binding free energy estimates for diosgenin and monohydroxy spirostanol is comparable to the reference drug, lapatinib. This study provides evidence that diosgenin and monohydroxy spirostanol may have the potential to act as dual suppressors of EGFR and HER2. Additional in vivo and in vitro research are needed to certify these results and assess their efficacy and safety as cancer therapy agents. The experimental data reported and these results are in agreement.

Keywords: bitter almond; EGFR; HER2; molecular docking; ADEMT; molecular dynamic; MM-PBSA

1. Introduction

Cancer is a leading cause of death worldwide, and traditional chemotherapy and radiation treatments can often have significant side effects [1]. This has led to a growing interest in alternative and complementary therapies for cancer [1]. In recent years, natural compounds have emerged as promising candidates for the treatment of cancer due to their ability to target specific signaling pathways involved in cancer progression [2]. There is a growing body of research exploring the use of natural compounds as alternative or complementary therapies for cancer [3].

Prunus amygdalus var. amara is a type of almond that contains a variety of phytocompounds that can be used to make essential oils with a potent fruity-almond aroma [4,5], as well as extracts and essential oils with potential healing properties [4,5]. Bitter almonds have been used to prevent and cure diseases for centuries [6], and recent research has associated the inclusion of almonds in the diet with elevating the levels of antioxidants, which can help protect against cancer [5]. A recent study suggested that bitter almond extract may possess anti-cancer properties by regulating the expression and immortality of MCF-7 (breast cancer cells) [4]. These extracts have been shown to exhibit anti-cancer properties, and their ability to target specific signaling pathways involved in cancer progression has received significant attention [4,6]. Despite these promising developments, it remains critical to further our knowledge of the molecular mechanisms of the action of these natural compounds as well as their efficacy in complex biological systems [6].

The anti-cancer activity of the Bitter almond active compounds demonstrated the anti-cancer impact of its active compounds in a diversity of cell lines, besides lung, breast, colon, and cervical cells [7–9]. The compounds induced apoptosis in a caspase-independent manner, with a dose much lower than other anti-cancer treatments [7–9]. In addition, these results show that the anti-cancer activity of the active compounds is dose-dependent and independent of the cell line tested, suggesting that the effect of these compounds may have a broad application to various cancer treatments [10].

Epidermal growth factor receptor (EGFR) and human epidermal growth factor receptor 2 (HER2) are two proteins that play a significant role in cancer proliferation [11,12]. EGFR is a transmembrane glycoprotein with an intracellular tyrosine kinase that serves as a receptor for extracellular protein ligands [12]. HER2 is a coreceptor that belongs to the human epidermal growth factor receptor family, which also includes EGFR, HER3, and HER4 [13]. HER2 works as an oncogene in several cancers, including breast cancer, manifesting its effect of carcinogenesis mainly by overexpression or due to gene amplification [13,14].

EGFR and HER2 are frequently overexpressed or mutated in solid tumors, such as carcinomas and gliomas [15]. EGFR drives metastasis in many ways, including paracrine loops comprising tumor and stromal cells that enable EGFR to fuel invasion across tissue barriers, survival of clusters of circulating tumor cells, and colonization of distant organs [11]. HER2 is overexpressed in 20% of breast cancer cases and is activated ligand-independently by homodimerization. In addition, HER2 is able to heterodimerize with EGFR, HER3, and HER4, which has been proposed as a mechanism of resistance to therapy for HER2 [16].

Anti-cancer drugs targeting either EGFR or HER2 have been clinically approved, but the emergence of drug resistance is nearly inevitable [11,16]. Therefore, it is important to consider the major evasion mechanisms, such as the heregulin-EGFR-HER3 autocrine signaling axis that can mediate acquired lapatinib resistance in HER2+ breast cancer models [11]. Understanding the roles of EGFR and HER2 in cancer proliferation is crucial for developing effective therapies that can target these proteins and overcome drug resistance [17–19]. TKIs (tyrosine kinase inhibitors) such as gefitinib, erlotinib, neratinib, and afatinib, are used to target EGFR/HER2 [17,20,21]. These four drugs have been associated with adverse impacts that can effectively influence patient health [17,20,21]. Lapatinib is a dual suppressor of EGFR and HER2 that has been used in clinical trials [19,22]. Lapatinib is an irreversible suppressor of chemotherapeutics [19,22] and was selected as a regarded drug in the current work.

The display investigation was initiated to evaluate the feasibility of new bioactive inhibitors as a means of addressing the limitations of clinically approved molecules for cancer treatment. There has been a growing interest in developing alternative cancer treatments and therapies that do not involve radiotherapy and chemotherapy, as these approaches can have negative effects on patients' health. In response, phytocompounds are gaining recognition as promising chemotherapeutic and chemopreventive agents in cancer therapy, as they can be derived from medicinal plants and exhibit the potential to treat and prevent cancer. The present study specifically focused on the characterization and examination of the phytochemical composition of Bitter almond seed, intending to identify a popular phytocompound dual suppressor for EGFR as well as HER2 that can demonstrate anti-cancer activity via molecular docking as well as dynamic simulation investigations [2,3,7,20]. This study expands upon previous research efforts aimed at uncovering new, naturally derived bioactive compounds with anti-cancer properties, and it will be expanded to show the anti-cancer activity of the crude extract as dose-dependent on 8 cancer cell lines (phase 2).

2. Results and Discussion

2.1. GC–MS Analysis of the Extract

The percentages of each component were determined using the Gas Chromatography (GC) technique. All identified peaks with area% greater than 0.812 were displayed, and unwanted peaks were integrated based on the standard material that was injected first. The relative percentage of each component was calculated and tabulated in Table 1 and illustrated in Figure 1.

The GC chromatogram revealed that the presence of the following unsaturated fatty acids predominates and represents (88.60%) while the saturated fatty acids represent only 11.39%: saturated fatty acids palmitic, and stearic, along withthe unsaturated fatty acids oleic, linoleic, arachidic, and palmitoleic. It is obvious that oleic acid was the major unsaturated fatty acid (52.04%) and oleic acid was the major saturated fatty acid (6.55%). The main essential fatty acids (linoleic, and arachidic) play an important role in the development of a baby's brain and prevent cancer [23].

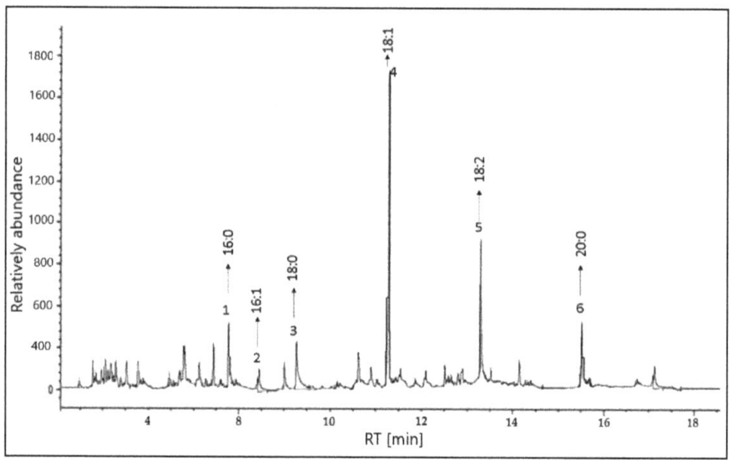

Figure 1. GC-MS chromatogram of *Prunus amygdalus var. amara* seeds.

Table 1. GC-MS phytoconstituents analysis of major *Prunus amygdalus var. amara* seeds compounds.

Peak no.	Retention Time (TR)	Type	Area %	Component Name	Percentage Contains %
1	7.832	(C16:0)	6.550	Palmitic	6.550
2	8.488	(C16:1)	0.812	Palmitoleic	0.812
3	9.267	(C18:0)	4.843	Stearic	4.843
4	11.316	(C18:1)	52.042	Oleic	52.042
5	13.233	(C18:2)	27.512	Linoleic	27.512
6	15.512	(C20:0)	8.241	Arachidic	8.241

2.2. HPLC Analysis of the Extract

The main idea of HPLC separation is based on the variation of the analyte (sample) between the mobile phase (eluent) as well as the stationary phase (fill material from the column). Depends primarily on the chemical composition of the analyte and the molecules lag while traversing the stationary phase. Identifies the specific interactions between sample molecules and packing materials at their respective times in the column. Hence, the different components of the sample are plotted at different times. Thus, the components of the sample are separated. We identify the indication unit of the analyst after finishing the column, and then the signals are transformed and recorded by a data administration system (computer program) and then displayed on a chromatogram (Figure 2A).

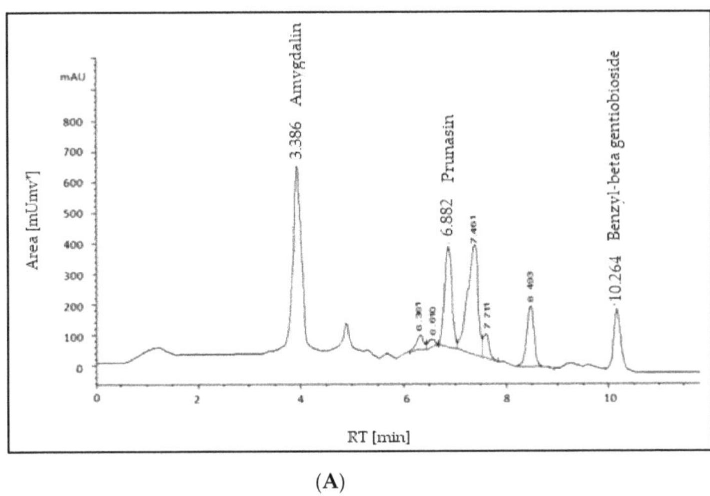

(A)

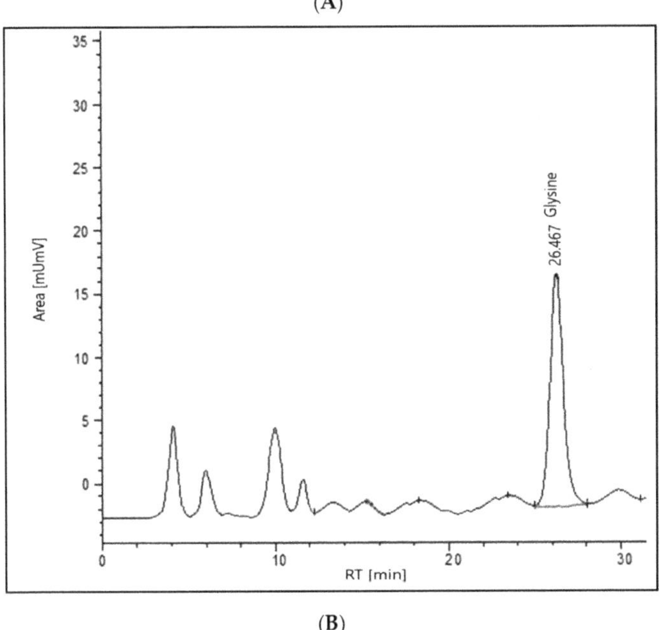

(B)

Figure 2. (**A**) HPLC-(UV-VIS) chromatogram of *Prunus amygdalus var. amara* seeds. (**B**) HPLC-(UV-VIS) chromatogram of *Prunus amygdalus var. amara* seeds.

2.2.1. Glycine

All the standard and sample solutions were injected three times, andthe average of the three readings was taken. The main active constituent, glycine, was appearing at a retention time of 26.467 min (Figure 2B). Chromatographic analysis showed glycine with a value of 0.285 mg/mL. Glycine helps the body make glutathione, which is an important antioxidant that protects the body from cell damage, resulting in cancer prevention [24].

2.2.2. Glycosides

The result of the determination of glycosides using HPLC showed the presence of the glycosides: amygdalin, prunasin, and benzyl-beta gentiobioside. All of these components appeared as follows for retention time: 3.386, 6.882, and 10.624 min, respectively. Amygdalin had the highest percentage (24.768 mg/mL), followed by prunasin (8.783 mg/mL) while benzyl-beta gentiobioside had the lowest (5.959 mg/mL). Two minor compounds, prunasin, and benzyl-beta gentiobioside, were identified along with the primary glycoside, amygdalin, and they were characterized as mandelic acid glycosides. The anti-tumor encouraging activity of these compounds was examined in both in vitro as well as in vivo assays. All the components had significant inhibition, and the Epstein-Barr virus early antigen stimulation was induced by the tumor promoter [25,26].

2.2.3. Flavonoids

All the standard and sample solutions were injected three times, and the average of the three readings was taken. The major component Kaempferol showed a retention time of 26.483 min, and the minor component centaureidin appeared at a retention time of 32.447 min, allowing kaempferol and centaureidin to calculate their percentages in the formulation as 0.9903 mg/g and 0.551 mg/g, respectively. Kaempferol, a well-characterized phytonatural flavonol, is found in 80% of plant-based food products, together with broccoli, tomatoes, grapes, beans, apples, strawberries, and some plant seeds or fruits. Thus, the importance appeared as anti-metastasis, anti-angiogenesis, and anti-proliferative [27].

2.2.4. Steroids

The method proceeded using the reported conditions mentioned according to the method used. All the standard and sample solutions were injected three times, and the average of the three readings was taken. Diosgenin was measured using peak area vs. concentration (mg/mL). The concentration of diosgenin was 3.087 mg/mL. Cleary showed a retention time of 8.866 min.

The steroidal diosgenin obtained from *Prunus amygdalus var. amara* seeds has been studied to execute anti-cancer activities in various human cancer cell lines [28].

2.3. LC-MS/MS Descriptions

The analysis of the value of energy had good flavonoids, phenolic acids, and their glycoside identifications, which led to a good understanding of the value of these compounds. The electrospray ionization in the +ve as well as the -ve ion mode, especially in combination with the MS/MS method, has quickly been the method of choice through sugar sequence evaluation. A positive ion mode electrospray ionization mass spectrum. The peak at m/z 456.6 corresponds to the [M+Na]$^+$, and m/z 460.3 corresponds to the [M+NH$_4$]$^+$. The peak at m/z 353.3 corresponds to the diglucoside ion generated by the loss of DL-mandelonitrile. the fragments and RT perspective to identify amygdalin or its derivatives. On the other hand, the peak at m/z 456.6, 459.4 and 460.3 corresponds to amygdalin and its metabolite compound, prunasin. Also, positive ion mode fragments were found based on the existence of the aglycone peak at m/z 610.3–611.4 correlating to [aglycone+H]$^+$, which suggested a saturated monohydroxy spirostanol skeleton [29]. In some cases, the aglycone peak seemed to be found at m/z 415, according to either [aglycone+H] or [aglycone+H-H$_2$O]$^+$, for the negative –ion mode The deprotonated ion was m/z 667.5 and 668.5 [M-H]$^-$, which corresponds to a cyanogenic glucoside known as thebenzyl-beta gentiobioside compound.

2.4. Molecular Docking Studies

In this investigation, molecular docking was utilized to predict the in silico molecular interactions between phytocompounds 1–14 and their targets, namely the epidermal growth factor receptor (EGFR) as well as the human epidermal growth factor receptor 2 (HER2). The binding free energy (ΔG) of each compound was determined and compared against reference controls comprising the co-crystallized ligand tak-285 and the commercially available drug lapatinib, both of which are known inhibitors of EGFR and HER2. The results of this analysis are described in Table 2. Our goal of this analysis is to identify hit phytocompounds with free binding energies substantially similar or lower than the reference controls, as they may have the potential to serve as effective and selective inhibitors of EGFR and HER2.

First, the AutoDock 4.2 software was used to re-dock the tak-285 co-crystallized ligand against the EGFR (3POZ.PDB) and HER2 (3RCD.PDB) proteins in order to validate the docking process parameters for the subsequent docking of 14 isolated phytocompounds. The RMSD of tak-285 was found to be 1.39 Å for EGFR (Figure S1) and 1.40 Å for HER2 (Figure S2), values that are within the acceptable range for using docking to predict the binding affinity of small molecules. These findings may demonstrate the reliability of the docking process parameters and support the use of docking as a tool for predicting the binding affinity of isolated phytocompounds against the EGFR and HER2 proteins.

Fourteen phytocompounds were compared to reference structures against EGFR and HER2. Diosgenin and monohydroxy spirostanol from this group showed EGFR binding energies of −9.77 kcal/mol as well as −9.74 kcal/mol, respectively, which were comparable to those of the reference drugs tak-285 and lapatinib. (Table 2). These values were similar to those of the reference drugs tak-285 (−9.71 kcal/mol) and lapatinib (−9.64 kcal/mol). For the HER2 receptor, diosgenin and monohydroxy spirostanol revealed the lowest binding energy values, −9.19 kcal/mol and −10.10 kcal/mol, respectively, as well as among the 14 phytocompounds (Table 2). These values were similar to those of the reference drugs tak−285 (−9.21 kcal/mol) and lapatinib (−8.90 kcal/mol). Among these compounds, diosgenin exhibited a slightly lower binding energy value than the reference-bound ligands for the HER2 receptor. These findings suggest that diosgenin and monohydroxy spirostanol may have the potential to be effective phytocompounds (inhibitors) of both EGFR and HER2 and warrant further investigation.

Table 2. Free binding energy (ΔG) of isolated phytocompounds **1–14** and reference controls against EGFR (3POZ) and HER2 (3RCD) targets.

#	Target	EGFR (3POZ.PDB) Docking Score (kcal/mol)	HER2 (3RCD.PDB) Docking Score (kcal/mol)
1	Amygdalin	−7.57	−6.15
2	Arachidic Acid	−6.46	−5.87
3	Benzyl-beta gentiobioside	−6.8	−6.03
4	Centaureidin	−8.26	−7.07
5	Diosgenin	−9.77	−10.1
6	Glycine	−5.03	−4.27
7	Kaempferol	−8.46	−7.1
8	Linoleic Acid	−6.99	−5.73
9	Monohydroxy spirostanol	−9.74	−9.19
10	Oleic Acid	−6.45	−5.84
11	Palmitic Acid	−5.99	−5.47
12	Palmitoleic Acid	−5.92	−5.5
13	Prunasin	−8.14	−6.14
14	Stearic Acid	−6.2	−5.53
	Tak-285 (control)	−9.71	−9.21
	Lapatinib (control)	−9.64	−9.76

Interaction Examines the Hit Phytocompounds

The potential of the hit phytocompounds as active compounds was evaluated through analysis of non-covalent interactions with target receptors. The best-docked pose for these compounds is depicted in Figure 3 for EGFR and Figure 4 for HER2. In addition, the interactions of these compounds were compared to those of tak-285 and lapatinib, reference drugs for EGFR and HER2, to further understand their potential mechanisms of action. Tables 3 and 4 compare the stability as well as interactions of diosgenin and monohydroxy spirostanol with amino acid residues at the active binding sites of EGFR and HER2 receptors via hydrogen bonding, Pi Sigma, and hydrophobic interactions. These findings are compared to those for the reference drug lapatinib and the original co-crystallized stability of tak-285.

Diosgenin and monohydroxy spirostanol displayed favorable docking scores with common amino acids in the active binding site of EGFR, with binding energies of -9.77 kcal/mol and -9.74 kcal/mol, respectively (Table 2).

The molecular docking results in Figure 3 and Table 3 suggest that both diosgenin and monohydroxy spirostanol may have favorable interactions with the EGFR receptor as evidenced by their hydrogen bond and pi-sigma bond formations, as well as their hydrophobic interactions with specific amino acid residues. These interactions may contribute to the affinity of these compounds for the EGFR receptor.

Diosgenin forms hydrogen bonds with LYS745 and MET793 at distances of 1.81 Å and 1.91 Å, respectively, and also forms a pi-sigma bond with PHE723. In addition, diosgenin has hydrophobic interactions with LEU718, VAL726, PHE723, CYS799, LEU844, and ALA743. Monohydroxy spirostanol forms a hydrogen bond with THR854 at a distance of 2.01 Å and has hydrophobic interactions with VAL726, ALA743, LYS745, MET766, CYS775, LEU777, LEU788, LEU844, PHE856, and LEU858. These interactions may contribute to the affinity of these compounds for the EGFR receptor. In comparison, the reference drugs tak-285 and lapatinib have less favorable interactions with the EGFR receptor.

Tak-285 forms hydrogen bonds with LEU777, THR790, and MET793 at distances of 3.45 Å, 3.60 Å, and 2.78 Å, respectively, and also forms pi-sigma bonds with LEU718 and LEU844. It has hydrophobic interactions with VAL726, ALA743, LYS745, PHE766, CYS775, LEU788, LEU792, PHE856, and LEU858. Some of these amino acid residues, such as LYS745, MET793, and LEU844, also interact with diosgenin and monohydroxy spirostanol. However, the interactions of tak-285 with these residues may be less favorable than those of the phytocompounds, as the distances of the hydrogen bonds are longer and tak-285 does not form any pi-sigma bonds.

Lapatinib does not form any hydrogen bonds, but it does have hydrophobic interactions with MET766, THR790, and LEU844. Some of these amino acid residues, such as MET793 and LEU844, also interact with diosgenin and monohydroxy spirostanol (see Figure 3 and Table 3). However, lapatinib does not form any pi-sigma bonds or hydrogen bonds, which may make its interactions with these residues less favorable than those of the phytocompounds.

A molecular docking analysis was conducted to compare the binding interactions of diosgenin, monohydroxy spirostanol, tak-285, and lapatinib with the HER2 protein. The results of the analysis, presented in Figure 4 and Table 4, provide insight into the molecular interactions among these compounds and the HER2 protein at the active binding site.

Diosgenin had significant hydrogen bond interactions with LYS753 and MET801, with distances of 2.87 Å and 2.72 Å, respectively. These interactions may be significant because they involve amino acid residues that have been identified as key binding sites in the HER2 protein. In addition, diosgenin exhibited hydrophobic interactions with LEU726, VAL734, ALA751, LEU785, LEU796, and LEU852. These hydrophobic interactions may also participate in the binding affinity of diosgenin for the HER2 protein.

Similarly, monohydroxy spirostanol had hydrogen bond interactions with THR798 and THR862, with distances of 2.32 Å and 2.54 Å, respectively. These interactions may be significant because they involve amino acid residues that have been previously identified as important for binding to the HER2 protein. Monohydroxy spirostanol also had hydrophobic interactions with LEU726, VAL734, ALA751, LYS753, MET774, LEU796, and LEU852. These hydrophobic interactions may contribute to the highbinding affinity of monohydroxy spirostanol for the HER2 protein.

The original co-crystallized pose of tak-285 had hydrogen bond interactions with THR798, MET801, and THR862, with distances of 3.17 Å, 2.69 Å, and 2.77 Å, respectively. These interactions involve amino acid residues that have been identified as important for binding to the HER2 protein. Tak-285 also had pi-sigma interactions with LEU800 and LEU862 and hydrophobic interactions with VAL734, ALA751, LYS753, LEU785, LEU796, and PHE864. These interactions may participate in the overall binding affinity of tak-285 for the HER2 protein.

The reference drug lapatinib had hydrogen bond interactions with LYS753 and MET801, with distances of 2.00 Å and 1.86 Å, respectively. These interactions involve amino acid residues that have been identified as key binding sites in the HER2 protein. Lapatinib also had pi-sigma interactions with LEU785 and LEU852, and hydrophobic interactions with ALA751, LYS753, LEU796, LEU800, CYS805, and LEU852. These interactions may contribute to the binding affinity of lapatinib for the HER2 protein.

The molecular docking analysis carried out in this study suggests that diosgenin and monohydroxy spirostanol may have a similar affinity for binding and molecular interactions with EGFR and HER2 proteins as the reference medicines tak-285 and lapatinib. However, to fully evaluate the potential of these compounds as therapeutic agents, it is necessary to consider not only their binding properties but also their pharmacological properties and safety. In silico ADMET analysis can provide valuable insights into the pharmacological profiles of diosgenin and monohydroxy spirostanol and help predict their potential as hit candidates. In addition, conducting molecular dynamics studies can give a more detailed understanding of the binding mechanisms of these ligands. Together, these in silico analyses can provide a comprehensive evaluation of the suitability of diosgenin and monohydroxy spirostanol as therapeutic agents.

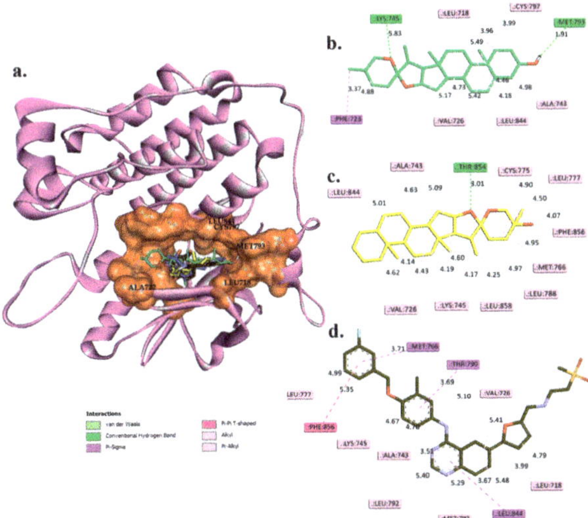

Figure 3. (a) The docked structures of diosgenin (coloured green C and red O), monohydroxy spirostanol (coloured yellow C and red O), lapatinib (coloured army green C, red O, stune N, orange S, and cyan F), and the original co-crystallized tak-285 (coloured dark blue C, red O, stune N, green CL, and cyan F) are superimposed into the active binding site (coloured rust) of EGFR (3POZ.PDB). (b–d) Two-dimensional interaction views of the key and surrounding amino acids with diosgenin, monohydroxy spirostanol, and lapatinib, respectively.

Table 3. Molecular interactions analysis between hit phytocompounds, controls, and EGFR (3POZ.PDB).

| Phytocompounds | Hydrogen Bond Interactions | | Pi-Sigma | Hydrophobic Interaction |
	Residues	Distances (Å)		
Diosgenin	LYS745 and MET793	1.81 and 1.91	PHE723	LEU718, VAL726, PHE723, CYS799, LEU844, and ALA743
Monohydroxy spirostanol	THR854	2.01	—	VAL726, LYS745, MET766, ALA743, LEU777, LEU844, CYS775, LEU788, PHE856, and LEU858
Tak-285 (control)	LEU777, THR790, and MET793	3.45, 3.60, and 2.78	LEU718 and LEU844	VAL726, ALA743, LYS745, PHE766, CYS775, LEU788, LEU792, PHE856, and LEU858
Lapatinib	—	—	MET766, THR790, and LEU844	LEU718, VAL726, ALA743, LYS745, LEU777, LEU792, MET793, LEU844, and PHE856

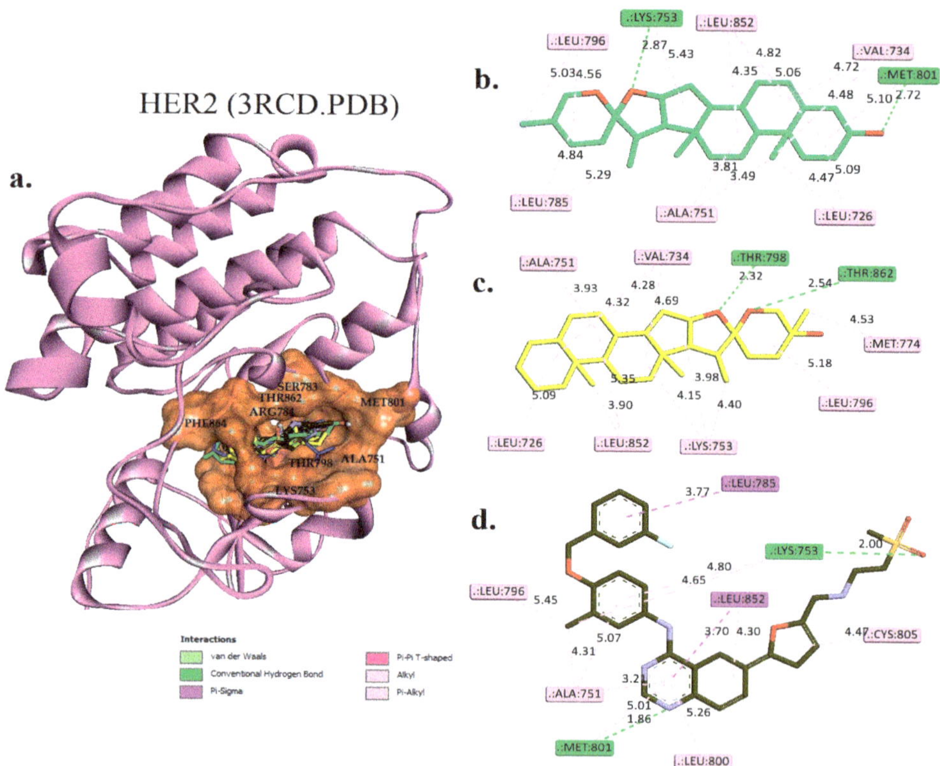

Figure 4. (**a**) The docked structures of diosgenin (colored green C and red O), monohydroxy spirostanol (colored yellow C and red O), lapatinib (colored army green C, red O, stune N, orange S, and cyan F), and the original co-crystallized tak-285 (colored dark blue C, red O, stune N, green CL, and cyan F) are superimposed into the active binding site (colored rust) of HER2 (3RCD.PDB). (**b–d**) Two-dimensional interaction views of the key and surrounding amino acids with diosgenin, monohydroxy spirostanol, and lapatinib, respectively.

Table 4. Molecular interactions analysis between hit phytocompounds, controls, and EGFR (3POZ.PDB).

| Phytocompounds | Hydrogen Bond Interactions | | Pi-Sigma | Hydrophobic Interaction |
	Residues	Distances (Å)		
Diosgenin	LYS745 and MET793	1.81 and 1.91	PHE723	LEU718, PHE723, VAL726, ALA743, CYS799, and LEU844
Monohydroxy spirostanol	THR854	2.01	—	VAL726, ALA743, MET766, LYS745, CYS775, LEU844, LEU777, LEU788, PHE856, and LEU858
Tak-285 (control)	LEU777, THR790, and MET793	3.45, 3.60, and 2.78	LEU718 and LEU844	VAL726, ALA743, LYS745, PHE766, CYS775, LEU788, LEU792, PHE856, and LEU858
Lapatinib	—	—	MET766, THR790, and LEU844	LEU718, VAL726, ALA743, LYS745, LEU777, LEU792, MET793, LEU844, and PHE856

2.5. ADMET Prediction

In Table 5, we present the ADMET and drug-likeness predictions of four compounds: diosgenin, monohydroxy spirostanol, TAK-285, and lapatinib. The predictions were made using the admetSAR 2.0 web-server tool, which employs several different algorithms to analyze various properties of the compounds [24,30].

As shown in the first column, diosgenin has an Fsp3 score of 0.926 and monohydroxy spirostanol has an Fsp3 score of 1, both indicating good hydrophobic properties similar to TAK-285 (Fsp3 score of 0.269) and lapatinib (Fsp3 score of 0.172), all compounds passing theLipinski Rule of five, which is considered a basic requirement for drug-like compounds. Furthermore, none of the compounds was flagged as PAINS (pan-assay interference compounds) or BMS (Bristol-Myers Squibb) rule violators, indicating that they have not been associated with poor pharmacological properties.

Regarding the absorption, our ligands diosgenin and monohydroxy spirostanol have similar poor Caco-2 Permeability (−4.805, −4.805 respectively) compared to TAK-285 (Caco-2 Permeability of −5.505) and lapatinib (Caco-2 Permeability of −5.707), and their Pgp-inhibitor and HIA predictions were relatively better than lapatinib (Pgp-inhibitor: 0.281, 0.993, 0.992, 0.999, HIA: 0.005, 0.002, 0.009, 0.006, respectively). Notably, TAK-285 is more likely to be a substrate for P-glycoprotein efflux pumps (Pgp-substrate of 0.973), which may lower its absorption efficiency. However, it has a higher BBB penetration (0.912) than the other three compounds, indicating a potential for brain-targeting drugs.

The predicted clearances (CL) for diosgenin, monohydroxy spirostanol, TAK-285, and lapatinib were 23.332, 22.718, 8.791, and 3.997 (unit: L/h/kg), respectively. The predicted half-life (T1/2) for diosgenin, monohydroxy spirostanol, TAK-285, and lapatinib were 0.023, 0.08, 0.59, and 0.066 (unit: h), respectively. These predictions indicate that diosgenin, monohydroxy spirostanol, and TAK-285 have a relatively longer half-life and faster clearance compared to lapatinib.

Regarding toxicity, the AMES toxicity, rat oral acute toxicity, and carcinogenicity predictions for diosgenin, monohydroxy spirostanol, TAK-285, and lapatinib were 0.053, 0.019, 0.632, and 0.536, 0.748, 0.67, 0.637, and 0.388, 0.188, 0.274, 0.108, and 0.022 (unitless), respectively. These values indicate that diosgenin and monohydroxy spirostanol have lower toxicity predictions compared to TAK-285 and lapatinib, indicating a lower potential for toxicity.

In general, the hit phytocompounds diosgenin and monohydroxy spirostanol may have good drug-like properties according to ADMET and drug-likeness predictions. They have good hydrophobic properties, passed the Lipinski rule, have no identified PAINS or BMS rule violators, have relatively better Pgp-inhibitor and HIA predictions, and have lower toxicity predictions compared to TAK-285 and lapatinib. However, further analysis, such as molecular dynamics simulations, is needed to fully understand the behavior and potential of these compounds as drugs. It is also important to note that the predictions made using the ADMET Predictor 2.0 web server are only a tool to aid in the discovery and development process and should not be the sole basis for decision-making. Further in vitro and in vivo studies are necessary to fully evaluate the safety and efficacy of these compounds as potential therapeutics.

Table 5. The ADMET and drug-likeness profiles of diosgenin, monohydroxy spirostanol, tak-285 and lapatinib were predicted using the admetSAR 2.0 web-server tool.

ADMET Prediction	Compound			
	Diosgenin	**Monohydroxy Spirostanol**	**Tak-285**	**Lapatinib**
Fsp3	0.926	1	0.269	0.172
Lipinski Rule	Accepted	Accepted	Accepted	Accepted
PAINS	0	0	0	0
BMS Rule	0	0	0	0
Caco-2 Permeability	−4.805	−4.805	−5.505	−5.707
Pgp-inhibitor	0.281	0.993	0.992	0.999
Pgp-substrate	0.001	0.001	0.973	0.995
HIA	0.005	0.002	0.009	0.006
BBB Penetration	0.701	0.187	0.912	0.043
CL	23.332	22.718	8.791	3.997
T1/2	0.023	0.08	0.59	0.066
AMES Toxicity	0.053	0.019	0.632	0.536
Rat Oral Acute Toxicity	0.748	0.67	0.637	0.388
Carcinogenicity	0.188	0.274	0.108	0.022

2.6. Molecular Dynamic Simulations

To further validate the association of diosgenin and monohydroxy spirostanol with the catalytic binding sites of EGFR and HER2, the stability of the docked complexes was investigated and compared to that of tak-285 and lapatinib. To accomplish this, 100 ns MD simulations were carried out by GROMACS 2016 for the four ligand complexes with their corresponding proteins. RMSD and RMSF of the protein, as well as ligand backbone atoms, were computed for each system to dictate their structural stability.

The average RMSD of the EGFR and HER2 complexes with tak-285, lapatinib, diosgenin, and monohydroxy spirostanol provides important insights into the structural stability and potential of these complexes as hit candidates.

As seen in Figure 5A, the EGFR-tak-285 complex reaches a stable state after 30 ns with an RMSD value of 4.2 Å and fluctuates within the range of 3.5–5.2 Å until the end of the simulation. In contrast, the EGFR-lapatinib complex starts the simulation with a lower RMSD value than the EGFR-tak-285 complex and reaches stability after 32 ns with an RMSD value of 3.1 Å, continuing to fluctuate within a narrow range of 2.7–4 Å until the simulation comes to an end.

The EGFR-diosgenin complex also reaches stability after 32 ns with a slightly lower RMSD value of 3.8 Å, slightly higher than the EGFR-lapatinib complex, and continues to fluctuate within a narrow range of 2.9–4.6 Å until the end of the simulation.

In contrast, the EGFR-monohydroxy spirostanol system takes slightly longer to reach the stable state, around 37 ns, with an average RMSD value of 4.3 Å. Notably, the system continued to fluctuate within a lower range than the EGFR-tak-285 system, with RMSD values ranging from 3.4 to 4.6 Å until the end of the simulation.

These results provide evidence for the robust binding of diosgenin and monohydroxy spirostanol to the active binding site of EGFR. The lower RMSD values of these complexes compared to the co-crystallized ligand tak-285 and the reference drug lapatinib suggest that they are more structurally stable and may have a higher potential as drug candidates. Additionally, the fact that the RMSD values of diosgenin and monohydroxy spirostanol fall within the same range as those of lapatinib suggests that they may have similar potential as hit candidates. It is important to note that the stability of the protein-ligand complex has a direct impact on the binding affinity and efficacy of a drug candidate, as a more stable complex is less likely to dissociate from the protein and therefore more likely to effectively inhibit its activity. Therefore, the results of this study offer valuable insights into the structural stability of these complexes, which can be further used to make predictions about the binding affinity and efficacy of these compounds as EGFR inhibitors.

In Figure 5B, it's clear that the HER2-tak-285 complex reaches a stable state after 33 ns with an average RMSD value of 3.7 Å as well as fluctuates within a range of 3.3–4.6 Å until the simulation is over. On the other hand, the HER2-lapatinib complex reaches stability after 33 ns with an average RMSD value of 3.6 Å and continues to fluctuate within a relatively narrow range of 3.1–4.6 Å throughout the simulation.

When comparing the structural stability of the HER2-diosgenin and HER2-monohydroxy spirostanol complexes to the co-crystallized ligand tak-285 and the reference drug lapatinib, it is observed that the HER2-diosgenin complex reaches stability after 47 ns with a lower RMSD value of 3.9 Å. However, the system continues to fluctuate within a relatively wide range of 3.8–4.8 Å until the end of the simulation. Similarly, the HER2-monohydroxy spirostanol complex reaches stability at around 37 ns with an average RMSD value of 3.8 Å and continues to fluctuate within a range of 3.3–4.4 Å throughout the simulation.

Overall, the findings show that although all the complexes are stable, the HER2-diosgenin and HER2-monohydroxy spirostanol complexes have slightly higher RMSD values than the co-crystallized ligand tak-285 and the reference compound lapatinib. Furthermore, the narrow RMSD range observed in the HER2-lapatinib complex suggests that it may exhibit a higher potential as a drug candidate when compared to the other complexes. Overall, the results of this study gave valuable insights into the average structural stability of these complexes and their potential as drug candidates against EGFR and HER2, and they highlights the importance of using MD simulation as a tool for evaluating the predictability of protein-ligand complexes and in the prediction of hit candidate molecules. This can be useful for identifying potential hit candidates among a pool of compounds and for optimizing the design of novel or new drugs. Furthermore, by comparing the simulation results to the experimentally determined binding data, it can be used as a tool for validating the results of computational studies. This can help to increase the reliability of the predictions made by computational methods and, thus, the identification of potential drug candidates that would be more likely to succeed in the clinic.

The utilization of RMSF analysis in MD simulations is a valuable tool for evaluating the structural stability and flexibility of protein-ligand complexes [30]. In this study, RMSF analysis was employed to further investigate the residual flexibility of the EGFR and HER2 structures after complex formation with tak-285, lapatinib, diosgenin, and monohydroxy spirostanol to gain important insights into the structural stability and potential of these complexes as hit candidates.

The average RMSF values of each residue's oscillation during the 100 ns MD simulation were computed and presented in Figure 6. The average RMSF plot in Figure 6A illustrates minimal fluctuation in certain loop places of the protein structure for the EGFR complex. It was observed that the EGFR protein structure after complexation with diosgenin and monohydroxy spirostanol displayed low flexibility, comparable to that of the co-crystallized ligand tak-285 and reference ligand lapatinib. This suggests that the interacting phytocompounds did not significantly affect the stability of the EGFR protein.

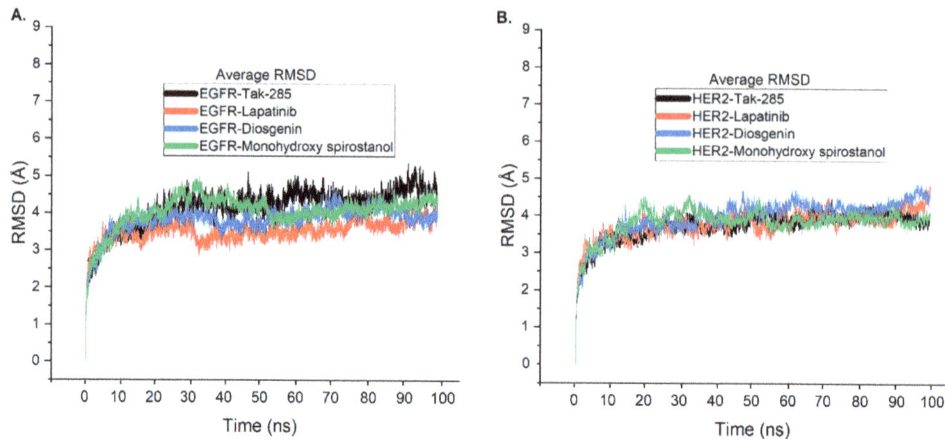

Figure 5. Comparison of the average RMSD values of EGFR and HER2 complexes with tak-285 (black), lapatinib (raspberry), diosgenin (sapphire), and monohydroxy spirostanol (fern). (**A**) RMSD values of EGFR complexes. (**B**) RMSD values of HER2 complexes.

In Figure 6B, it was noticed that the HER2 protein structure after complexation with diosgenin and monohydroxy spirostanol displayed slightly higher flexibility compared to that of the co-crystallized ligand tak-285 and the reference ligand lapatinib. However, the difference in flexibility is not significant and does not affect the stability of the HER2 protein.

Further, the study highlighted that the loop regions of the EGFR and HER2 proteins, which are known to take part in protein-ligand interactions, were relatively stable after complexation with diosgenin and monohydroxy spirostanol. This suggests that these compounds can form stable correlations with the key residues in the active site of the proteins. This is crucial for their potential as hit candidates. Furthermore, the findings of the RMSF examination were consistent with the findings of the RMSD analysis. This provides further evidence for the robust binding of diosgenin and monohydroxy spirostanol to the active binding sites of both EGFR and HER2.

It is worth noting that the RMSF values of lapatinib also fall in the same range as those of diosgenin and monohydroxy spirostanol for both EGFR and HER2. This suggests that lapatinib, diosgenin, and monohydroxy spirostanol are similarly stable in their interactions with EGFR and HER2, and thus, they may have similar potential as drug candidates.

The outcomes of this research provide valuable insights into the structural stability and flexibility of the EGFR and HER2 complexes with tak-285, lapatinib, diosgenin, and monohydroxy spirostanol. The RMSF analysis revealed that these compounds can form stable interactions with the active site of the proteins. In addition, they did not significantly affect the stability of the EGFR and HER2 proteins. These findings may be used to estimate the binding affinity and efficacy of diosgenin and monohydroxy spirostanol as dual EGFR/HER2 kinase inhibitors. They highlight the importance of using RMSF analysis as a tool in drug discovery.

The results of the MM-PBSA calculations, as presented in Table 6, provide valuable insights into the binding energies of the ligands to the active sites of the EGFR and HER2 receptors. The overall binding energies ($\Delta G_{Binding}$) for the ligands are within the range of -62.73 to -80.24 kJ/mol, indicating that all of the ligands have a strong binding affinity for the receptors. Furthermore, the energy contributions from different interactions can be analyzed to improve our understanding of the molecular mechanisms of bonding.

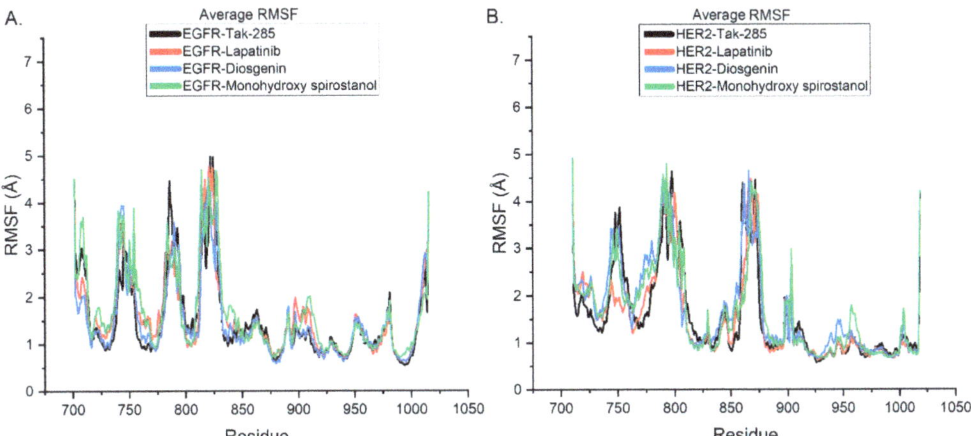

Figure 6. Comparison of the average RMSF values of EGFR and HER2 complexes with tak-285 (black), lapatinib (raspberry), diosgenin (sapphire), and monohydroxy spirostanol (fern). (**A**) RMSF values of EGFR complexes. (**B**) RMSF values of HER2 complexes.

It is clear from Table 6 that the major contributor to the binding energy for all the systems is the van der Waals interaction, which ranges from -50.93 to -78.99 kJ/mol. This suggests that the major driving force behind the action of ligands on receptors is the physical interaction between the atoms of the ligand and the receptor. Additionally, electrostatic interactions, which range from -28.05 to -13.74 kJ/mol, also make a significant contribution to the binding energy. This highlights the importance of electrostatic bindings in the binding of ligands to receptors.

The polar and non-polar solvation energies for the ligands are relatively low, as expected, and range from -18.59 to -11.33 and -25.98 to -14.23 kJ/mol, respectively. This suggests that the solvent does not play a key role in the binding of the ligands to the receptors. The data from the MM-PBSA calculations are in agreement with the RMSD and RMSF results, which indicate that diosgenin and monohydroxy spirostanol have strong binding interactions with both EGFR as well as HER2 receptors. The binding free energy values for diosgenin and monohydroxy spirostanol are comparable to those of the co-crystallized ligand tak-285 and reference ligand lapatinib, suggesting that they have similar binding affinities to both receptors. The electrostatic energy values for diosgenin and monohydroxy spirostanol are also similar to those of tak-285 and lapatinib, indicating that the ligands have similar interactions with the electrostatic potential of the receptors. However, the van der Waals energy values for diosgenin and monohydroxy spirostanol are slightly more negative than tak-285 and lapatinib, implying that they may have slightly different interactions with the van der Waals forces of the receptors. Overall, these results suggest that diosgenin and monohydroxy spirostanol may have the potential to act as dual inhibitors of both EGFR and HER2. Further studies, such as in vitro and in vivo assays, are required to confirm these findings. In addition, these studies are utilized to further quantify the binding affinity and efficacy of these compounds as EGFR and HER2 inhibitors. This study highlights the importance of using computational methods, such as RMSD, RMSF, and MM-PBSA, in the early stages of drug discovery to predict the structural stability and potential of protein-ligand complexes.

Table 6. MM-PBSA energies ($\Delta G_{Binding}$) for ligands binding at both active sites of EGFR (PDB ID: 3POZ) and HER2 (PDB ID: 3RCD) target receptors. All the energies units in kJ/mol.

System	$\Delta G_{Binding}$ (kJ/mol)	Electrostatic (kJ/mol)	Van der Waal (kJ/mol)	Polar Salvation (kJ/mol)	Non-Polar Salvation (kJ/mol)
EGFR-tak-285	-68.33 ± 0.16	-28.05 ± 0.16	-50.93 ± 0.34	29.98 ± 0.27	-11.33 ± 0.19
EGFR-lapatinib	-71.73 ± 0.24	-13.74 ± 0.18	-64.99 ± 0.31	25.59 ± 0.28	-18.59 ± 0.14
EGFR-diosgenin	-67.65 ± 0.13	-23.25 ± 0.33	-54.92 ± 0.23	26.98 ± 0.31	-16.46 ± 0.16
EGFR-monohydroxy spirostanol	-62.73 ± 0.31	-18.74 ± 0.34	-53.99 ± 0.19	24.23 ± 0.30	-14.23 ± 0.14
HER2-tak-285	-72.08 ± 0.23	-11.15 ± 0.26	-69.93 ± 0.32	34.98 ± 0.23	-25.98 ± 0.16
HER2-lapatinib	-80.24 ± 0.21	-7.72 ± 0.22	-78.99 ± 0.15	30.87 ± 0.19	-24.40 ± 0.15
HER2-diosgenin	-78.85 ± 0.33	-10.25 ± 0.16	-72.68 ± 0.24	27.76 ± 0.24	-23.68 ± 0.17
HER2-monohydroxy spirostanol	-69.31 ± 0.19	-10.87 ± 0.18	-65.36 ± 0.34	29.11 ± 0.28	-22.19 ± 0.16

3. Materials and Methods

3.1. Collection and Preparation of Prunus amygdalus var amara Seeds Extract

The *Prunus amygdalus var amara* seeds were obtained from Egypt. The plant has been characterized and matched with the voucher specimen (Eg-N. S42217) by the Cairo University Herbarium.

3.2. Instruments and Preparation of Prunus amygdalus var amara Seed Extraction

3.2.1. GC-MS Analysis

The plant material was obtained in a 100-mL conical flask as well as mixed with absolute ethanol using a solid/liquid ratio of 1:2 (m/v) for the extraction of the phytochemicals. Reflux was used during the extraction, which took place in a water bath at 34.4 °C. Following extraction, we used a vacuum rotating evaporator to evaporate the liquid extract at 50 °C in order to remove extra ethanol. The extract that resulted was dried completely before being stored in a desiccator [31].

An Agilent 6890 gas chromatograph with mass spectrometric detector was used with a direct capillary interface as well as fused silica capillary column PAS-5ms (30 m $\times$ 0.32 mm $\times$ 0.25 μm film thickness). The oil being investigated was injected under these conditions. Helium was utilized as the carrier gas at an estimated 1.0 mL/min in pulsed split-lowmode. The solvent incubation timewas 3 min, and the injection size has to be 1.0 μL. The mass spectrometric detector has been operated in electron effect ionization mode with anionization energy of 70 e.v. scanning via m/z 50 to 500. The ion supply temperature was 230 multiplier voltage (EM 5 voltage) and sustained at 1250 v out of auto-tune [31].

3.2.2. HPLC System-Glycine

For the purpose of obtaining of plant seed powder, one gram of the seeds in powder form was soaked in 100 mL of hexane in an evaporator for one hour. The soaked seeds have been extracted employing an ultrasound wave and 5 mL of an extracting solution (ethanol 0.2% metaphoric acid v/v) for 1 h from 0.5 g of ground up flesh. The resulting mixture was centrifuged at 10,000 rpm over 5 min at 4 °C, as well as the supernatant was obtained Utilizing a concentrator for 4 h, the 0.8 mL supernatant had been dried.The samples were transferred to an HPLC glass vial as well as securely sealed after being filtered through a 0.22 m nylon syringe filter. Finally, 0.5 μL of the obtained samples were then added to an HPLC [31].

The strategy of chromatography was accompanied by injection into an HPLC system along with a specific column (100 $\times$ 2.1 mm, 1.7 μm C18), thermostated at 16 °C. Data were monitored using the Chemstation (Agilent, Santa Clara, CA, USA) chromatography data processing system. The parameters of the mobile phase system have been used as follows:

Flow Rate 0.4 mL/min	A	B
Time	Methanol: Formic acid (10%: 0.1%)	Methanol: Formic acid (50%: 0.1%)
0–6.5	10–30	90–70
6.5–7	30–100	70–0
8–8.5	100–10	0–90
8.5–12.5	10	90

Fluorescence is detected using a detector by excitation at 335 nm and emission at 440 nm. Retention was used to distinguish amino acids [32].

3.2.3. Glycosides

The powdered seeds (0.5 g) were ground and weighed along with a conical flask (90 mL). After that, 20 mL of ethanol was added, and extractions were performed in a shaking water bath (37 °C) in terms of water extraction. Then, extracts were purified, and ethanol was evaporated from the filtrate by a rotary evaporator. Diethyl ether (5 mL) was added to the dried sample, as well as the mixture was vortexed 1 min at room temperature to precipitate the important phytonutrients (amygdalin, prunasin, and benzyl-beta gentio-bioside). The ether solvent was allowed to evaporate overnight in a fume hood, as well as the precipitated compounds were dissolved in 10 mL of water and organized for HPLC analysis.

The method of chromatography was placed on an OmniSpher C18-column (250 × 4.6 mm inner diameterand 5 μm, Varian-USA). The contents of the mobile phase were described as the following:

Flow Rate 0.8 mL/min	A %	B %
Time	0.1% phosphoric acid: water	Methanol 100% HPLC—Grade
0	95	5
0–0.5	5–25	95–75
0.5–2	80–90	20–10
2–4.5	10–60	90–40
4.5–8	50–60	50–40
8–14	0	100

The rate of flow was 0.8 mL/min. The volume of injection for samples as well as standards was 20 μL. The compounds were isolated at room temperature. Among individual runs, a 10-min re-equilibration period was used. UV/vis spectra were measured with a detection wavelength of 280 nm [33].

3.2.4. Flavonoids

The extraction procedure takes 5 g of the powdered seeds in a solvent, a combination mixture of 99% aqueous methanol as well as 1% hydrochloric acid, and an efficient collection of ultrasound (UAE) and microwave (MAE) assisted extraction. Moreover, 1 g of the lyophilized dehydrated powders was mixed with 4 mL of the extraction chemicals, which containing methanol cembined with hydrochloric acid (99: 1 (*v/v*), and after that, it was placed in a microwave, at 450 W for 15 s. Thereafter, each mixture was introduced in a vial protected against light and sonicated inside an ultrasound bath at 258 °C with a steady frequency of 35 kHz for 15 min. Following sonication, the lyophilized' solutions were left at room temperature for about 1 h, centrifuged at 3500 rpm for 20 min, and then each extract was deposited in a laboratory flask. The samples were then examined by an HPLC system (Waters 2996) along with a photodiode array detector. The reverse-phase Supelcosil™ LC-18 column that was used is 15 cm long, has a 4 mm internal diameter, and containsoctadecyl silane particles of 5 µm diameter [31,34].

3.2.5. Steroids

The powdered seeds (100 mg) were extracted in 200 mL of 70% methanol for 3 h at 60 °C using a magnetic stirrer. The extracted material was lyophilized, then dissolved in (1:1) methanol as well as filtered via a 0.22-µm nylon syringe filter, ChemLand-Poland, before HPLC assessment.

The Agilent 1200 HPLC device consisted of two LC-20AD pumps, degasser DGU-26A7, a micromixer along with 0.5–2.6 mL for HPLC-ELSD, with controller CBM-20A, also thermostat (CTO-20AC), an autosampler (SIL 20ACYR), in addition to an ELSD 3300 (Alltech Associates, Deerfield, IL, USA), a nitrogen generator, and an evaporative light scattering detector. Data was collected and handled by Chemstation software, version3.b32. The mobile phase is composed of A (99.9% water and 0.1% formic acid (v/v)) and B (99.9% acetonitrile and 0.1% formic acid (v/v)). Separation was first carried out on a Discovery C-18 column,150 mm 2.1 mm, 3 µm, using gradient program I: 0 min—20% B, 27 min—33.5% B, 45 min—100% B. The column temperature has to be 20 °C, and the flow rate has to be 0.2 mL/min. The volume of the injection was 1 µL [31,35].

3.3. Molecular Docking

3.3.1. Protein Structure Preparation

The 3D structures of the EGFR (PDB ID: 3POZ) [36] and HER2 (PDB ID: 3RCD) [37] complexes with the co-crystallized ligand tak-285 were selected as protein targets for further analysis. These structures were obtained from the Protein Data Bank (PDB) (http://www.rcsb.org, accessed on 8 January 2023) in PDB format [38]. The approved cancer treatment drug lapatinib, which is known to inhibit both EGFR and HER2 targets, was selected as a reference drug for a comparative study [39].

The 3D structures of the protein targets were preprocessed to prepare them for molecular docking studies. This process involved the elimination of heteroatoms and non-essential water molecules using the Biovia Discovery Studio Visualizer (Biovia, 2020) [40] and subsequently saving the structures in PDB format. In addition, missing amino acids in the target structures were incorporated using the YASARA web-server tool [41]. The ionization states of titratable amino acid groups were subsequently calculated at pH 7.4 using the H++ web-server tool [42]. The resulting output was then transformed into PDBQT format using the AutoDock Tools version 1.5.6 tools [43], which included adding polar hydrogen atoms and Kollman charges. The active binding site coordinates for the docking studies were identified from the potential ligand binding domain regions of the obtained crystal structures.

3.3.2. Ligand Preparation

In this study, the 2D structure of the reference drug lapatinib (PubChem ID: 208908) was taken from the PubChem database (https://pubchem.ncbi.nlm.nih.gov, accessed on 8 January 2023) to perform a molecular docking study. The structure of tak-285 was extracted from its respective protein structures as deposited in PDB, and its conformational change, if any, was taken into consideration. The 14 isolated compounds were drawn using the ChemDraw JS web page (https://chemdrawdirect.perkinelmer.cloud/js/sample/index.html, accessed on 8 January 2023) and saved in the structural data file (SDF) format. To attain the most stable conformation of each ligand, energy minimization was conducted by the Universal Force Field (UFF) and a Conjugate Gradient (CG) optimization algorithm with 1000 steps. The optimization process was carried out using the open-source babel software, and the resulting structures were saved in PDB format. Subsequently, using AutoDock tools version 1.5.6, Gasteiger charges were connected to the ligands, and the ligands were uploaded in PDBQT format, ready for molecular docking simulations.

3.3.3. Molecular Docking Preparation

The molecular docking analyses of the fourteen phytocompounds were conducted to evaluate their binding affinity and molecular interactions with the EGFR and HER2 proteins. The AutoDock 4.2 Release 4.2.6 program [43,44] was utilized for the docking calculations, and the compounds were docked against reference controls, including the co-crystallized ligand tak-285 and the commercially available drug lapatinib. The Lamarckian genetic algorithm was employed to optimize the binding poses of the compounds, and the ligands were set to be flexible while macromolecules were rigid.

The identified compounds were docked into the active binding sites of the EGFR and HER2, with the grid box focused on the center of the ligand in the original EGFR and HER2 structures. The grid box size was $40 \times 40 \times 40$ along with the X, Y, and Z axes for both enzymes, and the coordinates of the central grid point of the map have been set to be 18.74, 31.83, and 11.62 for EGFR and 12.48, 2.96, and 28.01 for HER2. The number of runs had to be set to 150, and the maximum number of evaluations was set to 25,000,000. The default values were utilized for all other parameters to ensure consistency in the calculations. The binding energies and properties of the different phytocompounds after docking were analyzed and studied to determine their potential as therapeutic agents.

3.4. ADMET Prediction

In this study, we used admetSAR 2.0 [45], a web-based tool for predicting ADMET (Absorption, Distribution, Metabolism, Excretion, and Toxicity) properties, to evaluate the potential of two hit phytocompounds, diosgenin and monohydroxy spirostanol, as candidates for drug development. The ADMET properties of interest were selected based on the common properties known to be important for oral bioavailability, such as oral absorption, blood-brain barrier penetration, and CYP450 metabolism. The reference compound used in the analysis was lapatinib, a commercially available drug that has been clinically used as a tyrosine kinase inhibitor.

The methodology for using admetSAR 2.0 consisted of the following steps: (1) the compounds of interest were uploaded to the web server in SMILES format, (2) the relevant ADMET properties were selected for prediction, and (3) the results were obtained in the form of predicted values along with their corresponding confidence levels. The predictions were generated using multiple algorithms and models available on admetSAR 2.0, which included multiple linear regression, decision trees, and artificial neural networks.

To validate the predictions, we compared the predicted ADMET properties of diosgenin and monohydroxy spirostanol against the reported values of lapatinib. Additionally, we also performed in silico toxicity and drug-likeness prediction using the same server. The results of these predictions were used to evaluate the potential of diosgenin and monohydroxy spirostanol as potential hit candidates and to identify potential areas for further optimization.

3.5. Molecular Dynamics

In this research, we aimed to assess the stability and binding behavior of selected phytocompounds in the active sites of EGFR and HER2 proteins using MD—dynamics simulations. We used the crystal structures of EGFR and HER2 complexed with tak-285 as the starting point for our simulations. The GROMACS software package (version 2016.3) and the Gromos96 54a7 force field [46] were employed to perform the MD simulations on a nanosecond time scale. The GROMOS96 54a7 force field has been shown to yield accurate results for investigating protein dynamics and ligand binding behavior, as reported in the literature [47]. This force field has been validated through simulations of the folding equilibrium of two β-peptides with distinct dominant folds using three different force fields, including GROMOS 54A7 [47].

To prepare the systems for simulation, we generated protein and ligand topology files with appropriate tools. The protein topology file was created by the GROMACS software, pdb2gmx, whereas the ligand topology file has been created by the PRODRG server ("http://davapc1.bioch.dundee.ac.uk/cgi-bin/prodrg, accessed on 15 December 2022"). The systems have been solvated by using the TIP3P (Transferable Intermolecular Potential along with Three Points) water model, as well as counterions could be added to neutralize the charge. The systems were then minimized by the steepest descent integrator to 50,000 maximum optimization process steps as well as a 0.01 energy step size. The v-rescale coupling technique was then used to equilibrate the designed to minimize processes for 100 ps at 310 K in the steady number of particles, volume, as well as temperature (NVT) outfit. A 100-ps equilibration period was then completed using the Berendsen pressure linkage method at 1.0 bar with a steady number of particles, pressure, and temperature (NPT) [48,49].

After the temperature and pressure equilibrations, MD simulation runs were performed for the models for 100 ns each at 1 bar and 310 K. The short-range non-bonded interactions cut-off was set at 1.2 nm, while long-range electrostatic interactions were treated using the Particle Mesh Ewald (PME) algorithm [50]. The LINCS algorithm was used to constrain the bonds with hydrogen atoms [51]. During the molecular dynamics (MD) simulations, a time step of 2 fs was utilized for all simulations. To ensure accurate and reliable results, the coordinates were reset at regular intervals of 5000 steps, which is equivalent to 10 ps, as a part of MD data processing. This approach was implemented to maintain the integrity of the simulations and obtain robust outcomes. To analyze the MD trajectories, we used various tools and techniques such as Root Mean Square Fluctuation (RMSF), Root Mean Square Deviation (RMSD), and hydrogen bond analysis to assess the strength and stability of the interactions between the phytocompounds and the proteins.

To visually represent the results, molecular graphics images were produced using Biovia Discovery Studio Visualizer (Biovia, 2020), and graphs were prepared using Origin Pro 2021 (version 9.8.0.200). These images and graphs provide a detailed representation of the systems and the interactions taking place, providing a deeper understanding of the results of the simulations.

3.6. Binding Free Energy Calculation Using MM/PBSA

In this study, we utilized the molecular mechanics Poisson-Boltzmann surface area (MM-PBSA) method [52], a widely used approach for calculating binding free energy from snapshots of molecular dynamics (MD) trajectories. The binding free energies of hit phytocompounds and controls against EGFR and HER2 were analyzed during the equilibrium phase of the MD simulations by taking snapshots at an interval of 100 ps from 90 to 100 ns, using the g_mmpbsa tool of Gromacs [53,54].

The binding free energy of the ligand-protein complex in solvent was calculated by subtracting the sum of the total energies of the separated protein ($G_{protein}$) and ligand (G_{ligand}) in solvent from the total free energy of the protein-ligand complex ($G_{complex}$) according to the following equation [54]:

$$\Delta G_{binding} = G_{complex} - (G_{protein} + G_{ligand})$$

The free energy for each state (complex, protein, and ligand) was calculated by adding the free energy of solvation ($G_{solvation}$) and the average molecular mechanic's potential energy in vacuum (EMM) [54]:

$$G_x = E_{MM} + G_{solvation}$$

The molecular mechanic's potential energy was calculated in a vacuum as the sum of bonded interactions (E_{bonded}) and non-bonded interactions ($E_{non-bonded}$), where E_{bonded}

included bond, angle, dihedral, and improper interactions and Enon-bonded included van der Waals (E_{vdw}) and electrostatic (E_{elec}) interactions [54]:

$$E_{MM} = E_{bonded} + E_{non\_bonded} = E_{bonded} + (E_{vdw} + E_{elec})$$

The solvation free energy ($G_{solvation}$) was estimated as the sum of electrostatic solvation-free energy (G_{polar}) and a polar solvation-free energy ($G_{non\text{-}polar}$) [54]:

$$G_{solvation} = G_{polar} + G_{non\text{-}polar}$$

The electrostatic solvation free energy (G_{polar}) was computed using the Poisson-Boltzmann equation [52], while the polar solvation-free energy ($G_{non\text{-}polar}$) was estimated from the solvent-accessible surface area (SASA) using the following equation:

$$Gnon\text{-}polar = \gamma SASA + b$$

where γ is a coefficient related to the surface tension of the solvent and b is a fitting parameter. The values for the coefficient and fitting parameter used in this study were: $\gamma = 0.02267$ Kj/mol/Å^2 or 0.0054 Kcal/mol/Å^2 and b = 3.849 Kj/mol or 0.916 Kcal/mol.

It is important to note that the ΔE_{bonded} was assumed to be zero in this calculation [55]. The results of this binding free energy calculation provide insight into the energetics of the protein-ligand interactions and can aid in the identification of potential hit candidates. These findings were experimentally validated in our previous study [56].

4. Conclusions

In conclusion, this study suggests that diosgenin and monohydroxy spirostanol may have the potential to act as dual suppressors of both EGFR and HER2. The molecular docking analysis conducted in this study reveals that these compounds may exhibit similar binding affinity and molecular interactions with EGFR and HER2 proteins as the reference drugs tak-285 and lapatinib. The binding free energy values for diosgenin and monohydroxy spirostanol were comparable to those of the co-crystallized ligand tak-285 and the reference ligand lapatinib, suggesting that they have comparable binding affinities for both enzymes.

Diosgenin and monohydroxy spirostanol had electrostatic as well as van der Waals energy values that were similar to those of tak-285 as well as lapatinib. This suggests that the ligands interact similarly with the electrostatic potential and van der Waals forces of the receptors.. In silico ADMET and molecular dynamics studies were also used to provide valuable insights into the pharmacological profile and interaction mechanisms of these compounds. The results indicate that diosgenin and monohydroxy spirostanol have good drug-like properties and strong binding interactions with EGFR and HER2 receptors. However, it is important to note that further in vitro as well as in vivo studies are necessary to fully evaluate their safety and efficacy as potential therapeutics. This study highlights the importance of using computational methods in the early stages of drug discovery to predict the structural stability and potential of protein-ligand complexes. The results of this study provide a promising starting point for further investigation of diosgenin and monohydroxy spirostanol as dual inhibitors of EGFR and HER2. These findings are consistent with the experimental data.

Supplementary Materials: The following supporting information can be downloaded at: https://www.mdpi.com/article/10.3390/ph16050704/s1. Figure S1. (a) Superimposition and (b) 2D Interaction analysis of the co-crystallized ligand TAK-285. (c) Re-docked Ligand (depicted in orange for carbon (C), red for oxygen (O), navy for nitrogen (N), and cyan for fluorine (F)) in the Crystal Structure of the Human EGFR Kinase Domain Complexed with TAK-285 (PDB ID: 3POZ). Figure S2. (a) Superimposition and (b) 2D Interaction analysis of the co-crystallized ligand TAK-285. (c) Re-docked ligand in the crystal structure of the human HER2 kinase domain complexed with tak-285 (PDB ID: 3RCD).

Author Contributions: Conceptualization, M.H.F.S. and G.M.A.-M.; methodology, G.M.A.-M. and M.H.F.S.; software, G.M.A.-M.; validation, A.A.A. and A.F.A.; writing—original draft preparation, M.H.F.S. and G.M.A.-M.; writing—review and editing, M.A.; project administration, M.H.F.S.; funding acquisition, A.A.A., A.F.A. and M.A. All authors have read and agreed to the published version of the manuscript.

Funding: This research work was funded by Institutional Fund Projects under the no. (IFP-A-2022-2-5-21). Therefore, authors gratefully acknowledge technical and financial support from the Ministry of Education and University of Hafr Al Batin, Saudi Arabia.

Institutional Review Board Statement: Not applicable.

Informed Consent Statement: Not applicable.

Data Availability Statement: Data is contained within the article and supplementary material.

Conflicts of Interest: The authors declare no conflict of interest.

References

1. Sharma, G.N.; Dave, R.; Sanadya, J.; Sharma, P.; Sharma, K. Various types and management of breast cancer: An overview. *J. Adv. Pharm. Technol. Res.* **2010**, *1*, 109. [PubMed]
2. Tewari, D.; Patni, P.; Bishayee, A.; Sah, A.N.; Bishayee, A. Natural products targeting the PI3K-Akt-mTOR signaling pathway in cancer: A novel therapeutic strategy. *Semin. Cancer Biol.* **2022**, *80*, 1–17. [CrossRef] [PubMed]
3. Singla, R.K.; Wang, X.; Gundamaraju, R.; Joon, S.; Tsagkaris, C.; Behzad, S.; Khan, J.; Gautam, R.; Goyal, R.; Rakmai, J. Natural products derived from medicinal plants and microbes might act as a game-changer in breast cancer: A comprehensive review of preclinical and clinical studies. *Crit. Rev. Food Sci. Nutr.* **2022**, 1–45. [CrossRef] [PubMed]
4. Abdolahi-Majd, M.; Hassanshahi, G.; Vatanparast, M.; Karimabad, M.N. Investigation of the Effect of *Prunus amygdalus amara* on the Expression of some Genes of Apoptosis and Immortality in Breast Cancer Cells (MCF-7). *Curr. Drug Res. Rev. Former. Curr. Drug Abus. Rev.* **2022**, *14*, 73–79.
5. Saati, S.; Dehghan, P.; Azizi-Soleiman, F.; Mobasseri, M. The effect of bitter almond (*Amygdalus communis* L. var. Amara) gum as a functional food on metabolic profile, inflammatory markers, and mental health in type 2 diabetes women: A blinded randomized controlled trial protocol. *Trials* **2023**, *24*, 35. [CrossRef] [PubMed]
6. Singh, D.; Gohil, K.J.; Rajput, R.T.; Sharma, V. Almond (*Prunus amygdalus* Batsch.): A Latest Review on Pharmacology and Medicinal uses. *Res. J. Pharm. Technol.* **2022**, *15*, 3301–3308. [CrossRef]
7. Moradi, B.; Heidari-Soureshjani, S.; Asadi-Samani, M.; Yang, Q. A systematic review of phytochemical and phytotherapeutic characteristics of bitter almond. *Int. J. Pharm. Phytopharm. Res.* **2017**, *7*, 1–9.
8. Keser, S.; Demir, E.; Yilmaz, O. Some Bioactive Compounds and Antioxidant Activities of the Bitter Almond Kernel (*Prunus dulcis* var. amara). *J. Chem. Soc. Pak.* **2014**, *36*, 922–930.
9. Guici El Kouacheur, K.; Cherif, H.S.; Saidi, F.; Bensouici, C.; Fauconnier, M.L. *Prunus amygdalus var. amara* (bitter almond) seed oil: Fatty acid composition, physicochemical parameters, enzyme inhibitory activity, antioxidant and anti-inflammatory potential. *J. Food Meas. Charact.* **2023**, *17*, 371–384. [CrossRef]
10. Mericli, F.; Becer, E.; Kabadayı, H.; Hanoglu, A.; Yigit Hanoglu, D.; Ozkum Yavuz, D.; Ozek, T.; Vatansever, S. Fatty acid composition and anticancer activity in colon carcinoma cell lines of Prunus dulcis seed oil. *Pharm. Biol.* **2017**, *55*, 1239–1248. [CrossRef]
11. Uribe, M.L.; Marrocco, I.; Yarden, Y. EGFR in cancer: Signaling mechanisms, drugs, and acquired resistance. *Cancers* **2021**, *13*, 2748. [CrossRef] [PubMed]
12. Murphrey, M.B.; Quaim, L.; Varacallo, M. *Biochemistry, Epidermal Growth Factor Receptor*; StatPearls Publishing: Treasure Island, FL, USA, 2023.
13. Rubin, I.; Yarden, Y. The basic biology of HER2. *Ann. Oncol.* **2001**, *12*, S3–S8. [CrossRef] [PubMed]
14. Oh, D.-Y.; Bang, Y.-J. HER2-targeted therapies—A role beyond breast cancer. *Nat. Rev. Clin. Oncol.* **2020**, *17*, 33–48. [CrossRef]
15. Schneider, M.R.; Yarden, Y. The EGFR-HER2 module: A stem cell approach to understanding a prime target and driver of solid tumors. *Oncogene* **2016**, *35*, 2949–2960. [CrossRef] [PubMed]
16. Weinberg, F.; Peckys, D.B.; de Jonge, N. EGFR expression in HER2-driven breast cancer cells. *Int. J. Mol. Sci.* **2020**, *21*, 9008. [CrossRef]
17. Riecke, K.; Witzel, I. Targeting the human epidermal growth factor receptor family in breast cancer beyond HER2. *Breast Care* **2020**, *15*, 579–585. [CrossRef] [PubMed]
18. Yu, X.; Ghamande, S.; Liu, H.; Xue, L.; Zhao, S.; Tan, W.; Zhao, L.; Tang, S.-C.; Wu, D.; Korkaya, H. Targeting EGFR/HER2/HER3 with a three-in-one aptamer-siRNA chimera confers superior activity against HER2+ breast cancer. *Mol. Ther. Nucleic Acids* **2018**, *10*, 317–330. [CrossRef] [PubMed]

9. Borrero-García, L.D.; del Mar Maldonado, M.; Medina-Velázquez, J.; Troche-Torres, A.L.; Velazquez, L.; Grafals-Ruiz, N.; Dharmawardhane, S. Rac inhibition as a novel therapeutic strategy for EGFR/HER2 targeted therapy resistant breast cancer. *BMC Cancer* **2021**, *21*, 652. [CrossRef] [PubMed]

0. Hsu, J.L.; Hung, M.-C. The role of HER2, EGFR, and other receptor tyrosine kinases in breast cancer. *Cancer Metastasis Rev.* **2016**, *35*, 575–588. [CrossRef]

1. Schlam, I.; Swain, S.M. HER2-positive breast cancer and tyrosine kinase inhibitors: The time is now. *NPJ Breast Cancer* **2021**, *7*, 56. [CrossRef]

2. Montemurro, F.; Valabrega, G.; Aglietta, M. Lapatinib: A dual inhibitor of EGFR and HER2 tyrosine kinase activity. *Expert Opin. Biol. Ther.* **2007**, *7*, 257–268. [CrossRef] [PubMed]

3. Lu, X.; Yu, H.; Ma, Q.; Shen, S.; Das, U.N. Linoleic acid suppresses colorectal cancer cell growth by inducing oxidant stress and mitochondrial dysfunction. *Lipids Health Dis.* **2010**, *9*, 106. [CrossRef] [PubMed]

4. Amelio, I.; Cutruzzolá, F.; Antonov, A.; Agostini, M.; Melino, G. Serine and glycine metabolism in cancer. *Trends Biochem. Sci.* **2014**, *39*, 191–198. [CrossRef] [PubMed]

5. Fukuda, T.; Ito, H.; Mukainaka, T.; Tokuda, H.; Nishino, H.; Yoshida, T. Anti-tumor promoting effect of glycosides from Prunus persica seeds. *Biol. Pharm. Bull.* **2003**, *26*, 271–273. [CrossRef] [PubMed]

6. Newmark, J.; Brady, R.O.; Grimley, P.M.; Gal, A.E.; Waller, S.G.; Thistlethwaite, J.R. Amygdalin (Laetrile) and prunasin beta-glucosidases: Distribution in germ-free rat and in human tumor tissue. *Proc. Natl. Acad. Sci. USA* **1981**, *78*, 6513–6516. [CrossRef]

7. Kashyap, D.; Sharma, A.; Tuli, H.S.; Sak, K.; Punia, S.; Mukherjee, T.K. Kaempferol–A dietary anticancer molecule with multiple mechanisms of action: Recent trends and advancements. *J. Funct. Foods* **2017**, *30*, 203–219. [CrossRef] [PubMed]

8. Arya, P.; Kumar, P. Diosgenin a steroidal compound: An emerging way to cancer management. *J. Food Biochem.* **2021**, *45*, e14005. [CrossRef]

9. El Sayed, A.M.; Basam, S.M.; Marzouk, H.S.; El-Hawary, S. LC–MS/MS and GC–MS profiling as well as the antimicrobial effect of leaves of selected Yucca species introduced to Egypt. *Sci. Rep.* **2020**, *10*, 17778. [CrossRef]

0. Shukla, R.; Tripathi, T. Molecular dynamics simulation of protein and protein–ligand complexes. In *Computer-Aided Drug Design*; Springer: Singapore, 2020; pp. 133–161.

1. Tautenhahn, R.; Böttcher, C.; Neumann, S. Highly sensitive feature detection for high resolution LC/MS. *BMC Bioinform.* **2008**, *9*, 504. [CrossRef]

2. Rodriguez-Garcia, M.; Surman, A.J.; Cooper, G.J.; Suárez-Marina, I.; Hosni, Z.; Lee, M.P.; Cronin, L. Formation of oligopeptides in high yield under simple programmable conditions. *Nat. Commun.* **2015**, *6*, 8385. [CrossRef]

3. Bolarinwa, I.F.; Orfila, C.; Morgan, M.R. Amygdalin content of seeds, kernels and food products commercially-available in the UK. *Food Chem.* **2014**, *152*, 133–139. [CrossRef] [PubMed]

4. Andreotti, C.; Ravaglia, D.; Ragaini, A.; Costa, G. Phenolic compounds in peach (*Prunus persica*) cultivars at harvest and during fruit maturation. *Ann. Appl. Biol.* **2008**, *153*, 11–23. [CrossRef]

5. Król-Kogus, B.; Głód, D.; Krauze-Baranowska, M. Qualitative and quantitative HPLC-ELSD-ESI-MS analysis of steroidal saponins in fenugreek seed. *Acta Pharm.* **2020**, *70*, 89–99. [CrossRef]

6. Aertgeerts, K.; Skene, R.; Yano, J.; Sang, B.-C.; Zou, H.; Snell, G.; Jennings, A.; Iwamoto, K.; Habuka, N.; Hirokawa, A. Structural analysis of the mechanism of inhibition and allosteric activation of the kinase domain of HER2 protein. *J. Biol. Chem.* **2011**, *286*, 18756–18765. [CrossRef] [PubMed]

7. Ishikawa, T.; Seto, M.; Banno, H.; Kawakita, Y.; Oorui, M.; Taniguchi, T.; Ohta, Y.; Tamura, T.; Nakayama, A.; Miki, H. Design and synthesis of novel human epidermal growth factor receptor 2 (HER2)/epidermal growth factor receptor (EGFR) dual inhibitors bearing a pyrrolo [3,2-d] pyrimidine scaffold. *J. Med. Chem.* **2011**, *54*, 8030–8050. [CrossRef]

38. Westbrook, J.; Feng, Z.; Chen, L.; Yang, H.; Berman, H.M. The protein data bank and structural genomics. *Nucleic Acids Res.* **2003**, *31*, 489–491. [CrossRef]

39. Voigtlaender, M.; Schneider-Merck, T.; Trepel, M. Lapatinib. In *Small Molecules in Oncology*; Springer International Publishing: Cham, Switzerlands, 2018; pp. 19–44.

40. Dassault Systèmes. *BIOVIA Discovery Studio 2020*; Dassault Systèmes: San Diego, CA, USA, 2019.

41. Land, H.; Humble, M.S. YASARA: A tool to obtain structural guidance in biocatalytic investigations. In *Protein Engineering: Methods and Protocols*; Humana: New York, NY, USA, 2018; pp. 43–67.

42. Gordon, J.C.; Myers, J.B.; Folta, T.; Shoja, V.; Heath, L.S.; Onufriev, A. H++: A server for estimating p K as and adding missing hydrogens to macromolecules. *Nucleic Acids Res.* **2005**, *33*, W368–W371. [CrossRef]

43. Morris, G.M.; Huey, R.; Lindstrom, W.; Sanner, M.F.; Belew, R.K.; Goodsell, D.S.; Olson, A.J. AutoDock4 and AutoDockTools4: Automated docking with selective receptor flexibility. *J. Comput. Chem.* **2009**, *30*, 2785–2791. [CrossRef]

44. Forli, S.; Olson, A.J. A force field with discrete displaceable waters and desolvation entropy for hydrated ligand docking. *J. Med. Chem.* **2012**, *55*, 623–638. [CrossRef]

45. Yang, H.; Lou, C.; Sun, L.; Li, J.; Cai, Y.; Wang, Z.; Li, W.; Liu, G.; Tang, Y. admetSAR 2.0: Web-service for prediction and optimization of chemical ADMET properties. *Bioinformatics* **2019**, *35*, 1067–1069. [CrossRef]

46. Schmid, N.; Eichenberger, A.P.; Choutko, A.; Riniker, S.; Winger, M.; Mark, A.E.; Van Gunsteren, W.F. Definition and testing of the GROMOS force-field versions 54A7 and 54B7. *Eur. Biophys. J.* **2011**, *40*, 843–856. [CrossRef] [PubMed]

47. Huang, W.; Lin, Z.; Van Gunsteren, W.F. Validation of the GROMOS 54A7 force field with respect to β-peptide folding. *J. Chem. Theory Comput.* **2011**, *7*, 1237–1243. [CrossRef] [PubMed]
48. Rühle, V. Pressure coupling/barostats. *J. Club* **2008**, 1–5.
49. Berendsen, H.J.; Postma, J.v.; Van Gunsteren, W.F.; DiNola, A.; Haak, J.R. Molecular dynamics with coupling to an external bath. *J. Chem. Phys.* **1984**, *81*, 3684–3690. [CrossRef]
50. Petersen, H.G. Accuracy and efficiency of the particle mesh Ewald method. *J. Chem. Phys.* **1995**, *103*, 3668–3679. [CrossRef]
51. Hess, B.; Bekker, H.; Berendsen, H.J.; Fraaije, J.G. LINCS: A linear constraint solver for molecular simulations. *J. Comput. Chem.* **1997**, *18*, 1463–1472. [CrossRef]
52. Kollman, P.A.; Massova, I.; Reyes, C.; Kuhn, B.; Huo, S.; Chong, L.; Lee, M.; Lee, T.; Duan, Y.; Wang, W. Calculating structures and free energies of complex molecules: Combining molecular mechanics and continuum models. *Acc. Chem. Res.* **2000**, *33*, 889–897. [CrossRef]
53. Kumari, R.; Kumar, R.; Consortium, O.S.D.D.; Lynn, A. *g_mmpbsa*—A GROMACS tool for high-throughput MM-PBSA calculations. *J. Chem. Inf. Model.* **2014**, *54*, 1951–1962. [CrossRef]
54. Verma, S.; Grover, S.; Tyagi, C.; Goyal, S.; Jamal, S.; Singh, A.; Grover, A. Hydrophobic interactions are a key to MDM2 inhibition by polyphenols as revealed by molecular dynamics simulations and MM/PBSA free energy calculations. *PLoS ONE* **2016**, *11*, e0149014. [CrossRef]
55. Homeyer, N.; Gohlke, H. Free energy calculations by the molecular mechanics Poisson–Boltzmann surface area method. *Mol. Inform.* **2012**, *31*, 114–122. [CrossRef]
56. Shalayel, M.H.F.; Al-Mazaideh, G.M.; Alanezi, A.A.; Almuqati, A.F.; Alotaibi, M. The Potential Anti-Cancerous Activity of *Prunus amygdalus* var. amara Extract. *Processes* **2023**, *11*, 1277. [CrossRef]

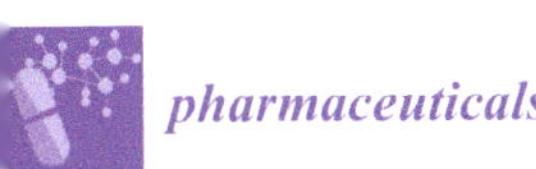 *pharmaceuticals*

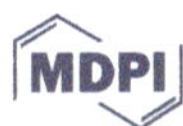

Article

Synthesis, Structural Elucidation and Pharmacological Applications of Cu(II) Heteroleptic Carboxylates

Shaker Ullah [1], Muhammad Sirajuddin [2,*], Zafran Ullah [2], Afifa Mushtaq [1], Saba Naz [1], Muhammad Zubair [1], Ali Haider [1], Saqib Ali [1,*], Maciej Kubicki [3], Tanveer A. Wani [4], Seema Zargar [5] and Mehboob Ur Rehman [6]

[1] Department of Chemistry, Quaid-i-Azam University, Islamabad 45320, Pakistan; shakirwazir23@gmail.com (S.U.); afifa_chemist@hotmail.com (A.M.); sabanaz20014@gmail.com (S.N.); zubairmarwatqau@gmail.com (M.Z.); ahaider@qau.edu.pk (A.H.)

[2] Department of Chemistry, University of Science and Technology Bannu, Bannu 28100, Pakistan; zafranmwt35@gmail.com

[3] Department of Chemistry, Adam Mickiewicz University in Poznan, 61-712 Poznan, Poland; maciej.kubicki@amu.edu.pl

[4] Department of Pharmaceutical Chemistry, College of Pharmacy, King Saud University, P.O. Box 2457, Riyadh 11451, Saudi Arabia; twani@ksu.edu.sa

[5] Department of Biochemistry, College of Science, King Saud University, P.O. Box 22452, Riyadh 11451, Saudi Arabia; szargar@ksu.edu.sa

[6] PIMS Cardiac Center, Islamabad 44000, Pakistan; drmehboobfcps@yahoo.com

* Correspondence: dr.sirajuddin@ustb.edu.pk (M.S.); drsa54@hotmail.com (S.A.)

Citation: Ullah, S.; Sirajuddin, M.; Ullah, Z.; Mushtaq, A.; Naz, S.; Zubair, M.; Haider, A.; Ali, S.; Kubicki, M.; Wani, T.A.; et al. Synthesis, Structural Elucidation and Pharmacological Applications of Cu(II) Heteroleptic Carboxylates. *Pharmaceuticals* **2023**, *16*, 693. https://doi.org/10.3390/ph16050693

Academic Editors: Halil İbrahim Ciftci, Belgin Sever and Hasan Demirci

Received: 30 March 2023
Revised: 28 April 2023
Accepted: 30 April 2023
Published: 3 May 2023

Abstract: Six heteroleptic Cu(II) carboxylates (**1–6**) were prepared by reacting 2-chlorophenyl acetic acid (**L^1**), 3-chlorophenyl acetic acid (**L^2**), and substituted pyridine (2-cyanopyridine and 2-chlorocyanopyridine). The solid-state behavior of the complexes was described via vibrational spectroscopy (FT-IR), which revealed that the carboxylate moieties adopted different coordination modes around the Cu(II) center. A paddlewheel dinuclear structure with distorted square pyramidal geometry was elucidated from the crystal data for complexes **2** and **5** with substituted pyridine moieties at the axial positions. The presence of irreversible metal-centered oxidation reduction peaks confirms the electroactive nature of the complexes. A relatively higher binding affinity was observed for the interaction of SS-DNA with complexes **2–6** compared to **L^1** and **L^2**. The findings of the DNA interaction study indicate an intercalative mode of interaction. The maximum inhibition against acetylcholinesterase enzyme was caused for complex **2** (IC$_{50}$ = 2 µg/mL) compared to the standard drug Glutamine (IC$_{50}$ = 2.10 µg/mL) while the maximum inhibition was found for butyryl-cholinesterase enzyme by complex **4** (IC$_{50}$ = 3 µg/mL) compared to the standard drug Glutamine (IC$_{50}$ = 3.40 µg/mL). The findings of the enzymatic activity suggest that the under study compounds have potential for curing of Alzheimer's disease. Similarly, complexes **2** and **4** possess the maximum inhibition as revealed from the free radical scavenging activity performed against DPPH and H$_2$O$_2$.

Keywords: substituted phenylacetic acid; Cu(II) carboxylates; DNA binding; enzymatic activity; antioxidant activity

1. Introduction

The use of metal-based drugs as a therapeutic agent is evident from ancient times, uncovered some 5000 years ago, and they also form the basis of modern pharmacology [1]. The fortuitous discovery of cisplatin, its potency, and related side effects led to an increased research interest for the synthesis of new metal-based drugs [2]. Moreover, the failure of the already-in-use antibiotics in controlling diseases caused by microbes is considered to be the one of the most important issues by WHO, putting a great responsibility on the researchers in biological science for the discovery of potent and safe metallodrugs [3]. Mostly, the present emphasis is on the synthesis of drugs that target the DNA responsible for biochemical processes occurring in cells. Cisplatin, which exerts its effect by interacting with DNA, is the most inspiring example of metal-based drugs. However, its efficacy is severely affected by its toxic side effects [4]. Similarly, the synthesis of drugs capable of inhibiting enzymes that may help in terms of health and disease treatment has also been the focus of current research. The most promising enzymes, whose inhibition is considered helpful in the pathology of Alzheimer's Disease (AD), may be acetylcholinesterase (AChE) and butyrylcholinesterase (BChE) [5]. AD is a major problem that is faced by developed countries with a high population of old age people [6]. Although there is no exact information as the possible causes of AD, an increase in the amount of acetylcholine as a result of inhibition of acetylcholinesterase is considered to be an effective strategy for the treatment of AD [7]. So, the drugs responsible for inhibition of these two enzymes are of growing interest; however, the already-in-use drugs are suffering from side effects and selective activities [7]. This puts a great demand on the researchers for the synthesis of effective, less toxic, and enzyme-targeting-drugs with a broad range of activities [6].

However, the synthesis of metal-based drugs with the required characteristics is not an easy task, as one has to be careful about the possible toxicity, the lethal effects of metal accumulation, unnecessary interaction with biomolecules and many more aspects [8]. Inspired from the natural biological macromolecules where a suitably organized complex architecture performs multitask functions, a huge amount of research has been focused on the synthesis of heteroleptic complexes, which offer great structural diversity [9]. The proper selection of metal and ligand is one of the most influential factors contributing towards the desired final geometry of complexes. The metal is considered to be the heart of coordination complexes, whereas the ligands exert their influence on physiochemical characteristics and applications as well [10].

Among the first row transition metals, Cu, which possesses biologically compatible chemistry, may be a good choice as metal center for the synthesis of complexes with a desired biological application. With the ability to adopt various easily accessible oxidation states, it is part of many enzymes involved in important biochemical processes in mammalian cells [11]. Moreover, being an essential trace metal, there is no fear of toxicity, and its concentration can be adjusted by the bio system. The use of copper for medicinal purposes is apparent from prehistoric times. It was used to sterilize wounds and water, treat chronic infections, kill fatal microbes and treat various diseases [12]. The complexation of copper with two different bioactive ligands can be enhanced further as of result of chelation and, hence, an increased lipophilic character [13,14].

The carboxylic acids are a good choice as a primary ligand and they can adopt a variety of interesting coordination modes, which assist complexes to adopt biologically suitable fascinating topologies. Besides this, other characteristic features such as acidity and the ability to develop electrostatic and hydrogen bonding allow them to interact with the target [15]. A number of carboxylic acids, especially the derivatives of aromatic carboxylic acids like phenyl acetic acid, already display their role as anti-inflammatory, antipyretic, and antitumor agents. The substituted phenylacetic acids are the natural ingredients of plant and fruits and are added in cosmetics and foods to induce flavors and fragrances. They also play important pharmacological roles, as they are used as precursors for the synthesis of clinically employed drugs, virostatic agents, pain-relieving agents, etc. [16]. However, there are limitations for the use of carboxylic acids as drugs due to lability, toxicity resulting from metabolism, and reduced bioavailability as a result of its restricted ability to cross the cell membrane [17]. The attached metal center and nitrogen donor heterocycling as an auxiliary ligand will not only help to overcome these limitations but also add to the coordination flexibility and structural diversity. These elements assist each other in order to achieve the desired qualities via extended π system, various supramolecular interactions and extended chelation [18].

Most of the commonly employed drugs such as Nonsteroidal anti-inflammatory agents (NSAIDs) are derivatives of carboxylic acids and, compared to free precursors, possess enhanced bioactivities on complexation with a suitable metal center and additional nitrogen donor co-ligand (such as pyridine and its derivatives [19–21]). With the introduction of auxochromes like –CN, -OH, and –NO$_2$, the electron acceptance and fluorescence properties can be readily tuned. Cyanopyridine moiety, which is the most versatile organic intermediate, possesses an electron-withdrawing cyano group over an electron-accepting pyridine ring. The heteroleptic Cu(II) carboxylates with nitrogen donor heterocycles acting as auxiliary ligands have been characterized and found to show enhanced pharmacological potency [22,23].

Keeping in view the current demand as well as the relationship between structural diversity and biological significance, six new heteroleptic Cu(II) carboxylates were synthesized by using substituted phenylacetic acid as the primary ligand and substituted pyridine as the auxiliary ligand. They were characterized structurally and were evaluated for their DNA binding interaction through multi-spectroscopic techniques as well as for other pharmacological applications.

2. Results and Discussion

The heteroleptic Cu(II) carboxylates derived from the substituted chlorophenyl acetic acid were obtained in a good yield and pure form reflected from the values of their melting points. The heteroleptic carboxylates show solubility in the DMSO, ethanol, and methanol.

2.1. FT-IR Study

The broad bands appearing around 3400–3000 cm^{-1} originating from the –OH of carboxylate moiety of ligand acids L^1–L^3 were absent in the spectra of synthesized Cu(II) carboxylates, thus indicating deprotonation of the acids (Table 1). The appearance of new peaks in the finger print region in the spectra around 500 cm^{-1} attributed to the Cu-O bond further support the deprotonation and complexation [24]. Bands of vibrational energy coming from the carboxylate moiety's C-O bond vanish, whereas bands originating from the COO bond break into two bands, which are then classified as symmetrical around the COO and asymmetrical around the other atoms [24]. These two peaks are of great significance in the vibrational spectra of carboxylates and the difference in their values, i.e., Δv, is indicative of possible coordination modes adopted by the carboxylate moiety. It has been suggested for a number of similar reported dinuclear Cu(II) carboxylates with paddle wheel structures that a Δv falling in between 170–250 cm^{-1} indicates bridging bidentate coordination [24]. Here, too, for all six complexes, the values of Δv fall in the range of 185 cm^{-1} to 215 cm^{-1}, suggesting the presence of a bridging bidentate coordination mode adopted by the carboxylate moiety. This suggestion is also supported from the single crystal XRD data of the complex **2** and **5**, where the existence of this kind of coordination results in a paddle wheel structure. The attachment of the substituted pyridine moieties in the complexes is evident from the appearance of vibrational bands responsible for Cu-N bond around 500–550 cm^{-1} [25]. Furthermore, the vibrational band around 2200 cm^{-1} attributed to the stretching of the cyano group (C≡N) of 3-CNPy and 4-CNPy also confirms the presence of these moieties [26]. The vibrational bands arising from the stretching of the Ar-Cl group appear in their respective region around 720–760 cm^{-1} in the spectra of all complexes without any shift, indicating the presence of ligand moieties and the non-involvement of the substituted Cl group in bonding [27].

Table 1. FTIR data of compounds **1**–**6**.

	FTIR (v in cm^{-1})							
Comp. #	OCO$_{asym}$	OCO$_{sym}$	Δv	C≡N	C=C	Ar-Cl	Cu-N	Cu-O
1	1623	1420	203	2100	1473	740	589	567
2	1623	1418	205	2112	1473	741	596	568
3	1591	1392	199	2123	1473	740	597	569
4	1614	1399	215	2200	1475	746	590	571
5	1623	1403	220	2212	1473	725	569	530
6	1586	1403	183	2120	1476	772	592	553

2.2. Single Crystal XRD Analysis

The essential experimental details for the crystals of complexes **2** and **5** are given in Table 2, whereas the data for selected bond lengths and bond angles are given in Table 3. Figures 1 and 2 show the solid-state structures of both complexes. Both **2** and **5** are C_i-symmetrical (occupying inversion centers in their space groups) neutral di-nuclear complexes, in which two Cu(II) ions are bridged by four *syn, syn-η^1:η^1:μ* carboxylates showing a paddle-wheel cage type structure. The coordination environment around each copper is a (CuNO$_4$) distorted square pyramid as suggested for previously reported similar complexes [28,29]. The values of Cu-O$_{eq}$ distance (Table 3), ranging from 1.962(1) to 1.975(1) Å in **2** and from 1.962(1) to 1.976(1) Å in **2**, are in close agreement as proposed for similar reported dinuclear Cu(II) carboxylates. The value of Cu ... Cu bond distances 2.6061(3) Å in **1** and 2.6236(4) Å in **2**, which is less than the sum of the van der Waal's radii of 2.8 Å, are also in close agreement with previously reported Cu(II) carboxylates coordinating to apical ligands which have an N-donor atom [29–32]. The Cu–N axial bond lengths are 2.159 Å in **1** and 2.165(2) Å in **2** and are attributed to the elongation of apical Cu–ligand bond distance as a consequence of repulsion exerted by the doubly occupied dz^2-orbital along this axis, i.e., the Jahn–Teller effect. The elongated Cu-N bonds as compared to the Cu-O are attributed to the bigger covalent radii of nitrogen leading to distortion [33]. The distortion in geometry is also evident from the values of cisoid and transoid angles which are in the range of 84.13(6)°–97.33(6)° and 169.28(6)°–171.22(5)° in **1** and 83.43(4)°–99.38(6)° and 168.93(6)°–174.85(5)° in **2**, respectively, deviating from the values of 90° and 180° as prescribed for the ideal square pyramidal geometry [29].

Table 2. Crystallographic data for complexes **2** and **5**.

Complex Code	2	5
M. Formula, weight (g/mol)	C$_{44}$H$_{32}$Cl$_4$Cu$_2$N$_4$O$_8$, 1013.61	C$_{44}$H$_{32}$Cl$_4$Cu$_2$N$_4$O$_8$, 1013.61
Crystal system, space group	Triclinic, P-1	Monoclinic, P2$_1$/c
Unit cell dimensions	9.6420(4), 11.0293(5), 11.4257(6) Å and 83.409(4), 71.832(4), 68.677(4)°	9.66853(19), 23.3053(3), 10.1454(2) Å and 90, 112.758(2), 90°
V, Z	1075.45(9) Å^3, 1	2108.07(7) Å^3, 2
ρ, μ, F(000)	1.57 mg/m^3, 3.998 mm^{-1}, 514	1.60 mg/m^3, 1.322 mm^{-1}, 1028
θ range for data collection	4.07–76.25	3.41–27.012
Reflections collected, R$_{int}$	8467, 4381	8983, 4233
Reflections with I > 2σ(I)	3990	3850
R1, wR2 (all reflections)	0.0334, 0.0793	0.0320, 0.0689
R1, wR2 (I > 2σ(I))	0.0301, 0.0818	0.0282, 0.0709
S on F^2	1.052	1.039
Largest diff. peak and hole	0.29/−0.48	0.50/−0.44
CCDC No.	2239713	2239714

Table 3. Selected bond lengths/Å and bond angles/° of complexes **2** and **5**.

Bond Lengths/Å					
	2	5		2	5
Cu1−N1A	2.1593(15)	2.1649(5)	Cu1−O81B	1.9747(13)	1.9730(13)
Cu1−O81C	1.9712(13)	1.9619(13)	Cu1−O82B ^{i}	1.9623(13)	1.9758(13)
Cu1−O82C ^{i}	1.9697(13)	1.9713(13)	Cu1⋯Cu1 ^{i}	2.6060(5)	2.6236(4)

Bond Angles/°					
N1A−Cu1−O81B	93.31(6)	99.38(6)	N1A−Cu1−O81C	99.45(6)	93.86(6)
N1A−Cu1−O82B ^{i}	97.33(6)	91.68(6)	N1A−Cu1−O82C ^{i}	91.25(6)	97.19(6)
O81B−Cu1−O81C	87.78(6)	87.38(6)	O81B−Cu1−O82B ^{i}	169.35(5)	168.93(5)
O81B−Cu1−O82C ^{i}	87.78(6)	91.34(5)	O81C−Cu1−O82B ^{i}	88.05(6)	91.44(6)
O81C−Cu1−O82C ^{i}	169.28(6)	168.93(5)	O82B ^{i}−Cu1−O82C ^{i}	91.29(6)	87.71(6)

Symmetry code: ^{i} −x,1-y,1-z for **2**, 1-x,1-y,1-z for **5**.

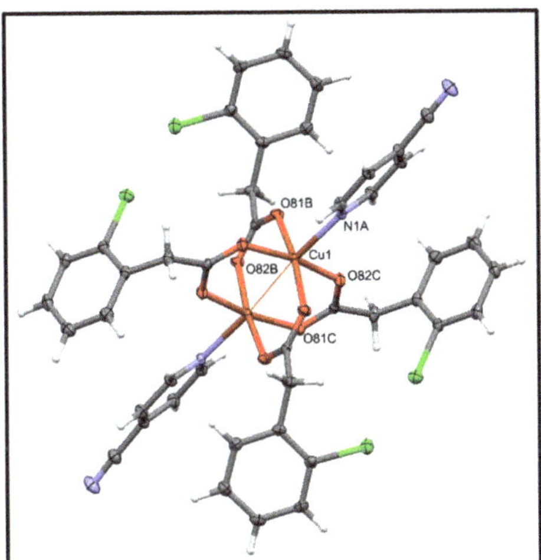

Figure 1. ORTEP diagram of complex **2** with 50% probability.

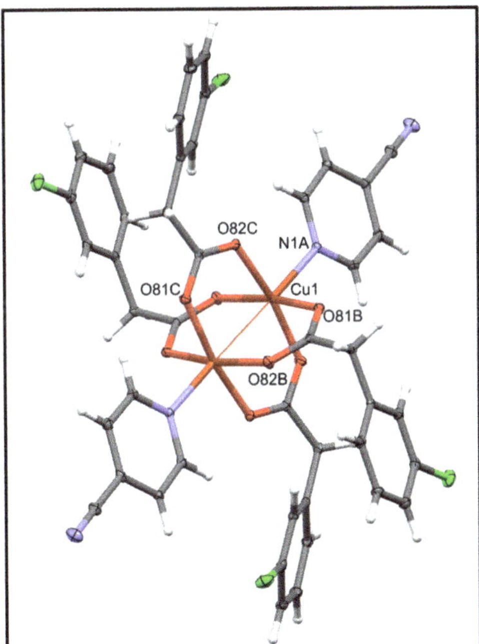

Figure 2. ORTEP diagram of complex **5** with 50% probability.

2.3. UV-Visible Absorption Spectroscopy

The UV–Visible spectroscopic study of the ligand **L^1**, **L^2** and complexes **1–6** was performed in absolute ethanol and the absorption spectra for representative **L^1**, and its complexes are given in Figure 3 whereas those for **L^2** and its complexes are given in Figure S1 of the Supplementary Data. The ligand acids **L^1** and **L^2** both show maximum absorption in the region 266–277 nm, owing to the intra-ligand π-π* transitions in the aromatic system. In complexes **1–6**, this ligand-based absorption maxima shows a shift in wavelength due to the increased conjugation resulting from the formation of new rings [34]. It is described in the single crystal XRD that the complexes possess a distorted octahedral geometry for which the highest energy orbital is $d_z{}^2$, so three different transitions, i.e., $d_z{}^2 \rightarrow d_x{}^2{}_{-y}{}^2$, $d_{xy} \rightarrow d_z{}^2$, $d_{xz}, d_{yz} \rightarrow d_{xy}$ are expected. However, the spectra of complexes **1–6** comprise only a single broad band. This is because all four *d* orbitals lie very close to each other and precise assignment of each d-d transition is a difficult task, as the order of d energy orbitals is controversial among several researchers. Here, too, the absorption peak only get broadened [35].

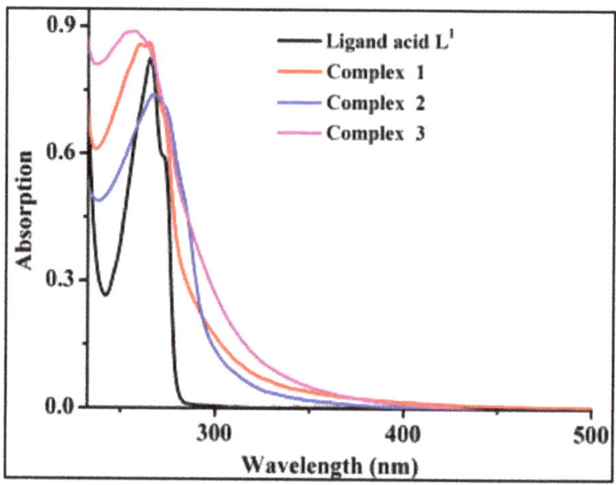

Figure 3. UV-Visible absorption spectrum of ligand **L^1** and complexes **1–3** in ethanol.

2.4. Electrochemical Study

A 3 mM solution of ligand acids **L^1**, **L^2** and their complexes **1–6** in DMSO were used to record their voltammograms at a scan rate of 100 mv/sec; the data are given in the Table S1 of the Supplementary Data. The cyclic voltammograms for complex **2** and **5** are given in Figure 4, whereas the cyclic voltammograms for **L^1**, **L^2**, **1**, **3**, **4**, and **6** are given in Figure S2. The voltammograms of the ligand acids indicate that the ligands were electrochemically silent at different scan rates. Meanwhile, the voltammograms of the complexes **1–6** reveal the presence of the redox couple, independent oxidation, and reduction peaks attributed to the presence of electroactive moieties present in the structural motifs of the complexes **1–6**. Here, for the complexes **2** and **5** with 4-cyanopyridine moiety as auxiliary ligand, two redox couples (in addition to one independent oxidation and one reduction potential) were observed. Similar behavior is observed for the rest of the complexes except that the second redox couple is missing and is replaced with two broad reduction peaks. The literature review concerning the substituted pyridine reveals that, in the case of 4-cyanopyridine, the complex gives a voltammogram with two redox couples, one at the positive side and other at the more negative side. Similarly, for 3-cyano pyridine, the first redox couple in the positive direction is dominant, whereas the second one on the negative side is diminished and left with only a broad reduction peak [36]. Similarly, dimeric Cu(II) carboxylates with the structural motifs similar to those described here produce electrochemical response with two redox couples: one attributed to inter-conversion of C(II)/Cu(III) and the second one originates from the reduction of Cu(II) to Cu(I) and vice versa [37–39]. So, based on the above description, it may be concluded that, for complexes **1–6**, the first very broad redox couple has originated as a result of overlap between the oxidation and reduction potentials associated with the metal center auxiliary ligands, i.e., substituted pyridine. In the voltammograms of the complexes **2** and **5**, an additional redox couple is observed at the very negative potential, which may be attributed to the 4-cyanopyridine moiety as per cited literature [36]. The other independent oxidation and reduction peaks in the voltammograms of the complexes may be attributed to the transition in heterocyclic moieties and may prove useful in the biological study [40].

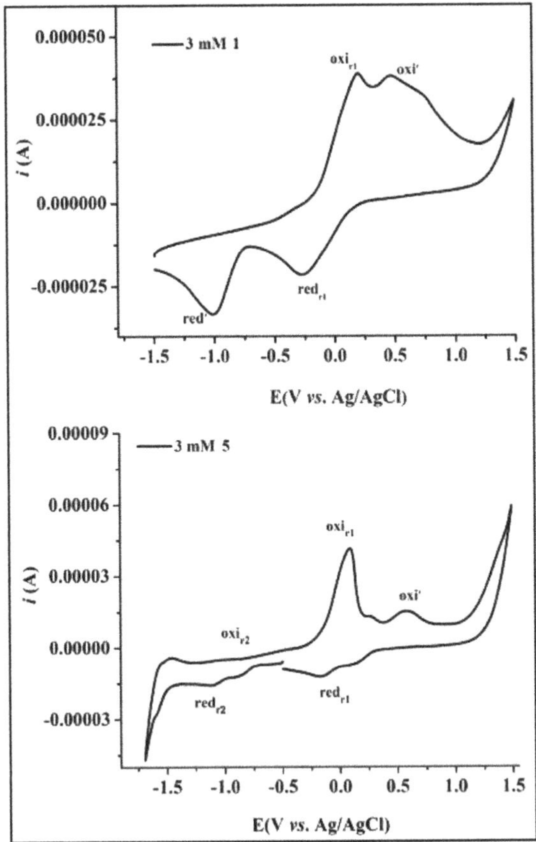

Figure 4. Cyclic voltammogram of complexes **1** and **5** recorded at 100 mv/s.

2.5. DNA Interaction

2.5.1. Through UV-Visible Absorption Spectroscopy

In order to get an idea about the mode and extent of interaction of the compounds with SS-DNA, the absorption spectra were recorded during the incremental addition of aqueous solution of DNA to the constant concentration of ligand acids and complexes. The representative absorption spectra of complexes **2** and **6** are given in Figure 5, whereas those of the L^1, L^2, **1**, **3**, **4** and **5** are given in Figures S3–S6 of the Supplementary Data. Mostly, the small molecules interact with DNA irreversibly through non-covalent interaction which may involve intercalation, electrostatic interaction, and surface binding through major or minor grooves. Modality of interaction was determined by monitoring absorption spectra for variations (hypo-, hyper-chromic effect, red, or blue shift) with the incremental addition of DNA. In the present study, for the ligand acid as well as for the synthesized complexes **1–6**, it was found that there was a significant hypochromic impact, along with a highly red shift of around 3 nm to 5 nm. This shift in absorption maxima and absorption intensity is the result of change in electronic transitions which depend on the number, alignment, and distance between the compounds under study and the chromophore of DNA. It is expected that the intercalating moieties sitting (insertion) in between the adjacent DNA base pairs, π–π stacking between the base pairs, and aromatic ring system stabilized this insertion. In order to avoid any expected distortion, space is provided to the intercalating moiety by the separation of base pairs of DNA to some extent, i.e., the DNA unwind, leading to an increased distance between adjacent phosphatase and thereby an increase in the length of DNA duplex [41]. This alters the absorption spectra and results in a bathochromic effect (red shift). This is because of decrease in π-π* electronic transition energies due to the overlap between orbitals of intercalating moiety and base pairs of DNA. Moreover, as π* of the compound is partially filled with electrons from DNA base pair, there is a decrease in electronic transition, which results in a decrease in absorption, i.e., hypochromism. Based on these changes, the intercalative mode of interaction is expected for the ligand acids L^1, L^2 and complexes **1–6**, which is also in accordance with the similar reported Cu (II) carboxylates. All of this is suggestive that the structural moieties of the compounds under study and DNA are in a direct bonding connection. They together with other structural changes are capable of altering the repairing process of DNA and hence prove to be effective against a disease [42].

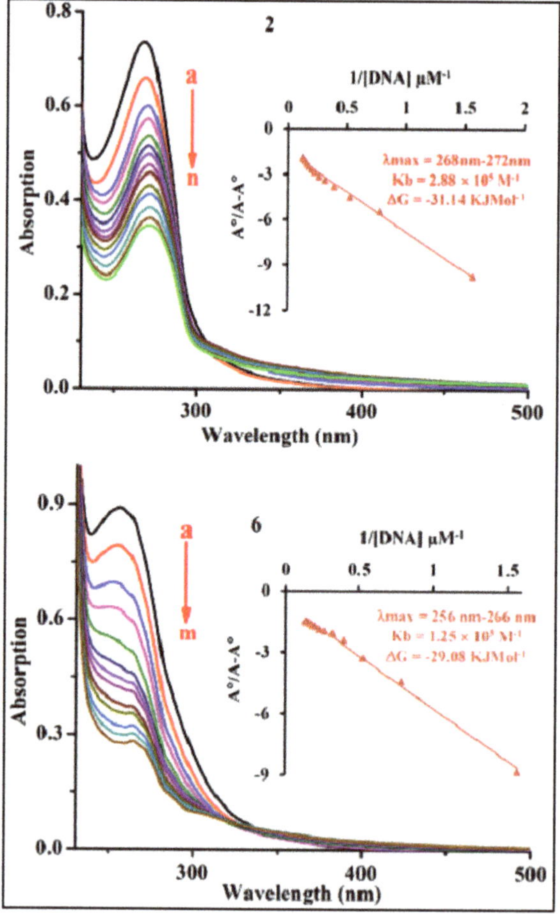

Figure 5. UV-visible absorption spectra of complexes **2** and **6** in the absence (a in each case) and in the presence of incremental addition, i.e., 0.63–8.19 µM (**2**) and 0.63–7.56 µM (**6**), respectively. Whereas the inside graph revels the values of K_b and ΔG calculated from graph plotted between the absorption and DNA concentration.

A plot between $A°/A\text{-}A°$ vs. $1/(DNA)$ of the Benesi–Hildebrand equation was used for the determination of binding constant. The intercept-to-slope ratio of these graphs was used to calculate binding constants K (M^{-1}), which are given in Table 4. The binding constant values are high compared to the already reported complexes and may be attributed to the planar moiety and active substituents on the aromatic ring.

Table 4. Binding parameters of the ligand acids and their complexes with SS-DNA.

Compound	λmax (nm)		K_b (M^{-1})	ΔG $(KJMol^{-1})$
	Before DNA	After DNA		
L^1	265	266	2.83×10^4	-25.39
1	262	264	7.14×10^4	-27.68
2	268	272	2.88×10^5	-31.14
3	255	262	9.29×10^4	-28.34
L^2	266	267	2.81×10^4	-25.37
4	263	264	9.03×10^4	-28.27
5	268	273	6.70×10^4	-27.53
6	256	266	1.25×10^5	-29.08

2.5.2. Through Cyclic Voltammetry

To corroborate the findings from UV-visible spectroscopy on the contact behavior of ligand acids and complexes with SS-DNA, an electrochemical study was conducted. The cyclic voltammograms of complexes (ligand acids were found to be electrochemically innocent) were recorded during an incremental addition of DNA (0.49, 0.99, 1.48, 1.96 μM) to the constant concentration of complexes (3 mM) under the electrochemical setup earlier explained in Section 3.3 (3 mM). The voltammograms of complexes **1**, **2**, **5**, and **6** are given in Figure 6, whereas those of the complexes **1**, **3**, **4**, and **6** are presented in Figure S7. Different scan rates (50–500 V) were used to record the electrochemical response. Recurring changes in the peak potential and intensification of the current are hallmarks of irreversible electrochemical processes. Because the DNA's stable helical form shields the bases that are susceptible to reduction, it is unable to generate an electrochemical reaction on its own [43]. A positive shift in the anodic and cathodic peak potential implies intercalation, while a negative shift suggests non-intercalation, i.e., electrostatic, hydrophobic, or groove binding. Another parameter, i.e., formal potential calculated as the average of anodic and cathodic peak potentials was also used in this regard to get an idea about the mode of interaction. For the intercalative mode of interaction of the compound with DNA, the formal potential shifts positively, while for the non-intercalative mode of interaction, the formal potential shifts negatively [44]. Here, very clear positive shifts given in Table S1 are observed in the electrochemical potential of the redox couple, independent oxidation, and reduction potentials as well as in the formal potential. Therefore, it may be deduced from the foregoing that the complexes interact with SS-DNA by means of intercalation. Voltammograms show that along with these alterations comes a reduction in current intensity. The development of heavy complex-DNA adducts, which diffuse slowly towards the electrode surface, is blamed for this shift because it lowers the concentration of the species responsible for the electrochemical reaction [44].

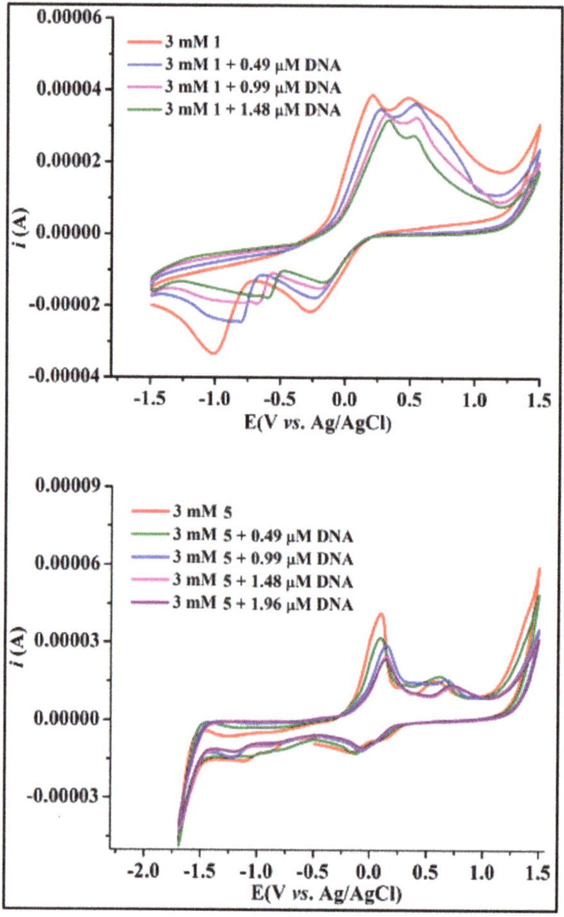

Figure 6. Cyclic voltammogram of complexes **1** and **5** recorded at 100 mv/s indicating the effect of DNA addition.

2.5.3. DNA Interaction Study through Viscometry

The interaction of SS-DNA with ligand acids and their heteroleptic Cu(II) carboxylates was also evaluated through viscometry, which is a hydrodynamic method capable of providing valuable information about interaction mode. Each kind of compound–DNA interaction induces its own specific hydrodynamic response. This method is sensitive to change in chain length which is directly relevant to the interaction mechanism. An intercalating compound sits in between the base pairs of DNA and causes separation and unwinding of the DNA double helical structure. This finally results in an increase in the viscosity of the SS-DNA [45]. The viscosity SS-DNA shows a gradual increase with the increasing concentrations of ligand acids L^1, L^2 and their heteroleptic Cu(II) carboxylates indicating the existence of intercalation [46]. The representative graph revealing this kind of changes is presented in Figure 7, strongly supporting the findings from the absorption and electrochemical methods, whereas those for ligand L^2 and complexes **4–6** are given in Figure S8 of the Supplementary Data.

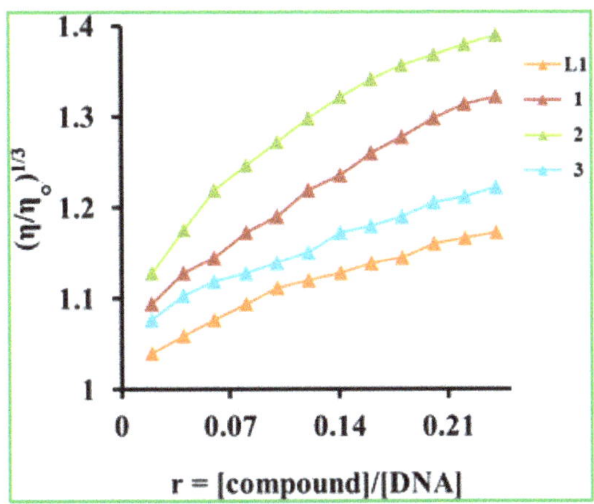

Figure 7. Graph presenting the effect on viscosity of DNA by the incremental addition of L^1 and its complexes **1–3**.

2.6. Antioxidant Activities

2.6.1. DPPH Scavenging Ability

The antioxidant potential of the free acids and their Cu(II) carboxylates was explored via the DPPH method using ascorbic acid as a reference. The DPPH, with a single unpaired electron, is capable of accepting a hydrogen or electron and gives a strong absorption at 517 nm. The absorption generally decreases when it accepts a hydrogen or electron from an antioxidant, forming a stable molecule. The results given in Table 5 indicate that the compounds under study show a moderate level of antioxidant potential. This activity may be attributed to the various structural and electronic factors like coordination geometry, redox properties, chelate ring size, degree of unsaturation, etc. [47]. The transfer of proton or electron from an antioxidant to DPPH results in the formation of species that undergo other reactions like coupling, fragmentation, and addition, which affect the rate and stoichiometry of the reaction. This leads to change in color from violet to yellow and hence a decrease in absorption at 517 nm which can be monitored UV-Visible spectrophotometer and the data indicate a direct activity concentration relationship [48]. The highest activity was observed for complex **2**.

2.6.2. Hydrogen Peroxide Scavenging Ability

In addition to DPPH the ligand acids and their complexes were also evaluated for their peroxide scavenging ability test. Hydrogen peroxide (H_2O_2) is a biologically important, non-radical reactive oxygen species (ROS) that can influence several cellular processes. It is a weak oxidizing agent and can inactivate a few enzymes directly, usually via oxidation of essential thiol (-SH) groups. It can cross cell membranes rapidly, and inside the cell, H_2O_2 probably reacts with Fe^{2+} (and possibly Cu^{2+}) ions to form the hydroxyl radical, which may be the origin of many of its toxic effects. It is, therefore, biologically advantageous for cells to control the amount of hydrogen peroxide that is allowed to accumulate [49]. A response was noted in terms of percentage scavenging ability and IC_{50} values and is presented in the Table 5. The data presented here indicate a direct relationship between the concentration of the antioxidant (compounds in the present study) and the percentage scavenging ability. The response in percentage ranges from 51.90 ± 1.16 to 87.63 ± 0.64 a little lower to compared to that of the reference used in the study. Again, the maximum activity was recorded for complex **2** followed by complex **3**.

Table 5. Antioxidant ability data of L^1, L^2, and complexes **1–6**.

Comp	Comp. Conc. (µg/mL) for DPPH Free Radical Scavenging Ability					
	1000	500	250	125	62.5	IC$_{50}$ (µg/mL)
L^1	73.08 ± 1.04 *	66.45 ± 0.90 *	60.58 ± 0.63 *	55.40 ± 0.20 *	45.80 ± 0.90 *	42.76
1	78.39 ± 0.49 *	73.47 ± 0.52 *	67.44 ± 0.55 *	61.40 ± 0.51 *	55.57 ± 0.84 *	17.69
2	95.20 ± 0.15 §	91.17 ± 0.53 §	86.98 ± 0.85 §	81.20 ± 0.65 ⧧	77.80 ± 0.37 ⧧	3.22
3	79.00 ± 0.16 *	74.66 ± 1.20 *	66.33 ± 0.33 *	62.50 ± 0.44 *	53.00 ± 0.57 *	21.72
L^2	71.27 ± 1.04 *	62.81 ± 0.90 *	59.35 ± 0.63 *	52.13 ± 0.20 ⧾	43.53 ± 0.30 *	44.63
4	83.17 ± 0.72 *	78.30 ± 0.64 *	73.34 ± 0.63 *	68.30 ± 0.64 *	61.93 ± 1.13 *	8.45
5	85.72 ± 0.79 *	77.68 ± 0.63 *	71.46 ± 0.53 *	64.78 ± 0.60 *	55.56 ± 0.52 *	20.29
6	80.85 ± 0.18 *	75.59 ± 0.30 *	68.75 ± 0.14 *	63.47 ± 0.49 *	58.12 ± 0.34 *	14.51
SD	95.85 ± 0.18	91.59 ± 0.30	87.75 ± 0.14	84.47 ± 0.49	81.12 ± 0.34	0.12
Comp	Comp. Conc. (µg/mL) for H$_2$O$_2$ free radical scavenging ability					
L^1	85.43 ± 1.26 *	78.83 ± 0.66 *	70.93 ± 0.90 *	63.26 ± 0.77 *	49.10 ± 0.95 *	50.30
1	80.30 ± 0.64 *	74.27 ± 0.57 *	70.32 ± 0.52 *	62.42 ± 0.57 *	53.50 ± 0.73 *	20.49
2	93.55 ± 0.40 §	89.37 ± 1.65 *	85.50 ± 0.40 *	79.60 ± 0.90 ⧾	74.17 ± 0.72 *	4.50
3	84.39 ± 0.60 *	78.58 ± 0.56 *	72.29 ± 0.43 *	66.37 ± 0.58 *	61.30 ± 0.52 *	11.47
L^2	85.43 ± 1.26 *	78.83 ± 0.66 *	70.93 ± 0.90 *	63.26 ± 0.77 *	49.10 ± 0.95 *	51.41
4	85.00 ± 0.30 ⧾	78.76 ± 0.58 *	73.67 ± 0.61 *	67.74 ± 0.61 *	63.47 ± 0.56 *	8.71
5	84.83 ± 0.62 *	80.76 ± 0.63 *	75.70 ± 0.62 *	66.65 ± 0.78 *	59.81 ± 0.65 *	27.35
6	83.53 ± 0.20 *	78.62 ± 0.17 *	73.42 ± 0.11 *	66.20 ± 0.15 *	61.35 ± 0.18 *	10.65
SD	97.53 ± 0.20	93.62 ± 0.17	88.42 ± 0.11	84.20 ± 0.15	81.35 ± 0.18	0.37

Data is presented as (mean ± S.E.M); TWO WAY ANOVA followed by Bonferoni test were followed, Values significantly different as compared to positive control; $n = 3$, ⧧ = $p < 0.05$, ⧾ = $p < 0.01$, * = $p < 0.001$, §; non-significant SD: Ascorbic acid.

2.7. Enzyme Inhibition Study

Acetylcholinesterase Inhibition

The synthesized compounds were evaluated for acetylcholinesterase (ACh) and butyrylcholinesterase (BCh) enzyme inhibitory activities. They were tested at five different concentrations (1000, 500, 250, 125, and 62.5 µg/mL) displayed varying degree of inhibition of enzyme acetylcholinesterase. The data are given in Table 6 for presenting percentage inhibition and IC$_{50}$ values. The ligand acids L^1 and L^2 were found to exhibit a lower degree of inhibition compared to the complexes and the standard drug glutamine used here as a reference. The complex **2** showed a highest percentage inhibition at the concentration of 1000 µg/mL with IC$_{50}$ 2 µg/mL. A drop in the activity was observed as the concentration was reduced from 1000 µg/mL to 500 µg/mL, 250 µg/mL, 125 µg/mL, and then to 62.5 µg/mL. The other complexes also showed their effect in a similar fashion with varying degree of inhibition.

Similar behavior has also been observed for the compounds under study when they were subjected to inhibition study of butyrylcholinesterase enzyme (Table 7). Enzyme inhibition and the concentrations of inhibitors were found to have a direct relationship However, they all possess a lower degree of activity compared to the standard drug used as reference. The order of activity was found to be **4** > **5** = **2** > **1** > **3** > **6**, which may be attributed to various structural and electronic factors. Similar reports are available for the previously reported Cu(II) complexes as per the cited data [50].

Table 6. Percentage inhibition data of enzyme L^1, L^2 and complexes **1–6**.

Comp	Comp. Conc. (µg/mL) for Inhibition of Acetylcholinesterase (%AChE Activity)					
	1000	500	250	125	62.5	IC_{50} (µg/mL)
L^1	65.39 ± 0.40 *	62.29 ± 0.32 *	57.34 ± 0.35 *	54.02 ± 0.24 *	50.35 ± 0.11 *	112
1	77.61 ± 0.77 *	72.60 ± 0.80 *	67.83 ± 0.56 *	62.69 ± 0.77 *	55.67 ± 0.61 *	39
2	87.50 ± 2.26 ⚘	83.01 ± 0.42 ‡	78.07 ± 0.62 ‡	73.70 ± 0.35 ⚘	71.73 ± 0.66 §	2
3	81.03 ± 0.35 *	77.08 ± 0.47 *	72.91 ± 0.88 *	67.90 ± 0.96 *	62.98 ± 0.72 *	17
L^2	65.39 ± 0.40 *	62.29 ± 0.32 *	57.34 ± 0.35 *	54.02 ± 0.24 *	50.35 ± 0.11 *	40
4	89.39 ± 0.60 §	83.39 ± 0.49 §	78.36 ± 0.49 ‡	72.34 ± 0.55 *	67.90 ± 1.16 *	6
5	89.20 ± 0.23 §	82.13 ± 0.20 ‡	76.87 ± 1.27 *	71.76 ± 0.61 *	69.91 ± 1.30 *	5
6	77.34 ± 0.98 *	72.32 ± 1.06 *	67.05 ± 0.75 *	62.70 ± 1.25 *	58.74 ± 0.68 *	33
SD	91.58 ± 1.12	87.65 ± 1.34	84.90 ± 0.96	79.03 ± 0.48	72.90 ± 0.48	2.10
Comp	Comp. Conc. (µg/mL) for inhibition of butyrylcholinesterase (% BChE activity)					
L^1	77.73 ± 0.03 *	73.42 ± 0.12 *	68.39 ± 0.35 *	63.36 ± 0.71 *	58.15 ± 0.22 *	44
1	81.79 ± 0.62 *	76.45 ± 0.49 *	71.75 ± 0.58 *	68.51 ± 0.77 *	64.53 ± 0.71 *	12
2	81.44 ± 0.09 *	76.87 ± 0.39 *	72.83 ± 1.07 *	67.23 ± 0.44 *	66.29 ± 0.43 *	04
3	76.8 ± 1.20 *	73.2 ± 0.98 *	68.2 ± 0.88 *	63.3 ± 1.10 *	60.2 ± 0.98 *	25
L^2	77.73 ± 0.03 *	73.42 ± 0.12 *	68.39 ± 0.35 *	63.36 ± 0.71 *	58.15 ± 0.22 *	40
4	86.47 ± 0.22 ‡	81.94 ± 0.45 *	77.61 ± 1.70 *	72.64 ± 0.16 *	68.52 ± 0.38 *	03
5	91.62 ± 0.74 §	86.86 ± 0.60 §	81.48 ± 0.64 §	76.54 ± 0.50 §	72.74 ± 0.61 §	04
6	75.33 ± 0.49 *	72.03 ± 0.23 *	65.00 ± 0.58 *	61.67 ± 0.89 *	57.00 ± 1.15 *	42
SD	93.33 ± 0.49	87.03 ± 0.23	83.00 ± 0.58	78.67 ± 0.89	71.00 ± 1.15	3.40

Two-way Anova followed by Bonferoni test were conducted, the values obtained were significantly different as compared to positive control; n = 3, ⚘ = $p < 0.05$, ‡ = $p < 0.01$, * = $p < 0.001$, §; non-significant, SD: Galantamine.

Table 7. Physical and FTIR data of the compounds **1–6**.

Comp. #	Formula	Yield (%)	M. P (°C)	Color and State
1	$Cu_2(2\text{-}ClC_6H_4COO)_4(3\text{-}CNPy)_2$	73	187–189	Light blue crystal
2	$Cu_2(2\text{-}ClC_6H_4COO)_4(4\text{-}CNPy)_2$	69	212–214	Blue amorphous solid
3	$Cu_n(2\text{-}ClC_6H_4COO)_4(4\text{-}OHPy)_2$	84	188–190	Light blue amorphous solid
4	$Cu_2(3\text{-}ClC_6H_4COO)_4(3\text{-}CNPy)_2$	77	202–204	dark blue crystalline solid
5	$Cu_2(3\text{-}ClC_6H_4COO)_4(4\text{-}CNPy)_2$	83	218–220	blue crystalline solid
6	$Cu_2(3\text{-}ClC_6H_4COO)_4(4\text{-}OHPy)_2$	76	228–230	blue shiny crystalline solid

3. Experimental

3.1. Materials and Instruments Used

The following chemicals were used: 2-chlorophenyl acetic acid (L^1), 3-chlorophenyl acetic acid (L^2), sodium bicarbonate, copper sulphate pentahydrate, 3-cyanopyridine, 4-cyanopyridine, and 4-hydroxypyridine were acquired from Fluka, Switzerland. Sodium salt of Salmon fish sperm DNA (SS-DNA) was purchased from Arcos, UK and was used as received. Analytical grade solvents were used as such. The following instruments were used: Electrothermal Gallenkamp (UK) serial number C040281 for melting point determination, Thermo Nicolet-6700 spectrophotometer for recording FTIR spectrum (4000–400 cm^{-1}), Shimadzu 1700 UV-Visible spectrophotometer for absorption measurement, Corrtest CS 300 electrochemical workstation for electrochemical behavior study.

3.2. Single Crystal XRD Analysis

Diffraction data were collected by the ω-scan technique, with two Rigaku four-circle diffractometers: SuperNova (Atlas CCD detector) for complex **2**, at 130(1) K with a mirror-monochromatized CuKα radiation source (λ = 1.54178 Å), and XCalibur (Eos CCD detector) for **5**, at 100(1) K with graphite-monochromatized MoK$_\alpha$ radiation source (λ = 0.71073 Å). The data were corrected for Lorentz-polarization as well as for absorption effects [51].

The structures were solved with SHELXT [52] and refined by a full-matrix least-squares procedure on F^2 employing SHELXL-2013 [53].

3.3. Synthesis of 2-Chlorophenyl Acetic Acid-Based Complexes 1–3

10 mL of an aqueous solution of $NaHCO_3$ (4.2 mg, 5 mmol) was added dropwise to the 10 mL solution of 2-chlorophenyl acetic acid (8.5 mg, 5 mmol) in doubly distilled water under constant stirring for 3–4 h at 25 °C to convert the ligand into its sodium salt. After that, the temperature was raised to 60 °C and 10 mL of $CuSO_4 \cdot 5H_2O_{(aq)}$ (6.2 g, 2.5 mmol) and 10 mL of 2.5 mmol methanolic solution of nitrogen donor heterocycle 3-cyanopyridine were added dropwise simultaneously and the reaction was further stirred for 3–4 h (complex **1**). The same synthetic procedure was used for 4-cyanopyridine (complex **2**) and 4-hydroxy pyridine (complex **3**) (Scheme 1). The precipitated products were washed with distilled water and then air dried. The equimolar solution (1:1) of DMSO and methanol was used for recrystallization of the product [22]. The physical and FTIR data are given in Table 7.

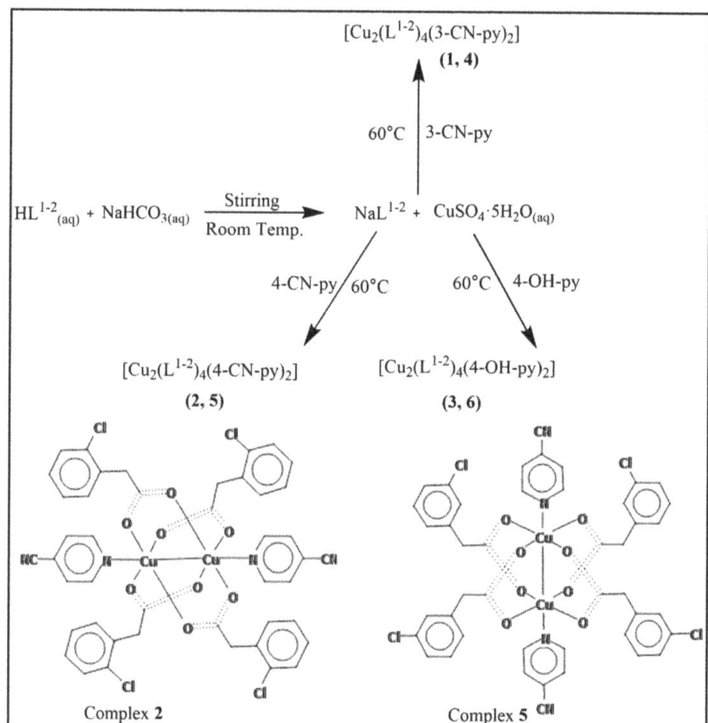

Scheme 1. Synthetic procedure for the synthesis of complexes **1–6**.

Synthesis of 3-Chlorophenyl Acetic Acid-Based Complexes 4–6

Similar procedure as described above (Scheme 1) was used for the synthesis of complexes **4–6**. The only difference is the use of 3-cholorophenyl acetic acid as a ligand in the first step of the synthesis.

3.4. Compound-DNA Interaction Study

The interaction ability of the ligand acids ($\mathbf{HL^{1-2}}$) and their synthesized Cu(II) carboxylates (**1–6**) was explored with SS-DNA. This study was carried out through UV-Visible absorption spectroscopy, viscometry, and cyclic voltammetry.

3.5. Compound-DNA Interaction Study through UV-Visible Absorption Spectroscopy

20 mg of SS-DNA was dissolved in 25 mL of double distilled water and the solution was left on stirring for 24 h at room temperature. Dilution of this stock solution was carried out and the final concentration was found to be 1.06×10^{-4} M using the molar absorptivity $\varepsilon = 6600$ M^{-1} cm^{-1}, $\lambda = 260$ nm, and the path length of cell, $l = 1$ cm. The nucleotide to protein ratio calculated by using the absorbance at A_{260}/A_{280} nm was found to be ~ 1.7, indicating that the solution is certainly free from protein. The solutions of the ligand acids and the complexes under study were made in ethanol having a concentration of 1 mM. The experiment was carried out by adding DNA to a constant concentration of compound in increments. During the experiment, identical amounts of DNA were introduced to both the reference and sample cells in order to neutralize the effect of DNA absorption [29].

3.6. Voltammetry-Based Analysis for Compound-DNA Interactions

Cyclic voltammetry was used to confirm the compound-DNA interaction study, and a Corrtest CS 300 (Potentiostat/Galvanostat) electrochemical workstation with a glassy carbon working electrode (diameter = 0.03 cm^2), a platinum wire working electrode, and a silver/silver chloride (Ag/AgCl) reference electrode were used in a continuous flow of argon. A glassy carbon electrode was polished on a nylon buffing pad with alumina and distilled water before each test to remove any absorbed contaminants. The cyclic voltammograms were taken when DNA was added in small increments while the quantities of the tested compounds were held constant [54].

3.7. Viscometry-Based Analysis for Compound-DNA Interactions

The purpose of the viscometric investigation was to document the shift in SS-DNA viscosity in response to the compounds. Ubbelohde viscometers were used to time the flow of DNA with and without ligand acids and their complexes and recorded using a digital stopwatch. The average reading was noted by repeating the experiment three times. Value of η_o was calculated by subtracting the flow time of pure solvent ethanol (t_o) from that of the SS-DNA solution (t). The η was determined by comparing the flow rates of pure DNA solution (t) and solutions containing various concentrations of compounds (t') in order to determine the effect of the compounds on the DNA solution flow rate. The graphs were drawn using the data $\sqrt[3]{\eta/\eta_o}$ vs. (compound)/(DNA) [29].

3.8. Antioxidant Activity

The synthesized compounds were subjected to DPPH (2,2-diphenyl-1-picrylhydrazyl) and H$_2$O$_2$ free radical scavenging ability test through procedures described in the following sections in order to get an idea about the antioxidant ability.

3.8.1. DPPH Scavenging Assay

The compounds under study were subjected to DPPH scavenging ability test as per cited literature [55]. A 0.004% solution of reagent DPPH was added to the different concentrations of tested compounds (i.e., 125, 250, 500 and 1000 µg/mL) and the reaction mixture was incubated subsequently for about thirty minutes in dark. Ascorbic acid was used as positive control. The UV-3000 O.R.I. Germany was used to record the change in absorption of the reaction mixture at 517 nm and the percentage scavenging ability of the compounds under study was determined using formula:

$$\% \text{ scavenging activity} = \frac{\text{Absorbance of control} - \text{Absorbance of compounds}}{\text{Absorbance of control}} \times 100$$

The experiments were repeated thrice. The GraphPad Prism$^{\circledR}$ (version 4.0, Sandiego, CA, USA) was used to calculate the IC$_{50}$ values.

3.8.2. Hydrogen Peroxide Scavenging Assay

The ligand acids and their Cu(II) carboxylates were further subjected to H_2O_2 scavenging ability test potential by following the procedure as per cited literature [56]. A 2 mM solution of H_2O_2 was made in 50 mM phosphate buffer having a pH 7.4. In the next step, 0.1 mL of the screened compounds was added to the 0.3 mL (50 mM) of phosphate buffer, then 0.6 mL of H_2O_2 was added and the solution was vortexed. After following the incubation period of 10 min, the absorption was 230 nm in comparison to the blank. Later on, these data were used to calculate the H_2O_2 free radical scavenging ability by applying the following equation:

$$\text{Hydrogen peroxide Scavenging ability} = \frac{1 - \text{absorbance of sample}}{\text{Absorbance of control}} \times 100$$

3.9. Enzyme Inhibition Study

The enzymes acetylcholinesterase (AChE) and butyrylcholinesterase (BChE) play an important role in the transfer of signals and physiological function. They assist acetylcholine to hydrolyze and produce choline and acetyl group in synaptic region. So, they are considered as targets in the management of Alzheimer's disease. Herein, the compounds under study were evaluated for their potential to inhibit acetylthiocholine iodide (AChI) and butyrylthiocholine iodide (BChI) enzymes.

The well-known Ellman's assay [57] was implemented to evaluate the inhibitory potential using acetylthiocholine iodide (AChI) and butyrylthiocholine iodide (BChI) as substrates, respectively. The basic principle of the assay is the hydrolysis of acetylthiocholine iodide and butyrylthiocholine iodide by their corresponding enzymes, resulting in the formation of 5-thio-2-nitrobenzoate anion. This anion is capable of forming a yellow color complex with 5,5-dithio-bis-(2-nitrobenzoic acid (DTNB), which shows absorption at 412 nm.

To carry out the assay, 0.1 M buffer solution with pH 8 was prepared as per the cited literature [58] where the pH was adjusted using KOH (potassium hydroxide). Using the freshly prepared buffer and following the dilution, final concentrations of 0.03 U/mL for AChE (518 U/mg solid) and 0.01 U/mL for BChE (7–16 U/mg) were obtained. Similar dilutions in methanol were also prepared for the galantamine which was selected as positive control. After that, the final solution of each of the AChE and BChE was prepared in distilled water in the presence of 2.27×10^4 M DTNB and were stored at 8 °C. The experiment was performed by taking 205 µL of inhibitor (tested compound) along with 5 µL of prepared solutions of enzymes, followed by the addition of 5 µL DTNB reagent. They were then incubated for about 15 min in a water bath at a temperature of 30 °C. Later on, 5 µL substrate solution was added to them which were subjected to absorption check at 412 nm. A 10 µg/mL galantamine was used as a positive control, whereas the other components in the solution other than the inhibitor acted as a negative control. The temperature of the spectrophotometer was adjusted at 30 °C and then, following the reaction time of 4 min, the absorbance values were noted after regular intervals. The experiment was repeated, and change in absorption with time was used to calculate the percentage activity of enzyme and enzyme inhibitor [59]. The p values, or calculated probability levels, are categorized as 5% ($p < 0.05$), 1% ($p < 0.01$) and 0.1% ($p < 0.001$). $p < 0.05$ means statistically significant and $p < 0.001$ means highly statistically significant.

4. Conclusions

Six new heteroleptic Cu(II) carboxylates were synthesized by using 2-chloro phenyl acetic acid and 3-chloro phenyl acetic acid as primary ligands and the substituted pyridine derivatives as auxiliary ligands. The complexes were characterized through FTIR spectroscopy which reveals the bridging bidentate mode of coordination for the ligands. Additionally, UV-visible absorption spectroscopy indicates the involvement of π-π^* transitions. The cyclic voltammograms indicate that the complexes are redox active compared to the ligands, which were silent electrochemically. The complexes **2** and **5** were also characterized through single crystal XRD and both the complexes are dinuclear and adopt a distorted square pyramidal geometry where each carboxylate moiety presents a bridging bidentate coordination with nitrogen donor auxiliary ligand sitting at the terminal position. The ligand acids and complexes were evaluated for their interaction study with SS-DNA through UV-visible absorption spectroscopy, cyclic voltammetry, and viscometry. The findings from each study support each other with the conclusion that all of the compounds interact with DNA through intercalation with a high binding affinity through a spontaneous process as determined by the negative ΔG value. The complexes were also found to exhibit a moderate level of antioxidant potential when tested for the DPPH and H_2O_2 free radical scavenging ability. They were found to be potent inhibitors of acetylcholinesterase and butyrylcholinesterase.

Supplementary Materials: The following supporting information can be downloaded at: https://www.mdpi.com/article/10.3390/ph16050693/s1, Figure S1: UV-Visible absorption spectrum of ligand L^2 and complexes **4–6** in ethanol. Figure S2: Cyclic voltammograms of Ligand L^1, L^2 and complexes **2–4** and **6**. Figure S3. UV-visible absorption spectra of ligand acids L^1 and L^2 in the absence (a in each case) and in the presence of incremental addition, i.e., 0.63–6.631 µM (L^1), and 0.63–4.41 µM (L^2), respectively. Figure S4. UV-visible absorption spectra of complexes **1** and **3** in the absence (a in each case) and in the presence of incremental addition, i.e., 0.63–8.19 µM (**1**), 0.63–5.67 µM (**3**, respectively. Figure S5. UV-visible absorption spectra of complexes **2** and **3** in the absence (a in each case) and in the presence of incremental addition, i.e., 0.63–8.19 µM (**2**), 0.63–5.04 µM (**3**, respectively. Figure S6. UV-visible absorption spectra of complexes **4** and **5** in the absence (a in each case) and in the presence of incremental addition, i.e., 0.63–5.04 µM (**4**) and 0.63–4.41 µM (**5**), respectively. Figure S7: Cyclic voltammograms of the complexes **2**, **3**, **C4** and **6** in the presence of DNA. Figure S8: Graph presenting the effect on viscosity of SS-DNA by the incremental addition of L^2 and its complexes **4–6**. Table S1. Electrochemical parameter for complexes **1–6** before and after DNA addition.

Author Contributions: Conceptualization, methodology, investigation, writing—original draft preparation, S.U., Z.U., A.M., S.N. and M.Z.; methodology, validation, data curation, project administration, A.H. and M.U.R.; software, formal analysis, M.K.; supervision, writing—review and editing, project administration, investigation, M.S. and S.A.; project administration, funding acquisition, writing—review and editing, T.A.W. and S.Z. All authors have read and agreed to the published version of the manuscript.

Funding: Researchers Supporting Project number (RSP2023R357), King Saud University, Riyadh, Saudi Arabia.

Institutional Review Board Statement: Not applicable.

Informed Consent Statement: Not applicable.

Data Availability Statement: Data will be available on request to corresponding authors.

Acknowledgments: The authors are thankful to Higher Education Commission Islamabad, Pakistan. The authors extend their appreciation to the Researchers Supporting Project number (RSP2023R357), King Saud University, Riyadh, Saudi Arabia, for funding this work. The authors are thankful to Higher Education Commission Islamabad, Pakistan.

Conflicts of Interest: The authors declare no conflict of interest.

References

1. Orvig, C.; Abrams, M.J. Medicinal inorganic chemistry: Introduction. *Chem. Rev.* **1999**, *99*, 2201–2204. [CrossRef]
2. Ranasinghe, R.; Mathai, M.L.; Zulli, A. Cisplatin for cancer therapy and overcoming chemoresistance. *Heliyon* **2022**, *8*, e10608. [CrossRef] [PubMed]
3. Vaou, N.; Stavropoulou, E.; Voidarou, C.; Tsigalou, C.; Bezirtzoglou, E. Towards advances in medicinal plant antimicrobial activity: A review study on challenges and future perspectives. *Microorganisms* **2021**, *9*, 2041. [CrossRef] [PubMed]
4. Ghosh, S. Cisplatin: The first metal based anticancer drug. *Bioorg. Chem.* **2019**, *88*, 102925. [CrossRef] [PubMed]

5. Ferreira, A.; Proença, C.; Serralheiro, M.; Araujo, M. The in vitro screening for acetylcholinesterase inhibition and antioxidant activity of medicinal plants from Portugal. *J. Ethnopharmacol.* **2006**, *108*, 31–37. [CrossRef]
6. Orhan, I.; Şener, B.; Choudhary, M.; Khalid, A. Acetylcholinesterase and butyrylcholinesterase inhibitory activity of some Turkish medicinal plants. *J. Ethnopharmacol.* **2004**, *91*, 57–60. [CrossRef]
7. Heinrich, M.; Teoh, H.L. Galanthamine from snowdrop—The development of a modern drug against Alzheimer's disease from local Caucasian knowledge. *J. Ethnopharmacol.* **2004**, *92*, 147–162. [CrossRef]
8. Zhang, C.X.; Lippard, S.J. New metal complexes as potential therapeutics. *Curr. Opin. Chem. Biol.* **2003**, *7*, 481–489. [CrossRef]
9. Pullen, S.; Clever, G.H. Mixed-ligand metal–organic frameworks and heteroleptic coordination cages as multifunctional scaffolds—A comparison. *Acc. Chem. Res.* **2018**, *51*, 3052–3064. [CrossRef]
10. Aleksandrov, H.A.; St Petkov, P.; Vayssilov, G.N. Computational Modeling of Coordination Chemistry of Transition Metal Cations in Zeolites and in Metal-organic Frameworks. *Curr. Phys. Chem.* **2012**, *2*, 189–199. [CrossRef]
11. Kaplan, J.H.; Maryon, E.B. How mammalian cells acquire copper: An essential but potentially toxic metal. *Biophys. J.* **2016**, *110*, 7–13. [CrossRef]
12. Ingle, A.P.; Paralikar, P.; Shende, S.; Gupta, I.; Biswas, J.K.; Silva Martins, L.H.d.; Rai, M. Copper in medicine: Perspectives and toxicity. In *Biomedical Applications of Metals*; Springer: Berlin/Heidelberg, Germany, 2018; pp. 95–112.
13. Panchal, P.K.; Parekh, H.M.; Pansuriya, P.B.; Patel, M.N. Bactericidal activity of different oxovanadium (IV) complexes with Schiff bases and application of chelation theory. *J. Enzyme Inhib. Med. Chem.* **2006**, *21*, 203–209. [CrossRef]
14. Dawar, N.; Devi, J.; Kumar, B.; Dubey, A. Synthesis, Characterization, Pharmacological Screening, Molecular Docking, DFT, MESP, ADMET Studies of Transition Metal (II) Chelates of Bidentate Schiff Base Ligand. *Inorg. Chem. Commun.* **2023**, *151*, 110567. [CrossRef]
15. Ballatore, C.; Huryn, D.M.; Smith III, A.B. Carboxylic acid (bio) isosteres in drug design. *Chem. Med. Chem.* **2013**, *8*, 385–395. [CrossRef]
16. Stuhr, A.; Hofmann, S.; Schlömann, M.; Oelschlägel, M. Investigation of the co-metabolic transformation of 4-chlorostyrene into 4-chlorophenylacetic acid in Pseudomonas fluorescens ST. *Biotechnol. Rep.* **2018**, *18*, e00248. [CrossRef]
17. Maag, H. Prodrugs of carboxylic acids. In *Prodrugs*; Springer: New York, NY, USA, 2007; pp. 703–729. [CrossRef]
18. Bardhan, D.; Chand, D.K. Palladium (II)-Based Self-Assembled Heteroleptic Coordination Architectures: A Growing Family. *Chem. Eur. J.* **2019**, *25*, 12241–12269. [CrossRef]
19. Psomas, G. Copper (II) and zinc (II) coordination compounds of non-steroidal anti-inflammatory drugs: Structural features and antioxidant activity. *Coord. Chem. Rev.* **2020**, *412*, 213259. [CrossRef]
20. Detsi, A.; Kontogiorgis, C.; Hadjipavlou-Litina, D. Coumarin derivatives: An updated patent review (2015–2016). *Expert Opin. Ther. Pat.* **2017**, *27*, 1201–1226. [CrossRef]
21. Abdolmaleki, S.; Ghadermazi, M.; Ashengroph, M.; Saffari, A.; Sabzkohi, S.M. Cobalt (II), zirconium (IV), calcium (II) complexes with dipicolinic acid and imidazole derivatives: X-ray studies, thermal analyses, evaluation as in vitro antibacterial and cytotoxic agents. *Inorg. Chim. Acta* **2018**, *480*, 70–82. [CrossRef]
22. Mushtaq, A.; Ali, S.; Iqbal, M.; Shahzadi, S.; Tahir, M.; Ismail, H. Supramolecular Heteroleptic Copper (II) Carboxylates: Synthesis, Spectral Characterization, Crystal Structures, and Enzyme Inhibition Assay. *Russ. J. Coord. Chem.* **2018**, *44*, 187–197. [CrossRef]
23. Muhammad, N.; Khan, I.N.; Ali, Z.; Ibrahim, M.; Shujah, S.; Ali, S.; Ikram, M.; Rehman, S.; Khan, G.S.; Wadood, A. Synthesis, characterization, antioxidant, antileishmanial, anticancer, DNA and theoretical SARS-CoV-2 interaction studies of copper (II) carboxylate complexes. *J. Mol. Struct.* **2022**, *1253*, 132308.
24. Iqbal, M.; Haleem, M.A.; Ali, S.; Shahid, K.; Abbas, S.M.; Tahir, M.N. Centro-symmetric paddlewheel copper (II) carboxylates: Synthesis, structural description, DNA-binding and molecular docking studies. *Polyhedron* **2021**, *208*, 115407. [CrossRef]
25. Muthukkumar, M.; Karthikeyan, A.; Kamalesu, S.; Kadri, M.; Jennifer, S.J.; Razak, I.A.; Nehru, S. Synthesis, crystal structure, optical and DFT studies of a novel Co (II) complex with the mixed ligands 3-bromothiophene-2-carboxylate and 2-aminopyridine. *J. Mol. Struct.* **2022**, *1270*, 133953. [CrossRef]
26. Heine, M.; Fink, L.; Schmidt, M.U. 3-Cyanopyridine as a bridging and terminal ligand in coordination polymers. *Cryst. Eng. Comm.* **2018**, *20*, 7556–7566. [CrossRef]
27. Madhavan, V.; Varghese, H.T.; Mathew, S.; Vinsova, J.; Panicker, C.Y. FT-IR, FT-Raman and DFT calculations of 4-chloro-2-(3, 4-dichlorophenylcarbamoyl) phenyl acetate. *Spectrochim. Acta A Mol. Biomol.* **2009**, *72*, 547–553. [CrossRef]
28. Jenniefer, S.J.; Muthiah, P.T. Synthesis, characterization and X-ray structural studies of four copper (II) complexes containing dinuclear paddle wheel structures. *Chem. Cent. J.* **2013**, *7*, 35. [CrossRef]
29. Iqbal, M.; Sirajuddin, M.; Ali, S.; Sohail, M.; Tahir, M.N. O-bridged and paddlewheel copper (II) carboxylates as potent DNA intercalator: Synthesis, physicochemical characterization, electrochemical and DNA binding studies as well as POM analyses. *Inorg. Chim. Acta* **2016**, *440*, 129–138. [CrossRef]
30. Motreff, A.; da Costa, R.C.; Allouchi, H.; Duttine, M.; Mathonière, C.; Duboc, C.; Vincent, J.-M. A fluorous copper (II)–carboxylate complex which magnetically and reversibly responds to humidity in the solid state. *J. Fluor. Chem.* **2012**, *134*, 49–55. [CrossRef]
31. Stephens, J.C.; Khan, M.A.; Houser, R.P. Copper (II) Acetate Complexes, [CuL m (OAc) 2] n (L= HNPPh3), Stable in the Solid State Either as a Dimer (m= 1, n= 2) or a Monomer (m= 2, n= 1). *Inorg. Chem.* **2001**, *40*, 5064–5065. [CrossRef]
32. Muhammad, N.; Ikram, M.; Perveen, F.; Ibrahim, M.; Ibrahim, M.; Rehman, S.; Shujah, S.; Khan, W.; Shams, D.F.; Schulzke, C. Syntheses, crystal structures and DNA binding potential of copper (II) carboxylates. *J. Mol. Struct.* **2019**, *1196*, 771–782. [CrossRef]

3. Sundberg, M.R.; Uggla, R.; Melník, M. Comparison of the structural parameters in copper (II) acetate-type dimers containing distorted square pyramidal CuO_4O and CuO_4N chromophores. *Polyhedron* **1996**, *15*, 1157–1163. [CrossRef]

4. Jomová, K.; Hudecova, L.; Lauro, P.; Simunkova, M.; Alwasel, S.H.; Alhazza, I.M.; Valko, M. A switch between antioxidant and prooxidant properties of the phenolic compounds myricetin, morin, 3′, 4′-dihydroxyflavone, taxifolin and 4-hydroxy-coumarin in the presence of copper (II) ions: A spectroscopic, absorption titration and DNA damage study. *Molecules* **2019**, *24*, 4335. [CrossRef]

5. Nishida, Y.; Kida, S. Splitting of d-orbitals in square planar complexes of copper (II), nickel (II) and cobalt (II). *Coord. Chem. Rev.* **1979**, *27*, 275–298. [CrossRef]

6. Brown, O.; Butterfield, R. Cathodic reductions of cyanopyridines in liquid ammonia. *Electrochim. Acta* **1982**, *27*, 1647–1653. [CrossRef]

7. Franco, E.; Lopez-Torres, E.; Mendiola, M.; Sevilla, M. Synthesis, spectroscopic and cyclic voltammetry studies of copper (II) complexes with open chain, cyclic and a new macrocyclic thiosemicarbazones. *Polyhedron* **2000**, *19*, 441–451. [CrossRef]

8. Fomina, I.; Dobrokhotova, Z.; Aleksandrov, G.; Bogomyakov, A.; Fedin, M.; Dolganov, A.; Magdesieva, T.; Novotortsev, V.; Eremenko, I. Influence of the nature of organic components in dinuclear copper (II) pivalates on the composition of thermal decomposition products. *Polyhedron* **2010**, *29*, 1734–1746. [CrossRef]

9. Iqbal, M.; Karim, A.; Ali, S.; Tahir, M.N.; Sohail, M. Synthesis, characterization, structural elucidation, electrochemistry, DNA binding study, micellization behaviour and antioxidant activity of the Cu (II) carboxylate complexes. *Polyhedron* **2020**, *178*, 114310. [CrossRef]

50. Bera, P.; Brandão, P.; Mondal, G.; Santra, A.; Jana, A.; Mokhamatam, R.B.; Manna, S.K.; Mandal, T.K.; Bera, P. An unusual iminoacylation of 2-amino pyridyl thiazole: Synthesis, X-ray crystallography and DFT study of copper (II) amidine complexes and their cytotoxicity, DNA binding and cleavage study. *Polyhedron* **2019**, *159*, 436–445. [CrossRef]

51. Andrezálová, L.; Országhová, Z. Covalent and noncovalent interactions of coordination compounds with DNA: An overview. *J. Inorg. Biochem.* **2021**, *225*, 111624. [CrossRef]

52. Zhong, W.; Yu, J.S.; Huang, W.; Ni, K.; Liang, Y. Spectroscopic studies of interaction of chlorobenzylidine with DNA. *Biopolymers* **2001**, *62*, 315–323. [CrossRef]

53. Zhou, C.-Y.; Zhao, J.; Wu, Y.-B.; Yin, C.-X.; Pin, Y. Synthesis, characterization and studies on DNA-binding of a new Cu (II) complex with N1, N8-bis (l-methyl-4-nitropyrrole-2-carbonyl) triethylenetetramine. *J. Inorg. Biochem.* **2007**, *101*, 10–18. [CrossRef] [PubMed]

54. Carter, M.T.; Rodriguez, M.; Bard, A.J. Voltammetric studies of the interaction of metal chelates with DNA. 2. Tris-chelated complexes of cobalt (III) and iron (II) with 1, 10-phenanthroline and 2, 2′-bipyridine. *J. Am. Chem. Soc.* **1989**, *111*, 8901–8911. [CrossRef]

55. Kellett, A.; Molphy, Z.; Slator, C.; McKee, V.; Farrell, N.P. Molecular methods for assessment of non-covalent metallodrug–DNA interactions. *Chem. Soc. Rev.* **2019**, *48*, 971–988. [CrossRef] [PubMed]

56. Revathi, N.; Sankarganesh, M.; Dhaveethu Raja, J.; Johnson Raja, S.; Gurusamy, S.; Nandini Asha, R.; Jeyakumar, T.C. Synthesis, spectral, DFT calculation, antimicrobial, antioxidant, DNA/BSA binding and molecular docking studies of bio-pharmacologically active pyrimidine appended Cu (II) and Zn (II) complexes. *J. Biomol. Struct. Dyn.* **2023**. [CrossRef]

57. Shakir, M.; Hanif, S.; Sherwani, M.A.; Mohammad, O.; Al-Resayes, S.I. Pharmacologically significant complexes of Mn (II), Co (II), Ni (II), Cu (II) and Zn (II) of novel Schiff base ligand,(E)-N-(furan-2-yl methylene) quinolin-8-amine: Synthesis, spectral, XRD, SEM, antimicrobial, antioxidant and in vitro cytotoxic studies. *J. Mol. Struct.* **2015**, *1092*, 143–159. [CrossRef]

58. Antonenko, T.; Shpakovsky, D.; Vorobyov, M.; Gracheva, Y.A.; Kharitonashvili, E.; Dubova, L.; Shevtsova, E.; Tafeenko, V.; Aslanov, L.; Iksanova, A. Antioxidative vs cytotoxic activities of organotin complexes bearing 2, 6-di-tert-butylphenol moieties. *Appl. Organomet. Chem.* **2018**, *32*, e4381. [CrossRef]

59. Corpuz, M.; Osi, M.; Santiago, L. Free radical scavenging activity of Sargassum siliquosum JG Agardh. *Int. Food Res. J.* **2013**, *20*, 291.

60. Mushtaq, A.; Ali, S.; Tahir, M.N.; Haider, A.; Ismail, H.; Iqbal, M. Mixed-Ligand Cu (II) Carboxylates: Synthesis, Crystal Structure, FTIR, DNA Binding, Antidiabetic, and Anti-Alzheimer's Studies. *Russ. J. Inorg.* **2019**, *64*, 1365–1378. [CrossRef]

61. Rikagu Oxford Diffraction. *CrysAlisPro*; Agilent Technologies Inc.: Yarnton, UK, 2018.

62. Sheldrick, G.M. SHELXT–Integrated space-group and crystal-structure determination. *Acta Crystallogr. A* **2015**, *71*, 3–8. [CrossRef]

63. Sheldrick, G.M. Crystal structure refinement with SHELXL. *Acta Crystallogr. C Struct. Chem.* **2015**, *71*, 3–8. [CrossRef]

64. Ramzan, S.; Shujah, S.; Holt, K.B.; Rehman, Z.-U.; Hussain, S.T.; Cockcroft, J.K.; Malkani, N.; Muhammad, N.; Kauser, A. Structural characterization, DNA binding study, antioxidant potential and antitumor activity of diorganotin (IV) complexes against human breast cancer cell line MDA-MB-231. *J. Organomet. Chem.* **2023**, *990*, 122671. [CrossRef]

65. Ayaz, M.; Junaid, M.; Ahmed, J.; Ullah, F.; Sadiq, A.; Ahmad, S.; Imran, M. Phenolic contents, antioxidant and anticholinesterase potentials of crude extract, subsequent fractions and crude saponins from *Polygonum hydropiper* L. *BMC Complement Altern. Med.* **2014**, *14*, 145. [CrossRef]

66. Ruch, R.J.; Cheng, S.-J.; Klaunig, J.E. Prevention of cytotoxicity and inhibition of intercellular communication by antioxidant catechins isolated from Chinese green tea. *Carcinogenesis* **1989**, *10*, 1003–1008. [CrossRef]

67. Ellman, G.L.; Courtney, K.D.; Andres, V., Jr.; Featherstone, R.M. A new and rapid colorimetric determination of acetyl-cholinesterase activity. *Biochem. Pharmacol.* **1961**, *7*, 88–95. [CrossRef]

58. Sadiq, A.; Mahmood, F.; Ullah, F.; Ayaz, M.; Ahmad, S.; Haq, F.U.; Khan, G.; Jan, M.S. Synthesis, anticholinesterase and antioxidant potentials of ketoesters derivatives of succinimides: A possible role in the management of Alzheimer's. *Chem. Cent. J.* **2015**, *9*, 31. [CrossRef]
59. Ovais, M.; Ayaz, M.; Khalil, A.T.; Shah, S.A.; Jan, M.S.; Raza, A.; Shahid, M.; Shinwari, Z.K. HPLC-DAD finger printing, antioxidant, cholinesterase, and α-glucosidase inhibitory potentials of a novel plant Olax nana. *BMC Complement Altern. Med.* **2018**, *18*, 1. [CrossRef]

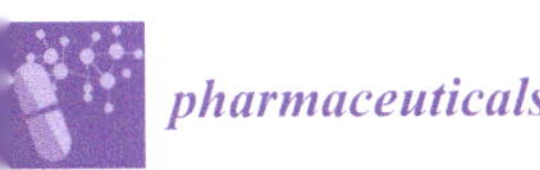
pharmaceuticals

MDPI

Article

Structure-Based Virtual Screening of Furan-1,3,4-Oxadiazole Tethered *N*-phenylacetamide Derivatives as Novel Class of hTYR and hTYRP1 Inhibitors

Ali Irfan [1], Shah Faisal [2], Sajjad Ahmad [3], Sami A. Al-Hussain [4], Sadia Javed [5], Ameer Fawad Zahoor [1,*], Bushra Parveen [1] and Magdi E. A. Zaki [4,*]

[1] Department of Chemistry, Government College University Faisalabad, Faisalabad 38000, Pakistan
[2] Department of Chemistry, Islamia College University Peshawar, Peshawar 25120, Pakistan
[3] Department of Health and Biological Sciences, Abasyn University, Peshawar 25000, Pakistan
[4] Department of Chemistry, College of Science, Imam Mohammad Ibn Saud Islamic University (IMSIU), Riyadh 11623, Saudi Arabia
[5] Department of Biochemistry, Government College University Faisalabad, Faisalabad 38000, Pakistan
* Correspondence: fawad.zahoor@gcuf.edu.pk (A.F.Z.); mezaki@imamu.edu.sa (M.E.A.Z.); Tel.:+92-3336729186 (A.F.Z.)

Abstract: Human tyrosinase (hTYR) is a key and rate-limiting enzyme along with human tyrosinase-related protein-1 (hTYRP1), which are among the most prominent targets of inhibiting hyper pigmentation and melanoma skin cancer. In the current in-silico computer-aided drug design (CADD) study, the structure-based screening of sixteen furan-1,3,4-oxadiazole tethered *N*-phenylacetamide structural motifs **BF1–BF16** was carried out to assess their potential as hTYR and hTYRP1 inhibitors. The results revealed that the structural motifs **BF1–BF16** showed higher binding affinities towards hTYR and hTYRP1 than the standard inhibitor kojic acid. The most bioactive lead furan-1,3,4-oxadiazoles **BF4** and **BF5** displayed stronger binding in affinities (−11.50 kcal/mol and −13.30 kcal/mol) than the standard drug kojic acid against hTYRP1 and hTYR enzymes, respectively. These were further confirmed by MM-GBSA and MM-PBSA binding energy computations. The stability studies involving the molecular dynamics simulations also provided stability insights into the binding of these compounds with the target enzymes, wherein it was found that they remain stable in the active sites during the 100 ns virtual simulation time. Moreover, the ADMET, as well as the medicinal properties of these novel furan-1,3,4-oxadiazole tethered *N*-phenylacetamide structural hybrids, also showed a good prospect. The excellent in-silico profiling of furan-1,3,4–oxadiazole structural motifs **BF4** and **BF5** provide a hypothetical gateway to use these compounds as potential hTYRP1 and hTYR inhibitors against melanogenesis.

Keywords: furan-1,3,4-oxadiazole; hTYR; hTYRP1; melanogenesis; molecular docking; MD simulations

Citation: Irfan, A.; Faisal, S.; Ahmad, S.; Al-Hussain, S.A.; Javed, S.; Zahoor, A.F.; Parveen, B.; Zaki, M.E.A. Structure-Based Virtual Screening of Furan-1,3,4-Oxadiazole Tethered *N*-phenylacetamide Derivatives as Novel Class of hTYR and hTYRP1 Inhibitors. *Pharmaceuticals* **2023**, *16*, 344. https://doi.org/10.3390/ph16030344

Academic Editors: Hasan Demirci, Halil İbrahim Ciftci and Belgin Sever

Received: 30 December 2022
Revised: 10 February 2023
Accepted: 12 February 2023
Published: 23 February 2023

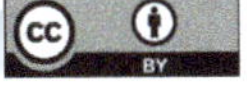

1. Introduction

Skin cancer is the one of the most common cancers which adversely affect humans. The main types of skin cancer include melanoma, basal cell carcinoma and squamous. Among them, melanoma is far less frequent than the other types. Melanoma cancer has a higher propensity to spread to other body areas by invading adjacent tissue [1]. Melanoma is the skin cancer that leads to the majority of fatalities, with an average increase of roughly one million new cases per year. Skin cancer has developed into the most prevalent malignant ailment, accounting for 4.5% of all new cancer cases, and it continues to be a fatal cancer that causes significant socioeconomic challenges [2–4]. When melanomas are in an advanced stage, they are required to be treated surgically and with adjuvant systemic therapies [5]. As with other malignancies, radiation can be used alone or in combination with surgery to treat melanoma. However, radiotherapy has a limited function in the treatment of melanoma since it is radio-resistant in comparison to other malignancies [6]. Thus, the development of drugs that specifically target cell-signaling pathways involved in this malignancy holds promise for the treatment of melanomas [7,8]. The enzyme human tyrosinase (hTYR) and human tyrosinase-related protein-1 (hTYRP1) are involved in the biosynthetic processes that produce the pigment melanin in the melanocytes. The hTYR and hTYRP1 have been shown to be sensitive melanoma biomarkers and these are also overexpressed during carcinogenesis [9–11]. Additionally, the melanin biosynthesis pathway produces powerful immunosuppressive intermediate species such as L-DOPA and other reactive quinines which further aggravate melanomas by negating the anti-melanoma actions of the immunotherapeutic medications that target these malignancies [12–15].

All the observations and factors link the elevated melanogenesis as a cause of the lethality of skin melanomas due to the increased activity and overexpression of hTYR and hTYRP1 [13,16]. Therefore, targeting the inhibition of crucial enzymes hTYR and hTYRP1 with suitable inhibitors prevents the formation of melanomas and may help in treating these cancers [13,17,18]. To date, several approaches of in-vivo studies targeting the melanin biosynthetic pathway for treating melanomas have been reported [19]. hTYR, hTYRP1 and the other related enzymes of the melanin biosynthetic pathway are possible molecular targets in the treatment of melanoma and other melanogenesis-related disorders due to their overexpression, which occurs during carcinogenesis primarily in the melanocytes [13,20,21].

The plethora of literature cited in previous studies revealed that numerous furans containing molecules, benzofurans (Figure 1), 1,3,4-oxadiazoles (Figure 1), furan-1,3,4-oxadiazoles and other furan moiety carrying scaffolds are effective inhibitors of mushroom and human tyrosinases. The origin of furan chemistry has been outlined by Partington and the furan first derivative pyromucic acid (furan-2-carboxylic acid) or simply 2-furoic acid (Figure 1) was obtained via dry distillation of mucic acid (Figure 1). In 1831, Johann Wolfgang Döbereiner reported another important derivative of furan called furfural (Figure 1) (furan-2-carbaldehyde), which was further characterized by John Stenhouse. Heinrich Limpricht isolated furan for the first time in 1870 from pine wood, called tetraphenol due to the presence of four carbon atoms and strong resemblance to phenol in many reactions, e.g., with bromine [22–25].

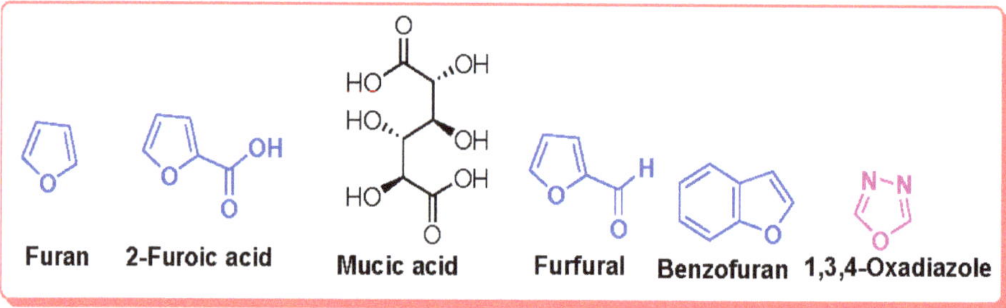

Figure 1. Structures of furan, mucic acid, 1,3,4-oxadiazole and furan-related compounds.

Furan, benzofuran and other nitrogen-oxygen heterocyclic structural motifs had demonstrated excellent medicinal and pharmacological profiles, and exhibited a wide spectrum of biological activities such as antibacterial, anti-fungal, anti-diabetic, anti-acetylcholine, anti-viral, anti-inflammatory, anti-parasitic, fluorescent sensor for analgesic, anti-HepG-2, anti-oxidative, bone anabolic agent and as bacterial tyrosinase inhibitors; they are also part of many natural and synthetic clinical drugs. In various research models, furan scaffolds have shown potent anti-tyrosinase actions which imply that these compounds are effective inhibitors of the melanin biosynthesis in the melanocytes and can be used in treating skin melanomas and other melanogenesis-related disorders, as depicted in Figure 2 [26–38].

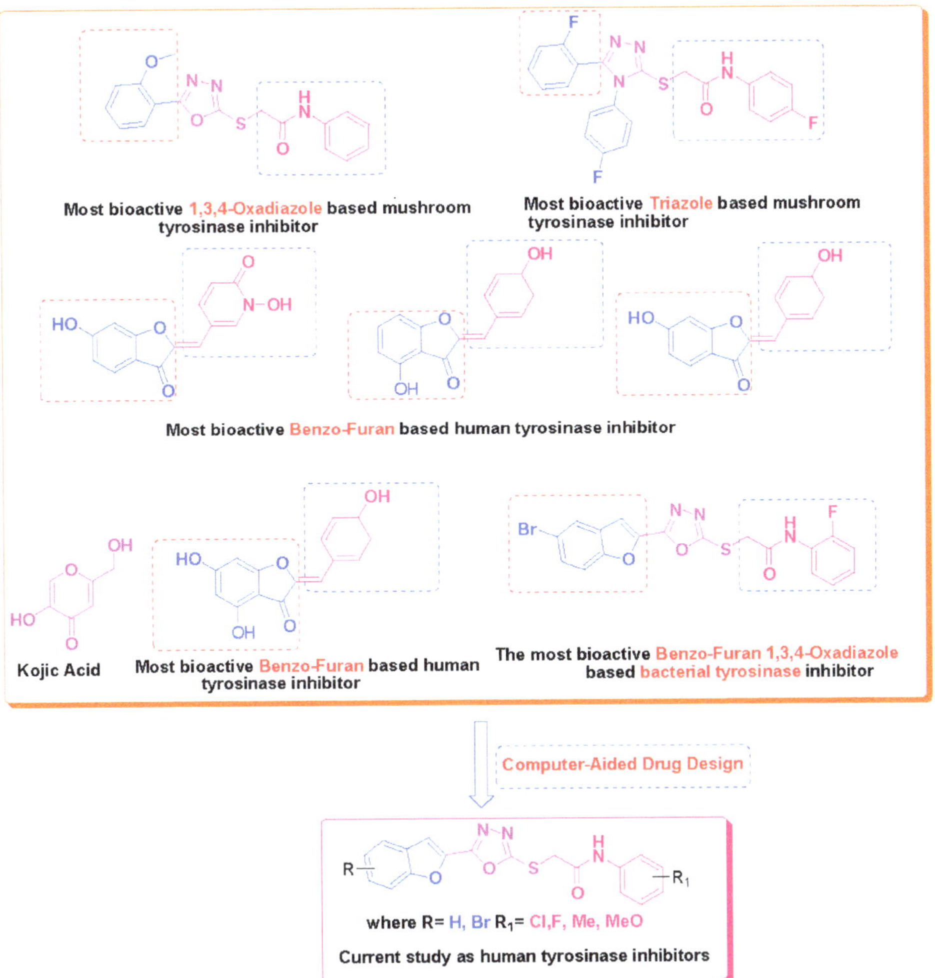

Figure 2. Bioactive tyrosinase inhibitors.

Our previous work reported the evaluation of benzofuran-1,3,4-oxadiazole tethered *N*-phenylacetamides as bacterial tyrosinase inhibitors and showed strong repressive activities of benzofuran compounds, which encouraged us to apply computer-aided drug discovery (CADD) approaches to assess the therapeutic potential of sixteen synthesized furan-1,3,4-oxadiazole tethered *N*-phenylacetamide structural hybrids, **BF1–BF16 [38,39]**, with different substituents to target the crucial enzymes hTYR and hTYRP1 of the melanin biosynthetic pathway.

The therapeutic potential of synthesized furan–oxadiazole scaffolds **BF1–BF16** was assessed utilizing a computer-aided drug design (CADD) workflow as displayed in Figure 3.

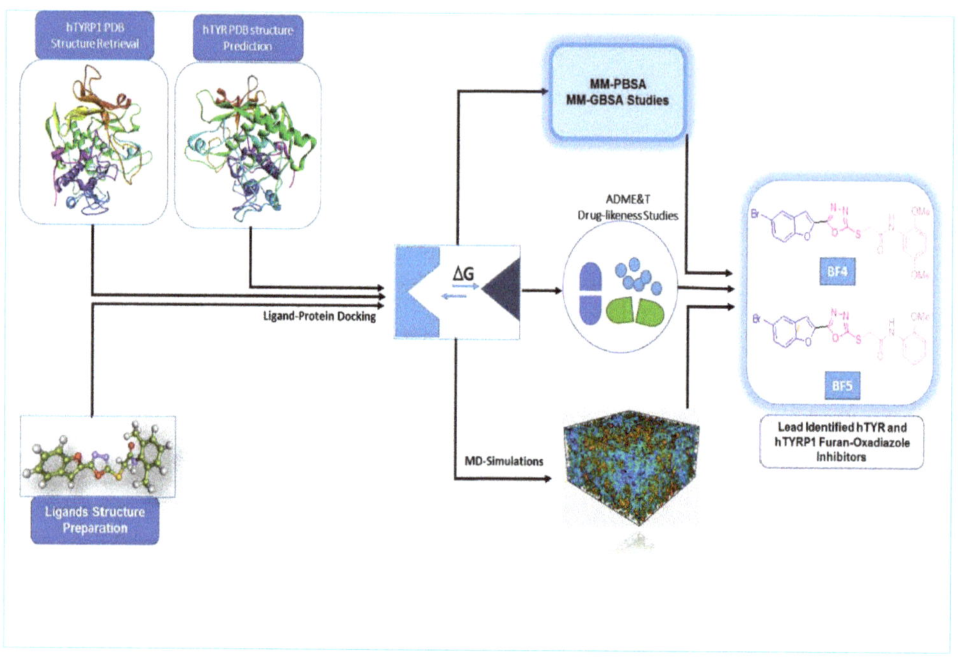

Figure 3. In silico work flow for discovery of novel hTYR and hTYRP1 inhibitors via CADD.

2. Results and Discussion

2.1. Computational Investigations of BF1–BF16 against hTYR and hTYRP1

Utilizing the in silico molecular docking approach, we evaluated furan-1,3,4-oxadiazoles synthesized compounds **BF1–BF16** using the molecular operating environment (MOE) against the hTYR and hTYRP1 of the melanin synthesis pathway and compared these results with the standard tyrosinase inhibitor drug kojic acid, which has been shown to repress these two enzymes (hTYR and hTYRP1) in various studies. The results of these investigations revealed that the anti-hTYR and hTYRP1 repressive agent kojic acid binds to the active site of the hTYR enzyme with a binding affinity score of −6.62 Kcal/mol, and it binds to the hTYRP1 with a binding affinity score of –8.90 Kcal/mol. Conformation analysis of the kojic acid inhibitor inside the active site pocket of hTYR revealed that it engaged multiple amino acids residues (ASN364, HIS367,and MET374) and made conventional-type and carbon–hydrogen-type hydrogen bonds with it; along with several other molecular interactions of Pi–Pi T-shaped and Pi–Alkyl-type interactions with HIS202 and VAL377 were also observed in the hTYR and kojic acid protein–ligand complex. Binding analysis of kojic acid with the hTYRP1 enzyme showed that it made conventional hydrogen bonds with the TYR362 and GLY389 active site residues and a Pi–Pi stacked interaction with the HIS381. The conformational poses of kojic acid with both enzymes are presented in Figure 4.

In comparison with the kojic acid inhibitor, some of the synthesized benzofuran compounds showed robust interactions and higher binding affinities with the hTYR and hTYRP1 enzymes of the melanin synthesis pathway. Out of the sixteen compounds, **BF1–BF16**, three compounds, **BF5**, **BF7**, and **BF15**, showed stronger affinities against the hTYR, while the other three, **BF4**, **BF5**, and **BF7**, showed stronger affinities against the hTYRP1 compared to the standard drug kojic acid. Analysis of the conformational pose and binding affinity of **BF5** showed that it binds to the hTYR active site with a binding affinity score of −13.30 Kcal/mol and forms multiple molecular interactions with the hTYR enzyme receptor residues. Hydrogen bonds of conventional and carbon–hydrogen types were noted between the benzofuran ring of **BF5** and HIS202, HIS367, GLN376, MET374 residues. Moreover, other interactions, such as Pi–Anion, Alkyl, and Pi–Alkyl interactions (with the VAL377), were also present between the 1,3,4-oxadiazole and benzofuran rings of this compound; in addition, several of the hTyrosinase receptor residues (ASP186 and ARG196) also made halogen molecular interactions with the bromine present on the benzofuran ring of this compound. These are diagrammatically presented in Figure 5.

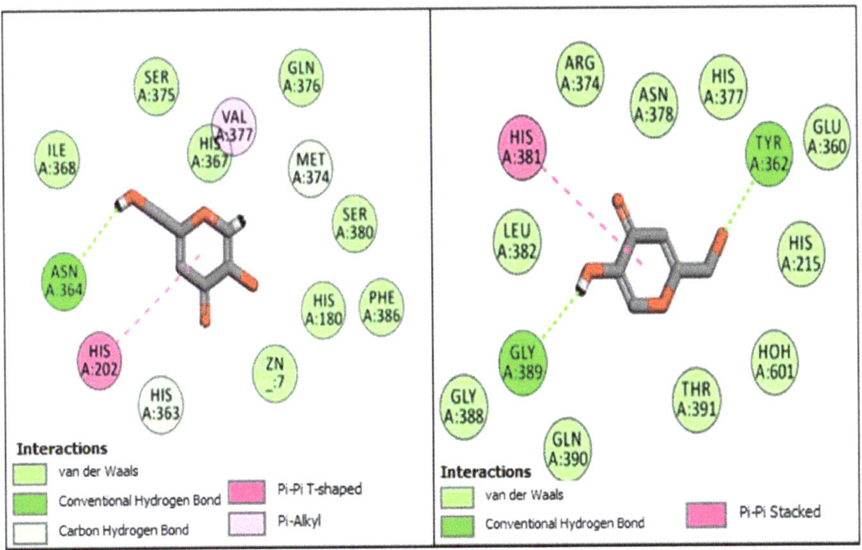

Figure 4. Conformational poses of kojic acid with hTYR (**Left panel**) and hTYRP1 (**Right panel**).

The two other compounds, **BF7** and **BF15,** were also able to bind to the hTyrosinase with higher binding affinities (−11.19 Kcal/mol and −11.88 Kcal/mol, respectively) compared to the kojic acid, which was able to bind to the hTYR with a binding affinity of −6.62 Kcal/mol. These two compounds were also able to engage multiple active site residues of hTYR via a different type of molecular interactions. Overall, the **BF7** compound showed a similar kind of binding conformation and interactions with the hTyrosinase enzyme; however, the sulfur atom of **BF7** made two more Pi–sulfur interactions with the HIS363, and HIS202 and the chlorine atom present on the phenyl ring of the **BF7** made two halogen interactions with the VAL377 and MET374 active site residues. Similarly, **BF15** also showed robust binding with the hTyrosinase by engaging the HIS363 with a carbon–hydrogen-type hydrogen bond, while PHE347 made a molecular contact via a Pi–sulfur interaction with the sulfur atom of **BF15**. Several other types of hydrophobic interactions were also observed between the benzofuran, 1,3,4- oxadiazole, and the phenyl ring of **BF15,** and they can be seen in Figure 6.

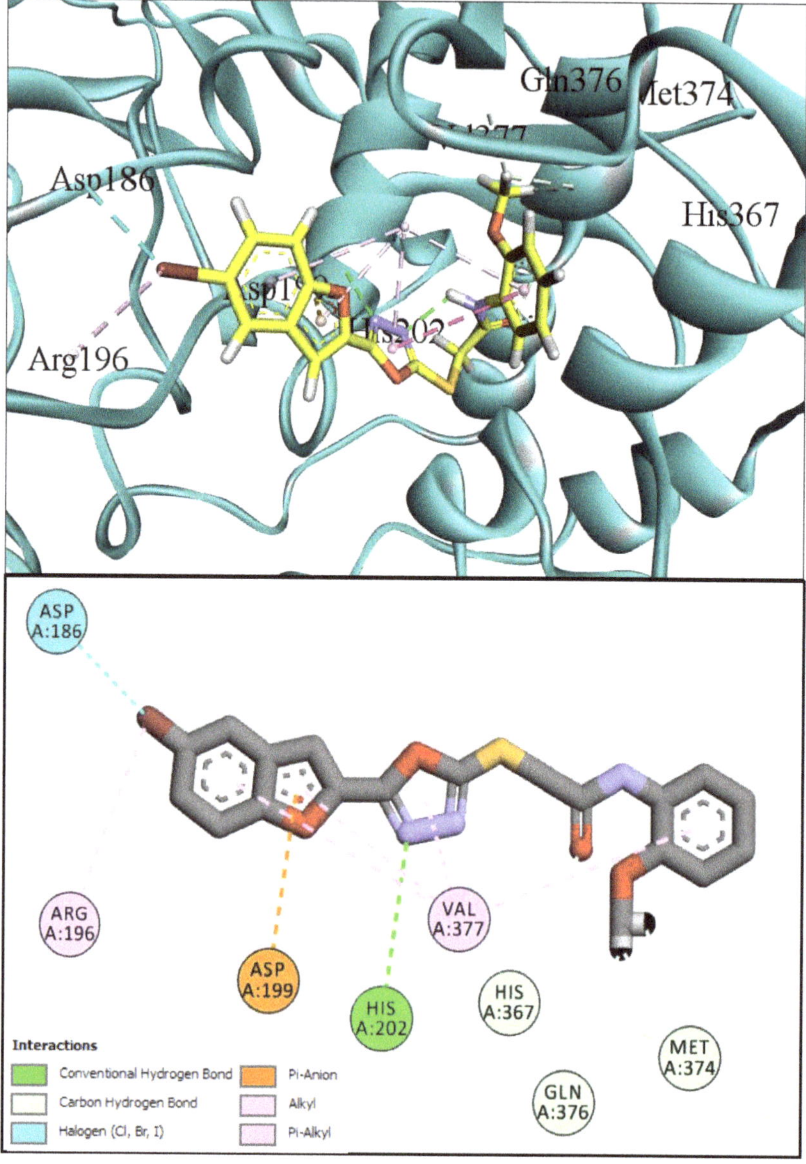

Figure 5. Three-dimensional conformational pose of BF5 with hTyrosinase (**Upper panel**) and two-dimensional pose (**Lower panel**).

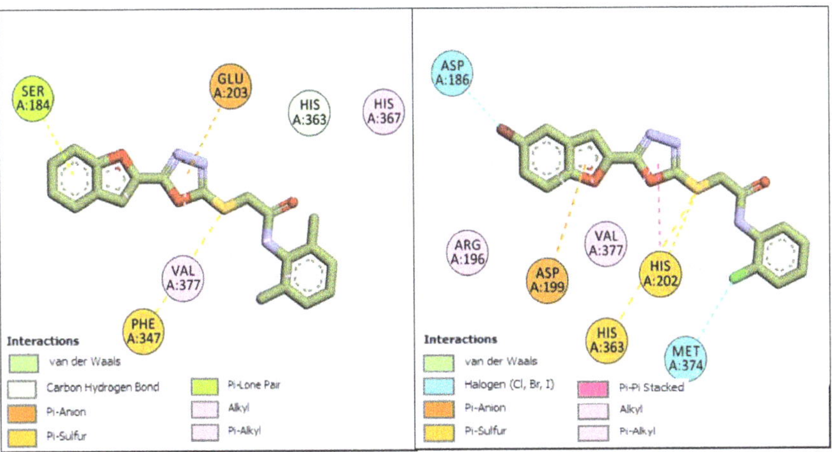

Figure 6. Two-dimensional conformational pose of **BF7** with hTyrosinase (**Right panel**) and two-dimensional conformational pose of **BF15** with hTyrosinase (**Left panel**).

The molecular docking investigations against the hTYRP1 enzyme also revealed that these newly synthesized compounds show superior binding and interactions with this important enzyme. The standard inhibitor kojic acid, as discussed in the previous paragraphs, binds to the hTYRP1 with a binding affinity score of –8.90 Kcal/mol; compared to kojic acid, some of these new furan-1,3,4-oxadiazoles (**BF4**, **BF5**, and **BF7**) have shown good binding affinities towards the hTYRP1 enzyme. The furan-1,3,4-oxadiazoles **BF4**, **BF5** and **BF7** were able to bind to the hTYRP1 with binding affinities of −11.50 Kcal/mol, −11.55 Kcal/mol, and −11.29 Kcal/mol, respectively. The conformational pose analysis of **BF4** in the active site of the hTYRP1 enzyme showed that it binds with the active pocket residues via different types of molecular interactions. The acetamide group, as well as the oxygen atom of the 1,3,4-oxadizole ring present in this compound, made conventional hydrogen bonds with the ARG374 and THR391 amino acids of the hTYRP1, and a carbon–hydrogen-type H-bond between the –OCH$_3$ and the SER394 amino acid was also present in this ligand–protein complex. The 1,3,4-oxadiazole ring of **BF4** also made another Pi–anion interaction with the GLU216 of the hTYRP1 active site, while the bromine atom on the benzofuran ring and the phenyl ring of BF-4 made Alkyl and Pi–Alkyl interactions with LEU293 and LYS198 residues of hTYRP1. **BF5**, which showed the highest binding affinity (−11.55 Kcal/mol) towards the hTYRP1 active site, also showed robust interactions of different types with this target enzyme. The phenyl ring of **BF-5** made a total of four interactions with the HIS381, GLN390, and HIS377 of Pi–Pi stacked, Pi-Pi T-shaped and amide–Pi stacked type along with a direct interaction with the zinc ion present in the active site of the hTYRP1. The 1,3,4-oxadiazole ring engaged the THR391 residue while the benzofuran ring made three Pi–anion interactions with the ASP212 and GLU216; however, the –OCH$_3$ present on the phenyl ring made a single carbon–hydrogen-type H-bond with the HIS215 of the hTYRP1 enzyme active site. Figure 7 shows the three and two-dimensional conformations of **BF5** inside the hTYRP1 active site.

The furan-1,3,4-oxadiazole **BF7** compound with a binding affinity of −11.29 Kcal/mol with the hTYRP1 also exhibited several different types of interactions with the LYS198, HIS215, HIS381, GLN390, and THR391 active sites. Figure 8 shows the two-dimensional poses of **BF4** and **BF7** with the hTYRP1 enzyme.

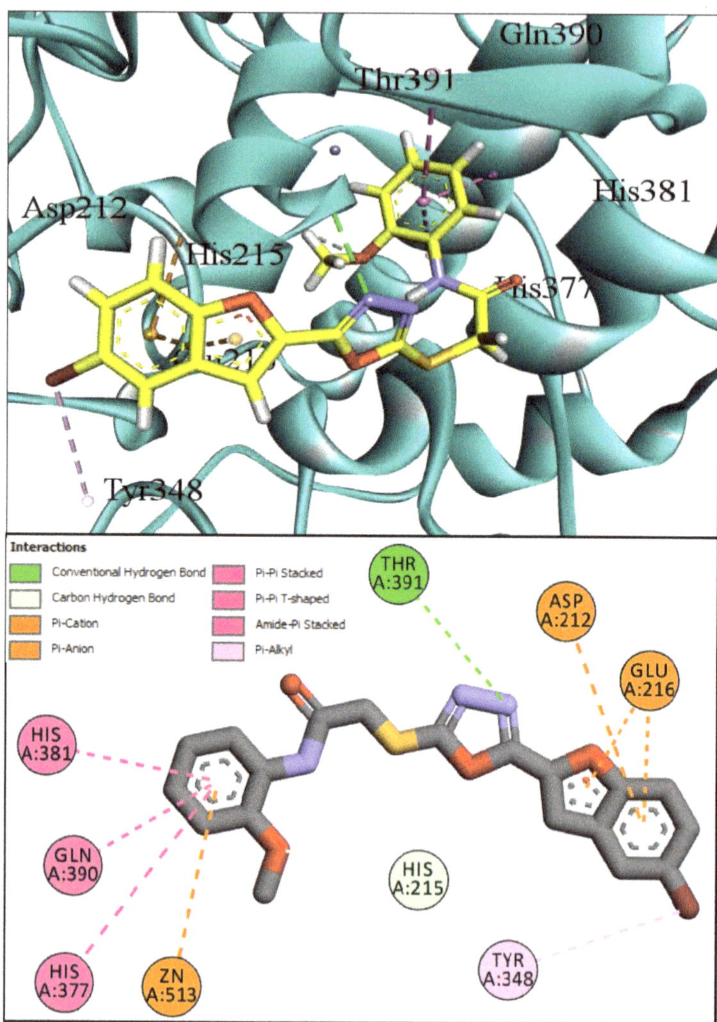

Figure 7. Three-dimensional conformational pose of **BF5** with human tyrosinase-related protein-1 (hTYRP1) (**Upper panel**) and its two-dimensional pose (**Lower panel**).

The binding affinities of the biologically active furan-1,3,4-oxadiazole compounds against hTYR and hTYRP1 are shown in Table 1.

Table 1. Binding affinities of the best binding compounds with the hTyrosinase and hTYRP1 enzymes.

Compound	Binding Affinity in (Kcal/mol) with hTYRP1	Binding Affinity in (Kcal/mol) with hTYR
BF4	−11.50 Kcal/mol	–
BF5	−11.55 Kcal/mol	−13.30 Kcal/mol
BF7	−11.29 Kcal/mol	−11.19 Kcal/mol
BF15	–	−11.88 Kcal/mol
Kojic acid (Standard)	−8.90 Kcal/mol	−6.62 Kcal/mol

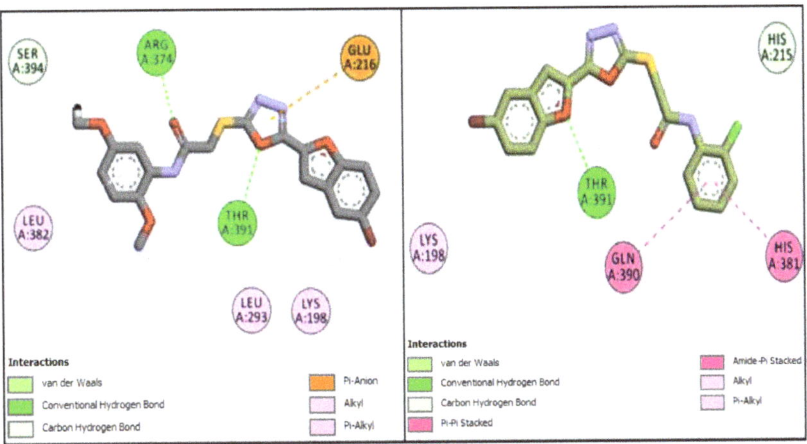

Figure 8. Two-dimensional conformational pose of **BF4** with hTYRP1 (**Left panel**) and two-dimensional conformational pose of **BF7** with hTYRP1 (**Right panel**).

2.2. ADMET and Drug-Likeness Predictive Studies

The pharmacokinetics, or, in short, the ADMET studies along with the drug-likeness in silico investigations, showed that the furan-1,3,4-oxadiazole compounds have significantly good GI-Tract absorption values and they were listed as HIA+. These compounds were listed to have acceptable lipophilic (iLogP) properties and also had good water solubility (LogS-ESOL) values. They were non-inhibitors of the P-gp protein and non-substrates of the CYP450-3A4 enzyme. They were non-inhibitors of renal (OCTs) and were found to be non-AMES toxic. Along with these good ADMET properties, these compounds also showed good medicinal chemistry profiles and accepted the Lipinski rule, Pfizer rule and Golden triangle rule. Table 2 has the different pharmacokinetic properties listed, while Table 3 contains the medicinal chemistry profiles of the best lead compounds identified in this investigation.

Table 2. ADMET profile of **BF4**, **BF5**, **BF7** and **BF15** furan-1,3,4-oxadiazole compounds.

Compounds	HIA+ Values	Lipophilicity (iLogP)	CYP450 3A4 Inhibitor/ Substrate	Water Solubility	P-gp Substrate	Carcinogenicity	Renal (OCTs)
BF4	1.0	3.99	Substrate	Moderately soluble	No	None	Non Inhibitor
BF5	1.0	3.75	Substrate	Moderately soluble	No	None	Non Inhibitor
BF7	1.0	3.66	Substrate	Poorly soluble	No	None	Non Inhibitor
BF15	1.0	3.57	Substrate	Moderately soluble	No	None	Non Inhibitor

Table 3. Drug-likeness profile of **BF4**, **BF5**, **BF7** and **BF15** furan-1,3,4-oxadiazole compounds.

Compounds	Bioavailability Score	PAINS Alerts	Brenk Alerts	Lipinski Rule	Pfizer Rule	Golden Triangle Rule	TPSA
BF4	0.55	None	None	Accepted	Accepted	Accepted	124.92 Å^2
BF5	0.55	None	None	Accepted	Accepted	Accepted	115.69 Å^2
BF7	0.55	None	None	Accepted	Accepted	Accepted	106.46 Å^2
BF15	0.55	None	None	Accepted	Accepted	Accepted	106.46 Å^2

2.3. Molecular Dynamics Stability Analysis of the Ligand-Protein Complexes

All atoms' molecular dynamic simulations were conducted for complexes in order to understand and interpret intermolecular dynamics and the stability of docked molecules with the receptor enzymes. As a bio-molecule function in dynamics inside the cells, it is important to evaluate the dynamic behavior rather than focusing on static nature. The trajectories of simulations were generated using the root mean square deviation (RMSD) statistical parameter. RMSD measure the all-atom carbon alpha mean deviation with respect to initial reference position versus time. Higher RMSD describes more structure deviations, while lower RMSD points to small structure changes. The RMSD plot for each complex is provided in Figure 9. The **BF4**-hTYRP1 (mean RMSD of 0.98 Å), **BF15** + hTYR (mean RMSD of 1.62 Å), **BF5** + hTYR (mean RMSD of 0.88 Å) and **BF7** + hTYRP1 (mean RMSD of 1.86 Å) were the most stable complexes that showed little structure deviations in the simulated time. The mean RMSD of these complexes was 1.2 Å. This stable nature of complexes enables the receptors' 3D structure to remain confined and fixed in the presence of compounds during simulation time. The **BF5** + hTYRP1, on the other hand, reported the highest RMSD, which touches almost five angstroms. It is very clear in the analysis that all complexes, after initial small deviation, attained considerable structure stability. The data showed that the compounds are stably docked inside the active pocket of enzymes, and the binding conformation, except for a few initial small adaptations, remained stable throughout the length of simulation time.

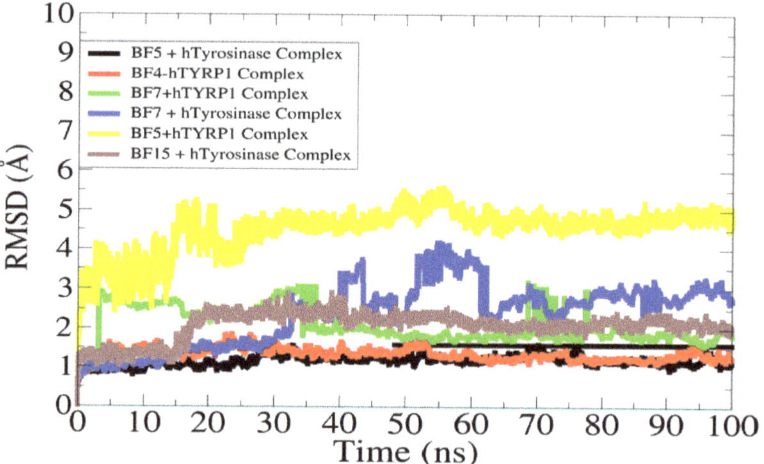

Figure 9. RMSD analysis of complexes to decipher their dynamic stability.

To obtain a further understanding of the residue level flexibility, root mean square fluctuation (RMSF) analysis was conducted. The mean RMSF of BF5 + hTyrosinase, BF7 + hTyrosinase, BF15 + hTyrosinase, BF4-hTYRP1, BF5 + hTYRP1, and BF7 + hTYRP1 is 1.1 Å, 2.2 Å, 0.8 Å, 1.8 Å, 2.7 Å, and 2.9 Å, respectively. All the systems reported stable fluctuations at the residue level with major deviations seen at loops. The RMSF of the complexes is shown in Figure 10.

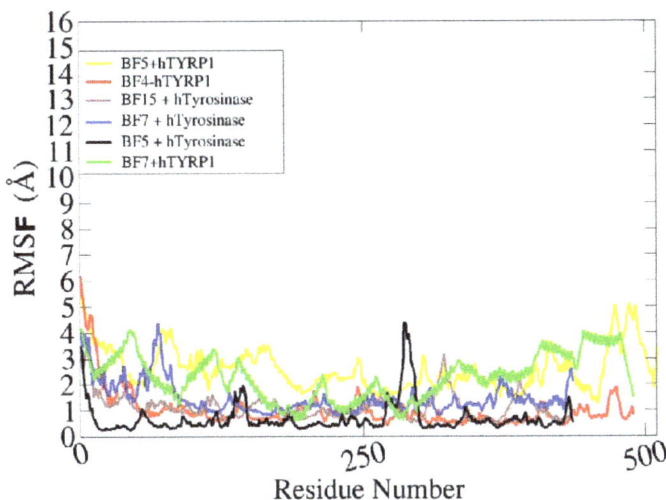

Figure 10. Residue level fluctuation of complexes.

2.4. MM-GBSA/MM-PBSA Binding Free Energy Analysis of Complexes

The binding free energies calculation using MMGBSA and MMPBSA is a significant approach to revalidate the docking results, as they are more reliable and use modest computational power. The order of complexes based on stable net-binding energy is in the following order: **BF4**-hTYRP1 > **BF4**-hTYRP1 > **BF7** + hTYRP1 > **BF5** + hTYR > **BF7** + hTYR > **BF5** + hTYRP1. Generally, the gas phase energy in all complexes was found to dominate the chemical interaction network between the docked molecules and enzymes' active pocket residues. Decomposing the gas phase energy, the van der Waals energy component was the most dominating, ranging from −55.01 kcal/mol for **BF4**-hTYRP1 and −48.62 kcal/mol for **BF5** + hTYRP1. In addition to that, electrostatic energy played a major role in intermolecular complex formation. The highest contribution was seen in the case of −31.74 kcal/mol for **BF4**-hTYRP1 and the lowest contribution was seen in the case of −22.17 kcal/mol for **BF5** + hTYRP1. The non-favorable contribution was reported from solvation energy, which was highest at 28.99 kcal/mol in **BF5** + hTYR and lowest at 23.59 kcal/mol in **BF7** + hTYRP1. The net-binding energy along with each energy parameter value (kcal/mol) is shown in Table 4.

Table 4. Different energy contribution to net binding energy of complexes.

Energy Parameter	BF5 + hTYR (SD)	BF7 + hTYR (SD)	BF15 + hTYR (SD)	BF4-hTYRP1 (SD)	BF5 + hTYRP1 (SD)	BF7 + hTYRP1 (SD)
MM-GBSA						
Van der Waals	−52.20(4.25)	−50.28 (3.68)	−52.62 (5.72)	−55.01 (5.07)	−48.62 (4.68)	−49.55 (5.21)
Electrostatic	−23.89(3.65)	−24.01 (3.56)	−28.21 (2.51)	−31.74 (4.68)	−22.17 (3.66)	−26.30 (4.22)
Delta G gas	−76.09(6.84)	−74.29 (5.38)	−80.83 (8.60)	−86.75 (6.81)	−70.79 (7.25)	−75.85 (6.38)
Delta G solv	28.99 (2.38)	27.68 (7.48)	24.86 (3.84)	25.08 (4.29)	28.64 (4.21)	23.59 (3.56)
Delta Total	−47.1 (5.52)	−46.61 (6.87)	−55.97 (5.69)	−61.67 (6.31)	−42.15 (6.11)	−52.26 (3.98)
MM-PBSA						
Van der Waals	−52.20(4.25)	−50.28 (3.68)	−52.62 (5.72)	−55.01 (5.07)	−48.62 (4.68)	−49.55 (5.21)
Electrostatic	−23.89(4.25)	−24.01 (3.56)	−28.21 (2.51)	−31.74 (4.68)	−22.17 (3.66)	−26.30 (4.22)
Delta G gas	76.09(6.84)	74.29 (5.38)	80.83 (8.60)	86.75 (6.81)	70.79 (7.25)	75.85 (6.38)
Delta G solv	25.60 (1.68)	25.07 (2.58)	28.61 (3.64)	24.01 (3.29)	27.64 (4.62)	24.50 (3.33)
Delta Total	−50.49(4.68)	−49.22 (5.28)	−52.22 (4.22)	−62.74 (2.67)	−43.15 (3.08)	−51.35 (2.67)

3. Material and Methods

3.1. Structures of Synthsized Furan-1,3,4-Oxadiazoles BF1–BF16

The structures of furan-1,3,4-oxadiazole structural motifs, which were synthesized by Irfan, A et al. [38,39], are shown in Table 5.

Table 5. Structures of synthetic furan-1,3,4-oxadiazoles **BF1–BF16**.

Compounds	Structures of Furan-1,3,4-Oxadiazssoles
BF1	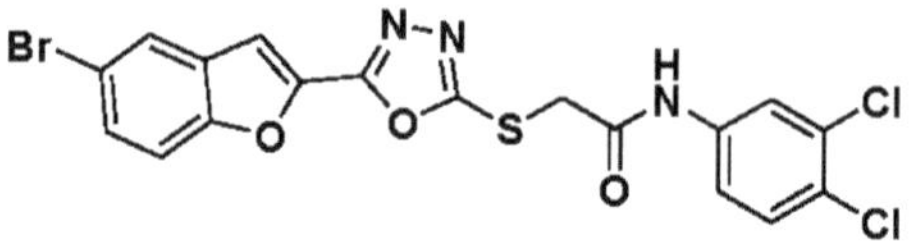
BF2	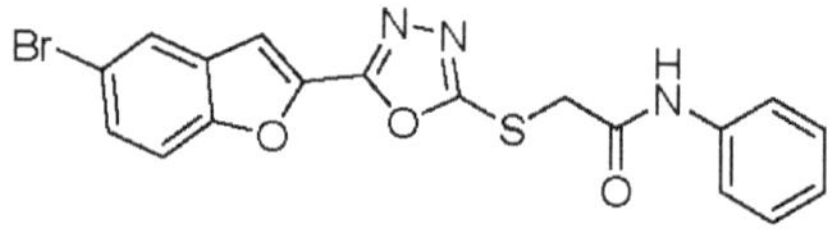
BF3	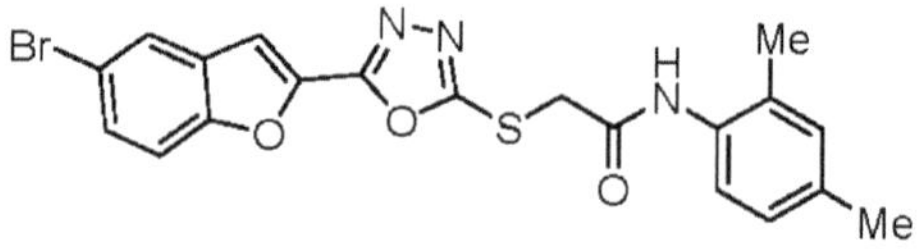
BF4	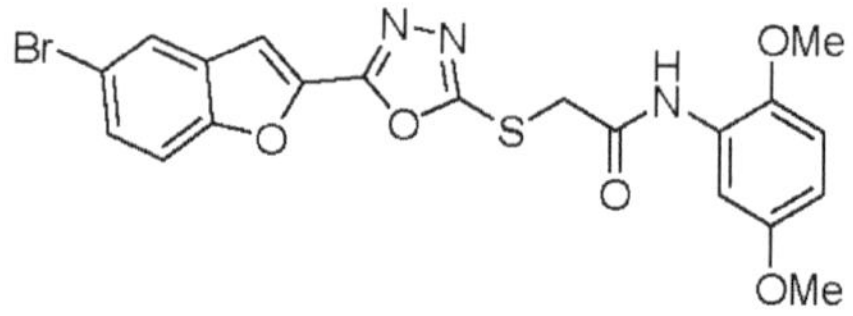
BF5	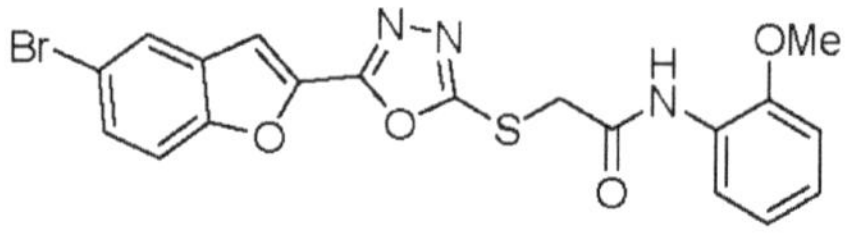
BF6	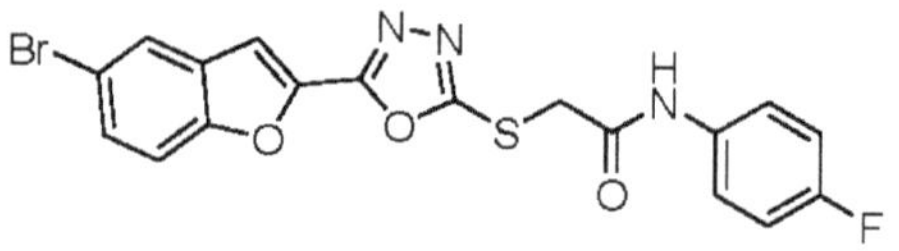
BF7	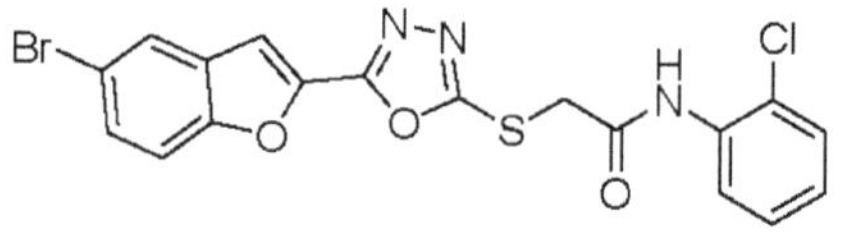
BF8	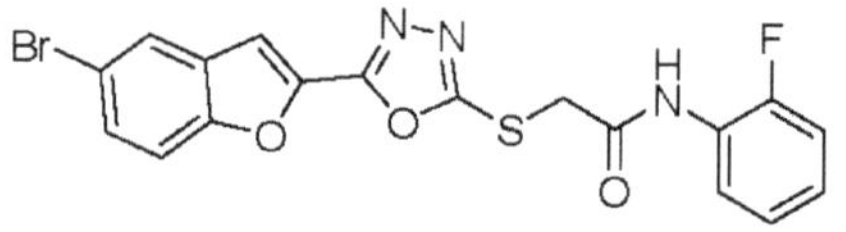

Table 5. *Cont.*

Compounds	Structures of Furan-1,3,4-Oxadiazssoles
BF9	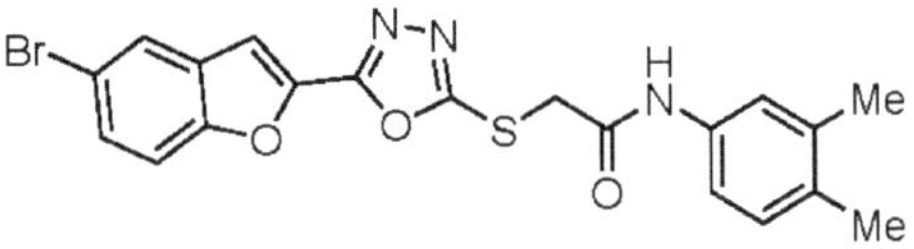
BF10	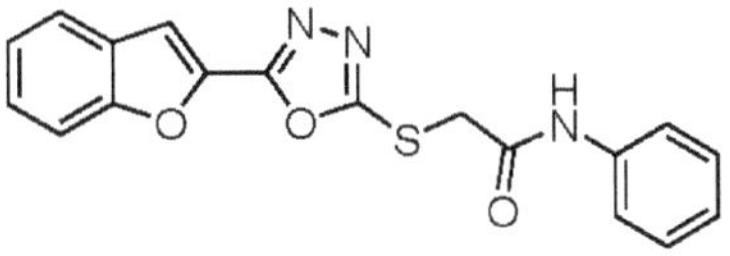
BF11	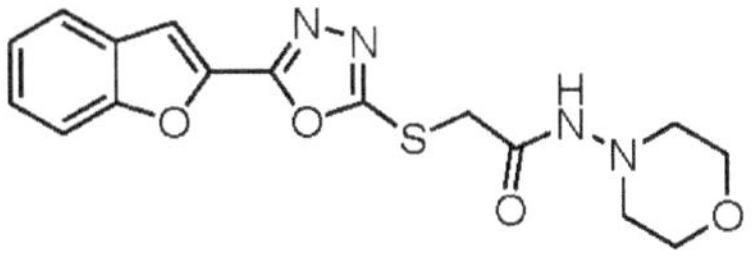
BF12	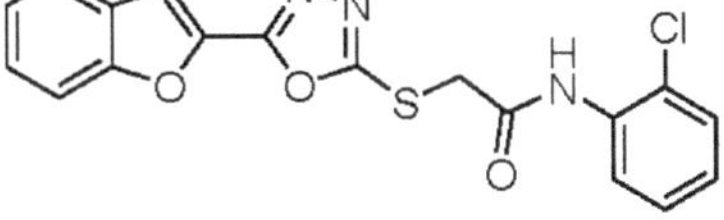
BF13	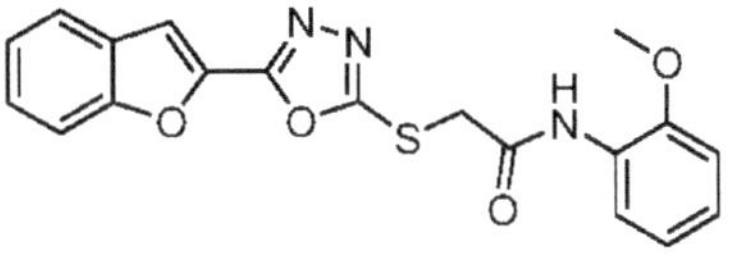
BF14	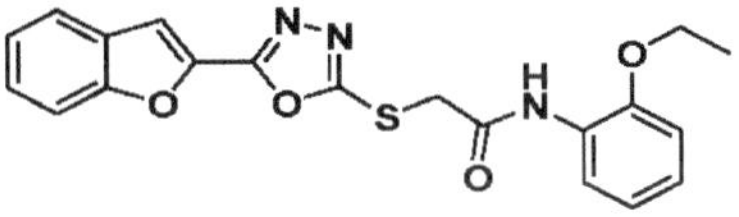
BF15	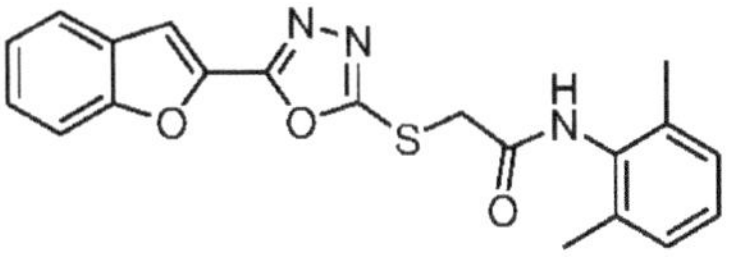
BF16	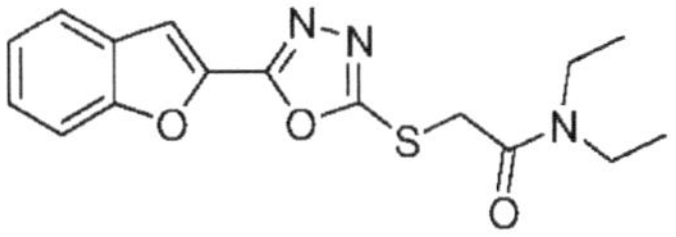

3.2. In Silico Biological Evaluation of Furan-1,3,4-Oxadiazoles BF1–BF16

3.2.1. Molecular Docking, ADME&T, Drug-Likeness, and Protein Homology Modeling Studies

The PDB structure of the target enzyme hTYR was predicted with homology modeling via the Swiss-Model prediction server using the fasta sequence of human tyrosinase with Uniprot ID = P14679 (because its resolved crystal structure is not available yet), while the structure of the hTYRP1 PDB ID-5M8M was accessed from the RCSB website for the computational investigations. The molecular docking investigations were performed via the Molecular Operating Environment (MOE) (Version-2009.10). Before docking, the protein structure of the hTYR and hTYRP1 enzyme was prepared for docking studies using the Biovia DS software. The structures of ligands **BF1–BF16** were prepared using the ChemDraw Professional. The (.mol) format structure of these ligands was imported into MOE, where the partial charges were added to them along with energy minimization of these compounds, which was performed using the MMFF94x –ff. In MOE, the protein structures were loaded and 3D-protonated; after that, its site-finder function was utilized for the active site identification. The triangle matcher technique and the London-dG scoring functions were used for the binding affinity estimations of these compounds against the target enzymes by the DOCK module of the MOE Software. Furthermore, the BIOVIA DS (Version-2017) software was utilized for the interaction analysis and visualization of the ligand–protein complexes [40–49]. The ADMET and drug-likeness investigation were carried out using the Swissadme and ADMETlab (Version 2.0) online servers, while the admetSAR (Version 1.0 and 2.0) online servers were utilized for the toxicity investigations of these compounds [50–53].

3.2.2. Molecular Dynamic Simulation Studies

For all docked complexes, the computer-based molecular dynamic simulations were performed employing AMBER (Version-20) simulation software. This analysis was important to conduct in order to understand protein–ligand's stability and dynamics in simulated time scale. In order to define parameters for the proteins and compounds, AMBER FF14SBand GAFF force fields were used, respectively. Charge assignment was carried out using the AMBER antechamber program. The placement of complexes into TIP3 simulation box was then accomplished by setting the distance between the molecules and box edge as 12 Å. Addition of counter ions was performed to obtain neutral systems. Long-range electrostatic interactions were evaluated using the Ewald summation method. The SHAKE algorithm was applied to constrain bounded hydrogen atoms, while to control temperature and pressure, Langevin and Berendson's barostats were run, respectively [54–60].

Prior to production, the complexes were minimized for energy in two stages; first by fast steepest descent for 10,000 steps followed by slow conjugate gradient for 15,000 steps. The complexes were then heated to 300 K. The equilibration of complexes was achieved using NPT and NVE ensembles with a collision frequency of 2. The production run was performed for 100 ns and the generated trajectories were evaluated through the CPPTRAJ tool [61]. The statistical plots were produced using XMGRACE (Version-5.1).

3.2.3. Estimation of Binding Energies and Interactions (MM-GBSA and MM-PBSA)

Estimation of binding interactions was carried out using the molecular mechanics Poisson–Boltzmann surface area (MM-PBSA) technique of AMBER (Version-20). This involves the calculation of continuum electrostatics, molecular mechanics, and solvent-accessible surface area [62,63]. Equation (1) was used for this calculation to describe the difference between the energy of the complex, receptor and ligand, as shown below (Equation (1)) [64,65].

$$\Delta G_{bind} = G_{complex} - G_{protein} - G_{ligand} = \Delta E_{MM} + \Delta G_{sol} - T\Delta S \tag{1}$$

The equation was performed on 1000 simulation frames and the net-binding energies were estimated as a sum of gas phase and solvation energies.

4. Conclusions

In conclusion, we have evaluated sixteen furan-1,3,4-oxadiazole tethered *N*-phenylacetamides, **BF1–BF16**, which were evaluated via in silico analysis for melanogenesis. We have screened out the most bioactive *N*-phenylacetamide-based furan-1,3,4-oxadiazole scaffolds, **BF4** and **BF5**, against hTYRP1 and hTYR, respectively. Among these promising molecules, 2,5-dimethoxy containing furan-1,3,4-oxadiazole, **BF4**, displayed stronger binding affinity (−11.50 kcal/mol) against hTYRP1, and 2-methoxy containing furan-1,3,4-oxadiazole, **BF5**, exhibited the best binding affinity (−13.30 kcal/mol) against hTYR compared to the binding in affinities of its standard inhibitor drug kojic acid. Furthermore, the MM-GBSA/MM-PBSA binding energy analysis also showed that these two compounds, **BF4** and **BF5**, bind strongly with the target enzymes hTYRP1 and hTYR. The molecular dynamics simulations stability analysis of the simulation trajectories of these complexes after the 100 ns simulation time provided insights into the stable bindings of these *N*-phenylacetamide-based furan-1,3,4-oxadiazole compounds (**BF4** and **BF5**) within the hTYRP1 and hTYR enzymes active sites. The furan-1,3,4-oxadiazole tethered *N*-phenylacetamide structural hybrids **BF4** and **BF5** also exhibited good ADMET and drug-likeness properties, which suggests the suitability of these compounds as potent inhibitory drug candidates against hTYRP1 and hTYR.

Author Contributions: Conceptualization, A.F.Z., M.E.A.Z. and A.I.; methodology, A.I.; software, S.F., A.I. and S.A.; validation, S.F., S.A. and A.I.; formal analysis, A.I., S.F., S.J. and S.A.; investigation, A.I. and S.F.; resources, A.F.Z. and S.A.A.-H.; data curation, S.A.A.-H., A.I. and S.J.; writing—original draft preparation, A.I.; writing—review and editing, A.I., B.P., S.F., A.F.Z. and M.E.A.Z.; visualization, S.F.; supervision, A.F.Z.; project administration, A.F.Z. and M.E.A.Z.; funding acquisition, S.A.A.-H. and M.E.A.Z. All authors have read and agreed to the published version of the manuscript.

Funding: This research was supported by the Deanship of Scientific Research, Imam Mohammad Ibn Saud Islamic University (IMSIU), Saudi Arabia.

Institutional Review Board Statement: Not applicable.

Informed Consent Statement: Not applicable.

Data Availability Statement: Data is contained within the article.

Acknowledgments: The authors acknowledge the Government College University Faisalabad for the research facilities provided to carry out this research work.

Conflicts of Interest: The authors declare no conflict of interest.

References

1. Zhang, W.; Zeng, W.; Jiang, A.; He, Z.; Shen, X.; Dong, X.; Feng, J.; Lu, H. Global, Regional and National Incidence, Mortality and Disability-Adjusted Life-Years of Skin Cancers and Trend Analysis from 1990 to 2019: An Analysis of the Global Burden of Disease Study 2019. *Cancer Med.* **2021**, *10*, 4905–4922. [CrossRef] [PubMed]
2. Ijaz, S.; Akhtar, N.; Khan, M.S.; Hameed, A.; Irfan, M.; Arshad, M.A.; Ali, S.; Asrar, M. Plant Derived Anticancer Agents: A Green Approach towards Skin Cancers. *Biomed. Pharmacother.* **2018**, *103*, 1643–1651. [CrossRef] [PubMed]
3. Apalla, Z.; Lallas, A.; Sotiriou, E.; Lazaridou, E.; Ioannides, D. Epidemiological Trends in Skin Cancer. *Dermatol. Pract. Concept.* **2017**, *7*, 1–6. [CrossRef] [PubMed]
4. Simões, M.C.F.; Sousa, J.J.S.; Pais, A.A.C.C. Skin Cancer and New Treatment Perspectives: A Review. *Cancer Lett.* **2015**, *357*, 8–42. [CrossRef]
5. Chummun, S.; McLean, N.R. The Management of Malignant Skin Cancers. *Surgery* **2017**, *35*, 519–524.
6. Testori, A.; Rutkowski, P.; Marsden, J.; Bastholt, L.; Chiarion-Sileni, V.; Hauschild, A.; Eggermont, A.M.M. Surgery and Radiotherapy in the Treatment of Cutaneous Melanoma. *Ann. Oncol.* **2009**, *20*, vi22–vi29. [CrossRef]
7. Shtivelman, E.; Davies, M.A.; Hwu, P.; Yang, J.; Lotem, M.; Oren, M.; Flaherty, K.T.; Fisher, D.E. Pathways and Therapeutic Targets in Melanoma. *Oncotarget* **2014**, *5*, 1701–1752. [CrossRef]
8. Gray-Schopfer, V.; Wellbrock, C.; Marais, R. Melanoma Biology and New Targeted Therapy. *Nature* **2007**, *445*, 851–857. [CrossRef]
9. Xu, X.; Zhang, P.J.; Elder, D.E.; Haupt, H.M.; Stern, J.B.; Multhaupt, H.A.B. Tyrosinase Expression in Malignant Melanoma, Desmoplastic Melanoma, and Peripheral Nerve Tumors. *Arch. Pathol. Lab. Med.* **2003**, *127*, 1083–1085. [CrossRef]
10. Bandarchi, B.; Ma, L.; Navab, R.; Seth, A.; Rasty, G. From Melanocyte to Metastatic Malignant Melanoma. *Dermatol. Res. Pract.* **2010**, *2010*, 583748. [CrossRef]
11. Kobayashi, T.; Urabe, K.; Winder, A.; Jiménez-Cervantes, C.; Imokawa, G.; Brewington, T.; Solano, F.; García-Borrón, J.C.; Hearing, V.J. Tyrosinase Related Protein 1 (TRP1) Functions as a DHICA Oxidase in Melanin Biosynthesis. *EMBO J.* **1994**, *13*, 5818–5825. [CrossRef]
12. Ghanem, G.; Fabrice, J. Tyrosinase Related Protein 1 (TYRP1/Gp75) in Human Cutaneous Melanoma. *Mol. Oncol.* **2011**, *5*, 150–155. [CrossRef] [PubMed]
13. Khalil, D.N.; Postow, M.A.; Ibrahim, N.; Ludwig, D.L.; Cosaert, J.; Kambhampati, S.R.P.; Tang, S.; Grebennik, D.; Kauh, J.S.W.; Lenz, H.J.; et al. An Open-Label, Dose-Escalation Phase I Study of Anti-TYRP1 Monoclonal Antibody IMC-20D7S for Patients with Relapsed or Refractory Melanoma. *Clin. Cancer Res.* **2016**, *22*, 5204–5210. [CrossRef] [PubMed]

14. Buitrago, E.; Hardré, R.; Haudecoeur, R.; Jamet, H.; Belle, C.; Boumendjel, A.; Bubacco, L.; Réglier, M. Are Human Tyrosinase and Related Proteins Suitable Targets for Melanoma Therapy? *Curr. Top. Med. Chem.* **2016**, *16*, 3033–3047. [CrossRef]
15. Mroz, P.; Huang, Y.; Szokalska, A.; Zhiyentayev, T.; Janjua, S.; Nifli, A.; Sherwood, M.E.; Ruzié, C.; Borbas, K.E.; Fan, D.; et al. Stable Synthetic Bacteriochlorins Overcome the Resistance of Melanoma to Photodynamic Therapy. *FASEB J.* **2010**, *24*, 3160–3170. [CrossRef] [PubMed]
16. Kameyama, K.; Sakai, C.; Kuge, S.; Nishiyama, S.; Tomita, Y.; Ito, S.; Wakamatsu, K.; Hearing, V.J. The Expression of Tyrosinase Tyrosinase-Related Proteins 1 and 2 (TRP1 and TRP2), the Silver Protein, and a Melanogenic Inhibitor in Human Melanoma Cells of Differing Melanogenic Activities. *Pigment. Cell Res.* **1995**, *8*, 97–104. [CrossRef] [PubMed]
17. Brożyna, A.A.; VanMiddlesworth, L.; Slominski, A.T. Inhibition of Melanogenesis as a Radiation Sensitizer for Melanoma Therapy. *Int. J. Cancer* **2008**, *123*, 1448–1456. [CrossRef]
18. Sharma, K.V.; Bowers, N.; Davids, L.M. Photodynamic Therapy-Induced Killing Is Enhanced in Depigmented Metastatic Melanoma Cells. *Cell Biol. Int.* **2011**, *35*, 939–944. [CrossRef]
19. Yan, J.; Tingey, C.; Lyde, R.; Gorham, T.C.; Choo, D.K.; Muthumani, A.; Myles, D.; Weiner, L.P.; Kraynyak, K.A.; Reuschel, E.L.; et al. Novel and Enhanced Anti-Melanoma DNA Vaccine Targeting the Tyrosinase Protein Inhibits Myeloid Derived Suppressor Cells and Tumor Growth in a Syngeneic Prophylactic and Therapeutic Murine Model. *Cancer Gene Ther.* **2014**, *21*, 507–517. [CrossRef]
20. Vargas, A.J.; Sittadjody, S.; Thangasamy, T.; Mendoza, E.E.; Limesand, K.H.; Burd, R. Exploiting Tyrosinase Expression and Activity in Melanocytic Tumors: Quercetin and the Central Role of P53. *Integr. Cancer Ther.* **2011**, *10*, 328–340. [CrossRef]
21. Jawaid, S.; Khan, T.H.; Osborn, H.M.I.; Williams, N.A.O. Tyrosinase Activated Melanoma Prodrugs. *Anticancer Agents Med. Chem.* **2012**, *9*, 717–727. [CrossRef] [PubMed]
22. Dean, F.M.; Sargent, M.V. 3.10-Furans and their Benzo Derivatives: (i) Structure. In *Comprehensive Heterocyclic Chemistry*; Elsevier: Amsterdam, The Netherlands, 1984; Volume 4, pp. 531–597. [CrossRef]
23. Rymbai, E.M.; Chakraborty, A.; Choudhury, R.; Biplab De, N.V. Review on Chemistry and Therapeutic Activity of the Derivatives of Furan and Oxazole: The Oxygen Containing Heterocycles. *Der Pharma Chem.* **2019**, *11*, 20–41.
24. Rodd, E.H. *Chemistry of Carbon Compounds: A Modern Comprehensive Treatise*; Elsevier: Amsterdam, The Netherlands, 1971.
25. Limpricht, H. Ueber das Tetraphenol C_4H_4O. *Ber. Der Dtsch. Chem. Ges.* **1870**, *3*, 90–91. [CrossRef]
26. Miao, Y.H.; Hu, Y.H.; Yang, J.; Liu, T.; Sun, J.; Wang, X.J. Natural source, bioactivity and synthesis of benzofuran derivatives. *RSC Adv.* **2019**, *9*, 27510. [CrossRef] [PubMed]
27. Vanjare, B.D.; Choi, N.G.; Mahajan, P.G.; Raza, H.; Hassan, M.; Han, Y.; Yu, S.M.; Kim, S.J.; Seo, S.Y.; Lee, K.H. Novel 1,3,4 oxadiazole compounds inhibit the tyrosinase and melanin level: Synthesis, in-vitro, and in-silico studies. *Bioorg. Med. Chem.* **2021**, *1*, 116222. [CrossRef]
28. Mann, T.; Gerwat, W.; Batzer, J.; Eggers, K.; Scherner, C.; Wenck, H.; Stäb, F.; Hearing, V.J.; Röhm, K.H.; Kolbe, L. Inhibition of Human Tyrosinase Requires Molecular Motifs Distinctively Different from Mushroom Tyrosinase. *J. Investig. Dermatol.* **2018**, *138*, 1601–1608. [CrossRef]
29. Roulier, B.; Pérès, B.; Haudecoeur, R. Advances in the Design of Genuine Human Tyrosinase Inhibitors for Targeting Melanogenesis and Related Pigmentations. *J. Med. Chem.* **2020**, *63*, 13428–13443. [CrossRef]
30. Koirala, P.; Seong, S.H.; Zhou, Y.; Shrestha, S.; Jung, H.A.; Choi, J.S. Structure–Activity Relationship of the Tyrosinase Inhibitors Kuwanon G, Mulberrofuran G, and Albanol B from Morus Species: A Kinetics and Molecular Docking Study. *Molecules* **2018**, *23*, 1413. [CrossRef]
31. Okombi, S.; Rival, D.; Bonnet, S.; Mariotte, A.M.; Perrier, E.; Boumendjel, A. Discovery of Benzylidenebenzofuran-3(2H)-One (Aurones) as Inhibitors of Tyrosinase Derived from Human Melanocytes. *J. Med. Chem.* **2006**, *49*, 329–333. [CrossRef]
32. Hu, X.; Wang, M.; Yan, G.R.; Yu, M.H.; Wang, H.Y.; Hou, A.J. 2-Arylbenzofuran and Tyrosinase Inhibitory Constituents of MorusNotabilis. *J. Asian Nat. Prod. Res.* **2012**, *14*, 1103–1108. [CrossRef]
33. Faiz, S.; Zahoor, A.F.; Ajmal, M.; Kamal, S.; Ahmad, S.; Abdelgawad, A.M.; Elnaggar, E.M. Design, synthesis, antimicrobial evaluation, and laccase catalysis effect of novel benzofuran–oxadiazole and benzofuran–triazole hybrids. *J. Heterocycl. Chem.* **2019**, *56*, 2839–2852. [CrossRef]
34. Hassan, M.; Ashraf, Z.; Abbas, Q.; Raza, H.; Seo, S.Y. Exploration of Novel Human Tyrosinase Inhibitors by Molecular Modeling, Docking and Simulation Studies. *Interdiscip. Sci. Comput. Life Sci.* **2018**, *10*, 68–80. [CrossRef] [PubMed]
35. Shahzadi, I.; Zahoor, F.A.; Rasul, A.; Mansha, A.; Ahmad, S.; Raza, Z. Synthesis, hemolytic studies, and in silico modeling of novel acefylline-1,2,4-triazole hybrids as potential anti-cancer agents against MCF-7 and A549. *ACS Omega* **2021**, *6*, 11943–11953. [CrossRef] [PubMed]
36. Lee, J.H.; Mei, H.C.; Kuo, I.C.; Lee, T.H.; Chen, Y.H.; Lee, C.K. Characterizing Tyrosinase Modulators from the Roots of Angelica Keiskei Using Tyrosinase Inhibition Assay and UPLC-MS/MS as the Combinatorial Novel Approach. *Molecules* **2019**, *24*, 3297. [CrossRef] [PubMed]
37. Waterhouse, A.; Bertoni, M.; Bienert, S.; Studer, G.; Tauriello, G.; Gumienny, R.; Heer, F.T.; De Beer, T.A.P.; Rempfer, C.; Bordoli, L.; et al. SWISS-MODEL: Homology Modelling of Protein Structures and Complexes. *Nucleic Acids Res.* **2018**, *46*, W296–W303. [CrossRef]

38. Irfan, A.; Zahoor, A.F.; Kamal, S.; Hassan, M.; Kloczkowski, A. Ultrasonic-Assisted Synthesis of Benzofuran Appended Oxadiazole Molecules as Tyrosinase Inhibitors: Mechanistic Approach through Enzyme Inhibition, Molecular Docking, Chemoinformatics, ADMET and Drug-Likeness Studies. *Int. J. Mol. Sci.* **2022**, *23*, 10979. [CrossRef]
39. Irfan, A.; Faiz, S.; Rasul, A.; Zafar, R.; Zahoor, A.F.; Kotwica-Mojzych, K.; Mojzych, M. Exploring the Synergistic Anticancer Potential of Benzofuran–Oxadiazoles and Triazoles: Improved Ultrasound- and Microwave-Assisted Synthesis, Molecular Docking, Hemolytic, Thrombolytic and Anticancer Evaluation of Furan-Based Molecules. *Molecules* **2022**, *27*, 1023. [CrossRef]
40. Lai, X.; Wichers, H.J.; Soler-Lopez, M.; Dijkstra, B.W. Structure of Human Tyrosinase Related Protein 1 Reveals a Binuclear Zinc Active Site Important for Melanogenesis. *Angew. Chem.* **2017**, *129*, 9944–9947. [CrossRef]
41. Burley, S.K.; Berman, H.M.; Bhikadiya, C.; Bi, C.; Chen, L.; Di Costanzo, L.; Christie, C.; Dalenberg, K.; Duarte, J.M.; Dutta, S.; et al. RCSB Protein Data Bank: Biological Macromolecular Structures Enabling Research and Education in Fundamental Biology, Biomedicine, Biotechnology and Energy. *Nucleic Acids Res.* **2019**, *47*, D464–D474. [CrossRef]
42. Vilar, S.; Cozza, G.; Moro, S. Medicinal Chemistry and the Molecular Operating Environment (MOE): Application of QSAR and Molecular Docking to Drug Discovery. *Curr. Top. Med. Chem.* **2008**, *8*, 1555–1572. [CrossRef]
43. Faisal, S.; Lal Badshah, S.; Kubra, B.; Sharaf, M.; Emwas, A.H.; Jaremko, M.; Abdalla, M. Computational Study of Sars-Cov-2 Rna Dependent Rna Polymerase Allosteric Site Inhibition. *Molecules* **2022**, *27*, 223. [CrossRef] [PubMed]
44. Dassault Systèmes. *BIOVIA Discovery Studio Visualizer, Release 2017*; Dassault Systèmes: Vélizy-Villacoublay, France, 2023.
45. Mills, N. ChemDraw Ultra 10.0 CambridgeSoft, 100 CambridgePark Drive, Cambridge, MA 02140. www.cambridgesoft.com. Commercial Price: $1910 for download, $2150 for CD-ROM; Academic Price: $710 for download, $800 for CD-ROM. *J. Am. Chem. Soc.* **2006**, *128*, 13649–13650. [CrossRef]
46. Shinu, P.; Sharma, M.; Gupta, G.L.; Mujwar, S.; Kandeel, M.; Kumar, M.; Nair, A.B.; Goyal, M.; Singh, P.; Attimarad, M.; et al. Computational Design, Synthesis, and Pharmacological Evaluation of Naproxen-Guaiacol Chimera for Gastro-Sparing Anti-Inflammatory Response by Selective COX2 Inhibition. *Molecules* **2022**, *27*, 6905. [CrossRef] [PubMed]
47. Mujwar, S.; Sun, L.; Fidan, O. In silico evaluation of food-derived carotenoids against SARS-CoV-2 drug targets: Crocin is a promising dietary supplement candidate for COVID-19. *J. Food Biochem.* **2022**, *46*, e14219. [CrossRef] [PubMed]
48. Fidan, O.; Mujwar, S.; Kciuk, M. Discovery of adapalene and dihydrotachysterol as antiviral agents for the Omicron variant of SARS-CoV-2 through computational drug repurposing. *Mol. Divers.* **2022**, *4*, 1–13. [CrossRef]
49. Kciuk, M.; Mujwar, S.; Szymanowska, A.; Marciniak, B.; Bukowski, K.; Mojzych, M.; Kontek, R. Preparation of Novel Pyrazolo[4,3-*e*]tetrazolo[1,5-b][1,2,4]triazine Sulfonamides and Their Experimental and Computational Biological Studies. *Int. J. Mol. Sci.* **2022**, *23*, 5892. [CrossRef] [PubMed]
50. Daina, A.; Michielin, O.; Zoete, V. SwissADME: A Free Web Tool to Evaluate Pharmacokinetics, Drug-Likeness and Medicinal Chemistry Friendliness of Small Molecules. *Sci. Rep.* **2017**, *7*, 42717. [CrossRef]
51. Xiong, G.; Wu, Z.; Yi, J.; Fu, L.; Yang, Z.; Hsieh, C.; Yin, M.; Zeng, X.; Wu, C.; Lu, A.; et al. ADMETlab 2.0: An Integrated Online Platform for Accurate and Comprehensive Predictions of ADMET Properties. *Nucleic Acids Res.* **2021**, *49*, W5–W14. [CrossRef]
52. Yang, H.; Lou, C.; Sun, L.; Li, J.; Cai, Y.; Wang, Z.; Li, W.; Liu, G.; Tang, Y. AdmetSAR 2.0: Web-Service for Prediction and Optimization of Chemical ADMET Properties. *Bioinformatics* **2019**, *35*, 1067–1069. [CrossRef]
53. Cheng, F.; Li, W.; Zhou, Y.; Shen, J.; Wu, Z.; Liu, G.; Lee, P.W.; Tang, Y. AdmetSAR: A Comprehensive Source and Free Tool for Assessment of Chemical ADMET Properties. *J. Chem. Inf. Model.* **2012**, *52*, 3099–3105. [CrossRef]
54. Case, D.A.; Cheatham, T.E., III; Darden, T.; Gohlke, H.; Luo, R.; Merz, K.M., Jr.; Onufriev, A.; Simmerling, C.; Wang, B.; Woods, R.J. The Amber Biomolecular Simulation Programs. *J. Comb. Chem.* **2005**, *26*, 1668–1688. [CrossRef]
55. Maier, J.A.; Martinez, C.; Kasavajhala, K.; Wickstrom, L.; Hauser, K.E.; Simmerling, C. Ff14SB: Improving the Accuracy of Protein Side Chain and Backbone Parameters from Ff99SB. *J. Chem. Theory Comput.* **2015**, *11*, 3696–3713. [CrossRef] [PubMed]
56. Wang, J.; Wolf, R.M.; Caldwell, J.W.; Kollman, P.A.; Case, D.A. Development and Testing of a General Amber Force Field. *J. Comput. Chem.* **2004**, *25*, 1157–1174. [CrossRef] [PubMed]
57. Wang, J.; Wang, W.; Kollman, P.A.; Case, D.A. Antechamber, An Accessory Software Package For Molecular Mechanical Calculations. *J. Am. Chem. Soc.* **2001**, *222*, 403.
58. Saunders, W.R.; Grant, J.; Müller, E.H. Long Range Forces in a Performance Portable Molecular Dynamics Framework. *Adv. Parallel Comput.* **2018**, *22*, 37–46. [CrossRef]
59. Paquet, E.; Viktor, H.L. Molecular Dynamics, Monte Carlo Simulations, and Langevin Dynamics: A Computational Review. *BioMed Res. Int.* **2015**, *2015*, 183918. [CrossRef]
60. Lin, Y.; Pan, D.; Li, J.; Zhang, L.; Shao, X. Application of BerendsenBarostat in Dissipative Particle Dynamics for Nonequilibrium Dynamic Simulation. *J. Chem. Phys.* **2017**, *146*, 124108. [CrossRef]
61. Roe, D.R.; Cheatham, T.E. PTRAJ and CPPTRAJ: Software for Processing and Analysis of Molecular Dynamics Trajectory Data. *J. Chem. Theory Comput.* **2013**, *9*, 3084–3095. [CrossRef]
62. Miller, B.R.; McGee, T.D.; Swails, J.M.; Homeyer, N.; Gohlke, H.; Roitberg, A.E. MMPBSA.Py: An Efficient Program for End-State Free Energy Calculations. *J. Chem. Theory Comput.* **2012**, *8*, 3314–3321. [CrossRef]

63. Sun, H.; Li, Y.; Shen, M.; Tian, S.; Xu, L.; Pan, P.; Guan, Y.; Hou, T. Assessing the Performance of MM/PBSA and MM/GBSA Methods. 5. Improved Docking Performance Using High Solute Dielectric Constant MM/GBSA and MM/PBSA Rescoring. *Phys. Chem. Chem. Phys.* **2014**, *16*, 22035–22045. [CrossRef]

64. Hou, T.; Wang, J.; Li, Y.; Wang, W. Assessing the Performance of the MM/PBSA and MM/GBSA Methods. 1. The Accuracy of Binding Free Energy Calculations Based on Molecular Dynamics Simulations. *J. Chem. Inf. Model.* **2011**, *51*, 69–82. [CrossRef] [PubMed]

65. Zhang, Y.; Qiu, Y.; Zhang, H. Computational Investigation of Structural Basis for Enhanced Binding of Isoflavone Analogues with Mitochondrial Aldehyde Dehydrogenase. *ACS Omega* **2022**, *7*, 8115–8127. [CrossRef] [PubMed]

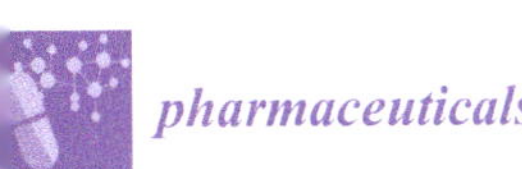

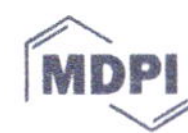

Article

In Silico Screening of Drugs That Target Different Forms of E Protein for Potential Treatment of COVID-19

Gema Lizbeth Ramírez Salinas [1,†], Alejandro López Rincón [2,3], Jazmín García Machorro [4], José Correa Basurto [1,*] and Marlet Martínez Archundia [1,*,†]

1 Laboratorio de Diseño y Desarrollo de Nuevos Fármacos e Innovación Biotecnológica (Laboratory for the Design and Development of New Drugs and Biotechnological Innovation), Escuela Superior de Medicina, Instituto Politécnico Nacional, México City 11340, Mexico
2 Utrecht Institute for Pharmaceutical Sciences, Division Pharmacology, Utrecht University, 3553 Utrecht, The Netherlands
3 Julius Center for Health Sciences and Primary Care, Department of Data Science, University Medical Center Utrecht, 3553 Utrecht, The Netherlands
4 Laboratorio de Medicina de Conservación, Escuela Superior de Medicina, Instituto Politécnico Nacional, México City 11340, Mexico
* Correspondence: corrjose@gmail.com (J.C.B.); marletm8@gmail.com or mtmartineza@ipn.mx (M.M.A.)
† These authors contributed equally to this work.

Abstract: Recently the E protein of SARS-CoV-2 has become a very important target in the potential treatment of COVID-19 since it is known to regulate different stages of the viral cycle. There is biochemical evidence that E protein exists in two forms, as monomer and homopentamer. An in silico screening analysis was carried out employing 5852 ligands (from Zinc databases), and performing an ADMET analysis, remaining a set of 2155 compounds. Furthermore, docking analysis was performed on specific sites and different forms of the E protein. From this study we could identify that the following ligands showed the highest binding affinity: nilotinib, dutasteride, irinotecan, saquinavir and alectinib. We carried out some molecular dynamics simulations and free energy MM–PBSA calculations of the protein–ligand complexes (with the mentioned ligands). Of worthy interest is that saquinavir, nilotinib and alectinib are also considered as a promising multitarget ligand because it seems to inhibit three targets, which play an important role in the viral cycle. On the other side, saquinavir was shown to be able to bind to E protein both in its monomeric as well as pentameric forms. Finally, further experimental assays are needed to probe our hypothesis derived from in silico studies.

Keywords: SARS-CoV-2; COVID-19; drug repositioning; in silico studies; E protein

Citation: Ramírez Salinas, G.L.; López Rincón, A.; García Machorro, J.; Correa Basurto, J.; Martínez Archundia, M. In Silico Screening of Drugs That Target Different Forms of E Protein for Potential Treatment of COVID-19. *Pharmaceuticals* **2023**, *16*, 296. https://doi.org/10.3390/ph16020296

Academic Editors: Halil İbrahim Çiftçi, Belgin Sever and Hasan Demirci

Received: 9 December 2022
Revised: 8 February 2023
Accepted: 8 February 2023
Published: 14 February 2023

1. Introduction

The coronavirus (CoV) belongs to the *Coronaviridae* family, subfamily *Coronavirinae*. They are RNA single-stranded and enveloped viruses. The subfamily *Coronavirinae* are divided in four genera: alpha, beta, gamma and delta coronavirus. The CoVs are able to infect different species of mammals, including human beings, mainly the beta coronavirus [1]. The first reports on endemic human CoV (HCoV) were published in the decade of 1960, when HCoV-OC43 and HCoV-229E were first described. Some years later, HCoV-NL63 and HCoV-HKU1 were discovered in 2004 and 2005 [2,3].

Some of the most known endemic CoVs in the last two decades include: (a) SARS-CoV that emerged in 2002 with about 8000 cases all over the world and with a mortality rate of 9.6%, (b) MERS-CoV that emerged in 2012 and infected about 2500 over the world and with a mortality rate of 40%, and (c) SARS-CoV-2 which shows a mortality of 6.9% [4], representing the lowest rate in comparison to other coronaviruses but with the highest efficiency of virus spread infecting 676,945,055 people and 6,777,045 of deaths (9 February 2023) [5], leading to an important social, economic and health problem all over the globe.

The disease originated by SARS-CoV-2 has been denominated COVID-19. The pathology of COVID-19 has been characterized by intense, rapid stimulation of the innate immune response that triggers activation of diverse proteins such as inflammasome (NOD-like receptor family, pyrin domain containing 3 (NLRP3), NOD-like receptor family and among others) [6].

The CoV genome codifies four main structural proteins: spike protein (S), nucleocapsid (N), membrane protein (M) and envelope protein (E). All these proteins are necessary to assemble the virus and to release new viruses in the human cells [7,8]. These structural proteins are conserved from a subgenomic RNA. From all these structural proteins, E protein is the least abundant protein of the mature viral particles and is also the smallest [9,10]. Specifically, for the CoV, the E protein is particularly expressed during the cellular infection stage although only a small portion of this protein is incorporated into the virions [10,11].

The E protein of the CoV is an integral membrane protein which consists of 76 to 109 amino acids and has a molecular size within 8.4 to 12 kDa [12,13]. This protein shows a short N-terminal segment of 7 to 12 residues followed by a hydrophobic transmembrane domain (TMD) of 25 residues and ending up with a large hydrophilic C-terminal segment (segment 38–75) [13,14]. The E protein shows palindromic transmembrane helical hairpin around a pseudo-center of symmetry. The hairpin deforms lipid bilayers by way of increasing their curvature, while playing a fundamental role in viral budding [15]. Some other critical functions of E protein include replication cycle, including virion assembly, budding, release, and pathogenesis processes [16] The TMD manifests ion channel activity, while the C-terminal segment and N-terminal region participate in protein–protein interactions [17].

1.1. Homopentamer

This E protein is viroporin. These viroporins are known to form membrane pores [14, 18,19]. It has been reported that during the viral infection, the viroporins oligomerize causing the disruption of the physiological homeostasis in the host cell while contributing the viral pathogenicity [20].

1.2. Ion Channel

The E protein of CoV is selective to cations which is related to its ionic channel properties, and it shows its preference for the cationic monovalent Na^+ and K^+. Moreover, E protein is essential and known for its role in the activation of the inflammatory NF-kB pathway [21]. The E protein also forms a calcium ion (Ca^{2+}) channel in the endoplasmic reticulum Golgi apparatus intermediate compartment (ERGIC)/Golgi membranes [21]. The changes in calcium homeostasis in the intracellular environment leads to activation of the cytosolic innate immune signaling receptor NLRP3 inflammasome [6].

The activation of the inflammasome for the E protein of SARS-CoV was identified for the first time in porcine reproductive and respiratory syndrome virus (PRRSV). The blockage of the activity of the ionic channel with amantadine significantly inhibited the activation of the inflammasome which suggests the role of the E protein in the inflammation processes [13]. Additionally, it has been shown the role of the E protein in Ca^{2+} transportation in SARS-CoV, which triggers activation of the inflammasome [21]. Interestingly, it has been associated to the decrease of inflammatory cytokines in the absence of activity of ionic channel E in CoV as well as the inhibition or deficiency of the E protein [13,17,22].

Additionally, the biochemical evidence proposes that the capability of the E protein of the CoV to form homo-oligomeric conformers depends on its TMD [13,23]. In addition, the capacity of the E protein of CoV to assemble homopentameric structures is clearly important in the formation of a functional viroporin [13]. Recently, some point mutations in the TMD such as N15A and V25F have been found to eliminate the capability of ionic canalization of the viroporin; on the other hand, these mutations seem to block the oligomerization of the E protein in SARS-CoV [13,23]. The appearance of monomers in response to V25F clearly suggests that this residue plays a crucial role in oligomerization—in contrast to the N15A mutant, which reduces the pentamer formation [13,23]. The assembly of the homopentamer of E protein is crucial for virus replication [23].

1.3. N-Terminal

It has been determined that the N-terminal segment of the E protein is responsible for the activation of TLR2 in macrophages, and thus in the inflammatory signaling pathways [24–26]. For all these reasons, the N-terminal segment has been considered a potential target for inhibition. Recently, different experiments have been employed in order to identify proteins that are associated with the uncontrolled production of proinflammatory cytokines which could lead to a serious infection of COVID-19 [24].

1.4. Monomeric

The C-terminal region of E protein interacts with several other proteins:

(1) Interaction with PALS1:

The E protein by PDZ-Binding Motif (PBM) interacts with syntenin proteins which triggers the activation of the p38 MAPK and leads to the overexpression of inflammatory cytokines [27,28]. Additionally, the C-terminal domain of the monomeric E protein affects host intracellular activities through interference with the Golgi endoplasmic reticulum and intermediate compartment ER-Golgi [29]. The E protein monomer modulates intracellular activities of the host through the C-terminal domain (segment 38–75) [13]. In the C-terminal domain, there is the PDZ-domain binding motif (DLLV), which binds to the Protein Associated with Lin Seven 1 (PALS1) [30]. The interactions of the E protein of SARS and PALS1 protein introduced the relocation of PALS1 in the assembly site of the virus and interrupted the narrow binding sites to promote virus propagation [31]. The increased virulence of SARS-CoV-2 compared to SARS-CoV may rely on the increased affinity of its E protein for PALS1 [31,32]. The residues of E protein of SARS-CoV-2 that are involved in the formation of the complex E protein-PALS1 are: Val75, Leu74, Leu73, Asp72, Pro71 and Val70 [33].

(2) Interaction with BET:

Of worthy interest is that Gordon and collaborators found that the transmembrane E protein, which is likely resident on the endoplasmic reticulum-Golgi intermediate compartment and Golgi membranes, binds to bromodomain-containing protein 2 (BRD2) and bromodomain-containing protein 4 (BRD4) proteins, which are members of the bromodomain and extra-terminal (BET) domain family [34]. The C-terminal region of E protein mimics the N-terminal segment of histone H3, which is a known interacting partner of bromodomains [35].

On the other hand, it has been suggested that the interaction between BET with E protein can cause important changes in the genetic expression within the host cell, and thus, is also important for the viral cycle. BET proteins are also known to regulate immunity and inflammation mechanisms [36,37].

(3) Interaction with M protein:

The C-terminal segment of the E proteins is known to be important for the interaction with the C-terminal domain of the M protein, which is located at the cytoplasmic side of the endoplasmic reticulum-Golgi intermediate compartment, the budding compartment of the host cell [38]. The mentioned interactions are known to be considered important drivers for the envelope formation [39]. The interaction of the E protein with both PALS1 and BET proteins leads to proinflammatory activation mechanism, while interaction with M protein modulates viral budding processes and the release of newly formed viruses.

COVID-19 is characterized by an excessive production of proinflammatory cytokines, yielding in some cases to acute pulmonary damage which is highly associated with the mortality of the patients. Even though innate immunity cells produce multiple inflammatory cytokines during the SARS-CoV-2 infection, Karki and collaborators found that the combination of TNF-α and IFN-γ induces inflammatory cellular death [40]. The SARS-CoV-2 infection causes cardiac dysfunction induced by proinflammatory cytokines. Additionally,

TNF has been also associated with cardiac dysfunction, while inducing systolic dysfunction [37].

Due to the strong evidence that the E protein is crucial in the modulation of diverse processes, in this work we propose diverse in silico approaches to study the binding of potential inhibitors on this protein. Moreover, here we propose to investigate different forms of the E protein, such as monomer as well as pentamer. We also considered different potential sites of inhibition (1) ionic channel (pentamer), (2) N-terminal (pentamer), (3) C-terminal (monomer).

It has been stated in the literature that the C-terminal region is a very flexible segment. Two conformations of the monomer have been denominated: the first one is where the C-terminal region shows the shape of a curve or harpin, and it is embedded in the membrane [41,42]; the second conformation of the C-terminal region is exposed to solvent [41]. In the present work, we have investigated both conformations as potential sites of inhibition. Due to the sanitary emergency of the COVID-19 pandemic, it became quite important to discover new potential drugs for the treatment of this disease, although it is known that drug discovery is a time-consuming and high-investment process [43]. Nowadays, drug repositioning represents an effective strategy to find new uses for existing and already probed drugs which makes it a highly efficient, low cost and riskless procedure [43]. In this work, we have considered an in silico strategy from a large database of compounds while using ADMET screening analysis in order to identify potential drugs that could inhibit different conformations of the E protein of SARS-CoV-2.

2. Results

2.1. Molecular Modeling of E Protein of SARS-CoV-2

Quaternary structures of the homopentamer and monomeric E protein of SARS-CoV-2 were modeled. Figure 1 shows the quaternary structure of this homopentamer and monomeric forms, and ionic channels, N-terminal and C-terminal. As stated in the Methodology (Section 4.1), the tri-dimensional model of the E protein of SARS-CoV2 was built by using the crystal structure of the E protein of SARS-CoV (PDB: 5 × 29) and employing Modeller 10.1 Software. Alignment of the query vs. template is shown in the Supplementary Materials (Figure S2).

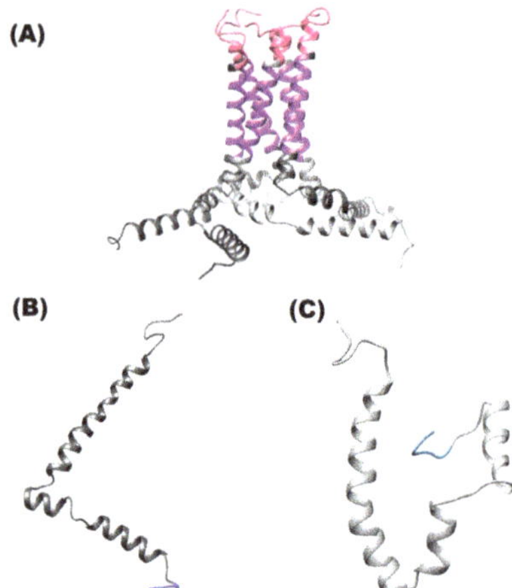

Figure 1. Structure of the E protein of SARS-CoV-2. (**A**) Shows the structure of homopentamer. (**B**) Three-dimensional structure of the protein is shown in ribbons and surface of the monomer C-terminal solvent-exposed. (**C**) Shows the ribbons of the monomer conformation (hairpin). Color pink (N-terminal site), color purple (ion channel) and color blue (C-terminal site).

2.2. In Silico ADMET Analysis

We screened 5852 compounds from the Zinc database through ADMET analysis, discarding the compounds that did not fulfill the safety requirements (3697 ligands). Furthermore, docking analysis was performed with the remaining 2155 compounds.

2.3. Molecular Docking Analysis on the Different Targets

Different docking analyses were carried out, considering different conditions: (a) homopentameric form as an ion channel itself and the N-terminal segment of this form, (b) monomer form which includes two binding sites: C-terminal solvent-exposed and hairpin. Four molecular docking studies were carried out, which are described (Tables S1–S4).

2.3.1. Molecular Docking Analysis on E Protein Form Homopentamer (Ionic Channel Region)

As can be seen in the Figure 2A, lumacaflor binds to E protein through Pi-Pi interactions which include the following residues: Phe26E, Phe26A y Phe23E, alkyl interactions with the residues Val29A, Val25A, Ala22E, Leu19E, Ala22C and Ala22B, halogen interactions with the residue Ala22D, and van der Waal's forces with the following residues: Phe23C, Phe26D, Phe26C, Phe26B, Val25D, Leu19C and Ala22A. Figure 2B shows that saquinavir binds to E protein through van der Waal's interactions by interacting with the residues Phe26B, Ala22B, Leu19A, Phe26C, Phe26D, Phe23C, Ala22D, Leu18D, Leu19C, Phe26A, Leu18E, Leu19D, Leu18B, Leu19E, Val25A, Phe23E, Leu18C, Asn15B, Leu21C and Pi-Sigma interaction with Ala22C, alkyl interactions with Ala 22A, Leu18A, Ala22E, Leu19B, and finally Pi-Pi interaction with Phe26E. In the Figure 2C is depicted that nilotinib interacts with E protein through diverse interactions such as: (a)van der Waal's interactions with the following residues: Leu28D, Leu27C, Val25D, Leu19A, Phe23A, Phe26B, Phe26A, Phe26D, Thr30C, Phe26E, Val29C, (b) Pi-sigma interactions with the amino acids: Ala22B and Ala22D, (c) Pi-Pi interactions with Phe26C, (d) Alkyl interactions with Ala22C, Leu19C, Ala22A and Val29D, and (e) Hydrogen bonds with Phe23C and Phe26C. The zafirlukast (Figure 2D) binds to E protein through Pi-Pi interactions which include the following residues: Phe26C, Phe26A, Phe26E and Phe23E, the amino acid Val29C forming Pi-sigma interactions, the van der Waal's interactions with Thr30C, Thr30B, Thr30E, Phe23C, Ile33C and Val29E, and these amino acids Val29D, Val29A, Val25D, Phe26B and Phe26D forming alkyl interactions.

2.3.2. Molecular Docking Studies on E Protein Form Homopentamer (N-Terminal Region)

The amino acids of the N-terminal region of E protein in the homopentamer form interact with alectinib (Figure 3) while showing the following interactions: Asn15D (Hydrogen bond), Glu8A (Salt Bridge), Thr11A, Glu7B (Pi-Sigma interactions), Val5B, Leu12A, (alkyl interactions), Thr11B (carbon hydrogen bond), Asn15E, Val14E, Thr11D, Asn15, Glu7B, Gly10B, Ser6B, Glu7A and Ser3B (van der Waal's forces).

2.3.3. Molecular Docking Analysis on E Protein Form Monomer (C-Terminal Solvent Exposed)

Figure 4A shows the molecular interactions between the E protein monomeric (with the solvent-exposed C-terminal region) and the compound irinotecan. The drug interacts with the E protein through van der Waal's interactions with the amino acids Leu51, Lys53, Phe56, Arg69, Ser67, Ser68 and Val70. while the amino acids Ser60 and Asn64 form hydrogen bonds, and finally Pi interactions are observed between the amino acids Tyr57, Lys63, Val75 and Asp72. The molecular interactions that form in the saquinavir-E-monomer complex are as follows (Figure 4B): Hydrogen bond (Ser60, Asn64 and Arg69), van der Waal's force interactions (Leu51, Lys53, Phe56, Tyr59, Lys63, Ser67, Ser68, Val70, Asp72 and Val75), Pi-alkyl interactions (Leu74) and Pi-Pi T-Shaped interactions (Tyr57). The amino acids (Figure 4C) that interact to form the dutasteride-E-monomer complex are the following: Phe56, Tyr59, Ser60, Lys63, Asn64, Ser67, Ser68, Leu74 (van der Waal's forces),

Arg69 (hydrogen bond and Pi interaction), Val70 (Pi-alkyl Interaction), Pro71, Asp72 and Val75 (halogen interaction).

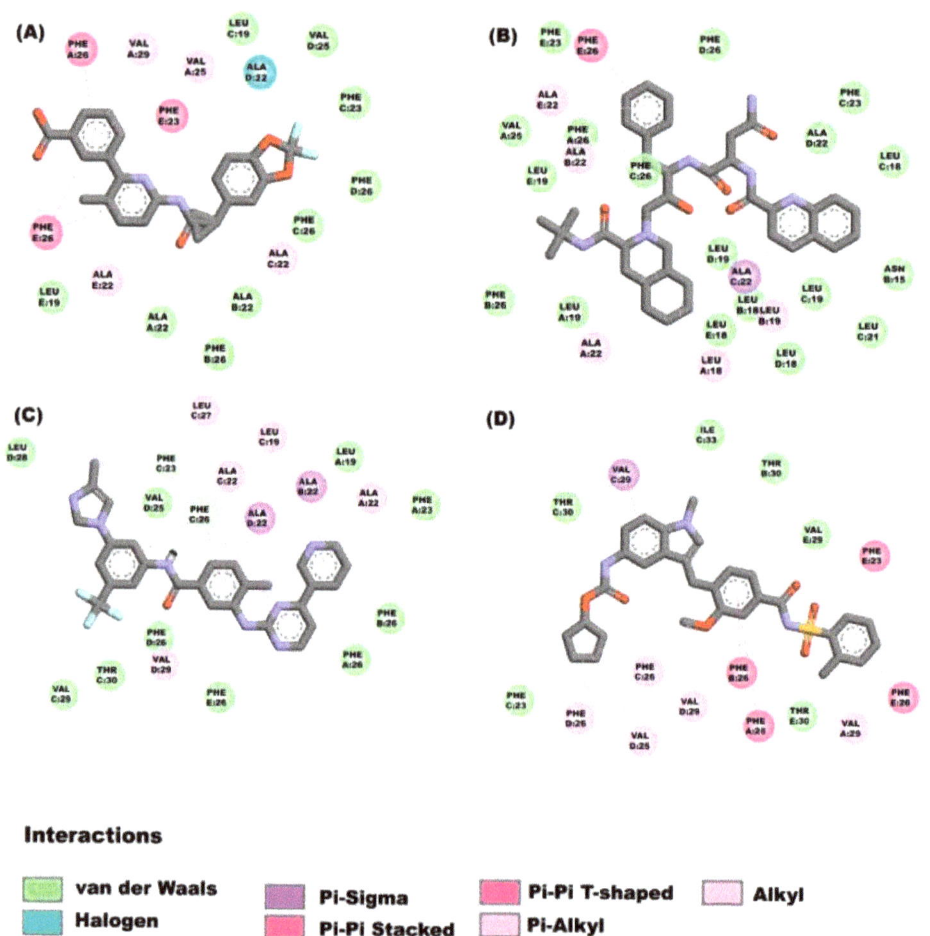

Interactions

Figure 2. Molecular interactions between some ligands and the E protein from SARS-CoV-2: The molecular interactions of the compounds (**A**) lumacaflor, (**B**) saquinavir, (**C**) nilotinib and (**D**) zafirlukast are observed.

2.3.4. Molecular Docking on E Protein Form Monomer (Harpin)

The drugs irinotecan, nilotinib, and saquinavir, bind to the E monomer in the hairpin conformations showing affinities of −8.2 kcal/mol, −8.2 kcal/mol and −7.7 kcal/mol respectively. Figure 5A shows the molecular interactions between irinotecan and the hairpin. Four main types of interactions are formed include: Pi-alkyl interactions (Ile46, Val49, and Leu51), hydrogen bonds (Ser55, Tyr57, and Tyr59), a carbon hydrogen bond (Val47) and van der Waal's (Phe20, Phe23, Leu27, Val58, Leu73 and Leu74). Nilotinib (Figure 5B) interacts with the following amino acids of the E protein: Leu51, Val58, Val62, Arg69, Val70, Pro71 (Pi-alkyl interaction), Ser55 (van der Waal's forces), Tyr57, Tyr59, Leu74, (hydrogen bonds) and Val75 (hydrogen bond and Pi-Sigma interaction). Figure 5C shows the interactions between saquinavir and the E monomer, the interactions that mediate this binding are hydrogen bonds (Ser55, Tyr57, Tyr59 and Val75), van der Waals forces (Val52, Phe56, Val58 and Pro71), Pi-alkyl interaction (Leu51, Arg61, Val70, and Leu74).

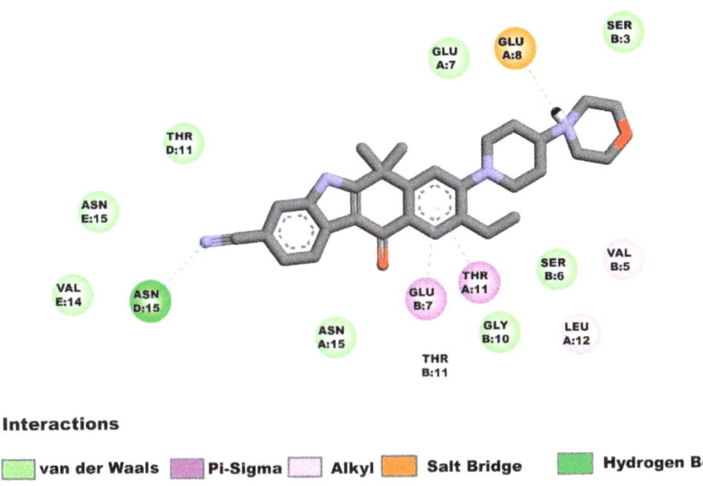

Figure 3. Molecular interactions between alectinib and the E homopentamer (N-terminal) from SARS-CoV-2: Molecular interactions of alectinib are shown.

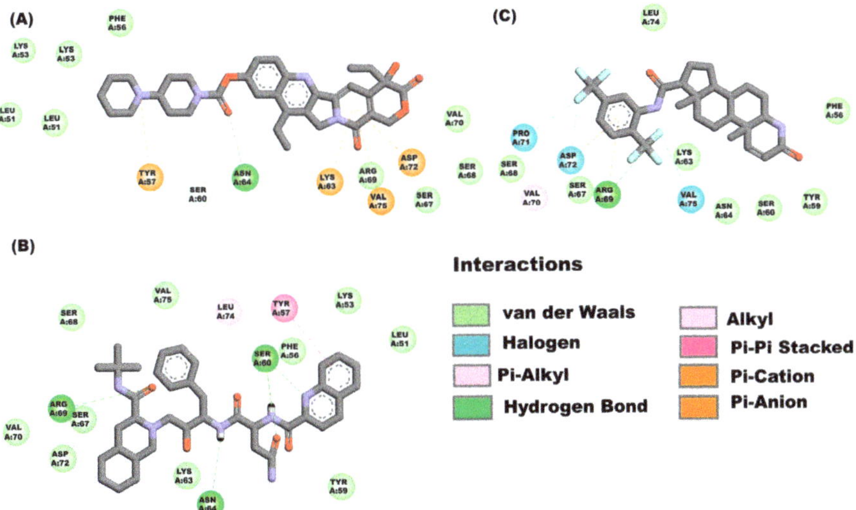

Figure 4. Molecular interactions between some drugs from the FDA subgroup and the E monomer from SARS-CoV-2: Molecular interactions of compounds (**A**) irinotecan, (**B**) saquinavir, and (**C**) dutasteride are observed.

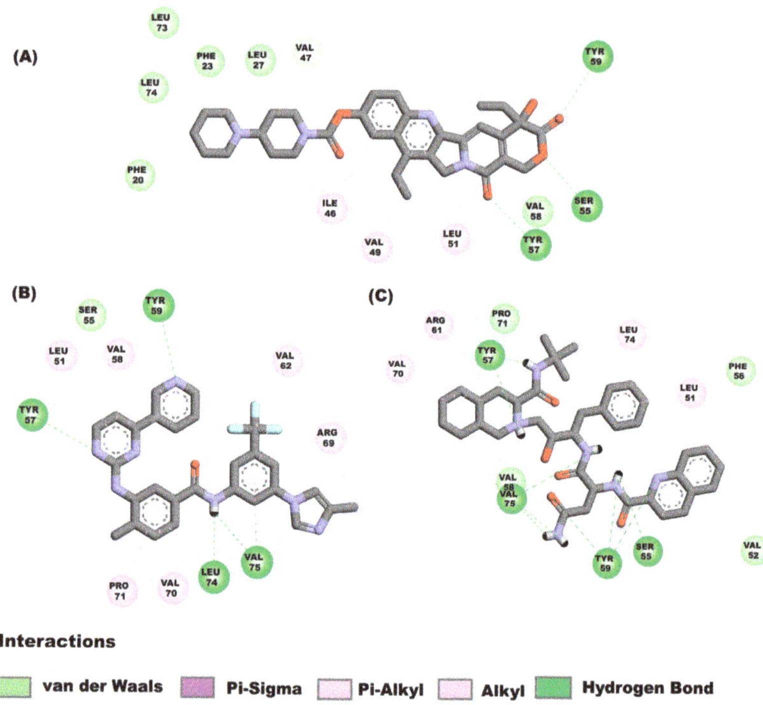

Figure 5. Molecular interactions between some drugs and the E monomer from SARS-CoV-2: Molecular interactions of compounds (**A**) irinotecan, (**B**) nilotinib, (**C**) saquinavir are shown.

After analyzing the molecular docking results, some compounds were selected based on the affinity criteria and considering critical residues at the site of interest. Table 1 shows the selected compounds with the respective affinity calculated from the dockings; the affinities are shown in bold. The selected complexes were selected to perform MD simulations.

Table 1. Binding affinities of some compounds and considering different forms (homopentameric and monomeric). Results from docking analysis are reported in the Table below. * lumacaftor and nilotinib were bound at the solvent-exposed C-terminal site although no critical residues were identified in the binding sites. Thus, for that particular site (monomeric structure), these compounds were not considered for molecular dynamics simulations studies.

	Binding Affinities of Some Compounds and Considering Different Forms			
	Homopentamer		Monomer	
	Binding Site			
Drugs	Ion Channel	N-terminal	C-terminal solvent-exposed	C-terminal Harpin
	ΔG (kcal/mol)			
lumacaftor	−10.9	−9.1	−7.6 *	−7.6
nilotinib	−10.8	−9.8	−7.5 *	−8.2
dutasteride	−10.6	−8.9	−7.7	−8.1
naldemedine	−10.5	−8.7	−7.4	−7.7
zafirlukast	−10.2	−9.1	−7.0	−7.3
irinotecan	−10.1	−9.0	−8.0	−8.2
saquinavir	−9.9	−9.3	−7.9	−7.7
alectinib	−9.4	−9.6	−7.0	−7.0

Pharmacokinetic properties of the compounds mentioned in Table S5 are shown in Supplementary Material.

2.4. Molecular Dynamics Simulations

Sixteen molecular dynamics (protein–ligand complexes) of 150 ns in total were performed, in which six are MD simulations of the homopentamer with compounds targeting the ion channel, which were named with the following nomenclature: lumacaftor (E-IC_lumacaftor), nilotinib (E-IC_nilotinib), dutasteride (E-IC_dutasteride), naldemedine (E-IC_naldemedine), zafirlukast (E-IC_zafirlukast) and saquinavir (E-IC_saquinavir), a MD simulation of the homopentamer without ligand (E-IC-Nt). Alectinib was selected for MD simulation targeting the N-terminal site of the E protein homopentamer (E-Nt_alectinib). For the case of dockings directed to the C-terminal site, simulations were explored in the two conformations. For the solvent-exposed C-terminal conformation, four MD simulations were performed: saquinavir (E-CtS_saquinavir), irinotecan (E-CtS_irinotecan), dutasteride (E-CtS_ dutasteride), and the MD simulation without ligand (E-CtS). Finally, the dynamics performed for the hairpin include: irinotecan (E-CtH_irinotecan), nilotinib (E-CtH_nilotinib), saquinavir (E-CtH_saquinavir) and the MD simulations without ligand (E-CtH). The results of the different MD simulations are described below. Figure 6A shows the RMSD results from the trajectories, from which it could be observed that simulations fluctuate in the range of 6 to 8 Å along the 150 ns MD simulations of the E protein (homopentamer form ion channel) and N-terminal site. RMSD results from the trajectories (Figure 6B), from which it could be observed that simulations fluctuate in the range of 8 to 11 Å along the 150 ns MD simulations of the E-monomer solvent-exposed C-terminal whereas in MD simulations where the ligands were directed to the hairpin show values range from 6 to 9 Å (Figure 6C). As we could observe from the RMSD results, the monomeric forms show higher values since they are known to be more flexible, whereas the homopentameric assembly form tends to be more stable. This observation is in agreement with previous studies published by Kuzmin and collaborators [41].

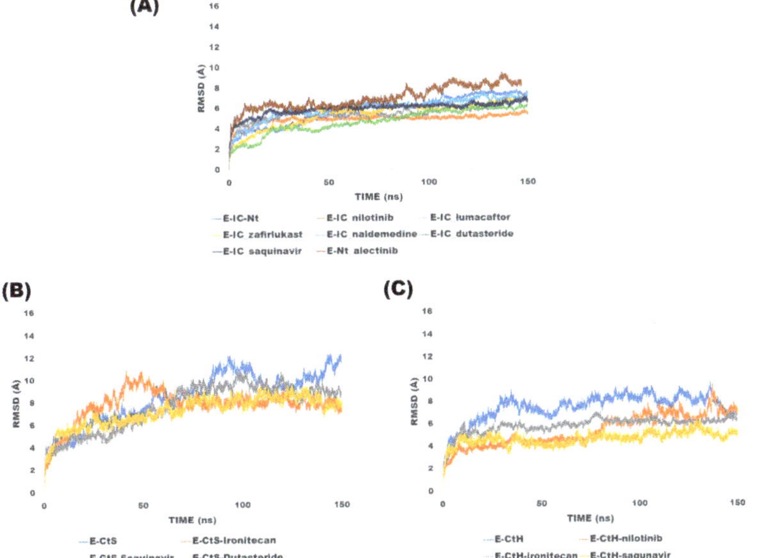

Figure 6. Root mean square deviations analysis of trajectories of the E protein simulations: (**A**) Ion channel and N-terminal, (**B**) C-terminal solvent-exposed and (**C**) hairpin: This figure shows the RMSD curves of each of the complexes.

2.5. Binding Free Energy Calculation Using MMPBSA Approach

The binding energy of E protein and the analyzed compounds were calculated. From these results, we could observe that saquinavir, nilotinib, dutasteride and alectinib bind with high affinity to the homopentamer form (Table 2).

Table 2. Binding Free energy MMPBSA for the E-Homopentamer complexes: This table shows free binding energies of complexes between E protein (pentameric form) and ligand. Highest energies are shown in bold.

Binding Free Energy MMPBSA for the E-Homopentamer			
Site Bind: Ion Channel			
Drugs	Complex Total (kcal/mol)	Receptor (kcal/mol)	Ligand (kcal/mol)	ΔG (kcal/mol)
Lumacaftor	−7885.9200	−7178.3400	−125.6700	−13.1500
Nilotinib	−7965.2763	−7537.2451	−404.9531	**−23.0781**
Dutasteride	−7392.0455	−7351.4972	−23.6330	**−16.9153**
Naldemedine	−7364.0697	−7341.7927	−15.1966	−7.0804
Zafirlukast	−7603.0986	−7358.9720	−241.1082	−3.0184
Saquinavir	−7582.0157	−7511.3579	−45.7430	**−24.9147**
Site bind: N-terminal			
Alectinib	−4203.9200	−4307.8700	−65.5600	**−116.6700**

In addition, dutasteride, irinotecan and saquinavir also bind to the monomer with the highest Gibbs free energy value in the C-terminal region (Table 3). Molecular interactions have been analyzed for the compounds marked in bold (Tables 2 and 3).

Table 3. Binding Free energy MMPBSA for the E-monomer complexes: This table shows free binding energies of complexes between E protein (monomeric form) and ligand. Highest energies are shown in bold.

Binding Free Energy MMPBSA for the E-Monomer			
Binding Site: Solvent Exposed C-Terminal			
Drugs	Complex Total (kcal/mol)	Receptor (kcal/mol)	Ligand (kcal/mol)	ΔG (kcal/mol)
Dutasteride	−2175.4155	−2058.9008	−105.8080	**−10.7068**
Irinotecan	−2111.4271	−2062.2341	−44.8761	−4.3169
Saquinavir	−2206.3300	−2245.6700	−50.1300	−2.1400
Binding site: Harpin			
Nilotinib	−2238.1565	−2071.3184	−163.2539	−3.5842
Irinotecan	−2114.7274	−2059.0421	−45.8114	**−9.8740**
Saquinavir	−2122.5089	−2073.9448	−36.6094	**−11.9547**

Diverse molecular interactions were tracked along the different MD simulations.

2.5.1. Monomeric Form

In the E-CtS_dutasteride complex we can observe different molecular interactions which include: Pi-alkyl interactions between residue Tyr59 and the ligand, additionally, this residue interacts with different rings of the ligand and the atoms C39 and C19. Furthermore, the residue Tyr59 shows a Pi-Sigma interaction with the atom HC, which is conserved in the MD simulation. Another alkyl interaction is formed between the atom CB of Val70 and the atom C39 of dutasteride, although this interaction is unstable. The interaction between irinotecan and the hairpin is towards one saline bridge formed between Val 75 (OT1) and H15 of the irinotecan; such an interaction is mostly conserved along the trajectory. On the other hand, in the binding of the ligand irinotecan on the hairpin, we could detect some important interactions which include: Leu74 (VdW), Leu73 (CHB) and Val75 (SB).

For the case of the complex E-CtH_saquinavir we could identify some hydrogen bonds that are stable along the trajectory, one of which is formed between Val75 (OT1) and the H89 of the drug. In addition, a hydrogen bond interaction was formed between the atom HG1 of Ser55 and the atom O43 of the ligand; such interaction is observed in almost half of the simulation. Another hydrogen bond that is formed between the atom HH of Tyr59 (E protein) and the atom O43 of saquinavir which is conserved half of the of the trajectory and it showed some other VdW interactions with the residues: Ile46, Tyr42 and Val58 Additionally, we could observe a saline bridge between the saquinavir and Val75 which is conserved mostly along the trajectory.

2.5.2. Homopentamer Form

In the complex E-IC_dutasteride it could be observed an alkyl interaction between Val17A (CB) of the pentameric form of the E protein and the atom C32 of the ligand dutasteride, which is mostly conserved along the trajectory. Additionally, other alkyl interaction is formed between Val12A (CB) and the atom C32 of the ligand, which is also conserved along the trajectory. Regarding the interactions between the compound alectinib and the homopentaric form of E protein, in which we could observe a saline bridge between the residue Glu8A, Pi-cation interaction with the amino acid Phe4B , and hydrogen bonds with the residues: Asn15D, Asn15E, and Asn15A. In the case of the binding of saquinavir on the homopentameric form it is mainly through van der Waal's interactions with the following residues: Asn15B, Asn15D, and Phe26C. All the mentioned interactions are shown constantly along the trajectories. Regarding the interactions of nilotinib with E homopentameric, it shows constant interactions with these residues: Phe26B (Pi-Pi stacking interaction), Phe26D (Pi-alkyl interaction), Phe26E (Pi-alkyl interaction) and Phe26A (van der Waals).

3. Discussion

E protein sequences from SARS CoV (NP_828854.1) and SARS CoV-2 (BCA87363.1) have an identity of 94.7% and sequence similarity of 97.4% [8]. Importantly, E protein is crucial in the viral replication cycle [44] such as assembly [45], virion release [45,46], and viral pathogenesis, [47,48] induction of membrane curvature, inflammation and even autophagy [49]. Additionally, the possibility of finding E protein in the Golgi and endoplasmic reticulum compartments has been described; where it can interact with bromodomain proteins such as BRD2 and BRD4 (proteins that bind to acetylated histones to regulate gene transcription) [50]. The C-terminal E protein binds to the PDZ domain, which induces immune-pathological reactions and causes overexpression of inflammatory cytokines. Indeed, E protein plays an important role in the release of inflammatory cytokines, which causes the acute respiratory syndrome, and it is considered the main cause of the death of patients with COVID-19 [51,52]. Thus, this protein can be considered as an interesting pharmacological target for potential antiviral drugs [16,17]. It has been also described that both the homopentamer and monomer forms play a role in the viral replication, as well as in the activation of pro-inflammatory signaling pathways, which in many cases are involved in the exacerbation of COVID-19. For all these mentioned ligands, targeting the C and N terminal of the ion channel has been considered [24,32,37].

From the binding energy simulations (MM–PBSA approach), we could identify the best evaluated compounds on the different forms of E protein (Tables 2 and 3).

Interactions between the monomeric and homopentameric forms are described below:

3.1. Monomeric

Considering the free binding energy simulations (MM–PBSA approach), we found that the compound dutasteride showed the highest energy on the C-terminal exposed to solvent; and for the hairpin, the most promissory compounds include irinotecan (−9.8740 kcal/mol) and saquinavir (−11.9547 kcal/mol). On the other side, considering the monomeric form, the compound irinotecan interacts with the residues: Leu73, Leu74 and Val75, and for the compound saquinavir, it shows interactions with Val75 and Leu74. The mentioned residues belong to the PBM of the E protein, which is known to be essential for the binding to the PDZ domain of the PALS1 protein [32,33]. The capacity of E protein to bind to the PDZ-binding domain has been associated with the virulence of the virus [13,41].

On the other hand, there is valuable information (protein interaction maps) about the involvement of C-terminal helical bundle as binding epitope for ligand binding, thus, corroborating our hypothesis regarding the potential role of a C-terminal helical bundle in the mediation of viral replication processes [52,53]. Interestingly the C-terminal region of E (can interact with bromodomains) is highly conserved in SARS and bat coronaviruses, which suggests that it has a conserved function [31,54]. This means that the compounds that interact in this region could have an effect on various coronaviruses.

3.2. Pentameric

We have performed diverse in silico studies which include docking analysis, MD simulations and free binding energy calculations (MM–PBSA) from which could depict the energy values of the following ligands: saquinavir -24.9147 kcal/mol, nilotinib -23.0781 kcal/mol, dutasteride -16.9153 kcal/mol and alectinib -116.67 kcal/mol showed the highest binding affinity to the homopentamer. Of worthy interest is that we could depict that alectinib showed the highest binding free energy (ΔG (-116.67 kcal/mol) from the molecular dynamics simulation studies in comparison to the other compounds. From the binding interactions, it could be observed that the mentioned ligand interacts with the residue Asn15 through hydrogen bond interactions, additionally it interacts with the segment of amino acid residues 7 to 12, which make it a very interesting target to inhibit the ionic channel and N-terminal at the same time. Additionally, it shows interactions with other residues which include: Glu8A and Phe4B.

Saquinavir seems to be an interesting ligand because it targets the spike protein and also 3C-like protease, as has been described previously [55,56]. Of worthy interest is that this ligand also binds to the E protein, and thus, it can be considered a multitarget ligand. Moreover, saquinavir is able to bind to both monomeric and homopentamer forms. Sarkar and collaborators reported that the homopentameric form interacts with the residues: Phe26 and Asn15 [57]. This fact would provide advantages over other compounds that only interact with one form (monomer or pentamer), since E protein could have conformational changes in the different steps of the viral replication cycle.

It has been reported that nilotinib appears to bind to the receptor binding domain RBD of the SARS-CoV-2 spike protein, and some in silico studies have been carried out to depict the interaction between tyrosine kinase inhibitors and SARS-CoV-2 protein. On the other side alectinib has been prescribed along antiviral treatment however clinical trials are needed in terms of treatment of cancer and treatment of COVID-19. Furthermore, it has been identified that the residue Phe26 is located in a key position better known as "bottleneck region" which is important for the function of the ion channel of the E protein [12,57]. On the other side, residues such as: Phe4, Glu8, Asn15, and Val25 which are known to be important for the function of E protein, Phe4 functions as a gate towards the ion channel and it has been suggested that residues Glu8 and Asn15 regulate the opening/closing of the channel [46,57,58]. Particularly, Val25 and Phe26 have been suggested as key residues in the binding for effective inhibitors for E protein [59]. In a general manner, nilotinib, saquinavir and alectinib are considered the most promising compounds that could effectively inhibit the homopentamer of the E protein. The blockage of ionic channels of E protein could significantly reduce viral pathogenicity [46].

Moreover, the primary sequence of E protein is quite conserved among the different coronaviruses, making it an interesting therapeutic target [32,34]. Despite the genome of SARS-CoV-2 having evolved constantly, while generating novel variants, E protein still shows a high global conservation grade of 99.98% in which mutations are extremely infrequent, and is present in less than 0.3% of total sequences [54] in comparison to other structural proteins, such as spike protein which shows 2671 changes in 1132 of the 1272 spike amino acids [54].

Nowadays, targeted drug repurposing represents a very useful strategy to identify libraries of pre-existing molecules or approved drugs that could prevent COVID-19 [60,61].

Of worthy interest is that the ligands we proposed in this work could also bind to different SARS-CoV-2 variants as well as another coronaviruses, meaning they can be considered as potential drugs for COVID-19 treatment.

4. Methods

4.1. Molecular Modeling

Based on the primary sequence of the E protein of SARS-CoV-2, it was possible to build the transmembrane region (TMD) of the E protein of this virus, by employing the crystal structure of E protein from SARS-CoV PDB: 5X29 as template [62]. The identity percentage between the sequence P0DTC4 [63] (sequence of the E protein of SARS-CoV-2), and the crystal structure is 89.0%. Alignment of the query vs. template is shown in the Supplementary Materials (Figure S2). The three-dimensional homology model of the homopentamer of the E protein of SARS-CoV-2 was built by using Modeller 10.1 Software [64]. The monomeric form of E protein was also modeled, for this purpose Modeler 10.1 Software [64] was employed, using the same template. Additionally, the scripts model-multichain-sym.py and model-loop.py were employed to obtain and refine the structure, yielding different 3D models which were built by means of the Modeller 10.1 program. Each of the models was first optimized with variable target function method (VTFM) with conjugate gradients (CG), and then, they were refined using molecular dynamics (MD) and simulated annealing (SA), while employing a slow refinement process of about 300 cycles during the whole optimization. CHARMM-22 parameters were employed to reproduce the protein geometry in the Modeller environment. Finally, the best evaluated model was selected using the discrete optimized protein energy (DOPE) method (GA341) [64–66].

4.2. Database Search and In Silico ADMET Analysis

We downloaded 5852 molecules from the Zinc database [67]. The molecules were obtained from the following subsets: FDA drugs (1604 FDA drugs, per Drug Bank), and world-not-FDA (4248 Other Drugs approved but not by the FDA).

In the process of virtual screening, software such as: DataWarrior program V5.5.0 [68] and SwissADME free web tool [69] were used to predict different drug-likeness parameters such as: physicochemical properties, solubility, and pharmacokinetics (absorption, distribution, metabolism, excretion and toxicity ADMET). From this analysis of 5852 drugs after some were discarded, the remaining 2155 compounds had to fulfill the following properties: high or medium lipophilicity(LogP > 1), bioavailability score (>0.11), Pains # Alert (0), Brenk # alert ($\leq$2), Lipinski # Violation ($\leq$2) and synthetic accessibility (<6.5) [70–72]. The filtered database is attached in Supplementary Materials.

4.3. Docking Analysis

Molecular docking studies of the 2155 ligands were carried out using Autodock Vina (version 1.2) program [73]. The docking procedure was validated by comparing the molecular interactions of amantadine on SARS-CoV-2 reported previously [74]. For all the docking simulations, the E protein was rigid and the ligands flexible. The drugs with the highest affinity and those that reach key amino acids that influence the E protein function were selected. Docking analyses were carried out on homopentameric and monomeric forms of E protein. For the case of homopentameric E protein, dockings were focused to the ionic channel (active site is formed by the following residues: Glu8, Thr11, Leu12, Val14, Asn15, Val17, Leu18, Leu19, Phe20, Leu21, Ala22, Phe23, Val24, Val25, Phe26, Leu27, Leu28, Val29, Thr30, Leu31, Ala32, Ile33, Leu34, Thr35, Ala36, Leu37, Arg38, Leu39, Ala40, Tyr42, Ala43, Ala44, Ile46, Val47, Val49, Leu51, Pro54, Val56, Tyr57, Ser60, Arg61, Lys63, Asn64 and Leu65) as well as the N-terminal region (residues 7 to 12). For both conformations of the monomeric form, dockings were focused to the C-terminal segment (residues 70 to 75). The docking process on the homopentamer (ionic channel) was carried out considering the following parameters: grid box (25.0 Å × 30.0 Å × 30.0 Å) centered at (40.0, 63.0, 55.0) Å and for the N-terminal: grid box (20.0 Å × 40.0 Å × 20.0 Å) centered at (20.0, 63.0, 55.0) Å. For the monomeric C-terminal harpin, grid box (25 Å × 25 Å × 25 Å) centered at (−20.0, 5.0, −1.0) Å, and finally for the C terminal region conformation (exposed to the solvent), a grid box (25 Å × 25 Å × 25 Å) centered at (−20.0, 5.0, −1.0) Å. For all the procedures, an implicit solvent function was employed, as well as the following parameters: num_modes = 100, energy_range = 6 and exhaustiveness = 25, and Monte Carlo force field. At the end of this procedure, the conformation that showed the highest Gibbs free energy was selected for further studies [75].

4.4. Molecular Docking Studies and Visualization of the Results

The process of selection was carried out by using a Perl script to obtain the binding affinity of each of 2155 compounds in just one file. Once docking simulations were finished, Discovery Studio Visualizer [76] and Chimera [77] programs were used to visualize the binding site of these ligands and their molecular interactions. Afterwards, ligands that showed the highest affinity (more negative) were selected. Additionally, surrounding residues could be detected from these theoretical studies.

4.5. Molecular Dynamics Simulations

Three E protein MD simulations (without a ligand) and sixteen MD simulations of E protein–ligand complexes were carried out by considering the results from docking analysis that showed the highest affinities and showed interactions with key residues. All these complexes were prepared by using Charmm-GUI Software [78,79] and embedded in a POPC membrane (1-palmitoyl-2-oleoyl-sn- glycero-3-phosphocholine) [80] which is native for this type of cell membrane. MD simulations were carried out by means of the NAMD program and using the known inputs for NAMD and standard scripts for MD simulations [81].

The method of particle-mesh Ewald (PME) was used for the calculation of the electrostatic potential energy. A no-bonded cutoff of 12 Å, switchdist of 10 Å and pairlistdist of 16 Å were implemented for these long-range interactions. MD simulations were solvated (TIP3 model) and neutralized up to a final concentration of 0.15 M NaCl in the equilibration step. The equilibration protocol consisted in six minimization steps, reaching a total of 2.5 ns of equilibration time; an NTV (constant volume and temperature) protocol was applied. For the production step an NTP (constant temperature and pressure) ensemble was maintained with a Langevin thermostat (310 K) and anisotropic Langevin barostat (1 atm). For these last two steps, an integration time step of 2 femtoseconds (fs) was used, with all the bond lengths involved, and used the CHARMM36 force field [78]. Finally, MD simulations were run 150 ns.

4.6. Structural Analysis of MD Simulations

Structural analysis of the E proteins (from the MD simulations) was carried out by employing the Carma program and considering the alpha atoms of the structure [80]. These structural analyses include calculation of the following parameters: RMSD (root mean square deviation) [82]. Additionally, we performed a structural comparison for each of the forms of the E protein: homopentamer, hairpin, C-terminal exposed to solvent (monomeric). For all the cases, the protein (without a ligand) conformation was used as a reference.

4.7. Binding Free Energy Calculations of the E Protein-Ligand Complexes

E protein–ligand complexes binding free energy (ΔG_{bind}) were estimated for the 100 ns MD simulation trajectories. A stride of 10 was considered for the calculations, resulting in about 100 frames for the ΔG_{bind} analysis. The estimations were carried out employing molecular mechanics combined with the Poisson–Boltzmann surface area (MM–PBSA) method. MM–PBSA was applied by the Calculation of Free Energy (CaFE) plugin [83] implemented to the VMD program [84–86]. For the MM–PBSA calculations, we have considered the most stable part of the trajectories, for each of the cases.

5. Conclusions

In this work we have employed in silico methods (docking analysis, molecular dynamics simulations and MM–PBSA calculations) to identify compounds with potential E protein interaction from SARS-CoV-2. From these studies, we could identify five compounds: irinotecan, alectinib, saquinavir, nilotinib and dutasteride which were best evaluated. Particularly, alectinib could inhibit the functions of the ion channel as well as avoiding the binding of other proteins involved in pro-inflammatory processes that could trigger the cytokines cascade, which in consequence could lead to a serious and mortal illness. On the other side, saquinavir, nilotinib and alectinib were also considered as a promising multitarget ligand because they seem to inhibit three targets, which play an important role in the viral cycle. Additionally, saquinavir was shown to be able to bind to E protein both in its monomeric as well as pentameric forms so it could act in different steps of the viral replication cycle. Finally, further experimental assays are needed to probe our hypothesis derived from in silico studies.

Consent for Publication

We give our consent to publish this manuscript.

Supplementary Materials: The following supporting information can be downloaded at: https://www.mdpi.com/article/10.3390/ph16020296/s1, Figure S1: Pipeline with goals. Figure S2: Alignment between the query (P0DTC4) and the template 5X29. Table S1: Molecular docking studies drugs on the E-homopentamer (Ion Channel). Table S2: Molecular docking studies drugs on the E-homopentamer (N-terminal). Table S3: Docking molecular from compounds on the E-monomer (C-terminal solvent exposed). Table S4: Docking molecular from compounds on the E-monomer (C-Terminal Harpin). Table S5: Pharmacokinetic properties. FDA_ADMET: Excelldatasheet. No_World_FDA_ADMET: Excelldatasheet.

Author Contributions: G.L.R.S. contributed in the conceptualization, writing and review of the manuscript. A.L.R. contributed in the methodology, validation and use of Software. J.G.M. contributed in the formal analysis. J.C.B. contributed in the review of the manuscript, and the Project administration and funding acquisition. M.M.A. contributed in the conceptualization, writing and review of the manuscript. She also participated in the administration and funding acquisition. All authors participated actively in the writing of the manuscript, analysis of the results, and in the review of the manuscript. All authors have read and agreed to the published version of the manuscript.

Funding: National Grants (Secretaria de Investigación y Posgrado (SIP) del Instituto Politécnico Nacional):20230833, 20230987, and 20230991. CONACYT: PAACTI 312807 and Instituto Politécnico Nacional (IPN).

Institutional Review Board Statement: Not applicable.

Informed Consent Statement: Not applicable.

Data Availability Statement: Data is contained within the article and Supplementary Materials.

Acknowledgments: The authors gratefully acknowledge the computing time granted by LANCAD and CONACYT on the supercomputer Yoltla/Miztli/Xiuhcoatl (Hector Manuel Oliver Hernandez) at LSVP UAM-Iztapalapa/DGTIC UNAM/CGSTIC CINVESTAV.

Conflicts of Interest: The authors declare no conflict of interest.

References

1. Corman, V.M.; Muth, D.; Niemeyer, D.; Drosten, C. Hosts and Sources of Endemic Human Coronaviruses. *Adv. Virus Res.* **2018**, *100*, 163–188. [CrossRef] [PubMed]
2. van der Hoek, L.; Pyrc, K.; Jebbink, M.F.; Vermeulen-Oost, W.; Berkhout, R.J.; Wolthers, K.C.; Wertheim-van Dillen, P.M.; Kaandorp, J.; Spaargaren, J.; Berkhout, B. Identification of a new human coronavirus. *Nat. Med.* **2004**, *10*, 368–373. [CrossRef] [PubMed]
3. Woo, P.C.; Lau, S.K.; Chu, C.M.; Chan, K.H.; Tsoi, H.W.; Huang, Y.; Wong, B.H.; Poon, R.W.; Cai, J.J.; Luk, W.K.; et al. Characterization and complete genome sequence of a novel coronavirus, coronavirus HKU1, from patients with pneumonia. *J. Virol.* **2005**, *79*, 884–895. [CrossRef] [PubMed]
4. Majumdar, P.; Niyogi, S. ORF3a mutation associated with higher mortality rate in SARS-CoV-2 infection. *Epidemiol Infect* **2020**, *148*, e262. [CrossRef] [PubMed]
5. Available online: https://www.worldometers.info/coronavirus/ (accessed on 9 February 2023).
6. Freeman, T.L.; Swartz, T.H. Targeting the NLRP3 Inflammasome in Severe COVID-19. *Front. Immunol.* **2020**, *11*, 1518. [CrossRef] [PubMed]
7. Hassan, S.S.; Choudhury, P.P.; Roy, B. SARS-CoV2 envelope protein: Non-synonymous mutations and its consequences. *Genomics* **2020**, *112*, 3890–3892. [CrossRef]
8. Yoshimoto, F.K. The Proteins of Severe Acute Respiratory Syndrome Coronavirus-2 (SARS CoV-2 or n-COV19), the Cause of COVID-19. *Protein J.* **2020**, *39*, 198–216. [CrossRef]
9. Duart, G.; García-Murria, M.J.; Grau, B.; Acosta-Cáceres, J.M.; Martínez-Gil, L.; Mingarro, I. SARS-CoV-2 envelope protein topology in eukaryotic membranes. *Open Biol.* **2020**, *10*, 200209. [CrossRef]
10. Malik, Y.A. Properties of Coronavirus and SARS-CoV-2. *Malays J. Pathol.* **2020**, *42*, 3–11.
11. Kuo, L.; Hurst, K.R.; Masters, P.S. Exceptional Flexibility in the Sequence Requirements for Coronavirus Small Envelope Protein Function. *J. Virol.* **2007**, *81*, 2249–2262. [CrossRef]
12. Satarker, S.; Nampoothiri, M. Structural Proteins in Severe Acute Respiratory Syndrome Coronavirus-2. *Arch. Med. Res.* **2020**, *51*, 482–491. [CrossRef] [PubMed]
13. Schoeman, D.; Fielding, B.C. Coronavirus envelope protein: Current knowledge. *Virol. J.* **2019**, *16*, 69. [CrossRef] [PubMed]
14. Yang, R.; Wu, S.; Wang, S.; Rubino, G.; Nickels, J.D.; Cheng, X. Refinement of SARS-CoV-2 envelope protein structure in a native-like environment by molecular dynamics simulations. *Front. Mol. Biosci.* **2022**, *9*, 1027223. [CrossRef]
15. Wong, N.A.; Saier, M.H., Jr. The SARS-Coronavirus Infection Cycle: A Survey of Viral Membrane Proteins, Their Functional Interactions and Pathogenesis. *Int. J. Mol. Sci.* **2021**, *22*, 1308. [CrossRef]
16. Park, S.H.; Siddiqi, H.; Castro, D.V.; De Angelis, A.A.; Oom, A.L.; Stoneham, C.A.; Lewinski, M.K.; Clark, A.E.; Croker, B.A.; Carlin, A.F.; et al. Interactions of SARS-CoV-2 envelope protein with amilorides correlate with antiviral activity. *PLoS Pathog* **2021**, *17*, e1009519. [CrossRef] [PubMed]
17. Ye, Y.; Hogue, B.G. Role of the Coronavirus E Viroporin Protein Transmembrane Domain in Virus Assembly. *J. Virol.* **2007**, *81*, 3597–3607. [CrossRef]
18. Ruch, T.R.; Machamer, C.E. A Single Polar Residue and Distinct Membrane Topologies Impact the Function of the Infectious Bronchitis Coronavirus E Protein. *PLOS Pathog.* **2012**, *8*, e1002674. [CrossRef]
19. Torres, J.; Maheswari, U.; Parthasarathy, K.; Ng, L.; Liu, D.X.; Gong, X. Conductance and amantadine binding of a pore formed by a lysine-flanked transmembrane domain of SARS coronavirus envelope protein. *Protein Sci.* **2007**, *16*, 2065–2071. [CrossRef]
20. De Diego, M.L.; Nieto-Torres, J.L.; Regla-Nava, J.A.; Jimenez-Guardeño, J.M.; Fernandez-Delgado, R.; Fett, C.; Castaño-Rodriguez, C.; Perlman, S.; Enjuanes, L. Inhibition of NF-κB-mediated inflammation in severe acute respiratory syndrome coronavirus-infected mice increases survival. *J. Virol.* **2014**, *88*, 913–924. [CrossRef]
21. Nieto-Torres, J.L.; Verdiá-Báguena, C.; Jimenez-Guardeno, J.M.J.; Regla-Nava, J.A.; Castaño-Rodriguez, C.; Fernandez-Delgado, R.; Torres, J.; Aguilella, V.M.; Enjuanes, L. Severe acute respiratory syndrome coronavirus E protein transports calcium ions and activates the NLRP3 inflammasome. *Virology* **2015**, *485*, 330–339. [CrossRef]
22. Nieto-Torres, J.L.; DeDiego, M.L.; Verdiá-Báguena, C.; Jimenez-Guardeño, J.M.; Regla-Nava, J.A.; Fernandez-Delgado, R.; Castaño-Rodriguez, C.; Alcaraz, A.; Torres, J.; Aguilella, V.M.; et al. Severe Acute Respiratory Syndrome Coronavirus Envelope Protein Ion Channel Activity Promotes Virus Fitness and Pathogenesis. *PLOS Pathog.* **2014**, *10*, e1004077. [CrossRef] [PubMed]
23. Rahman, M.S.; Hoque, M.N.; Islam, M.R.; Islam, I.; Mishu, I.D.; Rahaman, M.M.; Sultana, M.; Hossain, M.A. Mutational insights into the envelope protein of SARS-CoV-2. *Gene. Rep.* **2021**, *22*, 100997. [CrossRef] [PubMed]
24. Sariol, A.; Perlman, S. SARS-CoV-2 takes its Toll. *Nat. Immunol.* **2021**, *22*, 801–802. [CrossRef]
25. Zheng, M.; Karki, R.; Williams, E.P.; Yang, D.; Fitzpatrick, E.; Vogel, P.; Jonsson, C.B.; Kanneganti, T.D. TLR2 senses the SARS-CoV-2 envelope protein to produce inflammatory cytokines. *Nat. Immunol.* **2021**, *22*, 829–838. [CrossRef] [PubMed]
26. Rémi, P.; Jean-Baptiste, B.; Sofiane, T.; Lbachir, B.; Elmostafa, B. SARS-CoV-2 Envelope protein (E) binds and activates TLR2: A novel target for COVID-19 interventions. *bioRxiv* **2021**. bioRxiv:11.10.468173.
27. Caillet-Saguy, C.; Durbesson, F.; Rezelj, V.V.; Gogl, G.; Tran, Q.D.; Twizere, J.C.; Vignuzzi, M.; Vincentelli, R.; Wolff, N. Host PDZ-containing proteins targeted by SARS-CoV-2. *FEBS J.* **2021**, *288*, 5148–5162. [CrossRef]

38. Jimenez-Guardeño, J.M.; Nieto-Torres, J.L.; DeDiego, M.L.; Regla-Nava, J.A.; Fernandez-Delgado, R.; Castaño-Rodriguez, C.; Enjuanes, L. The PDZ-Binding Motif of Severe Acute Respiratory Syndrome Coronavirus Envelope Protein Is a Determinant of Viral Pathogenesis. *PLOS Pathog.* **2014**, *10*, e1004320. [CrossRef]

39. Li, Y.; Surya, W.; Claudine, S.; Torres, J. Structure of a Conserved Golgi Complex-targeting Signal in Coronavirus Envelope Proteins. *J. Biol. Chem.* **2014**, *289*, 12535–12549. [CrossRef]

40. De Maio, F.; Lo Cascio, E.; Babini, G.; Sali, M.; Della Longa, S.; Tilocca, B.; Roncada, P.; Arcovito, A.; Sanguinetti, M.; Scambia, G.; et al. Improved binding of SARS-CoV-2 Envelope protein to tight junction-associated PALS1 could play a key role in COVID-19 pathogenesis. *Microbes Infect* **2020**, *22*, 592–597. [CrossRef]

41. Shepley-McTaggart, A.; Sagum, C.A.; Oliva, I.; Rybakovsky, E.; DiGuilio, K.; Liang, J.; Bedford, M.T.; Cassel, J.; Sudol, M.; Mullin, J.M.; et al. SARS-CoV-2 Envelope (E) protein interacts with PDZ-domain-2 of host tight junction protein ZO1. *PLoS ONE* **2021**, *16*, e0251955. [CrossRef]

42. Toto, A.; Ma, S.; Malagrinò, F.; Visconti, L.; Pagano, L.; Stromgaard, K.; Gianni, S. Comparing the binding properties of peptides mimicking the Envelope protein of SARS-CoV and SARS-CoV-2 to the PDZ domain of the tight junction-associated PALS1 protein. *Protein Sci.* **2020**, *29*, 2038–2042. [CrossRef] [PubMed]

43. Javorsky, A.; Humbert, P.O.; Kvansakul, M. Structural basis of coronavirus E protein interactions with human PALS1 PDZ domain. *Commun. Biol.* **2021**, *4*, 724. [CrossRef] [PubMed]

44. Gordon, D.E.; Jang, G.M.; Bouhaddou, M.; Xu, J.; Obernier, K.; White, K.M.; O'Meara, M.J.; Rezelj, V.V.; Guo, J.Z.; Swaney, D.L.; et al. A SARS-CoV-2 protein interaction map reveals targets for drug repurposing. *Nature* **2020**, *583*, 459–468. [CrossRef] [PubMed]

45. Filippakopoulos, P.; Picaud, S.; Mangos, M.; Keates, T.; Lambert, J.-P.; Barsyte-Lovejoy, D.; Felletar, I.; Volkmer, R.; Müller, S.; Pawson, T.; et al. Histone Recognition and Large-Scale Structural Analysis of the Human Bromodomain Family. *Cell* **2012**, *149*, 214–231. [CrossRef]

46. Lara-Ureña, N.; García-Domínguez, M. Relevance of BET Family Proteins in SARS-CoV-2 Infection. *Biomolecules* **2021**, *11*, 1126. [CrossRef]

47. Mills, R.J.; Humphrey, S.J.; Fortuna, P.R.J.; Lor, M.; Foster, S.R.; Quaife-Ryan, G.A.; Johnston, R.L.; Dumenil, T.; Bishop, C.; Rudraraju, R.; et al. BET inhibition blocks inflammation-induced cardiac dysfunction and SARS-CoV-2 infection. *Cell* **2021**, *184*, 2167–2182. [CrossRef]

48. Corse, E.; Machamer, C.E. The cytoplasmic tails of infectious bronchitis virus E and M proteins mediate their interaction. *Virology* **2003**, *312*, 25–34. [CrossRef]

49. de Haan, C.A.; Vennema, H.; Rottier, P.J. Assembly of the coronavirus envelope: Homotypic interactions between the M proteins. *J. Virol.* **2000**, *74*, 4967–4978. [CrossRef]

50. Karki, R.; Sharma, B.R.; Tuladhar, S.; Williams, E.P.; Zalduondo, L.; Samir, P.; Zheng, M.; Sundaram, B.; Banoth, B.; Malireddi, R.K.S.; et al. Synergism of TNF-α and IFN-γ Triggers Inflammatory Cell Death, Tissue Damage, and Mortality in SARS-CoV-2 Infection and Cytokine Shock Syndromes. *Cell* **2020**, *184*, 149–168.e17. [CrossRef]

51. Kuzmin, A.; Orekhov, P.; Astashkin, R.; Gordeliy, V.; Gushchin, I. Structure and dynamics of the SARS-CoV-2 envelope protein monomer. *Proteins* **2022**, *90*, 1102–1114. [CrossRef]

52. Surya, W.; Li, Y.; Torres, J. Structural model of the SARS coronavirus E channel in LMPG micelles. *Biochim. Biophys. Acta (BBA)* **2018**, *1860*, 1309–1317. [CrossRef] [PubMed]

53. Tian, X.; Shen, L.; Gao, P.; Huang, L.; Liu, G.; Zhou, L.; Peng, L. Discovery of Potential Therapeutic Drugs for COVID-19 Through Logistic Matrix Factorization with Kernel Diffusion. *Front. Microbiol.* **2022**, *13*, 740382. [CrossRef] [PubMed]

54. Lim, K.P.; Liu, D.X. The missing link in coronavirus assembly. Retention of the avian coronavirus infectious bronchitis virus envelope protein in the pre-Golgi compartments and physical interaction between the envelope and membrane proteins. *J. Biol. Chem.* **2001**, *276*, 17515–17523. [CrossRef]

55. Ruch, T.R.; Machamer, C.E. The Coronavirus E Protein: Assembly and Beyond. *Viruses* **2012**, *4*, 363–382. [CrossRef] [PubMed]

56. Cao, Y.; Yang, R.; Lee, I.; Zhang, W.; Sun, J.; Wang, W.; Meng, X. Characterization of the SARS-CoV-2 E Protein: Sequence, Structure, Viroporin, and Inhibitors. *Protein Sci.* **2021**, *30*, 1114–1130. [CrossRef]

57. Chan, J.F.; Kok, K.H.; Zhu, Z.; Chu, H.; To, K.K.; Yuan, S.; Yuen, K.Y. Genomic characterization of the 2019 novel human-pathogenic coronavirus isolated from a patient with atypical pneumonia after visiting Wuhan. *Emerg. Microbes Infect* **2020**, *9*, 221–236. [CrossRef]

58. Weiss, S.R.; Navas-Martin, S. Coronavirus Pathogenesis and the Emerging Pathogen Severe Acute Respiratory Syndrome Coronavirus. *Microbiol. Mol. Biol. Rev.* **2005**, *69*, 635–664. [CrossRef]

59. Koepke, L.; Hirschenberger, M.; Hayn, M.; Kirchhoff, F.; Sparrer, K.M. Manipulation of autophagy by SARS-CoV-2 proteins. *Autophagy* **2021**, *17*, 2659–2661. [CrossRef]

60. Faivre, E.J.; McDaniel, K.F.; Albert, D.H.; Mantena, S.R.; Plotnik, J.P.; Wilcox, D.; Zhang, L.; Bui, M.H.; Sheppard, G.S.; Wang, L.; et al. Selective inhibition of the BD2 bromodomain of BET proteins in prostate cancer. *Nature* **2020**, *578*, 306–310. [CrossRef]

61. Alam, I.; Kamau, A.A.; Kulmanov, M.; Jaremko, Ł.; Arold, S.T.; Pain, A.; Gojobori, T.; Duarte, C.M. Functional Pangenome Analysis Shows Key Features of E Protein Are Preserved in SARS and SARS-CoV-2. *Front. Cell Infect Microbiol.* **2020**, *10*, 405. [CrossRef]

52. Duart, G.; García-Murria, M.J.; Mingarro, I. The SARS-CoV-2 envelope (E) protein has evolved towards membrane topology robustness. *Biochim. Biophys. Acta* **2021**, *1863*, 183608. [CrossRef]

53. Mukherjee, S.; Harikishore, A.; Bhunia, A. Targeting C-terminal Helical bundle of NCOVID19 Envelope (E) protein. *Int. J. Biol. Macromol.* **2021**, *175*, 131–139. [CrossRef] [PubMed]

54. Troyano-Hernáez, P.; Reinosa, R.; Holguín, Á. Evolution of SARS-CoV-2 Envelope, Membrane, Nucleocapsid, and Spike Structural Proteins from the Beginning of the Pandemic to September 2020: A Global and Regional Approach by Epidemiological Week. *Viruses* **2021**, *13*, 243. [CrossRef] [PubMed]

55. Ramírez-Salinas, G.L.; Martínez-Archundia, M.; Correa-Basurto, J.; García-Machorro, J. Repositioning of Ligands That Target the Spike Glycoprotein as Potential Drugs for SARS-CoV-2 in an In Silico Study. *Molecules* **2020**, *25*, 5615. [CrossRef] [PubMed]

56. Chiou, W.C.; Hsu, M.S.; Chen, Y.T.; Yang, J.M.; Tsay, Y.G.; Huang, H.C.; Huang, C. Repurposing existing drugs: Identification of SARS-CoV-2 3C-like protease inhibitors. *J. Enzym. Inhib. Med. Chem.* **2021**, *36*, 147–153. [CrossRef] [PubMed]

57. Sarkar, M.; Saha, S. Structural insight into the role of novel SARS-CoV-2 E protein: A potential target for vaccine development and other therapeutic strategies. *PLoS ONE* **2020**, *15*, e0237300. [CrossRef] [PubMed]

58. Dey, D.; Borkotoky, S.; Banerjee, M. In silico identification of Tretinoin as a SARS-CoV-2 envelope (E) protein ion channel inhibitor. *Comput. Biol. Med.* **2020**, *127*, 104063. [CrossRef] [PubMed]

59. Gupta, M.K.; Vemula, S.; Donde, R.; Gouda, G.; Behera, L.; Vadde, R. *In-silico* approaches to detect inhibitors of the human severe acute respiratory syndrome coronavirus envelope protein ion channel. *J. Biomol. Struct. Dyn.* **2021**, *39*, 2617–2627. [CrossRef] [PubMed]

60. Khataniar, A.; Pathak, U.; Rajkhowa, S.; Nath Jha, A. A Comprehensive Review of Drug Repurposing Strategies against Known Drug Targets of COVID-19. *COVID* **2022**, *2*, 148–167. [CrossRef]

61. Indari, O.; Singh, A.K.; Tiwari, D.; Jha, H.C.; Jha, A.N. Deciphering antiviral efficacy of malaria box compounds against malaria exacerbating viral pathogens-Epstein Barr virus and SARS-CoV-2, an in silico study. *Med. Drug Discov.* **2022**, *16*, 100146. [CrossRef]

62. Burley, S.K.; Bhikadiya, C.; Bi, C.; Bittrich, S.; Chen, L.; Crichlow, G.V.; Christie, C.H.; Dalenberg, K.; Di Costanzo, L.; Duarte, J.M.; et al. RCSB Protein Data Bank: Powerful new tools for exploring 3D structures of biological macromolecules for basic and applied research and education in fundamental biology, biomedicine, biotechnology, bioengineering and energy sciences. *Nucleic Acids Res.* **2021**, *49*, D437–D451. [CrossRef] [PubMed]

63. The UniProt Consortium. UniProt: The universal protein knowledgebase in 2021. *Nucleic Acids Res.* **2021**, *49*, D480–D489. [CrossRef] [PubMed]

64. Webb, B.; Sali, A. Comparative Protein Structure Modeling Using MODELLER. *Curr. Protoc. Bioinform.* **2016**, *54*, 5–6. [CrossRef] [PubMed]

65. Melo, F.; Sali, A. Fold assessment for comparative protein structure modeling. *Protein Sci.* **2007**, *16*, 2412–2426. [CrossRef] [PubMed]

66. Eramian, D.; Shen, M.-Y.; Devos, D.; Melo, F.; Sali, A.; Marti-Renom, M.A. A composite score for predicting errors in protein structure models. *Protein Sci.* **2006**, *15*, 1653–1666. [CrossRef]

67. Irwin, J.J.; Shoichet, B.K. ZINC—A Free Database of Commercially Available Compounds for Virtual Screening. *J. Chem. Inf. Model.* **2005**, *45*, 177–182. [CrossRef]

68. Sander, T.; Freyss, J.; Von Korff, M.; Rufener, C. DataWarrior: An open-source program for chemistry aware data visualization and analysis. *J. Chem. Inf. Model.* **2015**, *55*, 460–473. [CrossRef]

69. Daina, A.; Michielin, O.; Zoete, V. SwissADME: A free web tool to evaluate pharmacokinetics, drug-likeness and medicinal chemistry friendliness of small molecules. *Sci. Rep.* **2017**, *7*, 42717. [CrossRef]

70. Domínguez-Villa, F.X.; Durán-Iturbide, N.A.; Ávila-Zárraga, J.G. Synthesis, molecular docking, and in silico ADME/Tox profiling studies of new 1-aryl-5-(3-azidopropyl)indol-4-ones: Potential inhibitors of SARS CoV-2 main protease. *Bioorg. Chem.* **2021**, *106*, 104497. [CrossRef]

71. Durán-Iturbide, N.A.; Díaz-Eufracio, B.I.; Medina-Franco, J.L. In Silico ADME/Tox Profiling of Natural Products: A Focus on biofacquim. *ACS Omega* **2020**, *5*, 16076–16084. [CrossRef]

72. Zhang, Z.; Tang, W. Drug metabolism in drug discovery and development. *Acta Pharm. Sin. B* **2018**, *8*, 721–732. [CrossRef] [PubMed]

73. Trott, O.; Olson, A.J. AutoDock Vina: Improving the speed and accuracy of docking with a new scoring function, efficient optimization, and multithreading. *J. Comput. Chem.* **2010**, *31*, 455–461. [CrossRef] [PubMed]

74. Abreu, G.E.A.; Aguilar, M.E.H.; Covarrubias, D.H.; Duran, F.R. Amantadine as a drug to mitigate the effects of COVID-19. *Med Hypotheses* **2020**, *140*, 109755. [CrossRef] [PubMed]

75. Eberhardt, J.; Santos-Martins, D.; Tillack, A.F.; Forli, S. AutoDock Vina 1.2.0: New Docking Methods, Expanded Force Field, and Python Bindings. *J. Chem. Inf. Model.* **2021**, *61*, 3891–3898. [CrossRef] [PubMed]

76. *Discovery Studio Visualizer Software*, Version 4.0; BIOVIA: San Diego, CA, USA, 2012.

77. Pettersen, E.F.; Goddard, T.D.; Huang, C.C.; Couch, G.S.; Greenblatt, D.M.; Meng, E.C.; Ferrin, T.E. UCSF Chimera?A visualization system for exploratory research and analysis. *J. Comput. Chem.* **2004**, *25*, 1605–1612. [CrossRef] [PubMed]

78. Jo, S.; Kim, T.; Iyer, V.G.; Im, W. CHARMM-GUI: A web-based graphical user interface for CHARMM. *J. Comput. Chem.* **2008**, *29*, 1859–1865. [CrossRef]

79. Lee, J.; Cheng, X.; Swails, J.M.; Yeom, M.S.; Eastman, P.K.; Lemkul, J.A.; Wei, S.; Buckner, J.; Jeong, J.C.; Qi, Y.; et al. Charmm-GUI Input Generator for NAMD, GROMACS, AMBER, OpenMM, and CHARMM/OpenMM Simulations Using the CHARMM36 Additive Force Field. *J. Chem. Theory Comput.* **2016**, *12*, 405–413. [CrossRef]
80. Tan, H.; Zhao, Y.; Zhao, W.; Xie, H.; Chen, Y.; Tong, Q.; Yang, J. Dynamics properties of membrane proteins in native cell membranes revealed by solid-state NMR spectroscopy. *Biochim. et Biophys. Acta (BBA)* **2022**, *1864*, 183791. [CrossRef]
81. Phillips, J.C.; Braun, R.; Wang, W.; Gumbart, J.; Tajkhorshid, E.; Villa, E.; Chipot, C.; Skeel, R.D.; Kalé, L.; Schulten, K. Scalable molecular dynamics with NAMD. *J. Comput. Chem.* **2005**, *26*, 1781–1802. [CrossRef]
82. Glykos, N.M. Software news and updates carma: A molecular dynamics analysis program. *J. Comput. Chem.* **2006**, *27*, 1765–1768. [CrossRef]
83. Liu, H.; Hou, T. CaFE: A tool for binding affinity prediction using end-point free energy methods. *Bioinformatics* **2016**, *32*, 2216–2218. [CrossRef] [PubMed]
84. Humphrey, W.; Dalke, A.; Schulten, K. VMD: Visual molecular dynamics. *J. Mol. Graph.* **1996**, *14*, 33–38. [CrossRef] [PubMed]
85. Hsin, J.; Arkhipov, A.; Yin, Y.; Stone, J.E.; Schulten, K. Using VMD: An Introductory Tutorial. *Curr. Protoc. Bioinform.* **2008**, *24*, 5–7. [CrossRef] [PubMed]
86. Fernandes, H.S.; Sousa, S.F.; Cerqueira, N.M.F.S.A. VMD Store-A VMD Plugin to Browse, Discover, and Install VMD Extensions. *J. Chem. Inf. Model.* **2019**, *59*, 4519–4523. [CrossRef]

MDPI
St. Alban-Anlage 66
4052 Basel
Switzerland
www.mdpi.com

Pharmaceuticals Editorial Office
E-mail: pharmaceuticals@mdpi.com
www.mdpi.com/journal/pharmaceuticals

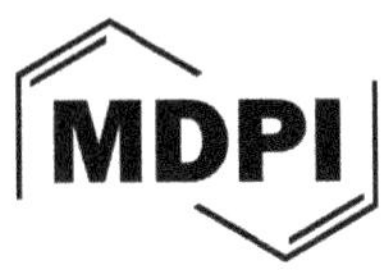